Other monographs in the series, Major Problems in Clinical Pediatrics:

Avery and Fletcher: *The Lung and Its Disorders in the Newborn Infant* — Third Edition, 1974

Bell and McCormick: *Increased Intracranial Pressure in Children* — Second Edition, 1978

Bell and McCormick: *Neurologic Infections in Children* — 1975

Brewer: *Juvenile Rheumatoid Arthritis* — 1970

Cornblath and Schwartz: *Disorders of Carbohydrate Metabolism in Infancy* — Second Edition, 1976

Dubowitz: *Muscle Disorders in Childhood* — 1978

Gryboski: *Gastrointestinal Problems in the Infant* — 1975

Hanshaw and Dudgeon: *Viral Diseases of the Fetus and Newborn* — 1978

Lubchenco: *The High Risk Infant* — 1976

Markowitz and Gordis: *Rheumatic Fever* — Second Edition, 1972

Oski and Naiman: *Hematologic Problems in the Newborn* — Second Edition, 1972

Rowe and Mehrizi: *The Neonate with Congenital Heart Disease* — 1968

Royer, et al: *Pediatric Nephrology* — 1974

Scriver and Rosenberg: *Amino Acid Metabolism and Its Disorders* — 1973

Smith: *Recognizable Patterns of Human Malformation* — Second Edition, 1976

Smith: *Growth and Its Disorders* — 1977

Solomon and Esterly: *Neonatal Dermatology* — 1973

Forthcoming Monographs

Belman and Kaplan: *Urologic Problems in Pediatrics*

Bluestone and Klein: *Otitis Media in Infants and Children*

Drash: *Juvenile Diabetes*

Glader: *Anemia in Children*

Griffin: *Children's Orthopaedics*

Harrison and Harrison: *Disorders of Calcium and Phosphate Metabolism in Childhood and Adolescence*

Solomon, Esterly, and Loeffel: *Adolescent Dermatology*

Wannamaker: *Streptococcal Infections*

MALIGNANT DISEASES OF INFANCY, CHILDHOOD AND ADOLESCENCE

by

Arnold J. Altman, M.D.
Associate Professor of Pediatrics and
Head, Division of Pediatric Hematology and Oncology
University of Connecticut Health Center
Farmington, Connecticut

Allan D. Schwartz, M.D.
Associate Professor of Pediatrics and
Head, Division of Pediatric Hematology and Oncology
University of Maryland School of Medicine
Baltimore, Maryland

Volume XVIII in the Series
MAJOR PROBLEMS IN
CLINICAL PEDIATRICS

ALEXANDER J. SCHAFFER
Consulting Editor
MILTON MARKOWITZ
Associate Consulting Editor

W. B. Saunders Company, Philadelphia, London, Toronto   1978

W. B. Saunders Company: West Washington Square
Philadelphia, PA   19105

1 St. Anne's Road
Eastbourne, East Sussex BN21 3UN, England

1 Goldthorne Avenue
Toronto, Ontario M8Z 5T9, Canada

Library of Congress Cataloging in Publication Data

Altman, Arnold.

Malignant diseases of infancy and childhood.

(Major problems in clinical pediatrics; v. 19)
Includes index.

1. Tumors in children.   I. Schwartz, Allan D.,
joint author.   II. Title. [DNLM: 1. Neoplasms—
In infancy and childhood. W1 MA492N v. 19 /
QZ200.3 A468m]
RC281.C4A44   618.9′29′94   77-79863
ISBN 0-7216-1212-1

Malignant Diseases of Infancy and Childhood   ISBN 0-7216-1212-1

© 1978 by W. B. Saunders Company. Copyright under the International Copyright Union. All rights reserved. This book is protected by copyright. No part of it may be reproduced, stored in a retrieval system or transmitted in any form or by any means, electronic, mechanical, photocopying, recording or otherwise, without written permission from the publisher. Made in the United States of America. Press of W. B. Saunders Company. Library of Congress catalogue card number 77-79863.

Last digit is the print number: 9   8   7   6   5   4   3   2   1

Dedication
to our parents,
who inspired and sustained us

to our wives, Cheri and Maria,
for their love and patience

to our sons, David and Michael,
who continually renew our hopes for the future

FOREWORD

We present this eighteenth volume in our series, *Major Problems in Clinical Pediatrics*, with pride. The practicing pediatrician does not find himself confronted with a new malignancy many times a year, but the possibility that such is present must be included in his differential diagnosis much more frequently than actual cases are found. Until the possibility becomes a probability and then a certainty, he is the primary physician, guiding the child through the various diagnostic procedures until no further doubt of the condition exists. He then must decide upon the proper course of therapy, aided now perhaps by a surgeon and ideally by an oncologist. Even at this point his work has barely begun, for now he must take on the tasks of supporting the child and his family emotionally for what may prove to be a seemingly interminable period of time, of acting as referee or mediator between consultants whose recommendations about further treatment may differ, and of watching with unflagging care for relapse, metastasis, or superimposed infection. Even if death of the child supervenes his work is not done.

All of these phases of action on the part of the primary physician are covered beautifully by the authors. Arnold J. Altman is a graduate of the Johns Hopkins Medical School, who trained at Yale, the U.S. Public Health Service in Atlanta, and the Children's Medical Center in Boston, then became Hematologist-Oncologist first in Indiana and now at the University of Connecticut Health Center in Farmington. His written work has focused largely upon the leukemias of childhood. Allen E. Schwartz received his M.D. degree from the University of Maryland; was trained at the Hopkins, Yale, and Los Angeles Children's Hospital; was Pediatric Hematologist-Oncologist at Yale and the Children's Memorial Hospital of Chicago and is now at the University of Maryland Hospital in Baltimore. His numerous communications deal with many aspects of both hematology and oncology.

Both men are exactly what we were looking for for this task—fine general pediatricians with very special training and experience in this field, who could delineate the proper paths the less well-trained generalists must follow in order to give ideal care to children afflicted with malignancy and to their equally sorely afflicted families.

ALEXANDER J. SCHAFFER, M.D.

PREFACE

To cure sometimes
To relieve often
To comfort always

    This fifteenth century French folk saying is an appropriate credo for the physician who cares for children afflicted with cancer. It aptly describes the commingling strains of hope, determination, anxiety, frustration, and compassion that characterize the field of pediatric oncology today. In moments of discouragement we might well derive some succor from the fact that this same quotation was once applied to another "hopeless" disease and may be found inscribed at the base of the statue of Dr. Edward Livingstone Trudeau on the site of his tuberculosis sanatorium at Saranac Lake, New York. Today, no one would find it necessary to refer to the therapy of tuberculosis in this manner. Indeed, statues are no longer being erected to honor tuberculosis specialists, and the sanatoria are either closed or diverted to the care of other diseases. The transformation of tuberculosis from a chronically debilitating and invariably fatal illness to one that is almost always easily cured on an outpatient basis should be an inspiration to all those involved in the care of patients with malignancy.

    Today the diagnosis of cancer, particularly in children, is still regarded in some circles as a death sentence, for malignant disease is second only to trauma as a killer of children above the age of one year. However, advances made in the field of pediatric oncology over the past few decades have resulted in markedly improved survival for many forms of childhood cancer; most noteworthy are the examples of Wilms' tumor, acute lymphocytic leukemia, histiocytosis X, rhabdomyosarcoma, and Hodgkin's disease, for which there is now a very real chance of cure for a significant portion of patients.

    Because of the increasing complexity and need for multidisciplinary coordination involved in the care of children with malignancy, the day has passed when the "compleat physician" can diagnose and manage cancer entirely on his own; optimum therapy requires a judicious blend of surgery, radiation therapy, chemotherapy, and possibly immunotherapy. Nonetheless, the primary physician still has a crucial role to play. Since most children with malignancy are initially seen by a pediatrician or family practitioner, it is essential that this primary physician be familiar with the presenting signs of malignancy and the life-threatening complications which may derive from the presence of malignancy or its therapy. Consequently, this book attempts to present the subspecialty of pediatric oncology in the perspective of the primary physician who is caring for children. Much emphasis is placed on diagnosis of malignancy, recognition and treatment of life-threatening complications, and the natural history of the major childhood neoplasms. Because the management of these illnesses is in a continual state of flux as new protocols are evaluated and new agents are developed, only those regimens which have become fairly standardized and successful are discussed in detail. It is to be hoped that the others will be rapidly outdated as new advances are made.

ARNOLD J. ALTMAN, M.D.
ALLAN D. SCHWARTZ, M.D.

ACKNOWLEDGMENTS

The authors would like to acknowledge with gratitude the efforts of our friends and colleagues who have reviewed portions of this manuscript. They include Drs. Robert Baehner, Thomas Ballantine, Mark Ballow, Bruce Camitta, Murray J. Casey, Lorraine Champion, Ronald Cooke, Ivan Damjanov, Herbert Felsenfeld, Bert Finklestein, Erwin Gelfand, Ronald Gold, George Klauber, Martha Lepow, Ruth Luddy, Scott Nystrom, Phillip Pizzo, John Quinn, Mark Seligman, and Dennis Shermeta.

We would also like to acknowledge the assistance of Mrs. Sandy Cutler, Mrs. Margaret Karasa, Mrs. Rita Rival, and Miss Liz Nawrocki in typing this manuscript. The long hours that Mrs. Margaret Hennessey spent checking references for the bibliography are also greatly appreciated.

The fact that the authors were able to devote sufficient time to finish this manuscript is largely attributable to the devoted and conscientious assistance in the care of our patients given by our fellows, Drs. Lorraine Champion, Luz Duque, Suppiah Pathmanathan, and Ali Talaizedeh.

CONTENTS

Chapter One
THE CANCER PROBLEM IN PEDIATRICS: EPIDEMIOLOGIC ASPECTS 1

Chapter Two
DIAGNOSIS OF CANCER IN CHILDHOOD 16

Chapter Three
CANCER CHEMOTHERAPY 57

Chapter Four
RADIOTHERAPY 89
William N. Brand, M.D.

Chapter Five
TUMOR IMMUNOLOGY AND IMMUNOTHERAPY 102

Chapter Six
PSYCHOLOGICAL AND SOCIAL SUPPORT OF THE PATIENT AND FAMILY 120
Julia M. Cotter and Allen D. Schwartz

Chapter Seven
ONCOLOGIC EMERGENCIES 128

Chapter Eight
THE LEUKEMIAS 169

Chapter Nine
HODGKIN'S DISEASE 234

Chapter Ten
NON-HODGKIN'S LYMPHOMAS 272

Chapter Eleven
THE HISTIOCYTOSES 289

Chapter Twelve
TUMORS OF THE CENTRAL AND PERIPHERAL NERVOUS SYSTEM ... 305
Maria Gumbinas and Allen D. Schwartz

Chapter Thirteen
TUMORS OF THE SYMPATHETIC NERVOUS SYSTEM 326

Chapter Fourteen
RETINOBLASTOMA 346

Chapter Fifteen
RENAL TUMORS 359

Chapter Sixteen
THE SOFT TISSUE SARCOMAS 380

Chapter Seventeen
PRIMARY BONE CANCERS 405

Chapter Eighteen
TUMORS OF GERM-CELL ORIGIN: EMBRYONAL CARCINOMAS, EXTRAEMBRYONAL TUMORS, AND TERATOMAS 427

Chapter Nineteen
TUMORS OF THE SEXUAL ORGANS 443

Chapter Twenty
LYMPHOEPITHELIOMA, SALIVARY GLAND TUMORS, AND THYROID TUMORS 475

Chapter Twenty-One
TUMORS OF THE LIVER 489

Chapter Twenty-Two
TUMORS OF THE GASTROINTESTINAL TRACT 502

INDEX.. 517

Chapter One

THE CANCER PROBLEM IN PEDIATRICS: EPIDEMIOLOGIC ASPECTS

Figure 1-1 shows the relative incidence of the major forms of cancer in U.S. white and black children. Malignant neoplasms of childhood differ markedly in clinical behavior, histology, and site of origin from those seen in adults. In adults the common malignancies usually arise within ectodermal or endodermal tissue (skin, breast, lungs, gastrointestinal tract, female genital tract); such tumors are known as *carcinomas*. Childhood tumors, on the other hand, frequently arise in mesodermal tissues (hematopoietic system, kidney, soft tissues) and are known as *sarcomas*; tumors of ectodermal origin may occur in the central nervous system or sympathetic nervous system (neuroblastoma) as well. Whereas most adult tumors appear to arise through dedifferentiation of cells within mature tissue, the

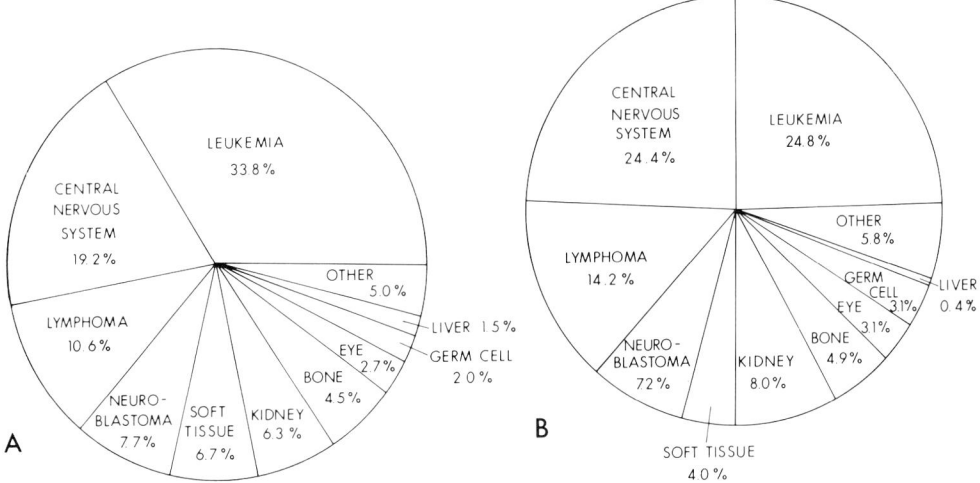

Figure 1-1 Relative incidence of major forms of cancer. A, U.S. white children. B, U.S. black children.

childhood tumors are frequently characterized by cellular features suggesting that they originate in abnormal embryogenesis.

AGE VARIATIONS

The distribution of the major forms of childhood cancer varies for different age groups (see Fig. 1–2). Many pediatric tumors have their peak incidence in children under 5 years of age—these include *acute lymphocytic leukemia, Wilms' tumor, neuroblastoma, retinoblastoma, presacral teratoma, rhabdomyosarcoma, glioma, medulloblastoma,* and *primary liver cancers;*[46, 51] the association of some of these tumors with various congenital defects or chromosomal anomalies (to be discussed later in this chapter) suggests prenatal influences in their genesis. Other neoplasms do not exhibit peak incidence in children under 5 years of age—these include *most brain tumors, gonadal tumors, lymphomas, bone sarcomas, thyroid cancer,* and *acute myelogenous leukemia.*[46, 51] These tumors may be pathogenetically related to postnatal (environmental) factors.

SEX VARIATIONS

In the United States and Britain the overall incidence of pediatric malignancies is more frequent in males by a ratio of approximately 1.2:1.[71a, 75] On the other hand, there appears to be no significant sexual variation in the incidence of malignant neoplasms in U.S. black children. Among the major pediatric tumor types, *acute lymphocytic leukemia, lymphosarcoma* (both Hodgkin's and non-Hodgkin's), and *central nervous system tumors* (particularly medulloblastoma) appear to be significantly more frequent in males;[75] *epithelial tumors* (skin, ovary) appear to be more frequent in females.[71a]

GEOGRAPHIC AND RACIAL VARIATIONS

Cancer is exceeded only by trauma as a killer of children between the ages of 1 and 15 years in nearly all developed countries. However, childhood cancer rates vary markedly among different countries and ethnic groups. The highest incidence is seen in Israel (30.6/100,000 in European- and American-born males) and Nigeria (22.1/100,000 males), whereas the lowest is in India (6.8/100,000 males) and Japan (10.2/100,000 males).[10] According to the Third National Cancer Survey (conducted over the 3-year period of 1969 to 1971), the annual incidence for all malignant tumors in U.S. children under 15 years of age is 12.45/100,000 whites and 9.78/100,000 blacks[75] (Table 1–1). Thus, there are approximately 6900 *new* cases of cancer in children annually in the United States (based on 1970 U.S. population figures).[75]

Of all the childhood cancers, none has a more uniform worldwide incidence than *Wilms' tumor* (approximately 1/15,000 births).[34] On the other hand, the incidence of *leukemia* varies widely, with high rates seen in Israel, Denmark, Japan, and U.S. whites, and low rates in Nigeria, India, and U.S. blacks.[10, 55] An extremely high frequency of *acute myelomonocytic leukemia with orbital chloroma* has been described in Ankara, Turkey,[49] and in Uganda.[55]

Lymphosarcoma (mainly Burkitt's lymphoma) has extremely high incidence in Nigeria, with peak rates at 5 to 9 years of age,[10, 55] whereas *intestinal lymphoma* is common in Israel. *Hodgkin's disease* has a high incidence rate in Colombia. Other tumors with uniquely high incidence in various areas are *liver cancer* (Far East), *retinoblastoma* (India), *neuroblastoma*

The Cancer Problem in Pediatrics: Epidemiologic Aspects

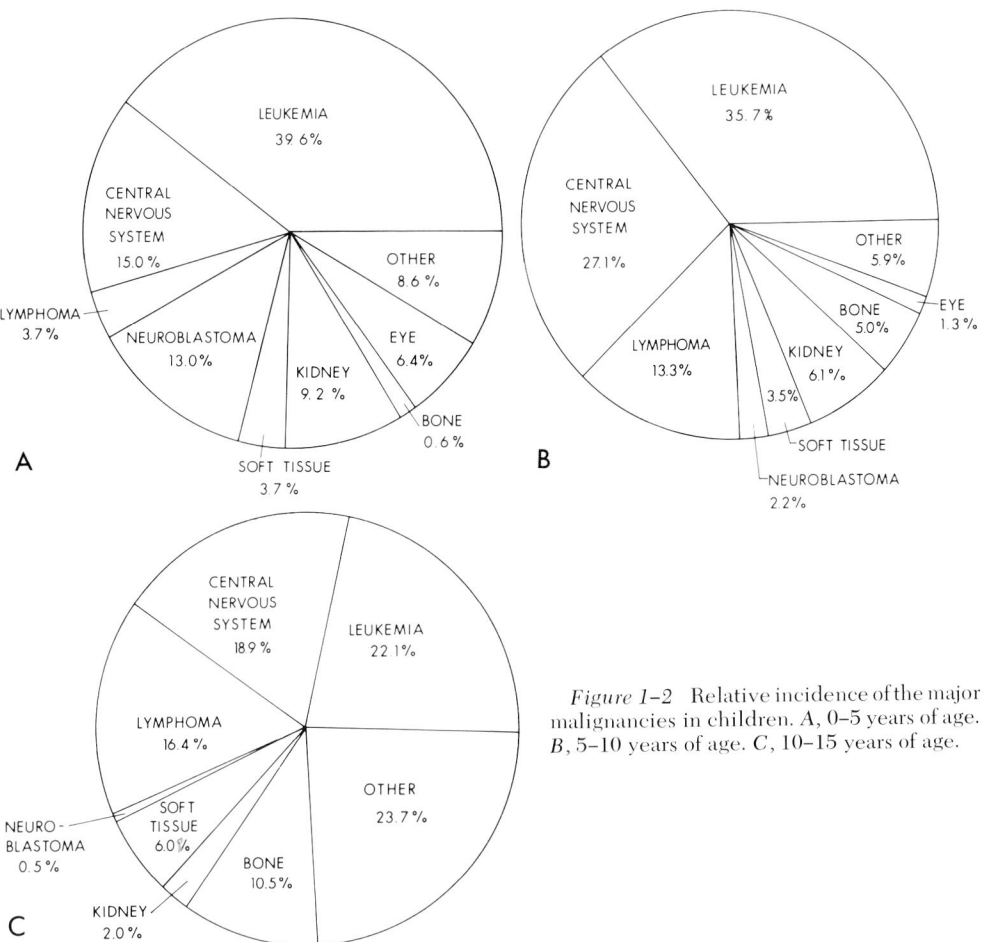

Figure 1-2 Relative incidence of the major malignancies in children. A, 0–5 years of age. B, 5–10 years of age. C, 10–15 years of age.

Table 1-1 Incidence of Malignant Tumors in U.S. Children[*][75]

Diagnosis	Rate (per 100,000 per year) Whites	Blacks
Leukemia	4.21	2.43
Central nervous system	2.39	2.39
Lymphoma	1.32	1.39
Neuroblastoma	0.96	0.70
Soft tissue sarcomas	0.84	0.39
Wilms' tumor	0.78	0.78
Bone tumors	0.56	0.48
Retinoblastoma	0.34	0.30
Gonadal and germ cell tumors	0.22	0.26
Liver tumors	0.19	0.04
Melanoma	0.07	—
Teratoma (nongonadal)	0.03	0.04
Miscellaneous	0.54	0.57
Total	12.45	9.78

* Total U.S. 1970 population of white children under 15 years of age was 49,001,683; total U.S. 1970 population of black children under 15 years of age was 7,989,935.

(western Europe), *pineal tumors* (Japan), and *skin cancer* as a complication of xeroderma pigmentosum (North Africa).[49]

A comparison of the incidence rates of the various childhood malignancies in the United States (Table 1–1) shows that many tumors have almost identical frequency in white and black children; however, there are some interesting variations between the races—for instance, the incidence of leukemia in whites is almost twice as high as it is in blacks, and certain other tumors (*melanoma, Ewing's sarcoma,* and *testicular cancers*) are absent or very rare in blacks.[17, 37, 75]

CHILDREN AT ABOVE AVERAGE RISK OF CANCER

Cancer does not occur as a random event in childhood. This has already been demonstrated by the marked racial, geographic, and age-related variations in the incidence of the various types of childhood cancer. Even within a given geographic or racial population, however, there are subgroups of children who have excessively high rates for specific forms of malignancy. Among the recognizable conditions which have been associated with a relatively high incidence of malignancy are the following:

- Hereditary cutaneous syndromes
- Hereditary neurocutaneous syndromes
- Hereditary and acquired gastrointestinal syndromes
- Hereditary chromosomal abnormalities
- Hereditary and acquired immunodeficiency syndromes
- Miscellaneous syndromes
- Sporadic congenital malformations
- Sibling with malignancy
- Prior episode of malignancy
- Prenatal insult
- Irradiation

CUTANEOUS SYNDROMES ASSOCIATED WITH TUMOR SUSCEPTIBILITY (Table 1–2)

These syndromes are all of a hereditary nature. For some (nevoid basal cell carcinoma syndrome, familial trichoepithelioma, and tylosis) the neoplasm appears as an integral part of a definable autosomal dominant clinical syndrome, whereas for others the malignancy arises with high frequency (but not consistently) from precursor

Table 1–2 Hereditary Cutaneous Syndromes Associated With Tumor Susceptibility

Syndrome	Tumor
Nevoid basal cell carcinoma syndrome	Basal cell carcinoma
	Medulloblastoma
Familial trichoepithelioma	Basal cell carcinoma
Tylosis (palmar-plantar-keratosis)	Esophageal carcinoma
Xeroderma pigmentosum	Basal and squamous cell carcinoma
	Melanoma
Albinism	Squamous cell carcinoma
Werner's syndrome (adult progeria)	Soft tissue sarcomas
	Carcinomas
Epidermodysplasia verruciformis	Basal and squamous cell carcinoma
Polydysplastic epidermolysis bullosa	Squamous cell carcinoma
Dyskeratosis congenita	Squamous cell carcinoma
	Mucous membrane carcinoma

lesions that are transmitted in an autosomal recessive fashion.[16]

Nevoid Basal Cell Carcinoma Syndrome. This syndrome is characterized by multiple basal cell skin hamartomas, skeletal anomalies (rib defects, spina bifida, kyphosis, scoliosis), central nervous system anomalies, jaw cysts, skin pits on palms and soles, hypertelorism, and soft tissue calcifications.[21, 28] The skin lesions tend to transform into frank *basal cell carcinoma* before age 15 (whereas ordinary basal cell carcinoma does not appear until after the age of 50). In addition, 20 per cent of children with this syndrome develop *medulloblastoma* at an early age.[7, 58]

Familial Trichoepithelioma (Multiple Benign Cystic Epithelioma). This syndrome develops as multiple and symmetrical tumors on the face and upper part of the body at puberty; the neoplasms often contain areas of *basal cell carcinoma*.[16, 19]

Tylosis. This is a rare syndrome which is characterized by keratosis of the palms and soles (in childhood) and *squamous cell carcinoma of the esophagus* (in middle age).[64]

Xeroderma Pigmentosum. This is a disorder of early childhood characterized by progressive skin atrophy, with dry, scaling, hyperpigmented lesions in areas exposed to the sun. *Basal cell* and *epidermoid carcinomas*, as well as *melanomas*, develop early in life (often by 3 to 4 years of age).[65] The propensity to cancer is apparently related to a defect in DNA repair which prevents repair of skin damaged by ultraviolet light.[8]

Albinism. Patients with this defect in skin pigmentation have a predisposition to *squamous cell carcinoma* in areas of heavy sun exposure.

Werner's Syndrome (Adult Progeria). These patients have scleroderma-like skin, soft-tissue calcification, growth retardation, cataracts, and shortened life span due to arteriosclerosis or cancer; various *sarcomas* and *carcinomas* have been reported.[13]

Epidermodysplasia Verruciformis. In this condition, multiple virus-induced warty lesions develop in early childhood; it is associated with a high frequency of *basal and squamous cell carcinomas*, particularly in areas with heavy sun exposure.[1]

Polydysplastic Epidermolysis Bullosa. This condition is characterized by bullous skin eruptions followed by erosion and delayed healing with tissue-paper–like scarring. Onset is at birth or shortly thereafter and involves mainly the extremities, being most pronounced about the joints and the acral and pressure areas. Well-differentiated solitary or multiple *squamous cell carcinomas* may appear in the scar tissue between the third and sixth decades.[72]

Dyskeratosis Congenita. This syndrome manifests the triad of skin pigmentation and atrophy, nail dysplasia, and leukoplakia of the mucous membranes; it may also show the stigmata of Fanconi's aplastic anemia and is associated with a high incidence of *squamous cell carcinoma* of the skin and mucous membranes.

NEUROCUTANEOUS SYNDROMES (PHAKOMATOSES) ASSOCIATED WITH TUMOR SUSCEPTIBILITY
(Table 1–3)

These conditions are considered hamartomatous; that is, they are characterized by structural defects of development with a localized growth excess of one or more tissues normally found in the affected part. Hamartomas are considered to be malformations, rather than benign neoplasms. Most of these conditions show autosomal dominant inheritance.

Neurofibromatosis (von Recklinghausen's disease) is characterized by multiple cutaneous neurofibromas and café-au-lait spots.[23] In about 2.4 to 29 per cent of patients the neurofibromas

Table 1-3 Hereditary Neurocutaneous Syndromes (Phakomatoses) Associated With Tumor Susceptibility

SYNDROME	TUMOR
Neurofibromatosis 2.5 - 29%	Sarcoma
	Glioma
	Meningioma
	Acoustic neuroma
	Pheochromocytoma
	Medullary thyroid carcinoma
Tuberous sclerosis 1-3	Brain tumors
Von Hippel-Lindau disease	Hypernephroma
	Pheochromocytoma
	Ependymoma

undergo *sarcomatous degeneration;* there is also an increased frequency of *cerebral and optic gliomas, menigiomas, acoustic neuromas, pheochromocytoma,* and *medullary thyroid carcinoma.*[22] Inheritance is as an autosomal dominant trait, with a high rate of penetrance.

Tuberous sclerosis consists of the triad of adenoma sebaceum, epilepsy, and mental retardation; in addition, hamartomas develop in the brain, retina, heart, lungs, and kidneys. About 1 to 3 per cent of patients develop *brain tumors.*

von Hippel-Lindau disease (angiomatosis of the retina and cerebellum) is associated with an increased incidence of *hypernephroma, pheochromocytoma,* and *ependymoma.*

GASTROINTESTINAL SYNDROMES ASSOCIATED WITH TUMOR SUSCEPTIBILITY (Table 1-4)

Polyposis Coli

Patients with this disorder have numerous adenomatous polyps of the colon and rectum; *adenocarcinoma* is present in the polyps of about 40 per cent of patients when they are initially diagnosed and develops in virtually all cases with advancing age.[16, 42, 53] The risk is of sufficient magnitude to warrant prophylactic colectomy in late childhood.[66] In *Gardner's syndrome*, a variant of polyposis coli, multiple soft tissue, or facial bone and skull tumors (osteomas, fibromas, lipomas, epidermal cysts, and fibrosarcomas) also develop;[18, 34] in addition to prophylactic

Table 1-4 Hereditary and Acquired Gastrointestinal Syndromes Associated With Tumor Susceptibility

SYNDROME	TUMOR
Polyposis coli	
Familial polyposis coli 40%	Carcinoma of colon
Gardner syndrome	Carcinoma of colon
	Skin, skull, and facial bone tumors
Turcot syndrome	Brain tumors
Peutz-Jeghers syndrome 2-3%	Ovarian tumors
	Duodenal cancer
Inflammatory bowel disease	
Ulcerative colitis	Colorectal carcinoma
Regional enteritis (Crohn's disease)	Colorectal carcinoma
	Small bowel carcinoma

colectomy, skull and facial x-rays should be taken at 5-year intervals.[12] *Turcot's syndrome* is an autosomal recessively transmitted disorder characterized by familial polyposis of the colon and *malignant brain tumors*.[68]

Peutz-Jeghers Syndrome (Hamartomatous Small Intestinal Polyps Accompanied by Melanin Spots on the Buccal Mucosa, Lip, and Digits)

Ovarian neoplasms occur in 5 per cent of women with this condition; there is also a 2 to 3 per cent risk of *gastrointestinal cancer*, often involving the duodenal region.[14]

INFLAMMATORY BOWEL DISEASE

Ulcerative Colitis

In patients with ulcerative colitis, four factors are associated with a high risk of subsequent development of cancer:[3] (1) extreme severity of the first attack; (2) universal involvement of the entire colon as judged radiologically; (3) continuous, rather than intermittent, symptoms; and (4) onset of the disease in childhood.

In Devroede's series, the incidence of carcinoma of the large bowel in a group of patients with chronic ulcerative colitis starting in childhood was about 3 per cent during the first 10 years and 20 per cent per decade after the first 10 years of the disease.[9] Michener found the susceptibility to carcinoma to begin between the ages of 5 and 9 years, with an incidence of 14.5 per cent once the disease has been present for 10 years.[43] Most cancers develop in the rectum and sigmoid and are extremely virulent; many have already metastasized by the time they are diagnosed. Consequently, in some centers a 10-year duration of disease is considered an indication for prophylactic colectomy, whereas in others, colonoscopy with serial biopsies is performed every 6 months.[23a]

Crohn's Colitis

The picture in Crohn's disease (regional enteritis) is less clear. However, in one study of patients with Crohn's disease of the colon in whom the onset was at 21 years of age or younger, the incidence of *colorectal cancer* was found to be 20 times greater than in a control population.[73] Likewise, carcinoma appears to occur with increased frequency in areas of the small bowel affected with regional enteritis;[59] frequently these patients have developed severe symptoms or complications of regional enteritis—particularly bowel obstruction—after a long quiescent period (4 or more years).[59, 69]

CHROMOSOME SYNDROMES ASSOCIATED WITH TUMOR SUSCEPTIBILITY (Table 1-5)

The probability that a child with *Down's syndrome* (trisomy 21) will develop *acute leukemia* is approximately 1/200—about 15 times the normal rate.[47] Both acute lymphocytic and acute myelogenous forms of leukemia are seen in these patients.

The *13q-syndrome* is accompanied by multiple malformations including mental and physical retardation, microcephaly, cardiac and eye defects, and various skeletal deformities (especially hypoplastic thumbs). In these patients, chromosome 13 may be in a ring or have deletions of the long arms. *Retinoblastoma* is a frequent feature of this syndrome.[54]

Klinefelter's syndrome is characterized by hypogonadism, sterility, gynecomastia, eunuchoid proportions, and a 47XXY karyotype. Such patients have an increased incidence of *breast carcinoma*.

Increased Chromosomal Fragility

Bloom's Syndrome. This syndrome consists of congenital telangiectatic erythema of the face, photosensitivity, short stature, and excessive chromo-

Table 1–5 Hereditary Chromosomal Abnormalities Associated With Tumor Susceptibility

Syndrome	Tumor
Trisomy 21 (Down's syndrome)	Acute leukemia
13 q−	Retinoblastoma
47XXY (Klinefelter's syndrome)	Breast carcinoma
46XY, 45X/46XY or other mosaic containing 46XY line (gonadal dysgenesis)	Gonadoblastoma (dysgerminoma)
Increased chromosome fragility	
Fanconi's anemia	Acute leukemia (myelomonocytic)
Bloom's syndrome	Acute leukemia
Ataxia-telangiectasia	Lymphoma
	Gastric carcinoma

somal fragility in cell culture. Among 50 patients with this autosomal recessive disorder, four *acute leukemias*, two *sigmoid carcinomas*, one *squamous cell carcinoma*, and one *reticulum cell sarcoma* have developed.[20]

Fanconi's Aplastic Anemia. These patients exhibit skeletal anomalies, growth retardation, renal anomalies, mental retardation, café-au-lait spots and other forms of abnormal pigmentation, bone marrow hypoplasia, and excessive chromsomal fragility in cell culture. *Leukemia* (usually acute myelomonocytic) develops in nearly 10 per cent of these patients, usually during *adolescence* or *early childhood*.[11, 45, 50]

Ataxia-Telangiectasia. This is a complex disorder in which an immunologic dysfunction is associated with progressive cerebellar dysfunction, telangiectasia of the bulbar conjunctiva and skin, and a very high incidence of malignancy (approximately 10 per cent), mainly *lymphoreticular* in nature. In vitro clones of lymphocytes with translocation have been described in this disorder.[24]

IMMUNODEFICIENCY SYNDROMES ASSOCIATED WITH TUMOR SUSCEPTIBILITY (Table 1–6)

The incidence of malignancy in children with various immunodeficiency syndromes is approximately 100 times that seen in the general population[31] and runs as high as 10 per

Table 1–6 Hereditary and Acquired Immunodeficiency Syndromes Associated With Tumor Susceptibility

Syndrome	Tumor
Congenital	
Wiskott-Aldrich syndrome	Lymphoreticular tumors
Bruton's disease (agammaglobulinemia)	Acute lymphocytic leukemia
Common variable immunodeficiency	Lymphoreticular tumors
Ataxia-telangiectasia	Gastric carcinoma
	Lymphoreticular tumors
IgA deficiency	Carcinoma of colon, lung, stomach, breast, skin
Acquired	
Transplant patients	Epithelial tumors
	Lymphoreticular tumors
Autoimmune diseases	
Dermatomyositis	Miscellaneous
Systemic lupus	Carcinoma of cervix

cent for patients with Wiskott-Aldrich disease and ataxia-telangiectasia. The major malignancies seen are *lymphoreticular* in nature. This subject is discussed further in Chapter Five.

SPORADIC CONGENITAL MALFORMATIONS ASSOCIATED WITH TUMOR SUSCEPTIBILITY (Table 1-7)

Cancers and certain sporadic congenital defects occur together more often than can be attributed to chance;[44] whether this association reflects gene mutation or environmental influences remains to be determined, however.

Among children with *Wilms' tumor* there is an increased frequency of *aniridia, hemihypertrophy, genitourinary tract abnormalities*, and probably *pigmented* or *vascular nevi*.[44, 51] When it occurs in the general population, aniridia is almost always due to the action of a dominant gene and, consequently, two of three aniridic children have an aniridic parent;[63] however, in children with coincident Wilms' tumor and aniridia, only one case in 30 has been familial.[50] This suggests that aniridia in children with Wilms' tumor is due to a mutation or to an environmental agent.

In addition to its association with *Wilms' tumor, hemihypertrophy* is also associated with *neoplasms of the adrenal gland* (mainly *adrenocortical carcinoma*) and of the *liver*.[44] Although the majority of the tumors were on the same side as the hemihypertrophy, in a significant number the tumor was on the opposite side; this suggests that there need be no anatomic connection between the hypertrophy and the tumor.

Beckwith's syndrome (gigantism, macroglossia, omphalocele or umbilical hernia, visceromegaly, adrenal cytomegaly, and mental retardation) may accompany hemihypertrophy and is also associated with a high incidence of *liver tumors, Wilms' tumors*, and *adrenal tumors*.[15]

Cryptorchid testes are found in 2 per cent of term male infants and have 33 times the normal risk for malignancy. The risk increases with degree of maldescent, being four times greater with abdominal than with inguinal testes.[54] In 20 to 25 per cent of patients with unilateral cryptorchidism, when neoplasm occurs, it appears in the properly descended testis.[54]

Gonadal dysgenesis has a 25 per cent incidence of *gonadoblastoma*[54] and accounts for the only instances when this tumor occurs in childhood.[46]

Enchondromatosis occurring as an isolated defect (Ollier's syndrome) or in association with hemangiomas (Maffucci's syndrome) is associated with *chondrosarcoma*.

Table 1-7 Sporadic Congenital Malformations Associated With Tumor Susceptibility

SYNDROME	TUMOR
Aniridia	Wilms' tumor
Hemihypertrophy	Wilms' tumor
	Liver tumors
	Adrenocortical carcinoma
Beckwith's syndrome	Wilms' tumor
	Liver tumors
	Adrenocortical carcinoma
Cryptorchidism	Testicular tumors
Gonadal dysgenesis	Gonadoblastoma
Enchondromatosis (Ollier's syndrome)	Chondrosarcoma

Table 1-8 Miscellaneous Syndromes Associated With Tumor Susceptibility

SYNDROME	TUMOR
Chediak-Higashi syndrome	Lymphoma
Multiple endocrine neoplasia	Medullary thyroid carcinoma
	Pheochromocytoma
Multiple exostoses	Chondrosarcoma
Tyrosinemia	Carcinoma of liver

MISCELLANEOUS SYNDROMES ASSOCIATED WITH TUMOR SUSCEPTIBILITY (Table 1-8)

Chediak-Higashi Syndrome. This is an autosomal recessive disorder. Patients so afflicted have partial albinism, neutropenia, large cytoplasmic inclusions (swollen lysosomes) in neutrophils and other granule-containing cells, and recurrent pyogenic infections. They have a high incidence of *malignant lymphoma*.[6]

Multiple Endocrine Neoplasia (Sipple's Syndrome). *Medullary carcinoma of the thyroid* (MCT) may occur in both sporadic and familial forms. The familial form is usually associated with multifocal bilateral involvement of the thyroid by the tumor and may be accompanied by pheochromocytoma and parathyroid hyperplasia.[27] Some patients may also have a characteristic physical appearance with a Marfanoid habitus, acromegaly-like facies, scoliosis, pectus excavatum, pes cavus, muscular hypotonia, and mucosal neuromas.[32] These entities are discussed further in Chapter Twenty.

Multiple exostoses (osteochondromas) at the surfaces of growing bones transform to chondrosarcoma in 5 to 11 per cent of patients.[16]

Tyrosinemia. This is an autosomal recessive disorder of tyrosine metabolism accompanied by nodular cirrhosis of the liver, hepatosplenomegaly, high plasma tyrosine levels, and renal tubular defects. Patients with tyrosinemia have an increased incidence of *carcinoma of the liver*.

SIBLINGS OF CHILDHOOD CANCER PATIENTS

There are a number of studies that suggest a familial element in the etiology of childhood cancer.[11a, 33, 40, 45, 60] Some tumors, such as retinoblastoma, are clearly associated with a hereditary pattern, whereas others (discussed above) have been associated with certain hereditary premalignant syndromes. Even when patients with these clearly hereditary conditions are excluded, the risk of developing cancer for the sib of an affected child is roughly twice that of the risk for the general pediatric population (one in 300 versus one in 600);[11a] the tumor in the second child is often, although not always, the same type as that in the first. Nonetheless, the actual magnitude of the risk for sibs is still relatively small, and the main conclusion to be drawn from these data is essentially a reassuring one for parents and pediatricians.

Li and colleagues, after reviewing records of over 5000 patients, have identified 38 families with cancer in two or more children; predisposition to cancer extended to parents and other relatives as well.[40] Likewise, Miller, after a review of death certificates in the United States, concluded that siblings of children with brain tumors have a tenfold increase in mortality rate from primary neoplasms of the brain, bone, and soft tissues.[48] Genetic susceptibility in both these studies could be related in some families to parental consanguinity or to an inherited disorder predisposing to cancer (e.g., von Recklinghausen's neurofibromatosis, multiple nevoid basal cell carcinoma syndrome), but in other instances no oncogenic factors were identified.[40]

Retinoblastoma is inherited as an autosomal dominant trait in 5 to 10 per cent of cases;[16, 33] bilateral involvement is more likely in these familial cases than in sporadic ones. A proportion of cases of Wilms' tumor (possibly 38 per cent) and neuroblastoma (possibly 20 per cent) are also considered to be hereditary and attributable to a dominant gene.[33, 60] Studies have shown increased susceptibility to acute leukemia among siblings of a leukemic child. The risk varies from 1 in 5 for identical twins (under the age of 5 years) and 1 in 720 for other siblings of leukemic children (versus approximately 1/2880 in the general pediatric population).[45]

For these tumors, as for other childhood tumors, there appear to be heritable and nonheritable subgroups; the genes responsible for the former increase tumor-specific risks by an order of magnitude of 10,000 to 100,000 times.[34] In general, the familial cancer syndromes have been characterized by:

1. A higher frequency of cancer within the family than seen in the general population.
2. The occurrence of malignant tumors in consecutive generations.
3. Occurrence of tumors several years or even decades earlier than the same neoplasm usually occurs in the general population.
4. A tendency to develop tumors at multiple sites in the same organ or bilaterally in paired organs.
5. A limited range of phenotypic expression. Affected family members either develop the same type of neoplasm in a single site or tissue system, a single histologic type of cancer in various sites or organs, or different types of tumors in one organ system.
6. Vertical transmission of cancer consistent with an autosomal dominant inheritance pattern.

As treatment for these cancers improves and more children survive to reach child-bearing age, it has been suggested that vertical transmission will become more apparent.[34] In one study of progeny of childhood cancer survivors, however, no cancers developed in the 90 offspring who survived the neonatal period and were followed for a median period of 4 years (range, 0 to 17 years).[38]

PRIOR EPISODE OF MALIGNANCY (SURVIVORS OF CHILDHOOD CANCER)

Long-term survivors of childhood cancer have a marked excess of new tumors, peaking at 15 to 19 years after initial diagnosis.[39] *The 20-year cumulative probability of developing a second cancer in this group of patients has been found to be 12 per cent.* Although the majority of these cases could be related to prior radiotherapy, host susceptibility may also play a role. Thus, approximately 1 per cent of survivors of bilateral retinoblastoma have developed osteosarcoma in an extremity *outside* the radiation field following a latent period ranging from 7 to 15 years.[7a] Late occurrence of second neoplasms emphasizes the need for *continued follow-up of all survivors of childhood cancer.*[39]

IRRADIATION

As already mentioned, a large proportion of the excess new tumors seen in survivors of childhood cancer may be attributed to radiotherapy. Children irradiated for therapy of benign diseases are also at increased risk for developing cancer.[25] This is especially true for those children who received radiation therapy to the neck and upper chest region for shrinkage of allegedly enlarged thymus glands, lymphangiomas, hemangiomas, and so forth; such patients have a fourfold increase in cancer cases over the expected rate, largely involving thyroid cancers, although excess cases of lymphoma, leukemia, fibrosarcoma, and nerve tissue tumors also developed.[25]

The incidence of induced malignant disease during the first 25 years after exposure in Japanese atomic bomb survivors irradiated postnatally has been in the range of 100 cases per million persons per rad exposure.[30, 52] The major malignancy seen in these patients has been leukemia.

PRENATAL INSULT

Prenatal Exposure to Diagnostic Irradiation

The incidence of malignancy appears to be higher for children exposed to diagnostic x-rays in utero. Several authors have found a 40 to 50 per cent increase in deaths from malignant disease before the age of 10 years in this group.[41, 52, 67] The risk appears to have been particularly great when exposure occurred during the embryonic phase of development (first trimester)[67] (Table 1-9). The risk also increases with increasing x-ray exposure, demonstrating a linear dose-response relationship of 57 cases per million per year per rad;[67] this sensitivity of fetal tissues is approximately 10 times that reported for many adult tissue exposures.[29]

Prenatal Exposure to Stilbestrol

The administration of stilbestrol to women during pregnancy has been associated with an increased incidence of vaginal and cervical adenocarcinoma in their daughters;[25a] in all cases the drug was started before the eighteenth week of pregnancy.[26] To date this is the only documented evidence of a direct relationship between in utero exposure to a drug and subsequent cancer.[56]

Prenatal Exposure to Certain Viruses

Muñoz has cited five epidemiologic studies which suggest an association between influenza during pregnancy and subsequent development of cancer in the offspring.[56] These report an increased risk of 1.8 to 7.1 times with leukemia and lymphoma accounting for most of the excess.

Chickenpox during pregnancy has also been reported to cause an excess incidence of cancer in the offspring (3.7 to 5.5 times expected incidence); leukemia and medulloblastoma also appear to be more frequent in these patients.[2, 5]

RELATIONSHIP BETWEEN CONGENITAL AND ENVIRONMENTAL FACTORS IN THE ETIOLOGY OF CANCER: THE "TWO-HIT" HYPOTHESIS

Knudson has proposed a mutation model of childhood cancer which is dependent upon two discrete mutational events to induce carcinogenesis.[34] These mutational events may be transmitted in a hereditary fashion or be produced de novo by radiation or by viral and chemical carcinogens. In this model, the first mutation would render the cell precancerous, but still capable of almost normal differentiation. The second mutation would then transform the cell into a cancer cell.

For individuals who carry a hereditary cancer mutation, the target tissue would already be in the precancerous state and require only a second mutation for the final carcinogenic transformation. On the other hand, individuals who do not carry such a mutation from the instant of fertilization may develop one postzygotically by the process of

Table 1-9 Relative Risk of Cancer for Children X-Rayed In Utero[67]

DATE OF X-RAY EXAMINATION	RELATIVE RISK OF CANCER
1st trimester	8.25
2nd trimester	1.49
3rd trimester	1.43
Overall	1.48

somatic mutation; however, in this case only a few cells in the target tissue would be susceptible to the second mutagenic transformation. As a result, there are two classes of individuals with respect to such mutations. One class carries a mutation from the moment of fertilization and develops a specific tumor with high frequency (usually at an earlier average age and at multifocal sites). The second class acquires the first mutation after fertilization and develops the specific tumor with low frequency, usually at a later age and in a unifocal site.

In view of the relatively high frequency of neoplastic transformation seen in hamartomas, developmental vestiges, and dysgenic tissues, it is likely that a primary teratogenic event in the fetus may somehow predispose a given tissue to a secondary mutational event in later life. One possibility is that the structures harbor a latent oncogenic agent, possibly a virus, which may have originally caused the congenital anomaly. Subsequent environmental events (radiation, chemicals, infection, or hormonal or metabolic changes) might result in activation of this agent and result in production of cancer.

REFERENCES

1. Aaronson, C. M., and Lutzner, M. A.: Epidermodysplasia verruciformis and epidermoid carcinoma. Electron microscopic observations. J.A.M.A. 201:775, 1967.
2. Adelstein, A. M., and Donovan, J. W.: Malignant disease in children whose mothers had chickenpox, mumps, or rubella in pregnancy. Brit. Med. J. 4:629, 1972.
3. Ament, M. E.: Inflammatory disease of the colon: ulcerative colitis and Crohn's colitis. J. Pediatr. 86:322, 1975.
4. Anderson, D. E.: Familial susceptibility to cancer. CA 26:143, 1976.
5. Bithell, J. F., Draper, G. J., and Gorbach, P. D.: Association between malignant disease in children and maternal virus infections. Brit. Med. J. 1:706, 1973.
6. Blume, R. S., and Wolff, S. M.: The Chediak-Higashi syndrome; studies in four patients and review of the literature. Medicine 51:247, 1972.
7. Bolande, R. P.: Neoplasia of early life and its relationship to teratogenesis. Perspectives in Pediatric Pathology 3:145, 1976.
7a. Chan, H., and Pratt, C. B.: A new familial cancer syndrome? A spectrum of malignant and benign tumors including carcinoma of the bladder and other genitourinary tumors, thyroid adenoma, and a probable case of multifocal osteosarcoma. J. Natl. Cancer Inst. 58:205, 1975.
8. Cleaver, J. E.: Defective repair replication of DNA in xeroderma pigmentosum. Nature 218:652, 1968.
9. Devroede, G. J., Taylor, W. F., Sauer, W. G., et al.: Cancer risk and life expectancy of children with ulcerative colitis. N. Engl. J. Med. 285:17, 1971.
10. Doll, R., Muir, C., and Waterhouse, J.: Cancer Incidence in Five Continents. Vol. II. New York, Springer-Verlag, 1970.
11. Dosik, H., Hsu, L. Y., Todaro, G. J., et al.: Leukemia in Fanconi's anemia: cytogenetic and tumor virus susceptibility studies. Blood 36:341, 1970.
11a. Draper, G. J., Heaf, M. M., Kinnier Wilson, L. M.: Occurrence of childhood cancer among sibs and estimation of familial risk. J. Med. Genet. 14:81, 1977.
12. Duncan, B. R., Dohner, V. A., and Priest, J. H.: Gardner syndrome: need for early diagnosis. J. Pediatr. 72:497, 1968.
13. Epstein, C. J., Martin, G. M., Schultz, A. L., et al.: Werner's syndrome: a review of its symptomatology, natural history, pathologic features, genetics, and relationship to the natural aging process. Medicine 45:177, 1966.
14. Erbe, R. W.: Inherited gastrointestinal-polyposis syndromes. N. Engl. J. Med. 294:1101, 1976.
15. Filipi, G., and McKusick, V. A.: The Beckwith-Wiedemann syndrome (The exophalos-macroglossia-gigantism syndrome). Report of two cases and review of the literature. Medicine 49:279, 1970.
16. Fraumeni, J. F., Jr.: Genetic factors. In Holland, J. F., and Frei, E., III, (eds.): Cancer Medicine. Philadelphia, Lea & Febiger, 1973.
17. Fraumeni, J. F., Jr., and Glass, A. G.: Rarity of Ewing's sarcoma among U.S. Negro children. Lancet 1:366, 1970.
18. Gardner, E. J., and Richards, R. C.: Multiple cutaneous and subcutaneous lesions occurring simultaneously with hereditary polyposis and osteomatosis. Amer. J. Hum. Genet. 5:139, 1953.
19. Gartler, S. M., Ziprkowski, L., Krakowski, A., et al.: Glucose-6-phosphate dehydrogenase mosaicism as a tracer in the study of hereditary multiple trichoepithelioma. Amer. J. Hum. Genet. 18:282, 1966.
20. German, J.: Bloom's syndrome. II. The prototype of human genetic disorders predisposing to chromosome instability

and cancer. *In* German, J. (ed.): Chromosomes and Cancer. New York, John Wiley & Sons, 1974.
21. Gorlin, R. J., Vickers, R. A., Kellen, E., and Williamson, J. J.: The multiple basal-cell nevi syndrome. Cancer *18*:89, 1965.
22. Gorlin, R. J., Sedano, H. O., Vickers, R. A., and Cervenka, J.: Multiple mucosal neuromas, pheochromocytomas and medullary carcinoma of the thyroid—a syndrome. Cancer *22*:293, 1968.
23. Griffith, B. H., McKinney, P., Monroe, C. W., and Howell, A.: Von Recklinghausen's disease in children. Plast. Reconstr. Surg. *49*:647, 1972.
23a. Gryboski, J.: Gastrointestinal Problems in the Infant. Philadelphia, W. B. Saunders Co., 1975.
24. Hecht, F., and McCaw, B. K.: Chromosomally marked lymphocyte clones in ataxia-telangiectasia. Lancet *1*:563, 1974.
25. Hempelmann, L. H., Hall, W. J., Phillips, M., et al.: Neoplasms in persons treated with x-rays in infancy. Fourth survey in 20 years. J. Natl. Cancer Inst. *55*:519, 1975.
25a. Herbst, A. L., Ulfelder, H., Poskanzer, D. C.: Adenocarcinoma of the vagina. Association of maternal stilbesterol therapy with tumor appearance in young women. N. Engl. J. Med. *284*:878, 1971.
26. Herbst, A. L., Robboy, S. J., Scully, R. E., and Poskanzer, D. C.: Clear cell adenocarcinoma of the vagina and cervix in girls: analysis of 170 registry cases. Am. J. Obstet. Gynec. *119*:713, 1974.
27. Hill, C. S., Jr.: Thyroid cancer—iatrogenic and otherwise. CA *26*:160, 1976.
28. Howell, J. B., Anderson, D. E., and McClendon, D. L.: Multiple cutaneous cancers in children: the nevoid basal cell carcinoma syndrome. J. Pediatr. *69*:97, 1966.
29. Hutchison, G. B.: Late neoplastic changes following medical irradiation. Cancer *37*:1102, 1976.
30. Jablon, S., and Kato, H.: Studies of the mortality of A-bomb survivors. 5. Radiation dose and mortality 1950–1970. Radiat. Res. *50*:649, 1972.
31. Kersey, J. H., Spector, B. D., and Good, R. A.: Cancer in children with primary immunodeficiency diseases. J. Pediatr. *84*:263, 1974.
32. Khairi, M. R. A., Dexter, R. N., Burzynski, N. J., and Johnston, C. C., Jr.: Mucosal neuroma, pheochromocytoma, and medullary thyroid carcinoma: multiple endocrine neoplasia type 3. Medicine *54*:89, 1975.
33. Knudson, A. G., Jr.: Mutation and cancer: statistical study of retinoblastoma. Proc. Natl. Acad. Sci. U.S.A. *68*:820, 1971.
34. Knudson, A. G., Jr.: Genetics and the etiology of childhood cancer. Pediat. Res. *10*:513, 1976.
35. Knudson, A. G., Jr., and Strong, L. C.: Mutation and cancer: a model for Wilms' tumor of the kidney. J. Natl. Cancer Inst. *48*:313, 1972.
36. Knudson, A. G., Jr., and Strong, L. C.: Mutation and Cancer: neuroblastoma and pheochromocytoma. Am. J. Hum. Genet. *24*:514, 1972.
37. Li, F. P., and Fraumeni, J. F., Jr.: Testicular cancers in children: epidemiologic characteristics. J. Natl. Cancer Inst. *48*:1575, 1972.
38. Li, F. P., and Jaffe, N.: Progeny of childhood-cancer survivors. Lancet *2*:707, 1974.
39. Li, F. P., Cassady, J. R., and Jaffe, N.: Risk of second tumors in survivors of childhood cancer. Cancer *35*:1230, 1975.
40. Li, F. P., Tucker, M. A., Fraumeni, J. F., Jr.: Childhood cancer in sibs. J. Pediatr. *88*:419, 1976.
41. MacMahon, B., and Hutchinson, G. B.: Prenatal x-ray and childhood cancer: A review. Acta Un. Int. Cancr. *20*:1172, 1964.
42. McKusick, V. A.: Genetic factors in intestinal polyposis. J.A.M.A. *182*:271, 1962.
43. Michener, W. M., Gage, R. P., Sauer, W. G., and Stickler, G. B.: The prognosis of ulcerative colitis in children. N. Engl. J. Med. *265*:1075, 1961.
44. Miller, R. W.: Relation between cancer and congenital defects in man. N. Engl. J. Med. *275*:87, 1966.
45. Miller, R. W.: Persons with exceptionally high risk of leukemia. Cancer Res. *27*:2420, 1967.
46. Miller, R. W.: Relation between cancer and congenital defects: an epidemiologic evaluation. J. Natl. Cancer Inst. *40*:1079, 1968.
47. Miller, R. W.: Neoplasia and Down's syndrome. Ann. N.Y. Acad. Sci. *171*:637, 1970.
48. Miller, R. W.: Deaths from childhood leukemia and solid tumors among twins and other sibs in the United States, 1960–67. J. Natl. Cancer Inst. *46*:203, 1971.
49. Miller, R. W.: Interim report: UICC international study of childhood cancer. Int. J. Cancer *10*:675, 1972.
50. Miller, R. W.: Etiology of childhood cancer. *In* Sutow, W. W., Vietti, T. J., and Fernbach, D. J. (eds.): Clinical Pediatric Oncology. St. Louis, C. V. Mosby Co., 1973.
51. Miller, R. W., Fraumeni, J. F., Jr., and Manning, M. D.: Association of Wilm's tumor with aniridia, hemihypertrophy, and other congenital malformations. N. Engl. J. Med. *270*:922, 1964.
52. Mole, R. H.: Antenatal irradiation and childhood cancer: causation or coincidence? Brit. J. Cancer *30*:199, 1974.
53. Morson, B. C., and Bussey, H. J. R.: Predisposing causes of intestinal cancer. *In* Current Problems in Surgery. Chicago, Year Book Medical Publishers, 1970.

54. Mulvihill, J. J.: Congenital and genetic diseases. *In* Fraumeni, J. F., Jr. (ed.): Persons at High Risk of Cancer. An Approach to Cancer Etiology and Control. New York, Academic Press, 1975.
55. Muñoz, N.: Geographical distribution of pediatric tumors. Tumori 62:145, 1976.
56. Muñoz, N.: Prenatal exposure and carcinogenesis. Tumori 62:157, 1976.
57. Myers, M. H., Young, J. L., Jr., Silverberg, E., and Herse, H. W.: Cancer incidence, survival and mortality for children under 15 years of age. American Cancer Society Professional Education Publication, 1974.
58. Neblett, C. R., Waltz, T. A., and Anderson, D. E.: Neurological involvement in the nevoid basal cell carcinoma syndrome. J. Neurosurg. 35:577, 1971.
59. Nesbit, R. R., Jr., Elbadawi, N. A., Morton, J. H., and Cooper, R. A., Jr.: Carcinoma of the small bowel. A complication of regional enteritis. Cancer 37:2948, 1976.
60. Pegelow, C. H., Ebbin, A. J., Powars, D., and Towner, J. W.: Familial neuroblastoma. J. Pediatr. 87:763, 1973.
61. Reed, W. B., Landing, B., Sugarman, G., et al.: Xeroderma pigmentosum; clinical and laboratory investigation of its basic defect. J.A.M.A. 207:2073, 1969.
62. Sawitsky, A., Bloom, D., and German, J.: Chromosomal breakage and acute leukemia in congenital telangiectatic erythema and stunted growth. Ann. Intern. Med. 65:487, 1966.
63. Shaw, M. W., Falls, H. F., and Neel, J. V.: Congenital aniridia. Am. J. Hum. Genet. 12:389, 1960.
64. Shine, I., and Allison, P. R.: Carcinoma of the oesophagus with tylosis (keratosis palmeris and planteris). Lancet 1:951, 1966.
65. Siegelman, M. H., and Sutow, W. W.: Xeroderma pigmentosum. J. Pediatr. 67:625, 1965.
66. Smith, D. W.: Recognizable Patterns of Human Malformation: Genetic, Embryologic and Clinical Aspects. Philadelphia, W. B. Saunders Co., 1976.
67. Stewart, A., and Kneale, G. W.: Radiation dose effects in relation to obstetric x-rays and childhood cancer. Lancet 1:1185, 1970.
68. Turcot, J., Després, J. P., and St. Pierre, F.: Malignant tumors of central nervous system associated with familial polyposis of the colon. Dis. Colon Rectum 2:465, 1959.
69. Tyers, J. F. O., Steiger, E., and Dudrick, S. J.: Adenocarcinoma of the small intestine and other malignant tumors complicating regional enteritis. Case report and review of the literature. Ann. Surg. 169:510, 1969.
70. U. S. Public Health Service, National Vital Statistics Division. Vital Statistics of the United States, 1969. Washington, D.C., U.S. Government Printing Office, 1973.
71. Valdés-Dapéna, M. A., Huff, D. S., and DiGeorge, A. M.: The association of congenital malformation and malignant tumors in infants and children. Ann. Clin. Lab. Science 4:363, 1974.
71a. Waterhouse, J. A. H.: Cancer Handbook of Epidemiology and Prognosis. Edinburgh, Churchill Livingstone, 1974.
72. Wechsler, H. L., Krugh, F. J., Domonkos, A. N., et al.: Polydysplastic epidermolysis bullosa and development of epidermal neoplasms. Arch. Derm. 102:374, 1970.
73. Weedon, D. D., Shorter, R. G., Ilstrup, D. M., et al.: Crohn's disease and cancer. N. Engl. J. Med. 289:1099, 1973.
74. Willis, R. A.: Hamartomas and hamartomatous syndromes. *In* The Borderland of Embryology and Pathology. 2nd Ed. Washington, D.C., Butterworths, 1962.
75. Young, J. L., Jr., and Miller, R. W.: Incidence of malignant tumors in U.S. children. J. Pediatr. 86:254, 1975.

Chapter Two

DIAGNOSIS OF CANCER IN CHILDHOOD

In its beginning the malady is easier to cure but difficult to detect, but later it becomes easy to detect but difficult to cure.
      NICCOLÒ MACHIAVELLI (1469–1527)

Machiavelli's sixteenth century aphorism about tuberculosis is to a large extent equally applicable to cancer in the twentieth century. The challenge facing the clinician is to be able to diagnose the disease "in its beginning," and thus it is incumbent on all physicians who care for children to be able to recognize the presenting signs and symptoms of malignancy. Cancer may be considered to present in one of three ways in childhood: (1) as a mass lesion, (2) with symptoms directly related to the tumor, or (3) with nonspecific symptoms related to the tumor.

In general, the presence of a *mass lesion* should alert the physician quickly to the possibility of malignancy, since there are only a few mass lesions which can be considered benign on the basis of location or physical appearance alone—among these are inflammatory lymph nodes, hemangiomas, thyroglossal duct cysts, fat necrosis, dermoid cysts of the eyebrow, prepubertal breast hyperplasia, lymphangiomas, and torticollis tumors.[63] Other mass lesions should not simply be followed in the hope that they will disappear, but should be biopsied to rule out malignancy.

Symptoms directly referrable to the tumor may include gastrointestinal bleeding, neurologic signs resulting from brain or spinal cord lesions, hematuria from a Wilms' tumor or bladder rhabdomyosarcoma, obstructive symptoms, or endocrinologic symptoms resulting from hormone production by the tumor.

Unfortunately, some cancers may present with very *nonspecific symptoms* which give no clue as to their nature or location. Such symptoms include weight loss, diarrhea, low-grade fever, failure to thrive, rheumatoid-like symptoms, and opsomyoclonus. These patients will frequently be followed until the underlying disease "declares itself" at which point it is usually too far advanced for any hope of good long-term control. The use of careful physical examination

Relationship of Tumor Volume to Time of Diagnosis

At the time of detection, the volume of a tumor reflects the duration of its period of growth and its rate of growth. It has been estimated that a single cancer cell 10 μm in diameter growing in a logarithmic fashion will produce a nodule 1 mm in diameter in 20 doublings.[16] (Figs. 2-1 and 2-2). A 1 cm nodule (the likely size for "early" diagnosis) will be achieved in 30 doublings and an additional 10 doublings would produce a nodule 8 cm in diameter weighing approximately 1 kg. Since another 10 doublings (if this were possible) would produce 1000 kg of cancerous tissue (Fig. 2-2), it becomes apparent that the time required for a malignancy to grow from a single cell to a lethal mass is of the order of 40 doublings, and that *half the doublings necessary to kill the patient occur in a period of undetected growth prior to the production of a clinically evident mass.* Thus, clinical diagnosis of even a small tumor nodule is a relatively late event.

The assumptions on which this model are based are not entirely valid for human neoplasms, for these tumors grow in cycles and only a portion of the cell population is growing at any given time. Their kinetic pattern is therefore more complex and variable than the simple logarithmic model. A more valid model, based on Gompertzian kinetics (discussed in Chapter Three), shows a slowing of the growth rate as the tumor becomes larger. Another fallacy of the logarithmic model is the fact that not all the tumor mass is

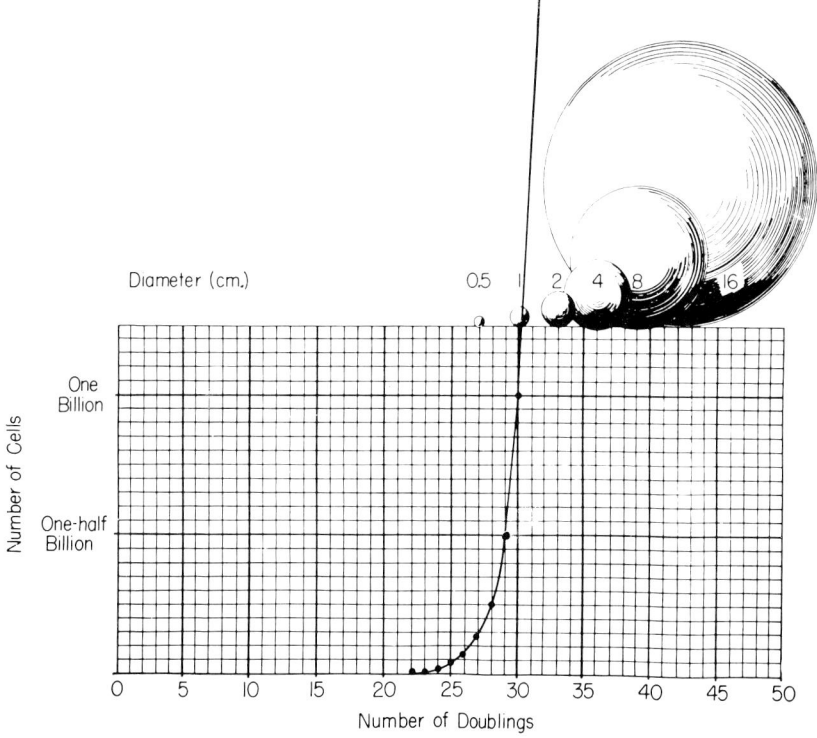

Figure 2-1 Growth curve of a hypothetical tumor on arithmetic coordinates. Note that as the tumor becomes larger, each doubling of cell number results in a progressively larger increase in the volume of the tumor. (From Collins, V. P.: Amer. J. Roentgenol. 76:98, 1956.)

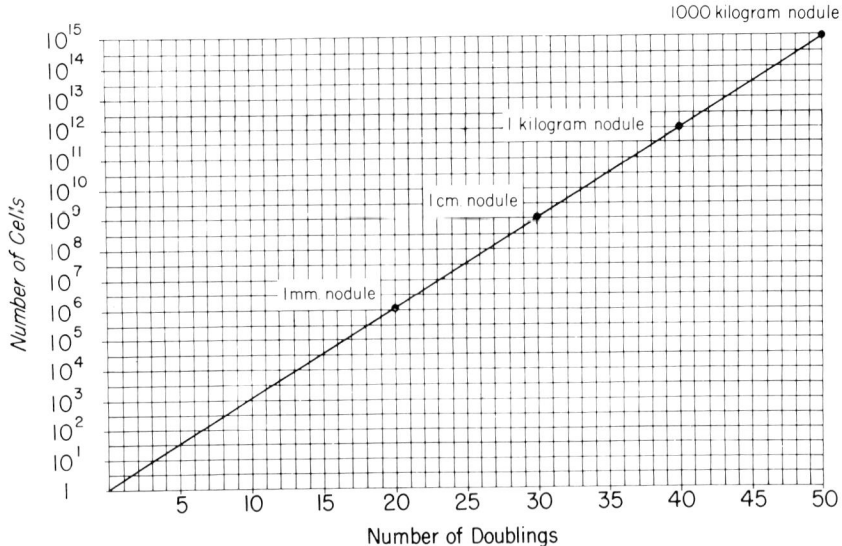

Figure 2–2 Growth curve of the hypothetical tumor in Figure 2–1 on semilogarithmic scale. (From Collins, V. P.: Am. J. Roentgenol. 76:988, 1956.)

composed of cellular elements, but part of it is stroma, secretions, and hemorrhage. Nonetheless, the logarithmic model does appear to be valid for the early stages of tumor growth and the determination of doubling time is generally accepted as the best available approach for estimating the duration of the preclinical stage of a tumor. On the basis of this model, it becomes apparent that in order for a tumor to be detected within the first 5 years of life, it must have a relatively rapid rate of growth (doubling time of less than 60 days), for tumors growing at a slower rate would require more than 5 years to reach clinically detectable size.[16]

A TOPOGRAPHIC APPROACH TO TUMOR DIAGNOSIS IN CHILDREN

Tumors of the Head and Neck
(Table 2–1)

Approximately 27 per cent of the malignant tumors of childhood occur in the region of the head and neck;[18, 77] the highest incidence of tumors in this anatomic region occurs in the orbit and brain. Tumors of the orbit are discussed below and in Chapter 14. Brain tumors are discussed in Chapter 12.

Jaffe and Jaffe have accumulated a series of 178 pediatric head and neck malignancies (excluding brain and orbit tumors) seen at the Children's Hospital Medical Center in Boston over a 10-year period. Their data are listed in Table 2–2; six tumor cell types—*lymphosarcoma, rhabdomyosarcoma, fibrosarcoma/neurofibrosarcoma, thyroid carcinoma, neuroblastoma,* and *squamous cell carcinoma (lymphoepithelioma)*—accounted for 80 per cent of the series, with the other 20 per cent of the cases being made up of a wide variety of miscellaneous tumor types.[53] These results are in general comparable with those found in other large series of pediatric head and neck tumors.[11, 18, 117]

Unlike adult tumors, which are usually epithelial in origin and easily visualized, pediatric head and neck tumors tend to occur in less superficial sites and to produce nonspecific signs and symptoms that commonly mimic those seen with more benign conditions. As a rule, symptoms depend more on the site of the tumor than on its histopathologic type.

Table 2-1 Head and Neck Masses in Childhood

	PRIMARY MALIGNANCY	METASTATIC MALIGNANCY	BENIGN LESIONS
HEAD			
Skull	*Histiocytosis X* Osteogenic sarcoma	*Neuroblastoma* Wilms' tumor	
Cranium	*Brain Tumors*	Wilms' tumor Neuroblastoma	*Abscess* *Hematoma* *Cysts* (congenital)
Orbit	*Retinoblastoma* *Rhabdomyosarcoma* *Histiocytosis X* Optic nerve glioma Teratoma Ewing's sarcoma	*Neuroblastoma* *Lymphoma* Chloroma	*Cellulitis* Thyrotoxicosis Hematoma Epidermoid cyst Lymphangioma
Nasopharynx	*Rhabdomyosarcoma* *Lymphoepithelioma* Histiocytic lymphoma Teratocarcinoma Esthesioneuroblastoma		*Polyps* *Papillomas* *Juvenile angiofibroma* Teratoma Glioma
Paranasal sinuses	*Rhabdomyosarcoma* Lymphosarcoma Fibrosarcoma		Fibroma
Oropharynx and oral cavity	*Lymphoepithelioma* *Histiocytosis X* *Rhabdomyosarcoma* *Lymphoma* (tonsil) Teratocarcinoma Fibrosarcoma Ameloblastoma		*Lymphangioma* (tongue) *Epulis* (gums) *Lingual thyroid* *Granuloma* (lip) Dermoid cyst
Salivary glands	*Mixed salivary tumor* Mucoepidermoid carcinoma	*Leukemia* *Lymphoma*	*Chronic Parotitis* Hemangioma Warthin's tumor
NECK			
Lymph glands	*Lymphoma*	*Neuroblastoma* Rhabdomyosarcoma Thyroid cancer Fibrosarcoma	*Inflammatory adenitis*
Other structures	*Neuroblastoma* *Rhabdomyosarcoma* Thyroid cancer Teratocarcinoma		*Thyroglossal duct cyst* *Branchial cleft cyst* *Cystic hygroma* *Torticollis tumor* Thyroid adenoma Thymic cyst Teratoma Epidermoid cyst

Table 2-2 Relative Frequency of Head and Neck Tumors in 178 Children[53]

CLASSIFICATION	FREQUENCY (PER CENT)	
1. Malignant lymphoid neoplasms		54.5
Hodgkin's disease	25.8	
Lymphosarcoma	24.2	
Reticulum cell sarcoma	3.9	
Burkitt's lymphoma	0.6	
2. Rhabdomyosarcoma		11.2
3. Fibrosarcoma/neurofibrosarcoma		6.1
4. Thyroid malignancies		5.1
5. Neuroblastoma		5.1
6. Squamous cell carcinoma (lymphoepithelioma)		3.9
7. Melanoma		2.2
8. Ewing's sarcoma		1.7
9. Osteogenic sarcoma/chondrosarcoma		1.1
10. Malignant hemangiopericytoma		1.1
11. Malignant histiocytoma		1.1
12. Malignant hemangioendothelioma		1.1
13. Parotid malignancies		1.1
14. Malignant Schwann cell tumor		1.1
15. Malignant teratoma		0.6
16. Miscellaneous		2.8

Tumors of the Orbit

Tumors of the orbit may be primary neoplasms or metastatic lesions, or may result from direct extension of tumor from adjacent anatomic areas. The most common primary malignancy in childhood arising within the orbit is the rhabdomyosarcoma. The tumor usually occurs during the first 5 years of life and histologically is of the embryonal variety. In most cases, it has not disseminated at the time of diagnosis. This neoplasm may sometimes be misdiagnosed as an orbital cellulitis because of its typically short history and signs suggestive of an inflammatory process.

About one third of optic nerve gliomas affect the infraorbital portion of the nerve. They usually present with proptosis, strabismus, or nystagmus. Many patients with optic nerve gliomas have evidence of von Recklinghausen's disease. Other primary malignant tumors, such as teratomas or Ewing's tumors, may also arise within the orbit, but are uncommon. Histiocytosis X may cause proptosis when the lesions involve the orbit. When this disease is present, there is usually evidence of typical punched-out defects of the skull with no evidence of bony reaction. Radiation-induced bone sarcomas occasionally arise years following treatment for another tumor. They may occur within the orbit or extend into the orbit from adjacent tissue.

The orbit is a common site for metastatic lesions from a neuroblastoma. The primary tumor usually is within the abdomen. The orbital lesions may be the first evidence of disease and are manifested by periorbital ecchymoses and proptosis. Leukemic or lymphoma deposits may also infiltrate the orbit and result in proptosis. Occasionally, rhabdomyosarcomas of the nasopharynx extend directly into the orbit. When diagnosed very late, a retinoblastoma may extend through the sclera to invade the orbit.

When the only obvious mass lesion is within the orbit, it is sometimes difficult to differentiate histologically among lymphoma, Ewing's tumor, metastatic neuroblastoma, and rhabdomyosarcoma. One must often rely on the detection of a primary lesion, the use of special histologic staining techniques, or evidence of elevated catecholamines or their metabolites in the urine to make the correct diagnosis.

Benign lesions of the orbit are much more common than malignant tumors and include infectious processes, exophthalmos due to thyrotoxicosis, hematomas, vascular abnormalities, epidermoid cysts, and lymphangiomas.

Tumors of the Nasopharynx and Paranasal Sinuses

Among the more common presenting signs associated with nasopharyngeal tumors are nasal obstruction, rhinorrhea (often blood-tinged), and a change in voice quality. If the eustachian tube is compressed or obstructed, symptoms related to the ear (tinnitus, hearing loss) may develop.

As the tumor progresses, it may lead to distinct neurologic signs, depending on its mode of spread; consequently, knowledge of the patterns of cranial nerve involvement is extremely useful for evaluation of the extent of disease and pattern of spread of nasopharyngeal tumors. Direct extension through the foramen lacerum into the cavernous sinus and middle fossa of the skull leads to involvement of cranial nerves III, IV, V, and VI, and the patient may complain of diplopia or hyperesthesia of the face or forehead; on the other hand, spread to the lateral pharyngeal nodes in and about the carotid jugular sheath may result in damage to cranial nerves IX, X, XI, and XII.[104] Usually cranial nerves VII and VIII are spared.

Since nasopharyngeal tumors may remain clinically silent for a relatively long period, their first symptoms may result from spread to cervical lymph nodes. Thus, small tumors in the nasopharynx may present with enlargement of nodes in the posterior cervical triangle or at the angle of the mandible (jugulodigastric node).

The differential diagnosis of obstructive nasopharyngeal symptoms includes such benign lesions as hypertrophied adenoids, choanal polyps, and juvenile angiofibroma. *Juvenile angiofibroma* occurs almost exclusively in young males 8 to 15 years old. It characteristically appears as a rounded, nonulcerated red mass. Since it is highly vascularized, it tends to bleed easily; diagnosis may be confirmed by arteriography. Although histologically benign, the tumor may behave in a clinically malignant fashion; complete resection is difficult because of the severe hemorrhage that the tumor may produce even after minimal manipulation.

Tumors of the paranasal sinuses grow silently for a long time before producing symptoms (unilateral nasal obstruction, bloody nasal discharge). If the superior wall of the antrum is involved, the orbital contents may be displaced and proptosis or diplopia may be evident; the tumor may also extend via the inferior portion of the antrum to the superior alveolar ridge and produce abnormal mobility of the teeth.

Tumors of the Ear

Earache, serous otitis media, or aural discharge may reflect extension of a nasopharyngeal malignancy through the eustachian tube or a primary malignancy of the mastoid sinus or middle ear. Malignant tumors may also arise in the external auditory meatus and produce aural discharge (often blood-tinged), a polypoid mass, or hearing loss. Trismus occurs if the temporomandibular joint is involved.

Tumors of the Oropharynx and Oral Cavity

Oropharyngeal tumors may produce unilateral tonsillar enlargement, dysphagia, trismus, or sore throat. A bulky tumor at the base of the tongue will interfere with speech and breathing. As with nasopharyngeal lesions, small tumors of the oropharynx may first present as metastatic lumps in the neck; the subdigastric and midjugular node groups are most frequently involved.

Tumors of the oral cavity most commonly occur in the cheek, lateral floor of the mouth, inferior gum, and lateral border of the tongue; early symptoms are difficulties with speech and swallowing or enlargement of the submaxillary and subdigastric lymph nodes.

Tumors of the Neck

Swellings in the neck are common in childhood and usually indicate benign inflammatory lymph node swellings or embryonal remnants. However, unilateral enlargement (especially greater than 3 cm) or the presence of a nontender, hard, single node much larger than any other should immediately suggest the possibility of malignancy.[52, 53, 56, 76] In the experience of Moussatos and Baffes, most solitary masses anterior to the sternomastoid muscle are benign, while about half of the solitary masses lying posterior to it are malignant; tumors lying both anterior and posterior to the sternomastoid are nearly always malignant.[84]

In the Children's Hospital series, malignant neck lesions in children varied in incidence according to age: in children from 0 to 6 years of age, the commonest tumor was neuroblastoma, followed by lymphosarcoma and rhabdomyosarcoma; in older children, Hodgkin's disease and lymphosarcoma were the leading tumors and neuroblastoma was unusual.[52] Since many cervical masses are metastatic, *surgical excision of an enlarged cervical lymph node for diagnosis should not be performed until a thorough search has been made to determine a possible primary site.* Careful examination of the ears, nose, upper respiratory and alimentary tracts, and particularly the nasopharynx (which was the primary site for 16 per cent of metastatic cervical nodes) is particularly useful.

Since 50 per cent of all malignant neck masses in children are due to lymphomas, a careful search for lymphadenopathy in other areas of the body (including chest x-ray for mediastinal enlargement) as well as for hepatosplenomegaly should be performed; peripheral blood count and bone marrow aspiration (with special attention to leukemic transformation) may also be helpful. Screening studies for VMA, HVA, metanephrine, and catecholamines in the urine should be performed, since 15 per cent of the neck masses are due to neuroblastoma; this is especially important in children under 6 years of age.

Embryonic Remnants and Other Benign Lesions of the Neck. Since the neck has so little free space, enlargement of a normal structure in almost any direction will produce a telltale bulge. Thus, embryonic remnants in the neck (for which no space is provided after birth) may persist and enlarge, producing characteristic mass lesions.

ECTOPIC THYROID. During embryogenesis, the thyroid gland normally migrates from the foramen cecum at the base of the tongue to its final position in the neck. Arrest of its descent at any level will result in an ectopically positioned thyroid, which may appear as a rounded midline mass lesion on the posterior aspect of the tongue (lingual thyroid), the neck region anterior to the hyoid bone (thyroglossal cyst), or over the thyroid isthmus. The thyroidal nature of these ectopic masses can be confirmed by demonstrating uptake of radioactive iodine. In these situations, palpation over the expected thyroid position yields a sensation of emptiness, and the carotid pulses are unusually easy to palpate.

THYROGLOSSAL DUCT CYST. This arises as a developmental remnant of the descent of the thyroid gland. As the thyroid anlage migrates downward, it forms a duct behind it, which usually becomes obliterated by the sixth to seventh week of fetal life; incomplete obliteration, however, may lead to the development of a thyroglossal duct cyst, which can appear anywhere in the midline between the foramen cecum and the suprasternal notch. The cyst is usually found at or below the level of the hyoid bone and retracts upon thrusting out of the tongue. Dermoid cysts and lymph nodes, which also can present as masses in this region, do not retract when the tongue is thrust forward. On rare occasions carcinoma may develop in a thyroglossal duct cyst;[105] however, a more important reason for removing this lesion is the high frequency of infectious complications.

BRANCHIAL CLEFT CYST. The branchial clefts arise as ectodermal invaginations between the branchial arches during embryogenesis; normally they become obliterated, but if obliteration fails to occur, various head and neck lesions may appear. Cysts of the first branchial cleft may present as cystic masses anterior and inferior to the ear lobe or as large cystic masses over the parotid gland and upper neck connected by a sinus tract to the external auditory canal. The more common second branchial cleft cyst presents as an intermittant or continuous swelling in the upper third of the neck, sometimes associated with a branchial sinus that opens as a small punctum at the anterior border of the sternomastoid muscle, from which mucus can be milked. Cysts of the third branchial cleft appear in the lower third of the neck; they are extremely uncommon.

PERSISTENT CERVICAL THYMUS. This is an infrequent cause of a neck mass, resulting from failure of embryologic descent of the third branchial pouch. The majority present as a unilateral or occasionally low midline mass that may become evident only when the child cries.

STERNOMASTOID TUMOR. This type of tumor is typically a hard, spindle-shaped mass found within the upper half of the sternomastoid muscle in infants from 2 to 5 weeks of age and accompanied by torticollis, faciocranial asymmetry, scoliosis, or thoracic asymmetry. The microscopic picture is that of degenerating muscle fibers and maturing fibroblasts.

LYMPH VESSEL SWELLINGS. These are hamartomas rather than true neoplasms. They range in size from small simple lymph cysts to lymphangiomas and finally to a cystic hygroma. The latter are frequently multilocular and unencapsulated; they may infiltrate around and through the roof of the neck, the cervical pleura, the axilla, or the floor of the mouth. Sudden enlargement may lead to respiratory embarrassment and necessitate emergency tracheotomy. The diagnosis is usually evident on physical examination by the diffuse, irregular, soft, compressible nature of the lesion which is also painless and can be transilluminated.

INTRATHORACIC MASSES (Table 2-3)

Pulmonary Neoplasms

Primary intrapulmonary neoplasms are very rare in childhood. The lungs, however, are a frequent site of metastasis; in general, tumors which metastasize by the hematogenous route appear in the pulmonary parenchyma, while those metastasizing by lymphogenous routes appear in the lymphoid tissue of the mediastinum. Probably the most common pediatric malignancy with early intrapulmonary metastases is Wilms' tumor, this occurring in approximately one-third of patients at the time of original diagnosis. Other tumors commonly metastasizing to the lung parenchyma are osteogenic sarcomas, Ewing's sarcomas (Fig. 2–3), thyroid tumors, hepatic tumors, soft tissue sarcomas, amelanotic melanomas, teratocarcinomas, and retinoblastomas. Neuroblastomas more commonly produce pleural (Fig. 2–4) and mediastinal node metastases, with intrapulmonary lesions uncommon except in the terminal phases.

Generally, metastatic pulmonary
Text continued on page 27

Table 2-3 Intrathoracic Masses in Childhood

	PRIMARY MALIGNANCY	METASTATIC MALIGNANCY	BENIGN LESIONS
Pulmonary parenchyma	Bronchial carcinoid tumor Anaplastic carcinoma	*Wilms' tumor* *Ewing's sarcoma* *Osteogenic sarcoma* *Thyroid tumors* *Melanoma (amelanotic)* *Rhabdomyosarcoma* *Ovarian tumors* *Retinoblastoma* *Neuroblastoma* *Hepatic tumors*	*Infection* Bronchial adenoma Hamartoma
Mediastinum Anterior mediastinum	*Lymphosarcoma* *Teratocarcinoma* Thymoma Thyroid cancer	*Leukemia*	*Enlarged thymus* Teratoma Lymphangioma Hemangioma Substernal goiter
Middle mediastinum	*Hodgkin's disease* Fibrosarcoma (bronchial)	*Hodgkin's disease* *Lymphosarcoma* *Leukemia* Neuroblastoma Testicular tumors	*Inflammatory adenitis* Bronchogenic cyst Angiomatous lymphoid hamartoma Cardiac myxoma Pericardial cyst
Posterior mediastinum	*Neuroblastoma* Neurofibrosarcoma		*Foregut duplication* Neurenteric cyst Neurofibroma Hemangioma

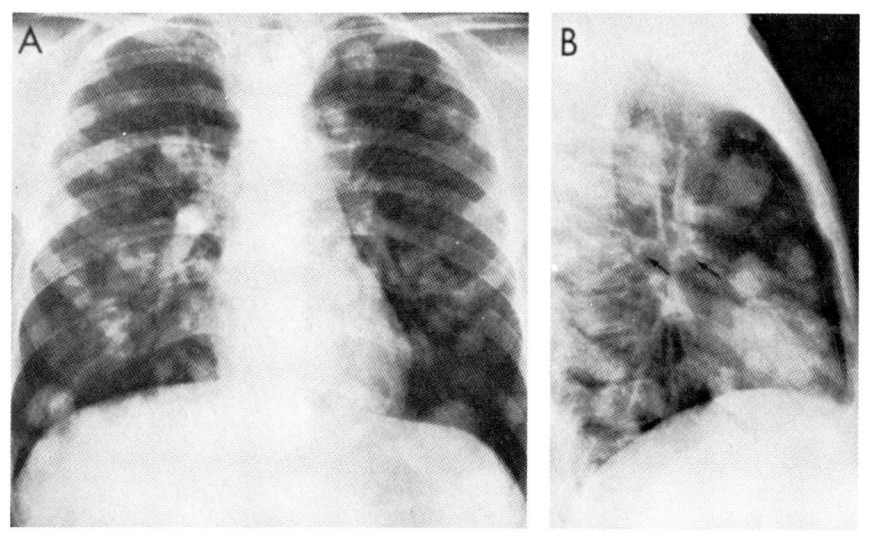

Figure 2-3 Metastatic pulmonary lesions from a Ewing's sarcoma of the ilium. (From Caffey, J. [ed.]: Pediatric X-ray Diagnosis. Chicago, Year Book Medical Publishers, 1972.)

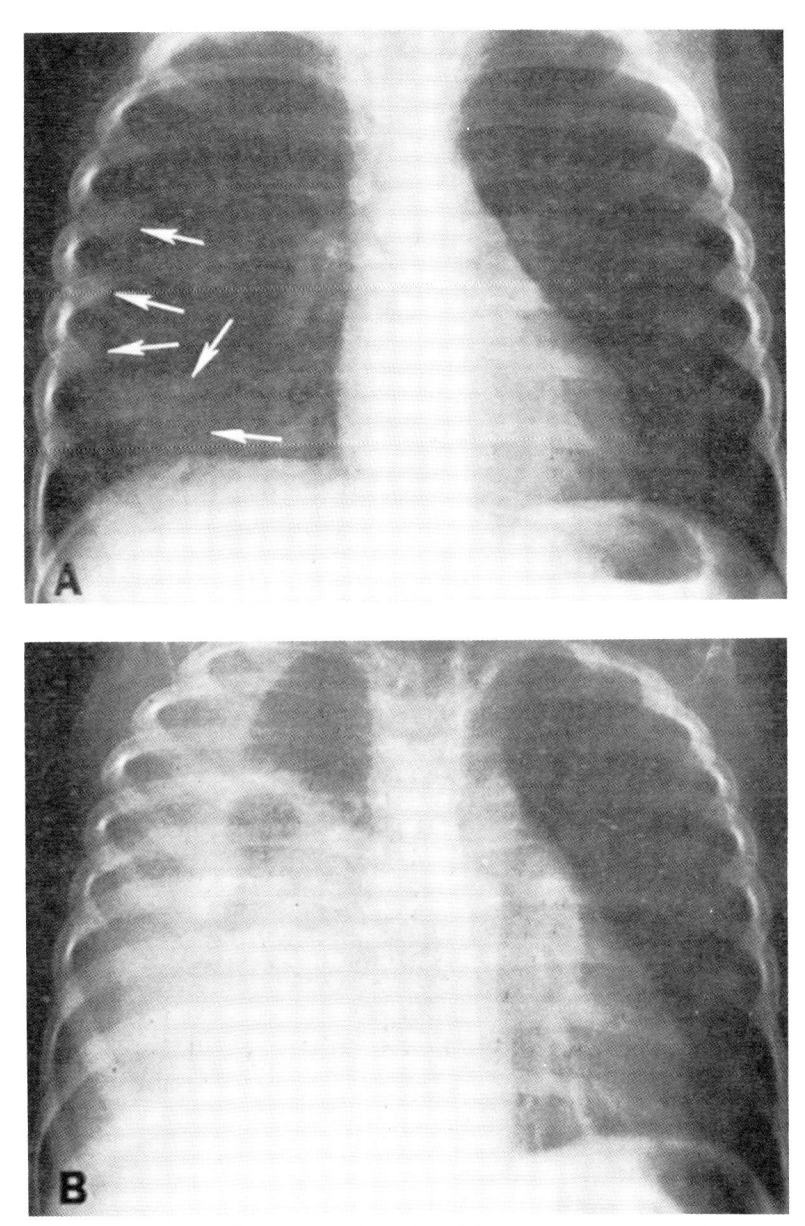

Figure 2-4 Metastatic neuroblastoma. *A*, Pleural nodules (arrows). *B*, Chest film two weeks later, demonstrating rapid accumulation of pleural fluid. (From Poole, C. A.: *In* Vuksanovic, M. M. (ed.): Clinical Pediatric Oncology. Mt. Kisco, N.Y., Futura Publishing Co., 1972.)

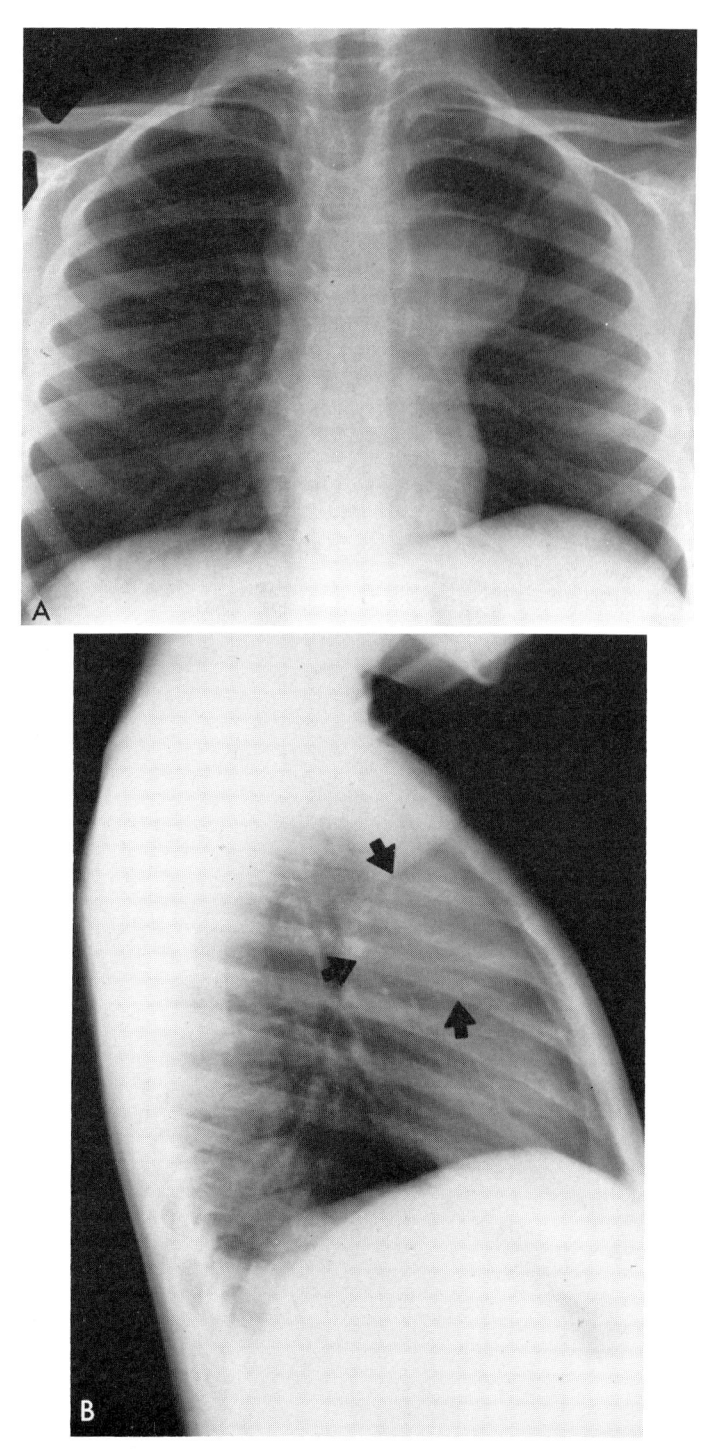

Figure 2–5   Anterior mediastinal mass in a 2 year old boy. *A*, Frontal projection. *B*, Lateral projection. The tumor was a benign cystic teratoma (uncalcified).

tumors can be distinguished radiologically from primary bronchial neoplasms because the latter tend to produce obstructive atelectasis and emphysema; however, metastatic lesions resemble each other so closely that it is impossible to distinguish between them, with the exception of those metastatic osteogenic sarcomas that contain enough bone to be radiographically opaque.

Mediastinal Neoplasms

A significant number of childhood malignancies occur in the mediastinum. These may be classified under three major headings:

1. Neurogenic (neuroblastoma, ganglioneuroblastoma, neurofibrosarcoma).
2. Lymphatic (malignant thymoma, lymphosarcoma, Hodgkin's disease).
3. Malignant germ cell tumors.

Frequently the anatomic location of a mediastinal mass will be very helpful in determining the nature of the lesion. Germ cell tumors occur in the anterior mediastinum (Fig. 2-5), lymphatic tumors in the anterior and middle mediastinum (Fig. 2-6), and neurogenic tumors in the posterior mediastinum (Fig. 2-7). These lesions must be distinguished from benign masses occurring in the same areas.

The presence of calcification in an anterior mediastinal mass usually suggests teratoma or some other germ cell tumor. However, a major diagnostic dilemma may result from the presence of an asymptomatic uncalcified anterior mediastinal mass in a young child. Differentiation of benign thymic hyperplasia from other masses in this location is sometimes difficult; one helpful finding, if present, is indentation of the anterior edges of the thymus

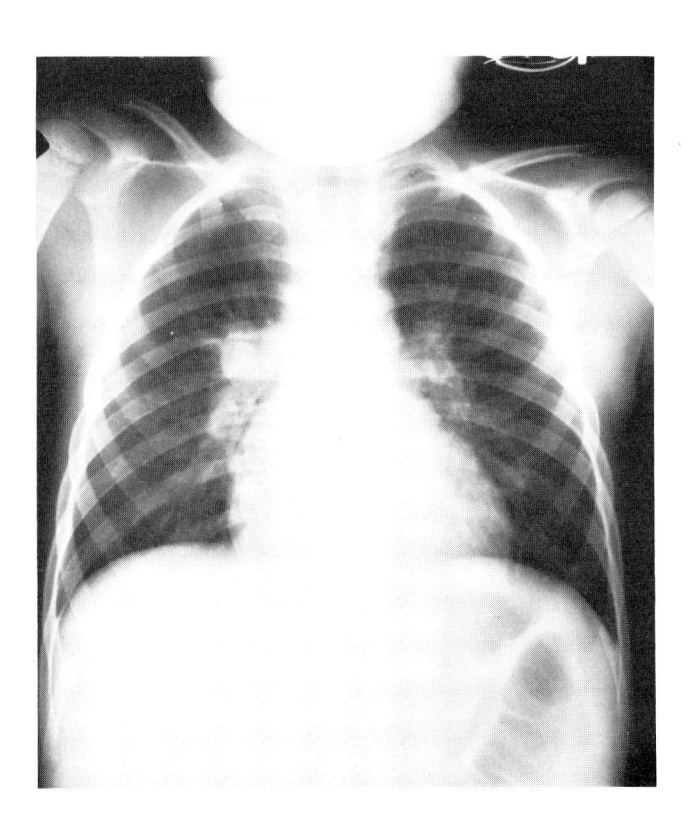

Figure 2-6 Middle mediastinal mass. Enlarged hilar nodes in a 4 year old boy with acute lymphoblastic leukemia.

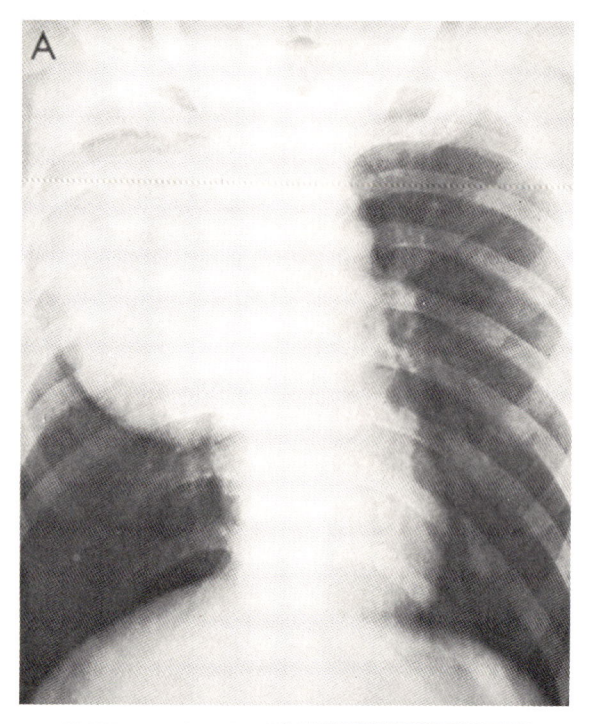

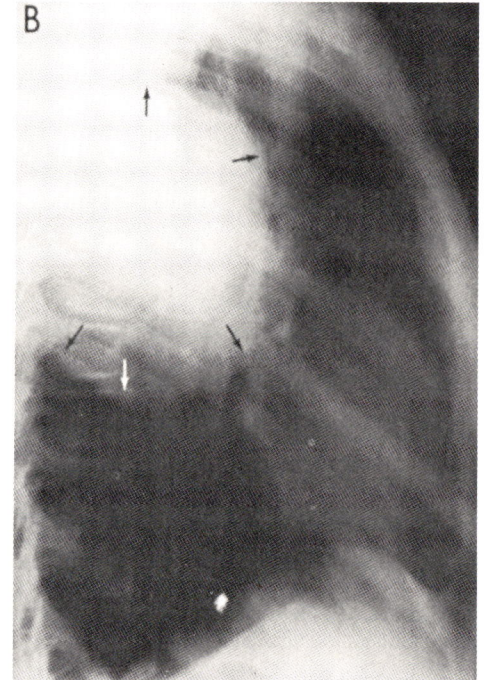

Figure 2-7   Posterior mediastinal mass. *A*, Frontal projection. *B*, Lateral projection. Tumor was a ganglioneuroma. (From Caffey, J. [ed.]: Pediatric X-Ray Diagnosis. Chicago, Year Book Medical Publishers, 1972.)

by the costal cartilages to produce a scalloped edge ("wave" sign). Haller and co-workers have recommended the use of a brief course of prednisone (1.5 mg/kg daily for 5 days) as a diagnostic test;[44] this treatment will cause rapid regression of benign thymic hyperplasia. However, this result should be interpreted with caution since lymphomatous masses may also show marked regression with steroid therapy. Chest fluoroscopy is also useful in distinguishing thymus from mass lesions, as the thymus is pliable and changes markedly in size and configuration with respiration.[43]

Lymphomatous lesions of the middle mediastinum, especially Hodgkin's type, are unusual in infants under 2 years of age. The most common middle mediastinal mass in this age group, bronchogenic cyst, frequently is not radiopaque but should be suspected in an infant with repeated episodes of respiratory distress and unilateral or bilateral emphysema. In older children, both Hodgkin's and non-Hodgkin's lymphomas are important causes of middle mediastinal mass lesions.

Calcification in a posterior mediastinal mass suggests neuroblastoma or other neurogenic tumors. Barium swallow may be useful in distinguishing foregut duplications and neurenteric cysts from posterior neurogenic tumors. Attention to the appearance of the vertebrae is also useful when a posterior mediastinal mass is present. Erosion of vertebral bodies and pedicles, separation of pedicles, and enlarged intervertebral foramina (on oblique views) may accompany intrathoracic neuroblastoma and provide an early clue to invasion of the spinal canal prior to the development of cord compression symptoms. Hemivertebrae may be indicative of neurenteric cyst with spinal cord involvement.

In the child, approximately 40 per cent of primary mediastinal masses are malignant (a figure two- to threefold higher than for adults);[40] moreover, initially benign lesions such as mature teratomas and neurofibromas may subsequently undergo malignant degeneration. Consequently, unless an adequate diagnosis can be made by other means, all primary mediastinal masses in childhood should be explored.[40]

ABDOMINAL, PELVIC, AND RETROPERITONEAL MASSES
(Table 2-4)

Every solid abdominal mass in an infant or child should be considered a potential malignancy until proved otherwise. Approximately half of solid abdominal masses in children can usually be diagnosed and managed without surgical intervention because they are of a "medical" nature, i.e., diffuse hepatomegaly and/or splenomegaly secondary to infectious problems, lipid storage diseases, leukemia, lymphoma, and so forth.[80] Of those masses that are "surgical" in nature, approximately half arise in the kidney and urinary tract. The common urologic masses are hydronephrosis (40 per cent), Wilms' tumor (30 per cent), and cystic renal disease (22 per cent).[80] Of those masses that do not arise in the urologic structures, approximately 39 per cent are intraperitoneal, and 61 per cent retroperitoneal (neuroblastoma, lymphomas, sarcomas, and so forth). Thus, when all childhood "surgical" abdominal masses are considered, 70 to 80 per cent arise in the retroperitoneal area.

To a certain extent the age of the patient is useful in determining the likelihood of malignancy in an abdominal mass and also the most probable type of neoplasm. In the neonate (discussed below) abdominal masses are much more likely to represent developmental renal lesions (hydronephrosis, cystic disease) than neoplasms, whereas palpable abdominal masses in children 1 to 2 years of age are much more likely to be neoplasms. Neuroblastoma and Wilms' tumor are most common between 6 months and 4 years of age.

Table 2-4 Abdominal Masses in Childhood

	PRIMARY MALIGNANCY	METASTATIC MALIGNANCY	BENIGN LESIONS
Intraperitoneal: Liver	*Hepatoblastoma* *Hepatocellular carcinoma*	*Wilms' tumor* *Neuroblastoma* Ovarian tumors	*Inflammatory diseases* *Metabolic diseases* *Cysts* (Intrahepatic) Abscess Hamartoma Hemangioendothelioma Choledochal cyst Adenoma
Gastrointestinal tract	*Lymphoma* Carcinoma (colon) Carcinoid (appendix) Multiple familial polyposis		*Juvenile polyps* Hemangioma Peutz-Jeghers syndrome
Spleen	*Lymphoma*	Leukemia	*Inflammatory diseases* Metabolic diseases Epidermoid cyst Pseudocysts Hemangioma Hamartoma
Retroperitoneal: Kidney	*Wilms' tumor*	Lymphosarcoma	*Hydronephrosis* *Multicystic kidney* *Polycystic kidney* Congenital mesoblastic nephroma Angiolipoleiomyoma (tuberous sclerosis)
Adrenal	*Neuroblastoma* Adrenal carcinoma		*Ganglioneuroma*
Lymph nodes	*Lymphoma*	*Multiple tumors*	
Other retroperitoneal	*Teratocarcinoma* Neuroblastoma		Teratoma Fetus in fetu

Neonatal Period. Fewer than 15 per cent of abdominal masses diagnosed in the first four weeks of life are malignant;[36,123] among these are neuroblastoma, fibrosarcoma, teratoma, reticulum cell sarcoma, leukemia, malignant histiocytosis, and primary liver tumors.[27,121]

More than half of neonatal masses arise in the kidney, with multicystic kidney and hydronephrosis accounting for almost 40 per cent of the total cases;[36] bilateral masses usually represent hydronephrotic kidneys, but polycystic kidneys can also present as bilateral masses. These lesions, as well as other masses of renal or adrenal origin, are located in the flanks and may be slightly movable; sometimes, however, renal masses may seem to be present surprisingly anteriorly on physical examination. Renal vein thrombosis should be considered if the infant has become severely dehydrated or gross hematuria is present.

Mobile anterior midline masses are usually due to intestinal duplication (enteric cyst), mesenteric cyst, or ovarian cyst; these cystic lesions, on transillumination, usually transmit

Table 2-4 (Continued) Pelvic Masses in Childhood

	PRIMARY MALIGNANCY	METASTATIC MALIGNANCY	BENIGN LESIONS
Ovary	*Teratocarcinoma* *Dysgerminoma* *Embryonal carcinoma* Lymphoma Arrhenoblastoma	*Lymphoma* Leukemia	*Teratoma* Gynandroblastoma Simple cysts Cystadenoma Fibroma
Testis	*Teratocarcinoma* *Embryonal carcinoma* *Rhabdomyosarcoma* Sertoli cell tumor Leydig cell tumor	*Lymphosarcoma* Leukemia	*Teratoma* Sertoli cell adenoma
Uterus and vagina	*Rhabdomyosarcoma* Infantile carcinoma Adenocarcinoma		*Papilloma* Hymeneal polyps Hydrocolpos Hydrometra
Bladder	*Rhabdomyosarcoma* Leiomyosarcoma		Leiomyoma Neurofibroma Inflammatory polyps
Sacrococcyx	*Teratocarcinoma* Neuroblastoma		*Teratoma* Ganglioneuroma Meningocele Lipoma
Bowel	Lymphosarcoma Carcinoma		Appendiceal abscess Fecal masses Polyps Duplication Cyst

light and have a smooth contour. A mass accompanied by symptoms of intestinal obstruction is most likely a distended loop of bowel due to meconium ileus, intestinal atresia, midgut volvulus, or a duplication derived from the midgut or hindgut.

A *fixed* midline mass arising in the pelvis or lower abdomen is usually an enlarged bladder, a hydrometra (massive distention of the uterus), or a hydrocolpos (massive distention of the vagina). These usually are found within the first 2 days of life.[36] The differential diagnosis of the enlarged bladder resulting from urinary retention due to obstruction at the bladder outlet deserves special mention, since it may be caused by both benign and malignant lesions. Conditions such as intrinsic urologic disease (urethral atresia, urethral valves, prolapsing ectopic ureterocele), extrinsic lesions which compress the bladder (pelvic neuroblastoma, presacral teratoma, sarcoma botryoides), and neurologic diseases (meningomyelocele) must be considered.

Physical Examination

Some differentiation between intraperitoneal and retroperitoneal masses can be made by palpation. Intraperitoneal masses (other than liver and spleen) may shift with manual pressure or change in the patient's position, while retroperitoneal masses are fixed and are felt deep in the renal fossa; malignant masses are usually hard while hydronephrosis is usually soft. Liver and spleen masses move with respiration, whereas retroperitoneal masses do not.

In the infant and child, bimanual examination (with the index finger of one hand in the patient's rectum) allows evaluation of renal and other retroperitoneal masses, pelvic masses, and lower abdominal masses to a far greater extent than in the adult. When examined by this technique, Wilms' tumors tend to have a regular outline (since they are expanding within Gerota's fascia) (Fig. 2-8), are more often mobile, and are usually (about 95 per cent) confined to one side of the midline.[19, 58] Neuroblastoma, on the other hand, tends to be more amorphous and unconfined in shape and is frequently nodular; it usually is not ballotable and tends to be fixed to surrounding structures.

Evaluation of hepatic and splenic size in childhood requires a knowledge of the normal range of variation of these organs. Unlike the situation for adults, projection of the liver and spleen edge below the costal margins does not necessarily indicate pathology of these organs in childhood. In a group of normal children studied by McNicholl,[79] the average projection of the liver edge below the right costal border (in the midclavicular line) was approximately 1 to 2 cm, with a range of 0 to 4 cm; 11.1 per cent of these children also had palpable spleens.

When a right upper quadrant mass is associated with obstructive jaundice and pain, the diagnosis of cystic dilatation of the common bile duct (choledochal cyst) should be considered. In 18 per cent of cases the diagnosis is made in the first year of life, and in 45 per cent it is made by the age of 10 years.[116]

Once the presence and location of an abdominal mass have been confirmed by *gentle* palpation by a single examiner, no further abdominal palpation should take place. The patient should *not* be used as a teaching exercise for house staff, medical students, nurses, and so forth, since any abdominal pressure increases the risk of dissemination of tumor emboli into efferent vessels or rupture of the tumor, or both, with resultant intraperitoneal dissemination. Meddling should be discouraged by means of a prominent sign stating: DO NOT PALPATE ABDOMEN.

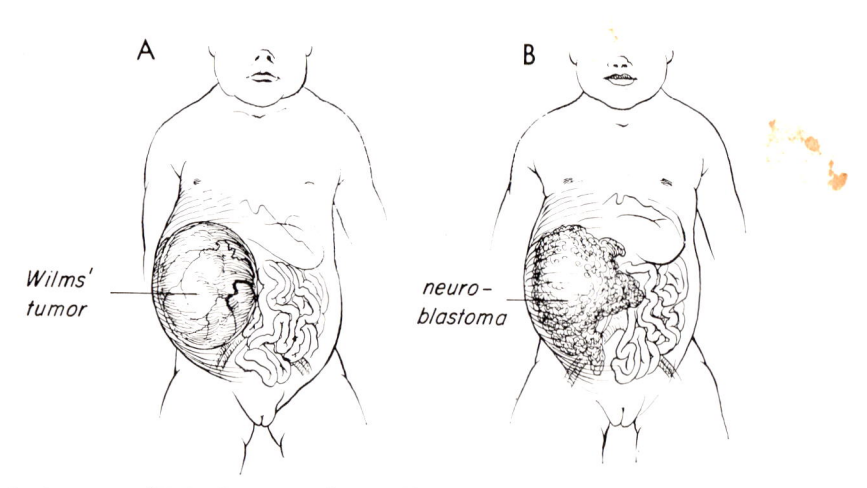

Figure 2–8 Anatomy of Wilms' tumor and neuroblastoma. The usual outline of Wilms' tumor is smooth and spherical while that of neuroblastoma is irregular and sometimes nodular, and often extends beyond the midline. (From Snyder, W. H., Hastings, T. N., and Pollack, W. F.: Retroperitoneal tumors. *In* Mustard, W. T., et al. [eds.]: Pediatric Surgery. 2nd ed. Copyright © 1969 by Year Book Medical Publishers, Inc. Chicago.)

Radiologic Evaluation

Radiologic evaluation of an abdominal mass can be considered to proceed in three phases:[87]

1. An attempt is made to determine if the mass is intraperitoneal or retroperitoneal.

2. If the mass is intraperitoneal, determine if it is intimately connected with the liver or spleen; if retroperitoneal, differentiate between renal, adrenal, and other masses.

3. Try to determine the exact location and nature of the mass; a search for the presence of calcification may be helpful in this regard (Table 2-5).

Retroperitoneal Masses. The retroperitoneal space contains fatty and areolar tissue, connective tissue, the kidneys, ureters, adrenal glands, elements of the autonomic and peripheral nervous systems, the lymphatic system, lymph nodes, blood vessels, the pancreas, and portions of the gastrointestinal tract (the duodenum, duodenojejunal junction, ascending colon, and descending colon) (Fig. 2-9).

Anterior displacement of retroperitoneal structures such as the duodenojejunal junction, ascending colon, or descending colon indicate that a mass has arisen in the retroperitoneal area (Fig. 2-10). Tumors in this region may also cause complete ureteral obstruction and displace intraperitoneal structures (e.g., stomach, small intestinal loops) in an anterior direction or to either side.

Intraperitoneal Masses. Intraperitoneal masses, on the other hand, never displace retroperitoneal structures anteriorly. When a mass arises in the liver, the pattern of displacement will depend upon whether a single hepatic lobe or the entire liver is involved: (1) when the right hepatic lobe is the predominant site of involvement (Fig. 2-11), the hepatic shadow is enlarged in the right upper quadrant of the abdomen; this shadow is located anteriorly when a lateral view of the abdomen is obtained. The stomach and duodenum are displaced to the left and the hepatic flexure of the colon is displaced downward; (2) enlargement of the left lobe of the liver (Fig. 2-12) results in an increased hepatic density in the left upper quadrant of the abdomen; the stomach fundus may be displaced to the left, downward, or posteriorly; (3) generalized hepatic involvement produces a combination of the above signs with displacement of the stomach, duodenum, small intestine, hepatic flexure, and transverse colon downward and to the left.

Splenic enlargement (Fig. 2-13) will indent the greater curvature of the stomach or depress the splenic flexure of the colon. There will also be a density visualized in the left upper quadrant of the abdomen.

Intrinsic gastrointestinal masses and other intraperitoneal masses may impinge upon or displace various intestinal loops. These usually are best visualized with contrast studies. When a child over 6 years of age presents with intussusception, the barium enema must be scrutinized carefully for evidence of lymphosarcoma of the ileum, the most common cause of intussusception in the older child;[122] if the barium enema is normal, an upper gastrointestinal series should be performed after the barium is evacuated.

Special Radiologic Studies

THE INTRAVENOUS PYELOGRAM AND ASSOCIATED STUDIES. Since the majority of abdominal masses of childhood arise in the kidney or its sur-

Table 2-5 Calcification in Abdominal Tumors

TUMOR	PERCENTAGE WHICH SHOW CALCIFICATION
Neuroblastoma	50[78]
Teratoma	50[17]
Primary liver tumors	20-25[41, 74]
Wilms' tumor	<10[94]
Lymphosarcoma	Rare, if ever
Rhabdomyosarcoma	Rare, if ever

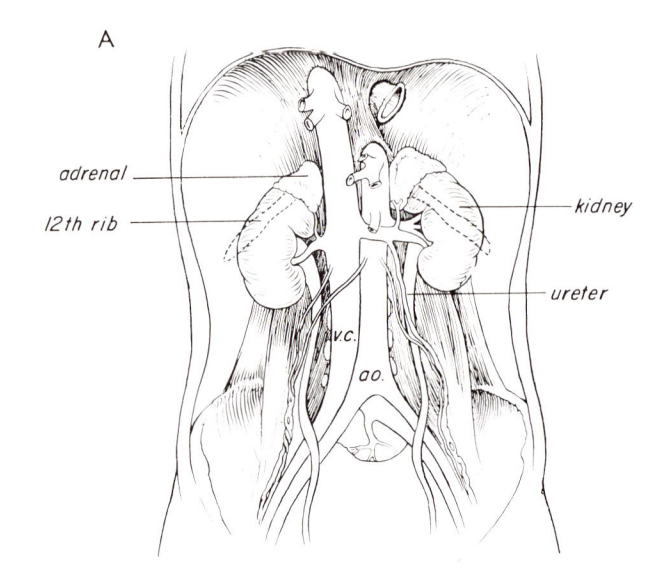

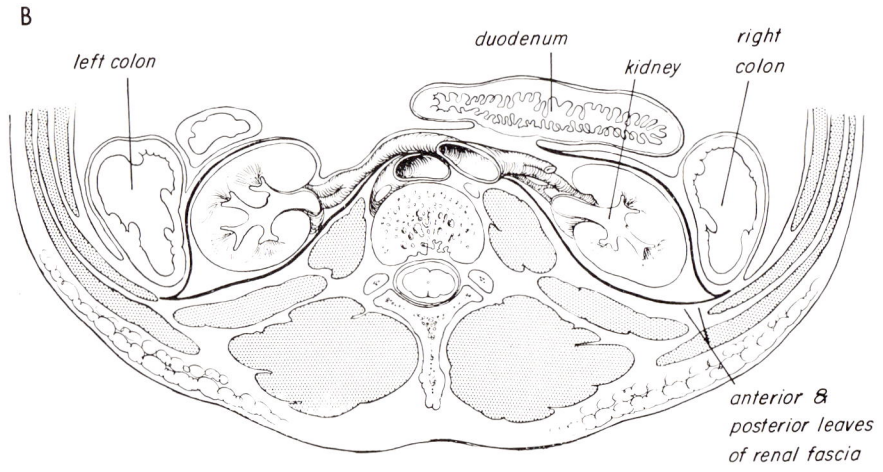

Figure 2–9 Anatomic relationships of the retroperitoneal space. *A*, Frontal view. *B*, Cross section at the level of the renal pedicles. (From Snyder, W. H., Hastings, T. N., and Pollack, W. F.: Retroperitoneal tumors. *In* Mustard, W. T., et al. [eds.]: Pediatric Surgery. 2nd ed. Copyright © 1969 by Year Book Medical Publishers, Inc., Chicago.)

DIAGNOSIS OF CANCER IN CHILDHOOD 35

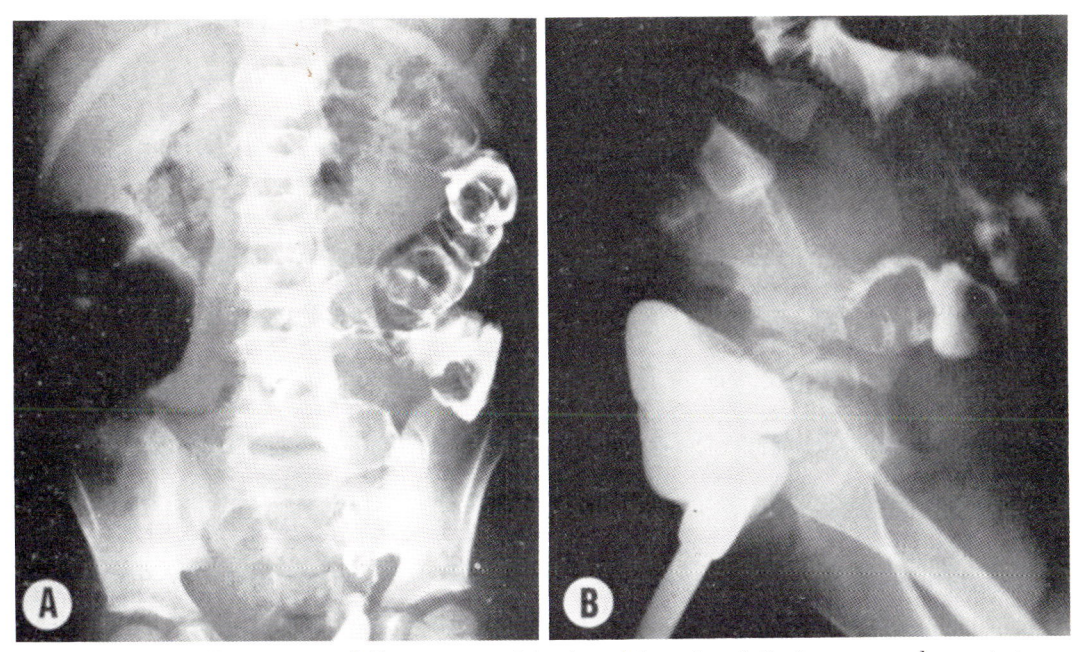

Figure 2–10 Retroperitoneal fibrosarcoma arising in pelvic region. *A,* Barium enema, demonstrating leftward displacement of rectosigmoid junction. *B,* Lateral views showing anterior displacement of rectosigmoid junction. (From Nice, C. M., et al.: Am. J. Roentgenol. 75:990, 1956.)

Figure 2–11 Hepatoma arising in the right lobe of the liver of a 1 day old female. Flocculent calcifications are seen in the mass, which is displacing the right kidney downward. (From Davis, L. A.: Pediatric Radiology. *In* Robbins, L. L. [ed.]: Golden's Diagnostic Radiology. © 1973. The Williams & Wilkins Co., Baltimore.)

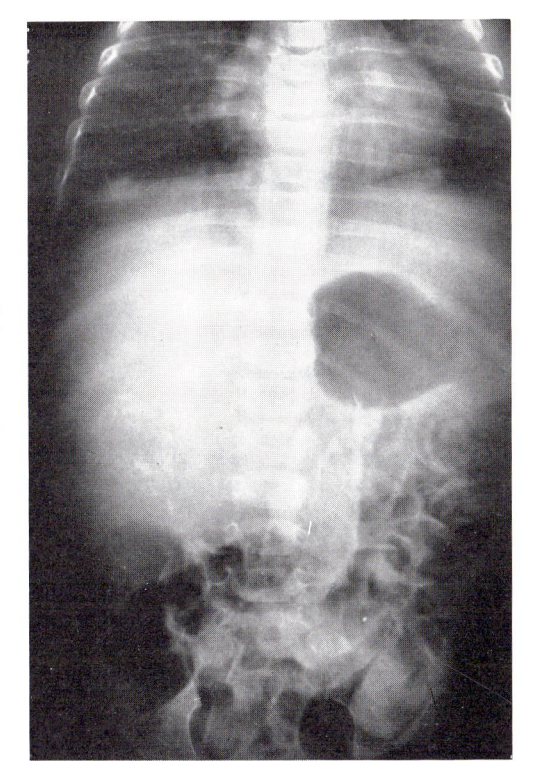

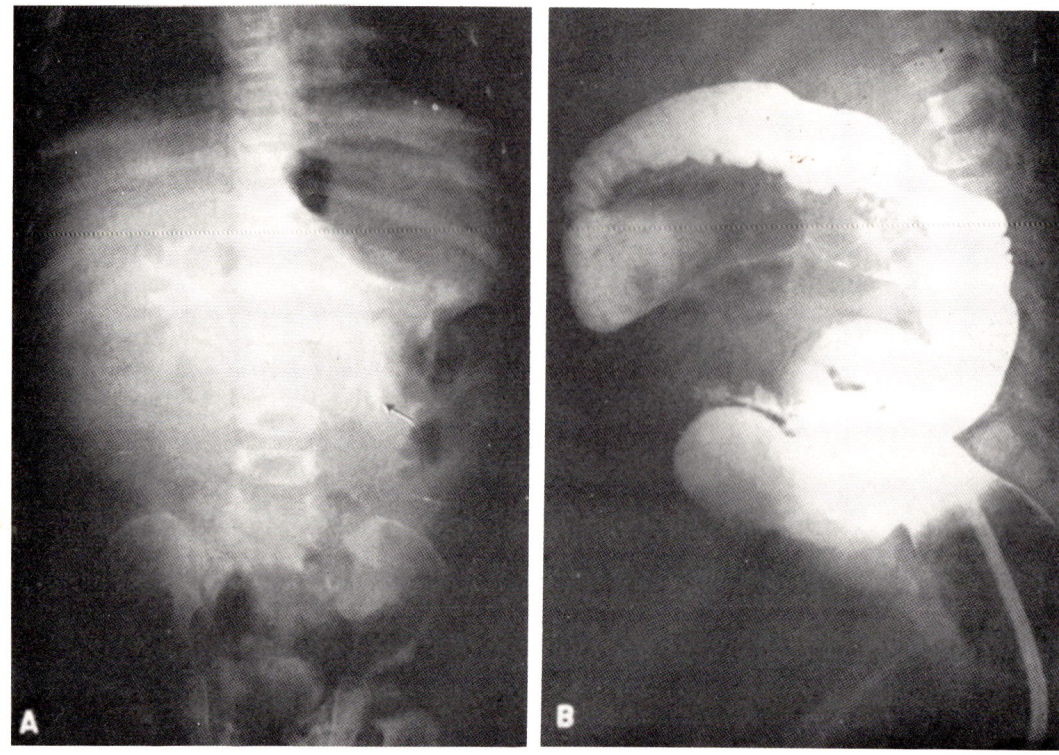

Figure 2–12 Primary carcinoma arising in the left lobe of the liver of a 7½ year old girl. *A*, Intravenous pyelography shows posterior compression and downward displacement of left kidney (arrow), as well as leftward displacement of the stomach. *B*, Barium enema (lateral view) demonstrates normal position of ascending and descending colon since they are retroperitoneal structures. The transverse colon, which is intraperitoneal, is wrapped around the mass. (From Margulis, A. R., et al.: Radiology 66:809, 1956.)

rounding structures, the initial special radiologic studies should be those which visualize this area; exceptions to this rule arise when it is apparent from physical examination or plain abdominal films that the mass is in the liver, spleen, or gastrointestinal tract.

The kidney, ureters, and bladder can be visualized by means of the intravenous pyelogram (IVP)—i.e., injection of a radiopaque substance which is concentrated in the kidneys and excreted via the urinary tract. Modifications of the IVP, such as the nephrotomogram, total body opacification, and inferior venacavography can sometimes add additional useful information to this basic study.

The IVP is most useful in distinguishing between the two most common abdominal malignancies of childhood: Wilms' tumor and neuroblastoma. Since Wilms' tumor arises within the kidney, the IVP changes are those of a large intrarenal parenchymal mass growing within a pseudocapsule of atrophic compressed renal cortex; the pelvocalyceal system is distorted, displaced, and stretched around the parenchymal mass (Fig. 2–14). While the tumor is generally confined to one portion of the kidney, it may occasionally diffusely infiltrate the entire kidney and result in nonopacification. Neuroblastoma, on the other hand, most commonly arises in the adrenal gland and is, therefore, an extrarenal tumor which displaces, but does not distort, the kidney. The picture is that of a kidney which is displaced inferiorly and perhaps anteriorly; it may also be rotated an-

DIAGNOSIS OF CANCER IN CHILDHOOD

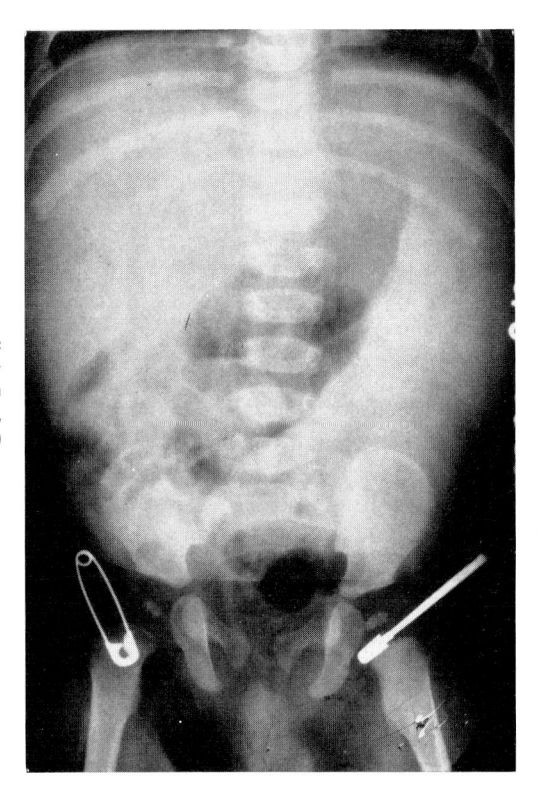

Figure 2–13 Splenic enlargement in a 6½ month old male with disseminated histoplasmosis. The stomach is displaced to the right. (From Davis, L. A.: Pediatric Radiology. *In* Robbins, L. L. [ed.]: Golden's Diagnostic Radiology. © 1973. The Williams & Wilkins Co., Baltimore.)

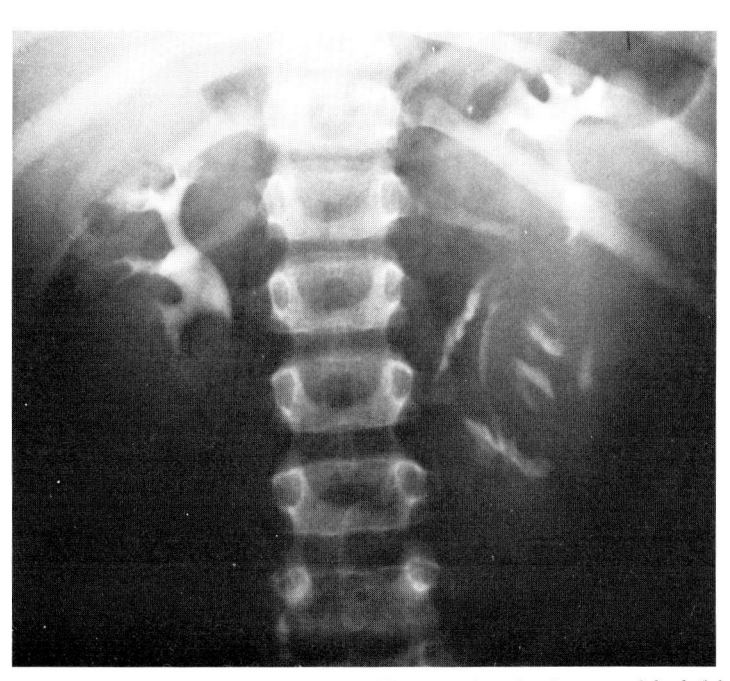

Figure 2–14 Intravenous pyelogram in a 5 year old boy with Wilms' tumor of the left kidney. There is distortion of the calyceal system of the involved kidney. (From Grossman, H.: Cancer 35:884, 1975.)

teriorly and laterally on its vertical axis (Fig. 2–15). Prone, oblique, and lateral views should be included as a routine part of the IVP in order to better define the nature of the renal displacement and rotation. Neuroblastoma can also arise from extra-adrenal sympathetic tissue; when such lesions arise medial to the kidney, they displace it laterally, while lesions arising below the kidney may displace the ureter laterally. Lesions arising in the pelvis may cause medial and anterior displacement of the bladder.

Other common causes of renal enlargement in childhood which must be differentiated from Wilms' tumor are hydronephrosis and unilateral multicystic kidney; these lesions have typical radiographic features which, if present, are very useful in defining the nature of the mass. For instance the unilateral multicystic kidney is usually discovered in the early neonatal period and its avascular nature results in failure of excretory function and a total body opacification effect during IVP. The cysts may be seen as round radiolucencies separated from each other by slightly opacified septa. The hydronephrotic kidney may either fail to opacify or may demonstrate a thin rim of compressed renal parenchyma outlining the hydronephrotic sac.

Rhabdomyosarcoma involving the genital and lower urinary tracts usually occurs in the first three to four years of life and may manifest signs of lower urinary tract obstruction or infection. IVP may demonstrate ureterovesical obstruction with diminished function as well as dilatation of ureters and renal pelvis. The bladder may show extrinsic displacement or a polypoid tumor mass (sarcoma botryoides) (Fig. 2–16) projecting into its base.

IVP is also useful in the localization of ovarian tumors and sacrococcygeal teratomas; common findings are hydronephrosis and obstruction of the ureters at the pelvic inlet.

Nephrotomography. Nephrotomography is a technique that combines intravenous pyelography with body section roentgenography (tomography) to permit a precise study of renal

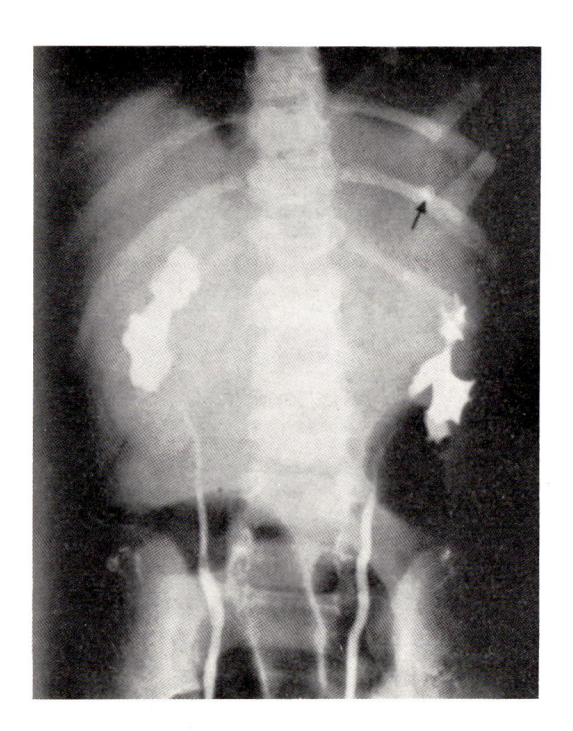

Figure 2–15 Neuroblastoma of left adrenal. Retrograde pyelogram demonstrating downward and lateral displacement of the left kidney by a calcified suprarenal mass (arrow). The mass extends across the midline and rotates the right kidney as well as displacing the ureteropelvic junction, producing hydronephrosis. (From Nice, C. M., Jr., et al.: Am. J. Roentgenol. 75:977, 1956.)

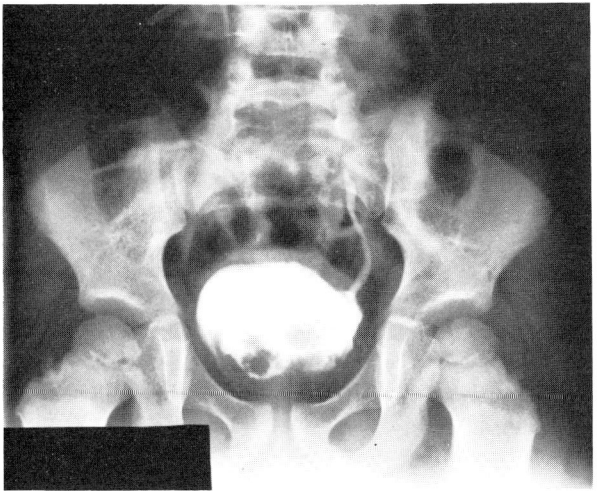

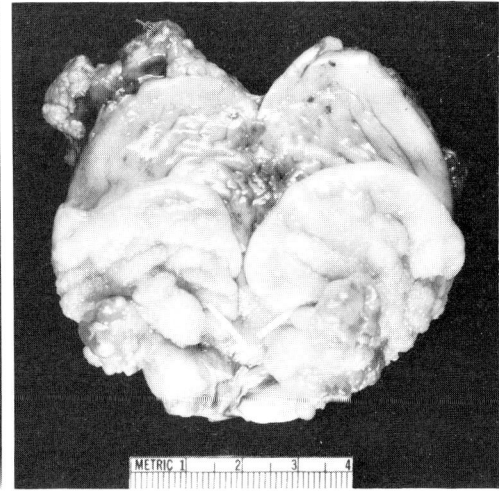

Figure 2-16 Rhabdomyosarcoma (sarcoma botryoides) of bladder. A, Excretory urogram showing lobulated filling defect in bladder. B, Surgical specimen showing fleshy lobules and surrounding submucosal spread. (From Tank, E. S., and Kelalis, P. P.: In Kelalis, P. P., et al. [eds.]: Clinical Pediatric Urology. Philadelphia, W. B. Saunders Co., 1976.)

morphology. The basic IVP study is modified by injecting a relatively large amount of contrast material rapidly via a peripheral vein; a tomogram is then taken which visualizes the midcoronal plane of the kidney.[24] This technique results in opacification of functioning renal parenchyma and eliminates the distortion produced by superimposed intestinal contents and gas. Renal size, renal outlines, and the calyceal system can be well defined, whereas nonfunctional renal masses such as cysts or tumors will be outlined by the more opaque functioning renal parenchyma. In contradistinction to cysts, tumors may be slightly opacified, but are not nearly as dense as the normally functioning surrounding renal tissue.

Total Body Opacification. The use of relatively large doses of contrast material may result in opacification of abdominal viscera other than those of the urinary tract.[90] Since the added radiodensity of an organ is proportional to the volume of blood it contains, solid structures with normal or increased vascularity will become selectively opacified while cystic structures, abscess cavities, and fat will remain radiolucent. In this manner liver, kidney, spleen, and bowel lesions may be visualized with better definition than seen in plain abdominal films. Since more than three quarters of neonatal abdominal masses are cystic or otherwise avascular, total body opacification is particularly useful in their differential diagnosis.[36]

Inferior Venacavography. Inferior venacavography is a special adaptation of the IVP which opacifies the inferior vena cava as well as the kidneys by injection of a bolus of contrast material into a suitable tributary in a *lower* extremity. There are numerous methods for doing this including injection into the femoral vein and saphenous vein via an intracath[51] or venous cutdown.[118] Although these give superior results, the technique may be technically difficult in young children and involves additional risk of morbidity. Koop and Kaufmann have advocated injection into a dorsal foot vein as a safe, reliable, and informative method.[63] This study, when performed at the time of IVP, may provide potentially important additional information in the evaluation of an abdominal mass, particularly a large or deep-seated one. Such information may help to localize the tumor, determine its extent, and establish whether or not vena cava invasion has occurred (Fig. 2–17). Proper interpretation of these studies, however, demands a thorough knowledge of congenital anomalies of the inferior vena cava, the effects of collateral channels, and the artefacts produced by heavy breathing, straining, or crying.

ANGIOGRAPHY. Angiography has proved to be a useful supplemental technique in the preoperative evaluation of the child with an abdominal mass. Although not usually necessary for diagnosis or evaluation of Wilms' tumor or neuroblastoma, angiography is now considered to be a routine part of the evaluation of liver masses and may also be useful in evaluating unusual renal masses.

Angiography (hepatic and celiac vessels) is currently the best method available for determining the extent, location, and nature of hepatic masses (Fig. 2–18), being particularly useful in determining whether a tumor has been confined to one hepatic lobe (in which case the mass may be treatable by partial hepatectomy). The nature of the mass can be determined to some extent by the contour of its margins — irregularly, poorly defined margins suggest malignancy, whereas smooth, well-defined margins are more likely to represent a benign lesion enclosed in a capsule or pseudocapsule. Other angiographic findings suggestive of malignancy are: large feeding vessels, tumor vessels, tumor "blush," and displacement or thrombosis of the portal vein.[89, 95]

Angiography is useful in evaluation of Wilms' tumor when there is nonvisualization on IVP or equivocal IVP findings, or when bilateral disease is suspected.[26] Since bilateral disease occurs in approximately 10 per cent of patients and may be subtle, some authors feel that this feature alone is indication for arteriography in cases of Wilms' tumor. The arteriographic fea-

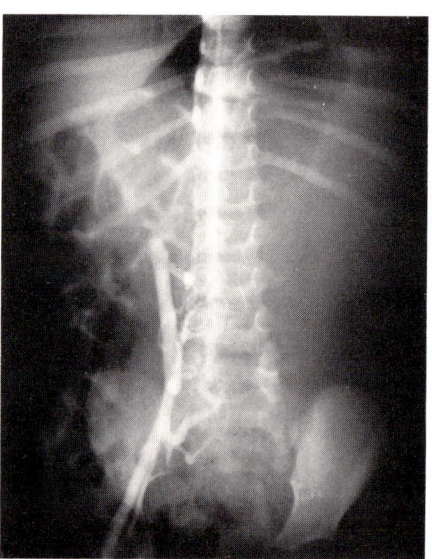

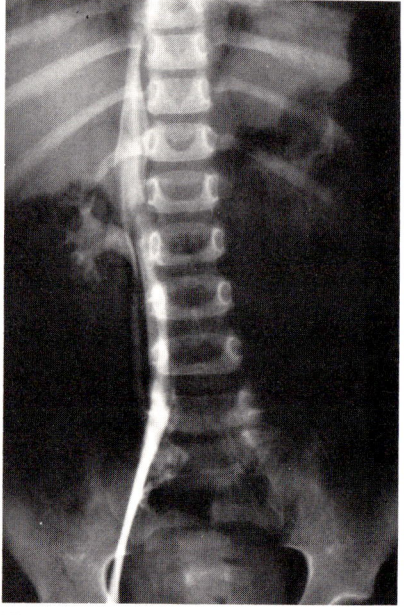

Figure 2–17 Inferior venacavogram in a 3 year old girl with Wilms' tumor of the right kidney. A, Obstruction of the inferior vena cava at the level of the renal veins. B, Inferior vena cava 1 year later, entirely free of obstruction. (From Tucker, A. S., and Izant, R. J., Jr.: *In* Kaufman, H. J. [ed.]: Progress in Pediatric Radiology. Vol. 3. Genito-Urinary Tract. Chicago, Year Book Medical Publishers, 1970.)

DIAGNOSIS OF CANCER IN CHILDHOOD

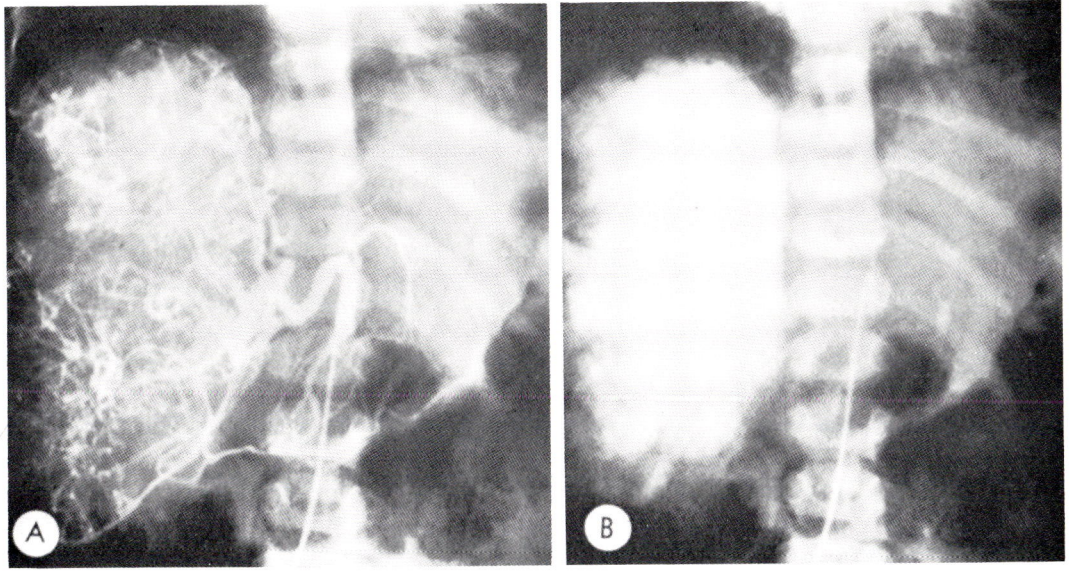

Figure 2–18 A, Selective hepatic angiogram demonstrating a large vascular mass in the right hepatic lobe. Large feeding vessels, absence of normal tapering of vessels, and tumor vascularity are evident. The left hepatic lobe does not appear to be involved. B, Late capillary phase showing dense homogeneous tumor stain in right hepatic lobe. (From Moss, A. A., et al.: Am. J. Roentgenol. *113*:61, 1971.)

tures of Wilms' tumor include distortion of intrinsic renal vessels[17] and some degree of neovascularity.[96]

Arteriography has also been useful in defining boundaries of malignant musculoskeletal tumors in order to help plan resection and to facilitate radiotherapy.

Radionuclide Scanning Techniques. The radionuclides used for scanning in patients with cancer can be divided into two major types:

1. Indirect agents: those which localize in normal parenchymal cells and depend upon displacement of normal tissue, disruption of normal physiologic mechanisms, or biologic reactions to tumor growth in order to detect the presence of tumor.

2. Direct tumor-scanning agents: those which localize in the tumors themselves.

INDIRECT AGENTS. Table 2–6 lists the agents which can be used to scan normal parenchymal organs. These agents are sensitive to the presence of disease, but generally are not specific for the diagnosis of cancer. They may be used to determine (1) organ size, and (2) distribution of radioactivity within the organ (homogeneous versus filling defects). These studies may be

Table 2–6 Radionuclides Which Localize in Normal Parenchymal Organs

RADIONUCLIDE	SITE OF LOCALIZATION	USEFUL IN SCANNING
^{99m}Tc-sulfur colloid	Reticuloendothelial cell	Liver and spleen
^{99m}Tc-polyphosphate	Sites of osteoblastic activity (? hydroxyapatite crystals)	Bone
^{99m}Tc-diphosphonate	Sites of osteoblastic activity	Bone
^{99m}Tc-albumin macroaggregates	Pulmonary capillary bed	Lung
^{131}I	Thyroid cells	Thyroid
^{131}I-rose bengal	Hepatocyte	Liver

performed to evaluate primary masses, to search for metastatic foci, to follow the patient's response to therapy, to screen for the appearance of new metastatic lesions during therapy, and to localize lesions for correct placement of biopsy needles or of radiation therapy portals.

Many of these studies utilize ^{99m}technetium* (^{99m}Tc) complexed to a variety of molecules. This radionuclide owes its current popularity to the fact that it is readily available, relatively inexpensive, and has a relatively short half-life ($T^{1/2} = 6.0$ hr). Since ^{99m}Tc itself has no organ specificity, the localizing properties of its complexes depend upon the nature of the molecule with which it is associated. Thus, attachment to sulfur colloid produces particles of sufficient size (0.1 to 1.0 mμm) to be phagocytized by the fixed macrophages of the liver and spleen, attachment to phosphate complexes results in deposition at crystal surfaces in immature bone, and attachment to macroaggregated albumin produces particles of sufficient size (10 to 90 μm) to be trapped in the pulmonary capillary bed.

Table 2–7 compares the absorbed radiation dosages from some common

---

*The notation "m" indicates that this isotope is metastable and decays to ^{99}technetium, giving off a gamma ray.

Table 2–7 Absorbed Doses From Common Roentgenographic Procedures[1]

	ABSORBED DOSE (MILLIRADS)		
		Gonads	
PROCEDURE	Bone Marrow	MALE	FEMALE
Skulls films (AP, lateral, base)	50	<10	<10
Chest films (PA, lateral)	40	<10	<10
Barium enema (PA, lateral, oblique)	600	200	800
Skeletal survey	700	3300	1200

Absorbed Doses From Common Nuclear Medical Scanning Procedures[1]
(70 kg. Adult)

	ABSORBED DOSE (MILLIRADS)				
	Bone Marrow	Gonads			
PROCEDURE		MALE	FEMALE	Organ of Greatest Exposure	
Brain scan (^{99m}Tc-pertechnetate) 15 mCi	450	350	400	Stomach	550
Lung scan (^{99m}Tc-albumin macroaggregates) 3.5 mCi	70	1	2	Lung	900
Liver/Spleen scan (^{99m}Tc-sulfur colloid) 3.5 mCi	200	50	75	Liver/Spleen	700
Bone scan (^{99m}Tc-polyphosphate) 10 mCi	300	375	400	Bladder*	3050

*No voiding assumed.

roentgenographic procedures with those associated with the common nuclear medicine scanning procedures.

Liver-Spleen Scanning. The most commonly used agent in liver scanning is ^{99m}Tc-sulfur colloid, which is taken up by the fixed macrophages of the liver (Kupffer cells). This radiocolloid is also accumulated by the fixed macrophages of the spleen, permitting evaluation of the size and functional activity of that organ as well.

Enlargement or displacement of the liver is an important clue to the presence of disease. In order to determine if the liver is enlarged, we must have standards of normal size for comparison. The normal adult liver is 17 ± 2 cm in length,[113] whereas in normal children liver length can be correlated with age and height; these relationships may be represented as follows:[113]

Liver length (cm) = 8.79 + 0.458 age (years)
Liver length (cm) = 2.07 + 0.090 height (cm)

In addition to liver size, the intrahepatic distribution of the scanning agent is of importance. Any mass lesion of the liver (primary and metastatic tumors, cysts, abscesses) will appear as a "filling defect" because of the absence of radioactivity in the region (Fig. 2–19A). Consequently, the scan is useful more for localizing a mass in the liver or detecting metastatic lesions to the liver than it is for determining the nature of the mass. Generally a focal lesion has to be at least 2 cm in diameter to be visible by this technique;[102] for this reason, some malignancies involving the liver (e.g., leukemia, Hodgkin's disease, non-Hodgkin's lymphoma) may produce only diffuse hepatomegaly on scan.

Determination of the spleen size is also useful in evaluating patients with potential malignancies. After birth the spleen is approximately 4.8 to 5.0 cm in length;[114] from ages 1 to 18.9 years, splenic length in normal children can be correlated with age and height according to the following formulae:

Splenic length (cm) = 5.7 + 0.31 age (years)
Splenic length (cm) = 2.3 + 0.05 height (cm)

Rose bengal labeled with ^{131}I is a scanning agent which is actively taken up by hepatocytes but not by fixed macrophages; consequently, the spleen is not visualized when this substance is used. It is, therefore, useful in distinguishing between liver and spleen when the ^{99m}Tc-sulfur colloid scan is confusing. ^{131}I rose bengal scanning may also be useful in differentiating choledochal cysts from liver tumors by demonstrating an obstructed excretion pattern and occasionally by concentrating in the cyst. In general, however, ^{131}I rose bengal is less commonly used than ^{99m}Tc-sulfur colloid because its rapid excretion often results in poor liver visualization.

Other scanning techniques (brain scan, bone scan) may be useful in detecting metastatic disease from an abdominal neoplasm. Sometimes the metastatic pattern is useful in determining the nature of an abdominal mass (e.g., skeletal metastases from neuroblastoma). These other organ scanning techniques are discussed in subsequent sections.

DIRECT TUMOR-SCANNING AGENTS. The observation that certain radioactive materials localize in certain tumors has produced a tendency to regard such agents as having a specific metabolic affinity for that tumor or for tumors in general ("tumor seekers"). In fact, these agents are not specific for tumors but may also be localized in areas of inflammation and certain phases of infarct development. Thus, the localization of these agents should be conceptualized in terms of the altered regional physiology attendant on the presence of the tumor.[125] These alterations include: (1) in-

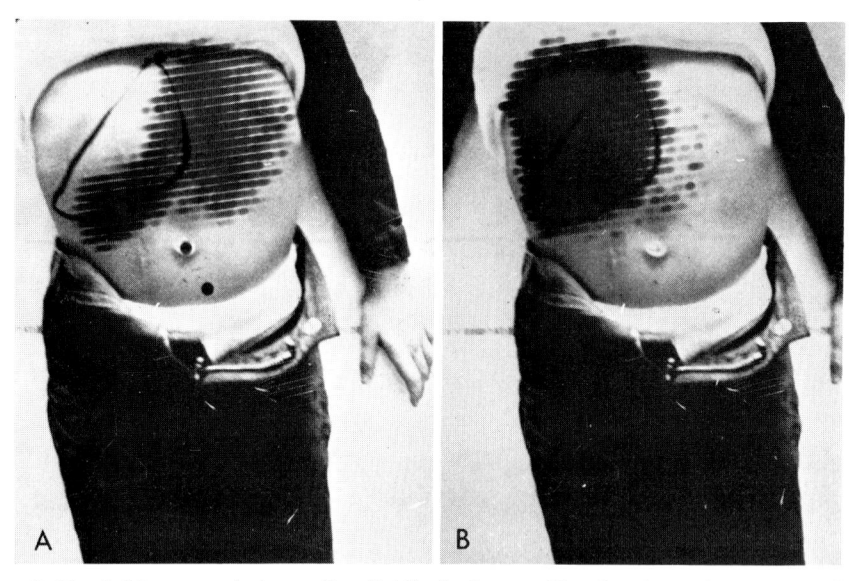

Figure 2–19 A, Liver scan (using radiocolloid) of a 5 year old girl with a right upper quadrant abdominal mass. A large "filling defect" is evident at the upper portion of the right hepatic lobe. B, ^{67}Ga scan of the same region, demonstrating selective uptake of the radionuclide in the region which was "cold" on liver scan. Metastatic Wilms' tumor was found in this region. (From Edeling, C. J.: Cancer 38:921, 1976.)

creased permeability of the capillary bed to macromolecules; (2) increased residence time of the macromolecules in the interstitial fluid space due to a delay in new lymphatic vessel growth; (3) increased macrophage activity associated with tissue necrosis; (4) altered cell membrane permeability to the scanning agent; or (5) receptor sites on the cell surface for the scanning agent.

The most commonly used tumor-scanning agent is the cation [67]gallium (^{67}Ga). The mechanism of uptake is unclear, but ^{67}Ga appears to accumulate primarily in lysosome-like cytoplasmic structures.[109]

[67]Gallium-citrate appears to have great affinity for the lymphomas, particularly Hodgkin's disease.[55] Also, virtually all hepatomas and half of metastatic hepatic tumors show increased ^{67}Ga uptake (Fig. 2–19, B), whereas hepatic cysts and cirrhotic nodules have no significant affinity for it. Other pediatric malignancies which have shown affinity for ^{67}Ga include Ewing's sarcoma, thyroid carcinoma, melanoma, testicular carcinoma, Wilms' tumor, brain tumors, and neuroblastoma.[10, 110, 119]

[67]Gallium is taken up by both leukemic myeloblasts and lymphoblasts[82] and appears useful in detecting both marrow and extramedullary foci of leukemia cells. One particularly useful application of this property may be the identification of chloromatous masses in the region of the spinal cord; if these masses could be localized before they caused cord compression symptoms, they could possibly be treated by radiotherapy with avoidance of laminectomy.[66, 85]

[67]Gallium-citrate scanning can, therefore, be of considerable diagnostic use in oncology patients, but only if certain precautions are exercised in its interpretation. It must be recognized that failure of ^{67}Ga to localize in a region does not rule out malignancy, nor does selective regional uptake necessarily mean the presence of tumor. Of particular clinical useful-

ness, however, is a diminution of ^{67}Ga concentration following therapy and a renewed uptake with recurrence of tumor.

A further application of ^{67}Ga scanning in patients with neoplasms would take advantage of its localization in site of inflammation such as abscesses and osteomyelitis[57, 82] by using it to detect occult infections as well as to monitor the response of the infection to antibiotic therapy.

Ultrasonography. Ultrasound is sound produced at frequencies above the hearing range of the normal human ear (18,000 cps). Ultrasonography is a technique whereby these high-frequency beams are propagated through tissue, reflected at soft tissue interfaces, and detected as echoes by an appropriate sensing device (transducer) which can convert them into an electrical signal that can be amplified and displayed on the screen of an oscilloscope. The amount and character of the echoes range from practically nonexistent (e.g., interior of cysts) to the increasing and variable patterns of various tumors or organs (Fig. 2–20). Complications of tumor growth such as localized pockets of fluid, general ascites,[35] hemorrhage or pus collections,[73] and displacement of adjacent structures can also be detected by ultrasound methods. Generally, a lesion has to be at least 1.5 to 2 cm in size to be reasonably detectable by ultrasonic means;[28] however, under suitable conditions, structures as small as 0.1 mm may be visualized.[8]

Ultrasonography has been found to be particularly useful in the detection, localization, and characterization of masses in the pelvis, abdominal cavity, and retroperitoneum. The procedure is noninvasive, painless, and associated with no known morbidity.[8, 9, 28] Since no ionizing radiation is involved, the examination may be repeated as frequently as necessary. *In the postpubertal female, ultrasonography should precede radiographic evaluation of an abdominal mass whenever pregnancy cannot be excluded.*

Lesions of the Female Pelvis. Generally ultrasonography permits satisfactory delineation of the bladder, vagina, uterus, neural and vascular bundles, and the iliopsoas muscles; masses arising in or from any of these organs (or the ovaries) can be detected (Fig. 2–21). Using this technique one can determine whether a pelvic mass is continuous with the uterus or separate from it and can also differentiate cystic from solid masses. Thus, benign ovarian cysts, for instance, present as echo-free extrauterine pelvic masses, whereas malignant ones have a mixed echo pattern.

Abdominal Organs. The size, shape, and position of the liver, spleen, kidneys, and major blood vessels, as well as the relationship of intraabdominal masses to these

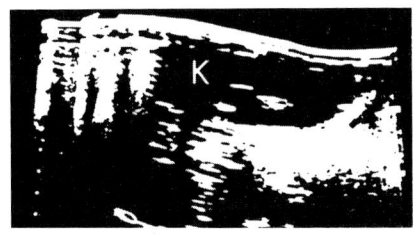

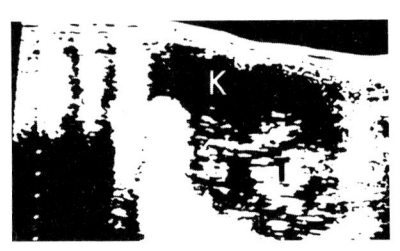

Figure 2–20 Ultrasonography of the kidneys of a patient with a left-sided abdominal mass. Right kidney is found to be of normal size while the left kidney is enlarged and contains echo-producing structures indicative of a solid tumor (*T*). Patient was found to have a Wilms' tumor. (From Grossman, H.: Cancer 35:884, 1975.)

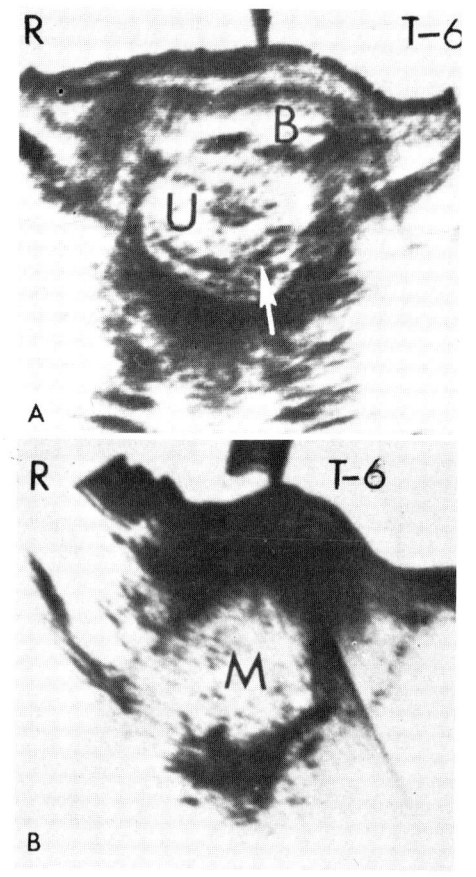

Figure 2-21 Ultrasonography of the pelvis of a 4 year old girl with a large pelvic rhabdomyosarcoma. *A*, Transverse sonogram showing a bulky nonhomogeneous mass in the region of the cervix and upper vagina; uterus is enlarged, probably due to retained secretions. *B*, Repeat sonogram 7 months after anterior exenteration with en bloc resection of the tumor was performed demonstrates recurrent tumor (*M*). (From Haller, J. O., et al.: Am. J. Roentgenol. *128*:425, 1977.)

tumors, may be measured precisely by ultrasonography. Liver metastases produce clearly different echo patterns from the normal fine echo pattern of the liver; most appear transonic in comparison to the liver tissue, and, if the lesions are calcified or necrotic, a scattering of internal echoes may also be present.

Neoplastic abdominal lymph node enlargement (particularly lymphoma) produces a very characteristic, highly transonic echo pattern which may prove capable of demonstrating 90 per cent of such lymph node enlargements.[5] Although lower extremity lymphangiography permits better visualization of the internal characteristics of lymph nodes then does ultrasonography, it is limited to those areas involved in the drainage of the lower extremity, whereas ultrasonography can identify lymph node enlargements in other lymphatic drainage areas of the abdomen as well. Although this technique cannot as yet be relied upon as a primary method of staging, it is most useful for repeated follow-up studies of patients with lymphoma.

Retroperitoneal Masses. Ultrasound is useful as an adjunct to the IVP in delineating solid renal tumors (e.g., Wilms') from multicystic kidney and hydronephrosis. It can also be useful in providing information regarding the presence or absence of a kidney, its size, gross configuration, and an idea of the pathology even when the kidney is nonfunctional on IVP; nonvisualization of a kidney occurs in approximately 3 to 10 per cent of patients with Wilms' tumor, and ultrasonography may demonstrate a solid tumor mass in such cases. Other retroperitoneal masses such as leiomyosarcomas, dermoid cysts, meningoceles, and hemorrhages can also be successfully identified.[69, 83]

Computerized Axial Tomography (CAT). Conventional radiographic studies project an image onto film which is the product of the proportion of the x-ray beam that is not absorbed (attenuated) by *all* tissues in its path. Computed tomography utilizes the x-ray as a primary tool but employs a computer to calculate the slight, but unique, differences in x-ray beam attentuation produced by various normal and diseased tissues and by this means can represent them separately in a recognizable anatomic pattern.[47] A very thin x-ray beam (16 to 26 mm mean width) is used to scan the desired area by multiple x-ray projections; in this manner, a scan sequence

Figure 2-22 Computed tomography of the abdomen of a patient with a huge left-sided Wilms' tumor (arrow). Residual left renal tissues are visible anteriorly and posteriorly. The normal right kidney and a vertebral body are also clearly visualized. (From Harwood-Nash, D. C., and Breckhill, D. L.: J. Pediatr. 89:343, 1976. Photograph by Dr. R. Alfidi, Cleveland.)

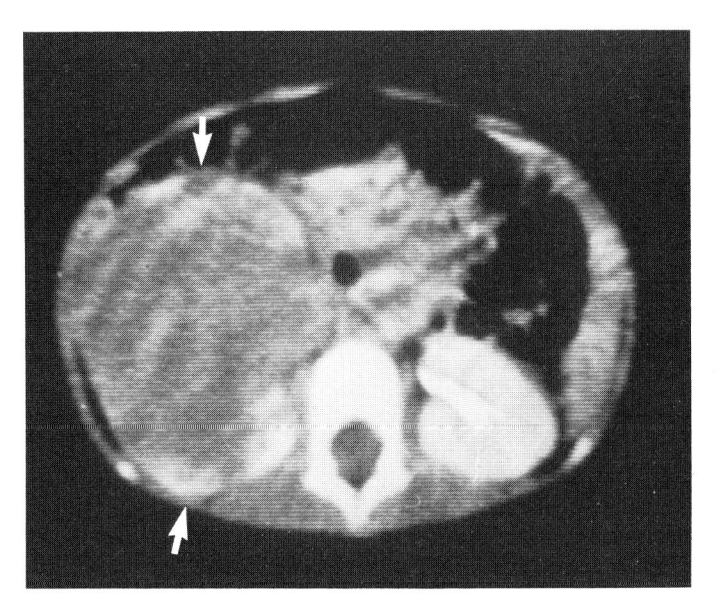

is obtained which views two contiguous "slices" of tissue on either side of a selected reference level. The readings from each "slice" are processed by the computer which then can calculate their absorption values and print out a picture which corrsponds to a direct visualization of the organ at the level selected.[86]

Although the initial application of this technique was for the study of cerebral structures, it has more recently been adapted to the study of the thoracic and abdominal organs[2] and for detection of enlarged lymph nodes in regions not accessible to lymphangiography.[64] The single most valuable function of CAT is to reveal the geography and characteristics of tissue structures within *solid* organs (Fig. 2-22). It may be used to confirm a clinically established lesion, determine the content of a mass lesion (edema, cystic, solid, lipid), demonstrate the cause of a nonspecific clinical sign or symptom, or follow the posttherapeutic or natural course of disease.

It has been estimated that the use of CAT in neuroradiology has decreased the necessity for "invasive" procedures such as angiography (by 15 to 20 per cent) and pneumoencephalography (by 60 per cent).[7] The disadvantages are the cost ($400,000 to $600,000 per machine; $120 to $300 per examination) and the necessity for prolonged immobilization (up to 40 min); heavy sedation or general anesthesia is sometimes necessary to prevent motion artefacts in young children.[47]

EXTREMITY LESIONS (Table 2-8)

Children with malignant limb lesions usually present with pain, nonspecific swelling, a lump, or a limp. The differential diagnosis ranges from cellulitis, arthritis, trauma, osteomyelitis, and other "benign" causes to the various neoplastic lesions of soft tissues and bones, both primary and metastatic.

Good quality radiographs of the bone and soft tissue are very useful in arriving at a presumptive diagnosis of a primary bone tumor. Thus, metaphyseal bone lesions, particularly when associated with new "tumor bone," are apt to suggest osteogenic sarcoma (Fig. 2-23), while diaphyseal lesions (in the tubular portion of the bone) are more compatible with Ewing's sarcoma

Table 2-8 Extremity and Soft Tissue Masses in Childhood

	Primary Malignancy	Metastatic Malignancy	Benign Lesions
Bone	*Osteogenic sarcoma* *Ewing's sarcoma* *Histiocytosis X* Lymphoma (histiocytic) Chondrosarcoma	*Neuroblastoma* *Osteogenic sarcoma* *Ewing's sarcoma* Lymphoma	*Osteochondroma* *Enchondroma* *Osteoid osteoma* Cysts Giant cell epulis
Lymph nodes	*Lymphoma*	Rhabdomyosarcoma Soft tissue sarcoma	Inflammatory adenitis
Soft tissue	*Rhabdomyosarcoma* *Fibrosarcoma* *Other sarcomas* *Melanoma* Neurofibrosarcoma	Neuroblastoma Lymphosarcoma Leukemia	*Neurofibroma* *Hemangioma* *Pigmented nevi* *Lipoma* *Fibroma* *Lymphangioma*

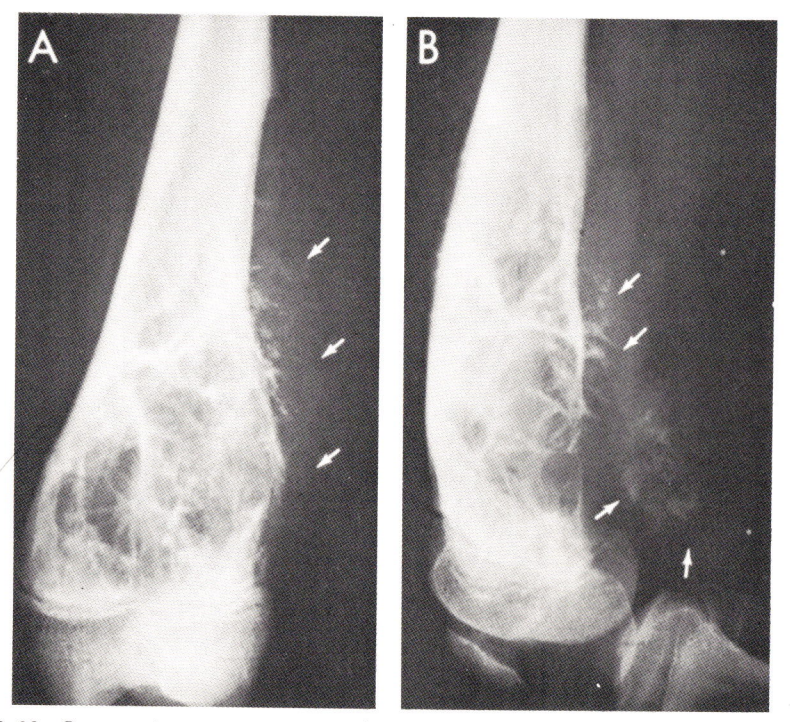

Figure 2-23   Osteogenic sarcoma arising in the epiphyseal region of the femur. *A*, Frontal projection. *B*, Lateral projection. The distal end of the femoral shaft is replaced by an irregularly radiolucent mass. The overlying cortex is partially destroyed on the medial posterior aspect and radial bony spiculation extends beyond the cortex into the extraosseous neoplastic mass. (From Caffey, J. [ed.]: Pediatric X-Ray Diagnosis. Chicago, Year Book Medical Publishers, 1972.)

(Fig. 2–24). Xeroradiograms may help define details of bone destruction or the outlines of a soft tissue mass.

Skeletal Survey. Because of the propensity of certain tumors to metastasize to bone, a careful search for evidence of bone lesions may provide useful information concerning the differential diagnosis, prognosis, and management of the patient with a suspected malignancy.

In childhood the most frequent primary lesion that metastasizes to bone is neuroblastoma; histiocytosis X, rhabdomyosarcoma, and retinoblastoma are less common sources of bone metastases. Wilms' tumor metastasizes to bone in approximately 10 per cent of cases. Primary bone tumors (osteogenic sarcoma, Ewing's sarcoma) also metastasize to other bones. Most metastatic childhood tumors produce lytic bone lesions, but bone metastases from Hodgkin's disease or osteogenic sarcoma may be sclerotic in nature.

The relationship between the clinical and roentgenographic findings in bone metastases depends upon the structure of the affected bone;[14]

1. Bones composed mainly of spongy material (vertebrae, ribs, pelvis, metaphyseal portions of long bones) do not demonstrate roentgenographic abnormalities until the lesion is far advanced. Metastases in these bones may produce clinical symptoms before they are radiologically visible *(roentgenographically occult metastases).*

2. Bones composed mainly of compact material (skull, diaphyseal portions of long bones) usually manifest roentgenographically visible lesions before they cause clinical symptoms *(clinically silent metastases).*

The standard roentgenogram is a relatively insensitive technique for visualizing metastatic disease, since a minimum of 30 to 50 per cent of bone mineral must be lost before a lesion becomes visible;[14] for reasons mentioned above, spinal metastases are even more difficult to demonstrate since they are not usually visible until

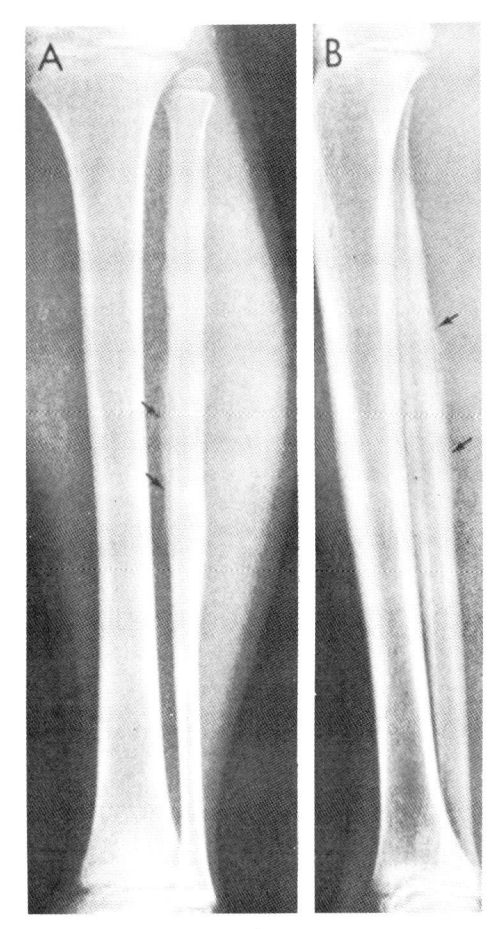

Figure 2–24 Ewing's sarcoma arising in metaphysis of left fibula. A long segment of the cortical wall of the proximal half of the fibula is irregularly thickened and there is peripheral marginal destruction as well. These changes are non-specific and may mimic those associated with inflammation or trauma. (From Caffey, J. [ed.]: Pediatric X-Ray Diagnosis. Chicago, Year Book Medical Publishers, 1972.)

50 to 75 per cent of the surrounding bone has been destroyed[6] and a destructive lesion greater than 1.5 cm in size has been produced.[20] Bone scanning techniques are more sensitive than conventional radiographs and are, therefore, superior for the detection of individual lesions. However, bone scanning, as will be discussed below, is a relatively nonspecific technique and must be supplemented with radiography to differentiate between

^{99}technetium (^{99m}Tc) with polyphosphate, diphosphonate, or pyrophosphate. These agents are deposited in proximity to sites of osteoblastic activity, apparently by adsorption onto the hydroxyapatite crystal surfaces of newly formed bone.[68] Since increased uptake of the scanning material reflects an abnormal degree of osteoblastic activity, any reactive bone change, including arthritis, fracture, osteomyelitis, primary bone tumor, or metastatic tumor, will be visualized as an area of increased activity on bone scan.

As bone scanning is a highly sensitive but nonspecific procedure, its major usefulness has been in the detection and follow-up of metastatic bone lesions (Fig. 2–25). In this regard the technique has been found to be superior to the radiologic skeletal survey. A recent prospective study comparing bone scanning with the conventional radiographic survey in 159 children with known primary neoplasm found 68 per cent of bone metastases to be demonstrable by bone scan alone;[30] generally a lesion on bone scan will predate the appearance on routine roentgenograms by 3 to 6 months. The percentage of false negatives with scanning techniques varies from 0 to 8 per cent;[30, 91] this usually occurs when the lesion is either highly anaplastic or very slow growing and reactive bone does not form around it.

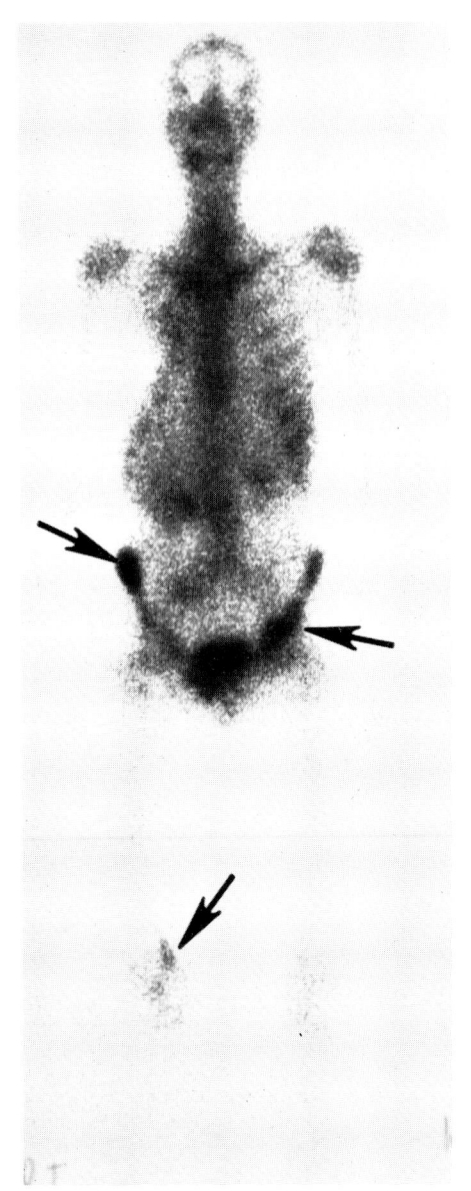

Figure 2–25 Bone scan of a patient with metastases in the pelvis and right knee (arrows). The midline pelvic density represents excretion of the radionuclide via the bladder. The patient's primary tumor was a Ewing's sarcoma of the right seventh rib, note post-thoracoplasty changes in right hemithorax. (Courtesy of Drs. Richard Spencer and Savita Puri.)

tumor and benign causes of increased radionuclide uptake.

Bone Scanning. The most commonly used bone scanning agents in current use are complexes of

ENDOCRINE SYNDROMES AS A PRESENTING FEATURE OF MALIGNANCY

A tumor arising in an endocrine gland may produce excessive amounts of the hormone normally made in that gland. Under some circumstances, a tumor arising in one endocrine gland may produce the hormone of another gland or a tumor arising in a nonendocrine tissue may synthesize and se-

Diagnosis of Cancer in Childhood

Table 2–9 Endocrine Syndromes Which May Result From Occult Neoplastic Hormone Production by Pediatric Malignancies

Syndrome	Hormone	Primary Synthesis	Ectopic Production
Cushing's	ACTH	Carcinoid	Neuroblastoma Pheochromocytoma Oat cell carcinoma (thymus) Islet cell carcinoma (pancreas)
Cushing's	Cortisol	Adrenal carcinoma	
Precocious puberty	Gonadotropin	Hypothalamic involvement by intracranial tumors	Hepatoblastoma Choriocarcinoma
Precocious puberty (male)	Androgen	Adrenal carcinoma Leydig cell tumor (testis)	
Virilism (female)	Androgen	Sertoli-Leydig cell tumor (ovary)	
Precocious puberty (female)	Estrogen	Adrenal carcinoma Granulosa cell tumor (ovary)	
Feminization (male)	Estrogen	Sertoli cell tumor (testis)	
Reactive parathyroid hyperplasia	Thyrocalcitonin	Medullary carcinoma (thyroid)	
Hypercalcemia	Parathormone		Hepatoblastoma Testicular carcinoma
Erythrocytosis	Erythropoietin		Wilms' tumor Pheochromocytoma Cerebellar hemangioblastoma
Hypoglycemia	? Insulin-like activity	Islet cell carcinoma (pancreas)	Large mesenchymal tumors*

*Most of the large abdominal and thoracic tumors (e.g., mesotheliomas, fibrosarcomas) that are associated with hypoglycemia apparently exert their effects through some mechanism other than the secretion of insulin (inordinate glucose consumption by the tumor, leakage from the tumors of nucleic acids with insulin-like activity, or production of a tryptophan derivative which inhibits hepatic gluconeogenesis).

crete substances with strong hormonal activity; this is known as *ectopic* hormone production.

Table 2–9 lists the various hormone abnormalities associated with pediatric malignancies. Knowledge of these various syndromes is useful because they can serve as diagnostic clues to the presence of an otherwise undetectable malignancy or may help in the clinical diagnosis of an apparent mass lesion.

Tumor Markers

Some fetal antigens, that is, antigens normally present in fetal life whose synthesis is repressed as mature, specialized histology is achieved, may reappear in the course of malignant transformation. This phenomenon may represent reactivation of "fetal" genes during the process of tissue dedifferentiation. Thus, the reappearance of fetal antigens has been proposed as a possible marker of the presence of tumor somewhere in the body.

An ideal tumor marker should: (1) permit early diagnosis of malignancy; (2) define the neoplasm; (3) describe its extent; and (4) be useful in following its progression or regression. Unfortunately, fetal antigens have not, as yet, proved to be consistent early guides to the presence of cancer. However, these tests have proved useful in following the progression or regression of disease and in establishing the presence of metastases.[106, 107] Consequently, they are most valuable when baseline values are obtained prior to therapy and serial determinations are subsequently made at regular intervals to follow the response to therapy. When used in this manner, a sudden increase in the titer of a given marker can be an early clue to recurrence of disease; likewise, failure of the titer to return to baseline values following surgery is indicative of persistent foci of tumor in the patient.

The fetal antigens most frequently used as tumor markers are alpha-fetoprotein (AFP), and carcinoembryonic antigen (CEA).

Alpha-Fetoprotein (AFP). Alpha-fetoprotein is an α_1-globulin which was first discovered in fetal calf serum and named Fetuin.[93] A similar α_1-globulin has been found in human fetal serum; this molecule disappears gradually during the third trimester of gestation and is usually absent at birth and throughout postnatal life.[31] It can reappear at high levels in the sera of patients with hepatocellular carcinoma[3] and entodermal sinus (yolk sac) tumors. This substance, however, is not specific for tumor cells, having also been detected in the sera of patients with hepatitis[61] and other non-neoplastic liver diseases;[12] indeed, with very sensitive radioimmunoassay techniques, small amounts of AFP can be detected in normal serum.[103]

Carcinoembryonic Antigen (CEA). CEA is a glycoprotein molecule originally extracted from a human colonic adenocarcinoma;[34] it has subsequently been found in normal human embryonic and fetal entodermally derived digestive organs (stomach, intestine, colon, liver, pancreas) during the first two trimesters of gestation and in all human cancers derived from these organs.[32, 33, 34]

Elevated CEA levels are also detectable in the serum of patients with gastrointestinal malignancies[32, 33] Although initially CEA was thought to be a specific indicator for cancer of entodermally derived structures, more recent studies have demonstrated elevated levels in a variety of benign conditions (ulcerative colitis,[75] biliary obstruction,[72] chronic heavy smoking[115]) as well as in some nonentodermally derived tumors (neuroblastoma,[99] head and neck tumors, bladder, and kidney tumors[75]).

REFERENCES

1. Adelstein, S. J.: Radiation risks. *In* Wagner, H. N., Jr. (ed.): Nuclear Medicine. New York, Hospital Practice, 1975.
2. Alfidi, R. J., Haaga, J., Meaney, T. F., et al.: Computed tomography of the thorax and abdomen: A preliminary report. Radiology *117*:257, 1975.
3. Alpert, M. E., Uriel, J., and De Nechaud, B.: Alpha 1 fetoglobulin in the diagnosis of human hepatoma. N. Engl. J. Med. *278*:984, 1968.
4. Altman, D. H., and Piccinini, M. T.: The radio-diagnostic follow-up of patients with Wilms' tumor. Progr. Pediatr. Radiol. *3*:312, 1970.
5. Asher, W., and Freimanis, A.: Echographic diagnosis of retroperitoneal lymph node enlargement. Am. J. Roentgenol. Radium Ther. Nucl. Med. *105*:438, 1969.
6. Bachman, A. L., and Sproul, E. E.: Correlation of radiographic and autopsy findings in suspected metastases to the spine. Bull. N. Y. Acad. Med. *31*:146, 1955.
7. Baker, H., Campbell, J., Houser, D., et al.: Computer assisted tomography of the head. Mayo Clin. Proc. *49*:17, 1974.
8. Baum, G.: Application of ultrasound. J.A.M.A. *229*:1065, 1974.
9. Bearman, S., Sanders, R. C., and Oh, K. S.: B-scan ultrasound in the evaluation of pediatric abdominal masses. Radiology *108*:111, 1973.
10. Berelowitz, M., and Blake, K. C. H.: [67]Gal-

lium in the detection and localization of tumors. S. Afr. Med. J. 45:1351, 1971.
11. Birdsell, D. C., and Lindsay, W. K.: Malignant tumors of the head and neck in children. Plast. Reconstr. Surg. 44:255, 1969.
12. Bloomer, J. R., Waldmann, T. A., McIntire, K. R., et al.: Serum alpha-fetoprotein levels in patients with non-neoplastic liver disease. Gastroenterology 65:530, 1973.
13. Boles, E. T., Jr., Hardacre, J. M., and Newton, W. A., Jr.: Ovarian tumors and cysts in infants and children. Arch. Surg. 83:580, 1961.
14. Borak, J.: Relationship between the clinical and roentgenological findings in bone metastases. Surg. Gynec. Obstet. 75:599, 1942.
15. Caffey, J.: Pediatric X-Ray Diagnosis. 6th Ed. Chicago, Year Book Medical Publishers, 1972.
16. Collins, V. P., Loeffler, R. K., and Tivey, H.: Observations on growth rate of human tumors. Am. J. Roentgenol. Radium Ther. Nucl. Med. 76:988, 1956.
17. Condon, V. R., and Nixon, G. W.: Pediatric neoplasms. In Holland, J. F., and Frei, E., III (eds.): Cancer Medicine. Philadelphia, Lea & Febiger, 1973.
18. Conley, J.: Tumors of the head and neck in children. In Concepts in Head and Neck Surgery. New York, Grune & Stratton, 1970.
19. Dibbins, A. W., and Wiener, E. S.: Retroperitoneal tumors in children. Current Problems in Surgery, October, 1973.
20. Edelstyn, G. A., Gillespie, P. J., and Grebbell, F. S.: The radiological demonstration of osseous metastasis. Experimental observations. Clin. Radiol. 18:158, 1967.
21. Editorial: A fetal serum protein in a new role. N. Engl. J. Med. 278:1016, 1968.
22. Edwards, C. L., Haynes, R. L., Nelson, B. M., and Tehranian, N.: Clinical investigation of ^{67}Ga for tumor scanning. J. Nucl. Med. 11:316, 1970.
23. Ellman, L.: Bone marrow biopsy in the evaluation of lymphoma, carcinoma, and granulomatous disorders. Amer. J. Med. 60:1, 1976.
24. Evans, J. E., Dubilier, W., Jr., and Monteith, J. C.: Nephrotomography. Am. J. Roentgenol. Radium Ther. Nucl. Med. 71:213, 1954.
25. Fanning, A., Dierich, H. C., and Lentle, B. C.: Bone scanning with technetium (^{99m}Tc) polyphosphate in tuberculosis osteomyelitis. Tubercle 55:227, 1974.
26. Fellows, K. E.: The uses and abuses of abdominal and peripheral arteriography in children. Radiol. Clin. North Am. 10:349, 1972.
27. Fraumeni, J. F., Jr., and Miller, R. W.: Cancer deaths in the newborn. Am. J. Dis. Child. 117:186, 1969.
28. Freimanis, A. K.: Ultrasonic imaging of neoplasms. Cancer 37:496, 1976.
29. Fuks, A., Banjo, C., Shuster, J. Freedman, S. O., and Gold, P.: Carcinoembryonic antigen (CEA): Molecular biology and clinical significance. Biochem. Biophys. Acta 417:123, 1974.
30. Gilday, D. L., Ash, J. M., and Reilly, B. J.: Radionuclide skeletal survey for pediatric neoplasms. Radiology 123:399, 1977.
31. Gitlin, D., and Boesman, M.: Serum alpha-fetoprotein, albumin, and gamma-G-globulin in human conceptus. J. Clin. Invest. 45:1826, 1966.
32. Go, V. L. W.: Carcinoembryonic antigen: Clinical application. Cancer 37:562, 1976.
33. Gold, P.: Circulating antibodies against carcinoembryonic antigens of the human digestive system. Cancer 20:1663, 1967.
34. Gold, P., and Freedman, S. O.: Specific carcinoembryonic antigens of the human digestive system. J. Exp. Med. 122:467, 1965.
35. Goldberg, B., Goodman, G., and Clearfield, H.: Evaluation of ascites by ultrasound. Radiology 96:15, 1970.
36. Griscom, N. T.: The roentgenology of neonatal abdominal masses. Am. J. Roentgenol. Radium Ther. Nucl. Med. 93:447, 1965.
37. Griscom, N. T., and Neuhauser, E. B. D.: Total body opacification. J. Pediatr. Surg. 1:76, 1966.
38. Grosfeld, J. L., and Baehner, R. L.: Mediastinal malignancy in children. Pediatrics Digest 15:37, 1973.
39. Grosfeld, J. L., O'Neill, J. A., Jr., and Clatworthy, H. W., Jr.: Enteric duplications in infancy and childhood: An 18-year review. Ann. Surg. 172:83, 1970.
40. Grosfeld, J. L., Weinberger, M., Kilman, J. W., and Clatworthy, H. W., Jr.: Primary mediastinal neoplasms in infants and children. Ann. Thorac. Surg. 12:179, 1971.
41. Grossman, H.: The evaluation of abdominal masses in children with emphasis on noninvasive methods. A radiologic approach. Cancer 35:884, 1975.
42. Grossman, H.: Evaluating common intraabdominal masses in children—a systematic radiographic approach. CA 26:219, 1976.
43. Gyepes, M. T., and Smith, L. E.: Pediatric neoplasms. In Steckel, R. J., and Kagan, A. R.: Diagnosis and Staging of Cancer. A Radiologic Approach. Philadelphia, W. B. Saunders Co., 1976.
44. Haller, J. A., Mazur, D. O., and Morgan, W. W.: Diagnosis and management of me-

diastinal masses in infants and children. J. Thorac. Cardiovasc. Surg. 58:385, 1969.
45. Han, T., Stutzman, L., and Rogue, A. L.: Bone marrow biopsy in Hodgkin's disease and other neoplastic diseases. J.A.M.A. 217:1239, 1971.
46. Hartfield, P. M., and Pfister, R. C.: Splenic and hepatic evaluation during infusion nephrotomography. Am. J. Roentgenol. Radium Ther. Nucl. Med. 119:687, 1973.
47. Harwood-Nash, D. C., and Breckbill, D. L.: Computed tomography in children: A new diagnostic technique. J. Pediatr. 89:343, 1976.
48. Heberman, R. B.: Tumor immunology and its application to the diagnosis of cancer. Ann. Clin. Lab. Science 4:323, 1974.
49. Hinman, F., Jr.: Non-obstructive anomalies of the kidney. In Benson, C. D., et al. (eds.): Pediatric Surgery. Chicago, Year Book Medical Publishers, 1962.
50. Hoffer, P. B., and Gottshalk, A.: Tumor scanning agents. Semin. Nucl. Med. 4: 305:1974.
51. Holtz, S., and Powers, W. E.: Inferior vena cavograms. Radiology 78:583, 1962.
52. Jaffe, B. F.: Pediatric head and neck tumors. Laryngoscope 83:1644, 1973.
53. Jaffe, B. F., and Jaffe, N.: Head and neck tumors in children. Pediatrics 51:731, 1973.
54. Jaffe, N., Cassady, R., Petersen, R., Traggis, D.: Heterochromia and Horner syndrome associated with cervical and mediastinal neuroblastoma. J. Pediatr. 87: 75, 1975.
55. Johnston, G., Benua, R. S., Teates, C. D., et al.: [67]Ga citrate imaging in untreated Hodgkin's disease. Preliminary report of cooperative group. J. Nucl. Med. 15:399, 1974.
56. Jones, P. G.: Swellings in the neck in childhood. Med. J. Aust. 1:212, 1963.
57. Kaplan, W. D., and Adelstein, S. J.: The radionuclide identification of tumors. Cancer 37:487, 1976.
58. Kasper, T. E., Osborne, R. W., Jr., Semerdjian, H. S., and Miller, H. C.: Urologic abdominal masses in infants and children. J. Urol. 116:629, 1976.
59. Kaufman, S. L., and Stout, A. P.: Lipoblastic tumors of children. Cancer 12:912, 1959.
60. Kaufmann, S. L., and Stout, A. P.: Congenital mesenchymal tumors. Cancer 18:460, 1965.
61. Kew, M. C., Puves, I. R., and Bersohn, I.: Serum alpha-fetoprotein levels in acute viral hepatitis. Gut 14:939, 1973.
62. Koch, K.: Clinical manifestations and differential diagnosis of malignant solid tumors of childhood. In Vuksanovic, M. M. (ed.): Clinical Pediatric Oncology. Mt. Kisco, N. Y., Futura Publishing Co., 1972.
63. Koop, C. E., and Kaufmann, H. J.: The diagnosis of cancer in children. Semin. Oncol. 1:5, 1974.
64. Kreel, L.: The EMI whole body scanner in the demonstration of lymph node enlargement. Clin. Radiol. 27:421, 1976.
65. Kurlander, G. J., and Smith, F. E.: Total-body opacification in the diagnosis of Wilms' tumor and neuroblastoma. A note of caution. Radiology 89:1075, 1167.
66. Larson, S. M., Graff, K. S., Tretner, I., et al.: Positive gallium 67 photoscan in myeloblastoma. J.A.M.A. 222:321, 1972.
67. Lavender, J. P., Lowe, J., et al.: Gallium-67 citrate scanning in neoplastic and inflammatory lesions. Brit. J. Radiol. 44: 361, 1971.
68. Lentle, B. C., Russell, A. S., Percy, J. S., et al.: Bone scintiscanning updated. Ann. Intern. Med. 84:297, 1976.
69. Leopold, G. R., and Asher, W. M.: Diagnosis of extra-organ retroperitoneal space lesions by B-scan ultrasonography. Radiology 104:133, 1972.
70. Leyton, B., Halpern, S., Leopold, G., and Hagen, S.: Correlation of ultrasound and colloid scintiscan studies of the normal and diseased liver. J. Nucl. Med. 14:27, 1973.
71. Lomas, F., Dibos, P., and Wagner, H. N., Jr.: Increased specificity of liver scanning with the use of 67-gallium citrate. N. Engl. J. Med. 286:1323, 1972.
72. Lurie, B. B., Lowenstein, M. S., and Zamcheck, N.: Elevated carcinoembryonic antigen in benign biliary obstruction. Clin. Res. 22:363A, 1974.
73. Maklad, N., Doust, B., and Baum, J.: Ultrasonic diagnosis of postoperative intra-abdominal abscess. Radiology 113: 417, 1974.
74. Margulis, A. R., Nice, C. M., Jr., and Rigler, L. G.: Roentgen findings in primary hepatoma in infants and children: Analysis of eleven cases. Radiology 66:809, 1956.
75. Martin, E. W., Jr., Kibbey, W. E., DiVecchia, L., et al.: Carcinoembryonic antigen. Clinical and historical aspects. Cancer 37:62, 1976.
76. Martin, H. F.: Cancer of the head and neck in children. J. Pediatr. 15:363, 1939.
77. May, M.: Neck masses in children: Diagnosis and treatment. Pediatr. Ann. 5:517, 1976.
78. McAlister, W. H., and Koehler, P. R.: Disease of the adrenal. Radiol. Clin. North Am. 5:205, 1967.
79. McNicholl, B.: Palpability of the liver and spleen in infants and children. Arch. Dis. Child. 32:438, 1957.
80. Melicow, M. M., and Uson, A. C.: Palpable abdominal masses in infants and chil-

dren: A report based on a review of 653 cases. J. Urol. 81:705, 1959.
81. Melki, G.: Ultrasonic patterns of tumors of the liver. J. Clin. Ultrasound 1:306, 1974.
82. Milder, M. S., Glick, J. H., Henderson, E. S., and Johnston, G. S.: ^{67}Ga scintigraphy in acute leukemia. Cancer 32:803, 1973.
83. Morley, P., and Barnett, E.: The use of ultrasound in the diagnosis of pelvic masses. Brit. J. Radiol. 43:602, 1970.
84. Moussatos, G. H., and Baffes, T. G.: Cervical masses in infants and children. Pediatrics 32:251, 1963.
85. Muss, H. B., and Moloney, W. C.: Chloroma and other myeloblastic tumors. Blood 42:721, 1973.
86. New, P. F. J., Scott, W. R., Schnur, J. A., Davis, K. R., and Taveras, J. M.: Computerized axial tomography with the EMI scanner. Radiology 110:109, 1974.
87. Nice, C. M., Jr., Margulis, A. R., and Rigler, L. G.: A simple approach to the roentgen diagnosis of abdominal tumors in infants and children. Am. J. Roentgenol. Radium Ther. Nucl. Med. 75:977, 1956.
88. Nixon, G. W., and Condon, V. R.: Bone tumors. In Holland, J. F., and Frei, E., III (eds.): Cancer Medicine. Philadelphia, Lea & Febiger, 1973.
89. Novy, S., Wallace, S., Medellin, H., and McBride, C.: Angiographic evaluation of primary malignant hepatocellular tumors in children. Am. J. Roentgenol. Radium Ther. Nucl. Med. 120:353, 1974.
90. O'Connor, J. F., and Neuhauser, E. B. D.: Total body opacification in conventional and high dose intravenous urography in infancy. Am. J. Roentgenol. Radium Ther. Nucl. Med. 90:63, 1963.
91. O'Mara, R. E.: Skeletal scanning in neoplastic disease. Cancer 37:480, 1976.
92. Omenn, G. S.: Ectopic hormone syndromes associated with tumors in childhood. Pediatrics 47:613, 1971.
93. Pedersen, K. O.: Fetuin, new globulin isolated from serum. Nature 154:575, 1944.
94. Poole, C. A.: Roentgenographic aspects of the most frequent abdominal malignancies in children. In Vuksanovic, M. M. (ed.): Clinical Pediatric Oncology. Mt. Kisco, N. Y., Futura Publishing Co., 1972.
95. Poole, C. A.: Special procedures in roentgen diagnosis of abdominal tumors in infancy and childhood. In Vuksanovic, M. M. (ed.): Clinical Pediatric Oncology. Mt. Kisco, N. Y., Futura Publishing Co., 1972.
96. Portsmann, W.: Renal angiography in children. Progr. Pediatr. Radiol. 3:51, 1970.
97. Raffensperger, J., and Abousleiman, A.: Abdominal masses in children under one year of age. Surgery 63:514, 1968.
98. Reynoso, G.: Biochemical tests in cancer diagnosis. In Holland, J. F., and Frei, E., III (eds.): Cancer Medicine. Philadelphia, Lea & Febiger, 1973.
99. Reynoso, G., Chu, T. M., Holyoke, D., et al.: Carcinoembryonic antigen in patients with different cancers. J.A.M.A. 220:361, 1972.
100. Rodriguez, V., Burgess, M., and Bodey, G. P.: Management of fever of unknown origin in patients with neoplasms and neutropenia. Cancer 32:1007, 1973.
101. Rosen, G.: The development of an adjuvant chemotherapy program for the treatment of osteogenic sarcoma. In Voath, J. (ed.): Frontiers of Radiation Therapy and Oncology. Vol. 10. Basel, Karger, 1975.
102. Rosenfield, N., and Treves, S.: Liver-spleen scanning in pediatrics. Pediatrics 53:692, 1974.
103. Rouslahti, E., and Seppala, M.: Alpha-fetoprotein in normal human serum. Nature 235:161, 1972.
104. Rubin, P. R.: Cancer of the head and neck. Nasopharyngeal cancer. J.A.M.A. 220:390, 1972.
105. Saharia, P. C.: Carcinoma arising in the thyroglossal duct remnant: case reports and review of the literature. Brit. J. Surg. 62:689, 1975.
106. Schwartz, M. K.: Biochemical procedures as aids in diagnosis of different forms of cancer. Ann. Clin. Lab. Science 4:95, 1974.
107. Schwartz, M. K.: Laboratory aids to diagnosis—enzymes. Cancer 37:542, 1976.
108. Schwartz, M. K., Fleisher, M., and Bodansky, O.: Clinical applications of phosphohydrolase measurements in cancer. Ann. N. Y. Acad. Sci. 166:775, 1969.
109. Schwartzendruber, D. C., Nelson, B., and Hayes, R. L.: Gallium-67 localization in lysosomal-like granules of leukemic and nonleukemic murine tissues. J. Natl. Cancer Inst. 46:941, 1971.
110. Silberstein, E. B.: Cancer diagnosis. The role of tumor-imaging radiopharmaceuticals. Am. J. Med. 60:226, 1976.
111. Snyder, W. H., Hastings, T. N., and Pollock, W.: Retroperitoneal tumors. In Benson, C. D., et al. (eds.): Pediatric Surgery. Chicago, Year Book Medical Publishers, 1962.
112. Spencer, R. P.: Radionuclide liver scans in tumor detection. Current concepts. Cancer 37:475, 1976.
113. Spencer, R. P., and Banever, C.: Growth of the human liver: A preliminary scan study. J. Nucl. Med. 11:660, 1970.
114. Spencer, R. P., Pearson, H. A., and Lange, R. C.: Human spleen: Scan studies on growth and response to medications. J. Nucl. Med. 12:466, 1971.
115. Stevens, D. P., and Mackay, I. R.: Increased

carcinoembryonic antigen in heavy cigarette smokers. Lancet 2:1238, 1973.
116. Strole, W. E., Jr.: Case records of the Massachusetts General Hospital, Case 6-1977. N. Engl. J. Med. 296:328, 1977.
117. Sutow, W. W., and Montague, E. D.: Pediatric tumors. In MacComb, W. S., and Fletcher, G. H. (eds.): Cancer of the Head and Neck. Baltimore, Williams & Wilkins Co., 1967.
118. Tucker, A. S., and Izant, J. B.: Inferior vena cavography. Progr. Pediatr. Radiol. 3:82, 1970.
119. Vaidya, S. G., Chaudhri, M. A., Morrison, R., et al.: Localization of gallium-67 in malignant neoplasms. Lancet 2:911, 1970.
120. Vinciguerra, V., and Silver, R. T.: The importance of bone marrow biopsy in the staging of patients with lymphosarcoma. Blood 41:913, 1973.
121. Vinik, M., and Altman, D. H.: Congenital malignant tumors. Cancer 19:967, 1966.
122. Wayne, E. R., Campbell, J. B., Koloske, A. M., and Burrington, J. D.: Intussusception in the older child — suspect lymphosarcoma. J. Pediatr. Surg. 11:789, 1976.
123. Wedge, J. J., Grosfeld, J. L., and Smith, J. P.: Abdominal masses in the newborn: 63 cases. J. Urol. 106:770, 1971.
124. Williams, L. E., Fisher, J. H., Courtney, R. A., and Darling, D. B.: Preoperative diagnosis of choledochal cyst by hepatoscintigraphy. N. Engl. J. Med. 283:85, 1970.
125. Winchell, H. S.: Mechanisms for localization of radiopharmaceuticals in neoplasms. Semin. Nucl. Med. 6:371, 1976.

Chapter Three

CANCER CHEMOTHERAPY

In the past three decades chemotherapeutic agents have become a powerful addition to the physician's armamentarium against cancer. In order to use these agents appropriately, the therapist must understand not only their potential beneficial effects but also their deleterious effects and the limits of their ability to combat the disease.

Stephens has symbolized the four broad uses of cancer chemotherapy by the acronym CRAB:[103]

Curative

Relief of symptoms

Adjuvant care: To prevent peripheral occult disease from developing after localized bulk tumor has been controlled by surgery or radiotherapy, or both.

Basal: To reduce the size, viability, and peripheral extent of large localized tumor masses in preparation for definitive surgical or radiotherapeutic endeavors.

Ideally, a chemotherapeutic regimen should be capable of totally eradicating both manifest bulk tumor and its occult metastases and thereby cure the patient; however, for most cancers, this rarely occurs. Since chemotherapy is much more effective against occult microscopic foci of tumor than against large tumor masses, it has found its major usefulness in relief of symptoms, adjuvant care, and basal treatment.

CELL POPULATION KINETICS

The basis for all forms of chemotherapy is a differential sensitivity of the offending organism and the normal host cells to the toxic effects of a given drug. In the case of bacterial infections, the metabolism of the bacteria is sufficiently different from that of mammalian cells to allow for treatment by agents with a good deal of selectivity. In the case of cancer, where the "offending organisms" are the host's own transformed cells, metabolic differences are much more subtle and difficult to exploit.

Most cancer chemotherapeutic agents appear to exert their cytotoxic effects by virtue of the relative kinetic vulnerability of neoplastic cells. Table 3–1 lists a group of pediatric malignancies which are highly responsive to chemotherapy. In general, these tumors are distinguished by a very rapid growth rate (doubling time = several days), whereas nonresponsive tumors generally have a much slower growth rate (doubling time = several months).[123]

The major determinants of any tissue's growth rate are: (1) the speed with which the individual cells replicate themselves (*generation time*), (2) the proportion of cells in the population which are actively dividing at any one time (*growth fraction*), and (3) the

Table 3-1 Pediatric Malignancies That Are Highly Responsive to Chemotherapy

---

Acute lymphocytic leukemia
Burkitt's lymphoma
Choriocarcinoma
Ewing's sarcoma
Hodgkin's disease
Embryonal testicular cancer
Lymphosarcoma
Rhabdomyosarcoma
Retinoblastoma
Wilms' tumor

---

cell death rate. Thus cell population kinetics covers two related fields of study: (1) the various stages or phases of the cell replication cycle, and (2) the dynamic characteristics of cell populations, including rates of cell proliferation, cell migration, and cell death.

THE CELL CYCLE

The cell cycle (Fig. 3-1) represents the sequence of events that occur during the growth and division of cells. These events center on the synthesis of DNA for chromosome replication and the separation of the chromosomes by mitosis.

When preparing for DNA synthesis and chromosome replication, actively proliferating cells enter a G_1 (Gap 1) phase during which RNA and protein synthesis as well as other molecular events occur. This is followed by the phase of DNA synthesis (S), during which the DNA content of the cells is doubled. The S phase is followed by a G_2 (Gap 2) phase consisting of RNA and protein synthesis in preparation for mitosis. The M (mitotic) phase is that time during which cell division actually occurs, resulting in the formation of two "daughter" cells. Following mitosis cells may either enter another G_1 phase and continue the events which will lead to replication, or enter a "resting" (G_0) or prolonged G_1 phase, during which they retain proliferative capacity but do not actively prepare for division unless appropriately stimulated.

DYNAMIC CHARACTERISTICS OF CELL POPULATIONS

The most important factor conditioning a tumor's responsiveness to cytotoxic agents is its growth fraction. In tumors with a large growth fraction a majority of the cells are making DNA and undergoing mitosis (i.e., they are in the cell cycle). Most active anticancer drugs have their major inhibitory activity during DNA synthesis or during mitosis; it therefore stands to reason that tissues (normal and neoplastic) with a high proportion of cells in the cell cycle will be the more vulnerable to these agents. Thus, a tissue with 95 per cent of its cells

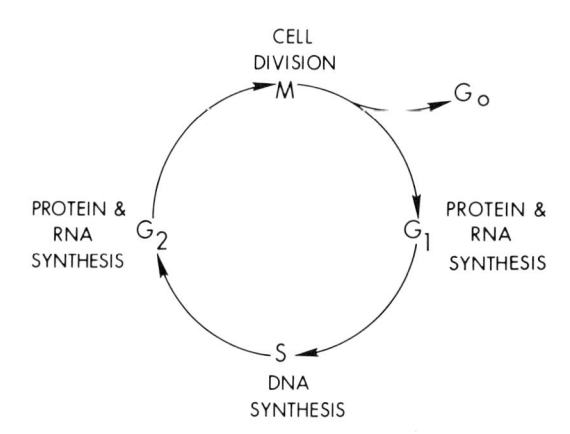

Figure 3-1 The cell cycle.

replicating will be seriously damaged by inhibitors of DNA synthesis, while a tissue with only 5 per cent of its cells in the cell cycle will be scarcely affected. Since most normal tissues (central nervous system, lung, kidneys) have very small (or nonexistent) growth fractions, they are relatively resistant to cancer chemotherapy; however, some normal tissues (hematopoietic precursor cells, gastrointestinal epithelium, hair follicles) have a high growth fraction and frequently are adversely affected along with the tumor cells.

Tissue repopulation after damage by cytotoxic agents will originate from the surviving stem cells. As shown in Figure 3-2, the life cycle of many normal tissues begins with a population of resting stem cells; for reasons currently unknown, some of these cells begin to proliferate and to respond to inductive stimuli by developing into functional, differentiated cells. Although chemotherapy can damage a high proportion of the dividing cells, the resting stem cell population remains relatively unaffected and is capable of resuming proliferation and maturation when the drug is no longer present.

The tumor population likewise appears to be derived from stem cells with unlimited proliferative potential, some of which are in a resting (G_0) state. For reasons stated below, the larger the tumor bulk, the higher the fraction of resting stem cells is likely to be, and the therapeutic effectiveness of chemotherapy is limited by the fact that these cells reenter the proliferating pool after therapy, so that tumor growth resumes.

Gompertzian Kinetics

One of the difficulties in treating the tumor-bearing host effectively is that a large fraction of the malignant cells may be out-of-cycle and thus insensitive to the majority of the chemotherapeutic agents. This is because a large number of animal tumors (and presumably human tumors as well) follow what is known as Gompertzian* growth kinetics. When they are small, their growth fraction is high and their size increases logarithmically with the passage of time (Fig. 3-3); it is at this point (when most of the cells are proliferating) that a tumor is most susceptible to chemotherapeutic agents. However, when the tumor reaches a larger size, its growth rate slows and may reach a steady state in which the mass does not show a further increase; coincident with this, an increasing number of tumor cells enter a nonproliferating state. Since most clinically apparent tumors are relatively large (a nodule measuring 1 cm in diameter contains approximately 10^9 cells), their growth fractions are usually relatively low (approximately 10 per cent), and as might be expected, they have become relatively refractory to chemotherapy.

The reduction in growth fraction of an enlarging tumor is not uniform throughout its entire mass, but instead is related to the geometry of the tumor. In solid tumors the proliferative fraction is characteristically higher in the

---

*Gompertz was a nineteenth century mathematician who originally derived the equation describing this relationship.

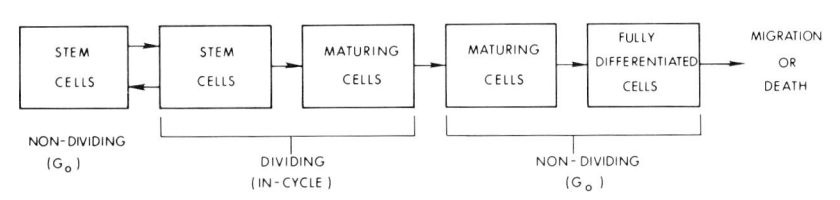

Figure 3-2 Cell kinetics of normal tissues.

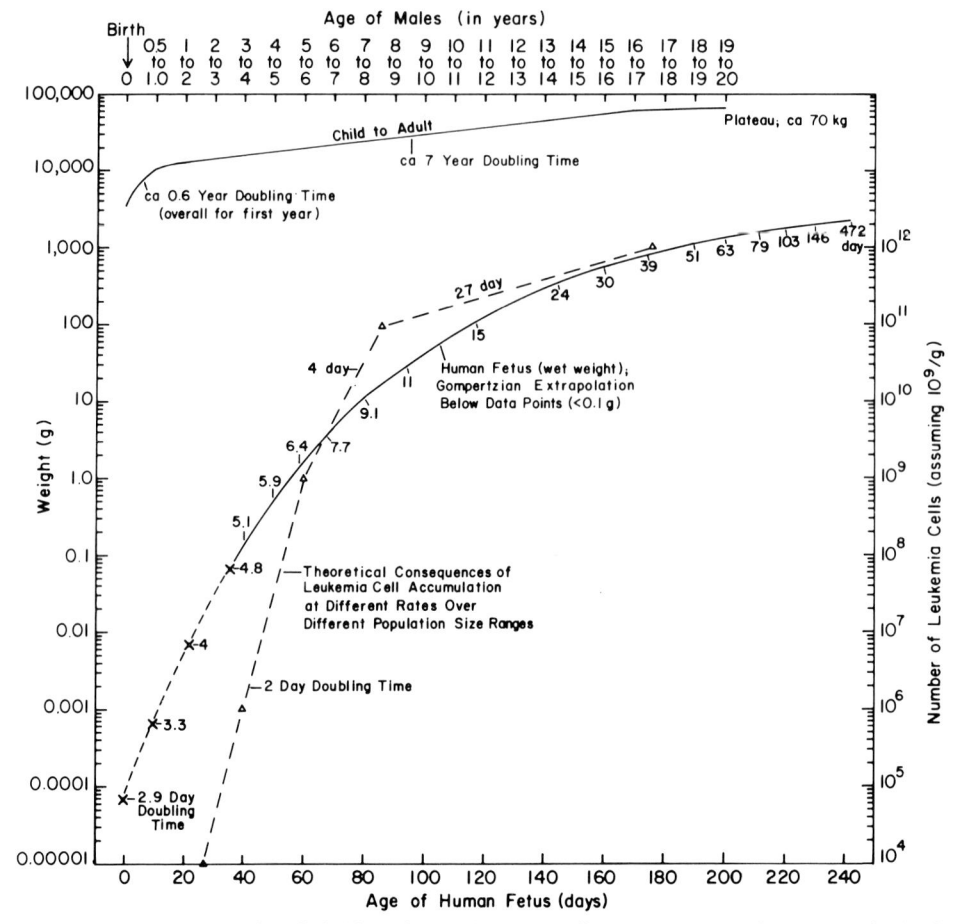

Figure 3-3 Human fetal and childhood growth expressed as Gompertzian functions. The broken line shows that the theoretical consequences of the accumulation of leukemic cells can also be visualized on the same plot. Note that the growth rates in all these systems are maximal initially and decline with increasing mass. (From Skipper, H. E., et al.: Cancer Res. *30*:1883, 1970.)

peripheral portions than in the center; this apparently reflects the critical role of vascularization, since the growth fraction of tumor cells decreases progressively with increasing distance from the blood vessels. Without being vascularized, most solid tumors are unable to grow larger than about 2 to 3 mm in diameter, after which simple diffusion of nutrients (and wastes) is insufficient to allow further enlargement.[51] Folkman has isolated from both animal and human tumors a "tumor-angiogenesis" factor that stimulates new capillary formation and has suggested that it might be possible to inhibit tumor growth and metastatic spread by inhibiting this factor.[38]

KINETICS OF DRUG ACTION

Destruction of tumor cells by chemotherapeutic agents follows first-order kinetics—*a given dose of drug will destroy a constant fraction (usually 99 to 99.99 per cent) of susceptible cells, not a fixed number of cells.*[100] Thus, a treatment dose which reduces a tumor cell population from 10^{12} (one trillion) to 10^9 (one billion) cells will result in a kill of 99.9 per cent of the cells (999 billion cells killed). A subsequent treatment dose (assuming no regrowth during the interval between treatments) will reduce the cell population to 10^6 (one million) cells, again a kill of 99.9 per cent, but this time only 999 million cells were killed. With each subsequent treatment 99.9 per cent of the residual population is killed, but 0.1 per cent remains. Theoretically, it should be possible to treat the patient until less than one cell remains, at which point most patients should be cured. However, in practice, this does not usually occur, for the following reasons:

1. Intervals between treatment must be spaced widely enough (usually 2 to 3 weeks) to allow the bone marrow to recover from the effects of the previous treatment. This length of time may permit significant regrowth of the tumor population, and if tumor is allowed to return to its original size, it can never be eradicated by this form of treatment.

2. Resistance to the drug may develop in the residual tumor population.

3. Not all of the tumor cells are actively proliferating; therefore, a significant number may not be susceptible to the drug. As the tumor bulk is reduced by the effects of chemotherapy, these cells may resume active proliferation and regenerate the tumor during the intervals between treatment or after treatment has been stopped.

4. Anatomic barriers may prevent the drug from entering certain tissues (e.g., brain, meninges, gonads, liver, spleen, kidneys) in sufficiently toxic concentrations to eradicate tumor cells.

Consequently, in order to completely eradicate a tumor population with chemotherapy, it is necessary either to increase the dose of drug within limits tolerable to the host, to combine drugs with different mechanisms of action or toxicity, or to start treatment when the number of cells is small and the growth fraction is high.[28] In humans, the latter situation is possible only when all clinically recognizable bulk tumor has been eradicated by surgery or radiotherapy; *adjuvant* chemotherapy can then be given to eradicate microscopic residual local and metastatic foci of disease. It is also possible that immunologic mechanisms might be able to eliminate small residual tumor foci.

Combination Chemotherapy

Single agents with known biochemical effect can produce lethal blockade of metabolic pathways; however, unless this blockade is sufficient to reduce the end product to levels below which a cell cannot survive, effective restriction of tumor growth will not occur.[30] Drug combinations, on the other hand, can produce different biochemical lesions by attacking multiple sites in biosynthetic pathways or inhibiting several processes involved in maintenance and function of essential macromolecules.[30] This may occur as the result of any of the following mechanisms:

1. *Sequential blockade*:[84] Inhibition of different enzymatic steps in a biochemical pathway leading to the production of an essential metabolite. Example: blockage of de novo purine biosynthesis at different steps by azaserine and methotrexate.

2. *Concurrent blockade*:[35] Inhibition of two different pathways, both leading to a common end product. Example: blockage of DNA synthesis as a result of interference with purine and pyrimidine biosynthesis by 6-thioguanine and cytosine arabinoside.

3. *Complementary inhibition*:[96] Repair of the damage done by one agent is inhibited by a second agent. Example: use of an alkylating agent to cross-link strands of DNA in combina-

tion with antimetabolites that inhibit DNA synthesis and may prevent repair.[30]

4. *Metabolic sensitization:*[105] One agent acts to increase the sensitivity of the cell to the damaging effects of a second agent. Example: administration of bromodeoxyuracil (BUDR), which then enhances the sensitivity of cells to a subsequent dose of irradiation.

5. *Relapse prevention.*[105] After treatment with a single agent, a subpopulation of drug-resistant cells may persist and give rise to recurrent tumor. The chances for development of a drug-resistant line will be less if two or more drugs of dissimilar modes of action are used.

Unlike single-agent chemotherapy, which developed as a result of their demonstrated efficacy in experimental tumor systems, most of the drug combinations currently in use have been designed empirically. The general rationale for combination of various chemotherapeutic agents is based on the following principles:[18]

1. Each drug in the combination should be active when used alone against the tumor.

2. The drugs should have different mechanisms of action.

3. The toxic effects of the drugs should not overlap, so that each can be given at or near its maximum tolerated level.

GUIDELINES FOR ADMINISTRATION OF CHEMOTHERAPEUTIC AGENTS

Most cancer chemotherapeutic agents are poisons; the only justification for using them is that they are more toxic to neoplastic cells than they are to normal ones. However, in order to achieve maximum therapeutic effects the dosages must be such that significant and even life-threatening toxicity to normal tissues must also occur. Errors in dosage or route of administration frequently result in disastrous consequences. Consequently, the utmost in precautions must be taken to ensure accuracy.

1. All drug dosages should be calculated and recorded in the chart by the physician in charge of the child's care and independently calculated by at least one other physician, preferably a member of the oncology service. This calculation should include: (1) desired dose per kilogram body weight (or per square meter surface area), (2) the patient's weight (or surface area), (3) the total dose, the concentration of the drug, and the volume to be administered. The example for vincristine is shown at the bottom of the page.

2. Administration of the drug should be supervised by a physician who is familiar with the drug and its side effects.

3. When drugs are given intravenously, care should be taken to avoid extravasation into the soft tissues since many chemotherapeutic agents can cause severe and painful burns and sloughing of skin. Toward this end, a double syringe technique is used, with one syringe being used to start the intravenous injection and to flush the medication through with saline and the other to inject the medication itself (Fig. 3–4).

CANCER CHEMOTHERAPEUTIC AGENTS

Anticancer drugs are classified into groups that share either a common source or a common mechanism of

---

Dosage	Surface Area		Total Dose		Concentration		Volume
1.5 mg/m^2	× 0.8 m^2	=	1.2 mg	×	10 ml/1 mg	=	12 ml

CANCER CHEMOTHERAPY 63

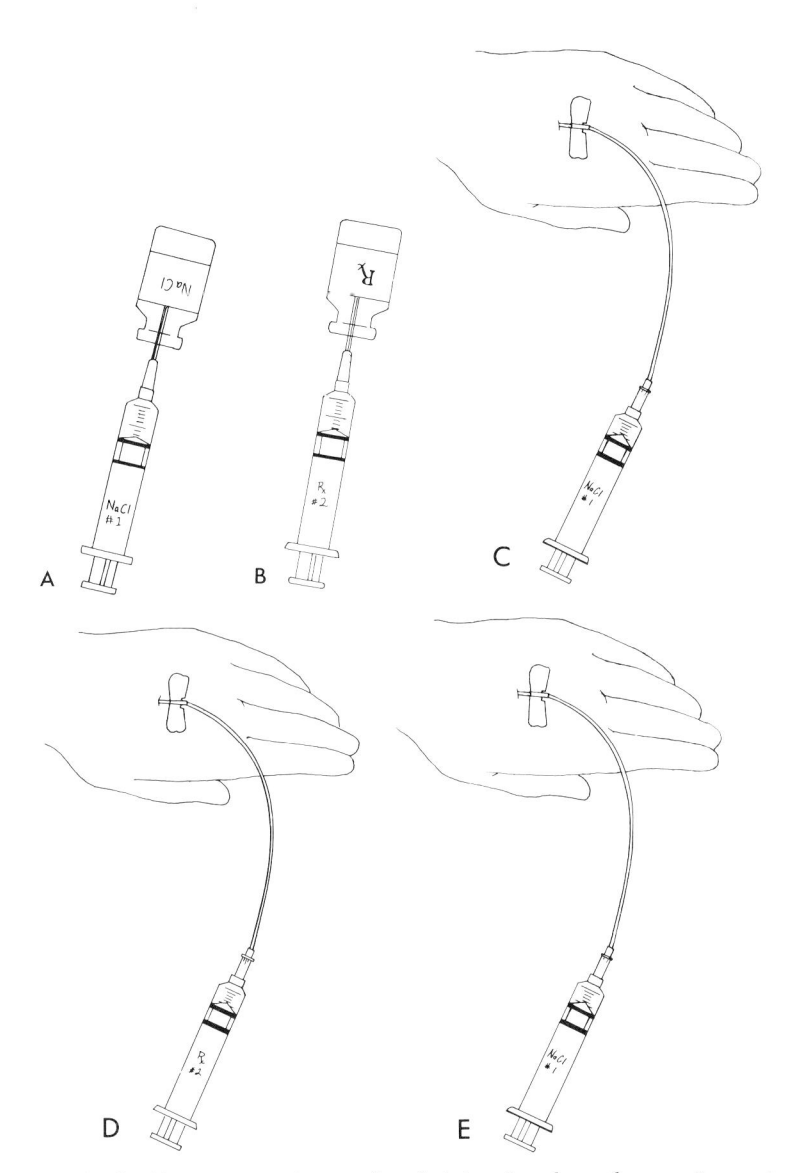

Figure 3-4 The double syringe technique for administering chemotherapeutic agents. *A*, Normal saline is drawn up into syringe #1. *B*, Medication is drawn up into syringe #2. *C*, Attach syringe #1 (saline) to a 23 gauge scalp vein needle, fill tubing with saline and insert into vein. Flush vein with saline. *D*, After ascertaining that there is good blood return and no extravasation of saline, remove syringe #1 and attach syringe #2 (medication). Inject medication slowly with constant monitoring for evidence of extravasation. *E*, Reattach syringe #1 (saline) to I.V. tubing and flush the remaining medication from the tubing with saline, then remove needle from vein.

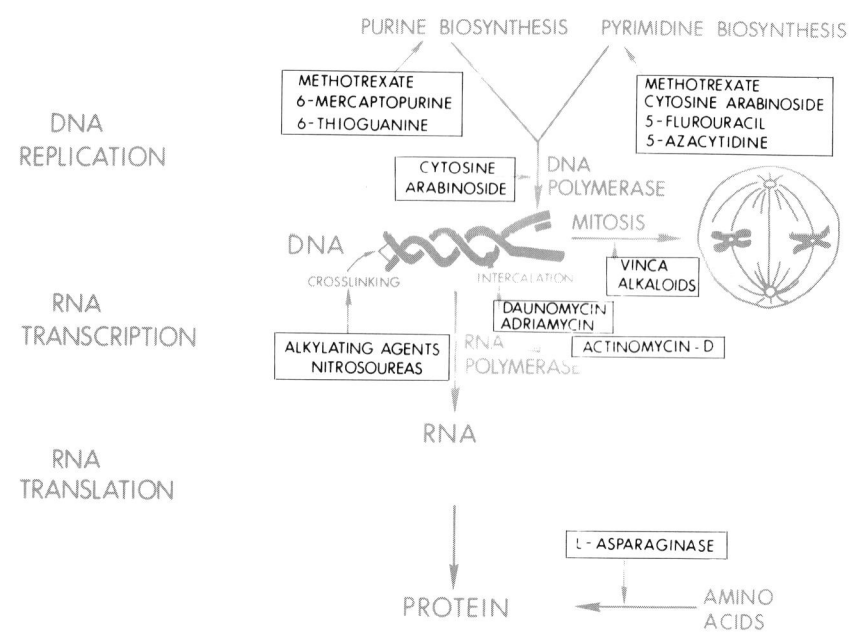

Figure 3-5 Sites of action of cancer chemotherapeutic agents.

action. The general classes of agents are:
1. Alkylating agents
2. Antimetabolites
3. Antibiotics
4. Vinca alkaloids
5. Miscellaneous

As shown in Figure 3-5, these agents interfere with the complex biochemical machinery of the cell at specific sites. Thus DNA replication may be blocked by interference with the synthesis of its precursor nucleotides by various antimetabolites or by inhibition of the enzyme DNA polymerase by cytosine arabinoside. The Vinca alkaloids arrest cell division by blocking formation of the mitotic spindle. Alkylating agents and nitrosoureas damage the DNA molecule by cross-linking its component strands, and the antibiotic agents bind to the DNA molecule, with subsequent inhibition of RNA transcription as well as DNA replication. Hydrolysis of L-asparagine by the enzyme L-asparaginase makes this amino acid unavailable for protein synthesis. These mechanisms will be discussed in further detail in subsequent sections.

Those chemotherapeutic agents which interfere primarily with DNA replication require the target cells to be actively proliferating in order to exert their toxic effect and thus are classified as *cell-cycle specific* (Table 3-2). *Cell-cycle nonspecific* agents, on the other hand, will damage resting (G_0) cells as well as those that are in active cell cycle (Table 3-3).

ALKYLATING AGENTS

The alkylating agents are very reactive compounds that combine readily with nitrogen, sulfur, or oxygen atoms of biologically important molecules. In doing so they substitute alkyl groups (R—CH—CH$_2^+$) for H$^+$ atoms; in the case of DNA this results in breaks in the molecule and cross-linking of DNA strands, thereby interfering with DNA replication and RNA transcription.

Cancer Chemotherapy

Table 3-2 Cell-Cycle Specific Agents

Drug	Mechanism of Action	Cycle Phase
Antimetabolites		
Methotrexate	Inhibits dihydrofolate reductase	S
6-Mercaptopurine	Inhibits purine synthesis	S
6-Thioguanine	Inhibits purine synthesis	S
Cytosine arabinoside	Inhibits DNA polymerase	S
Vinca Alkaloids		
Vincristine	Precipitate microtubular	M
Vinblastine	protein and block formation of mitotic spindle	M
Miscellaneous		
Hydroxyurea	Inhibits ribonucleoside phosphate reductase	S

Since similar effects can be produced by certain types of ionizing radiation, alkylating agents are considered to be "radiomimetic."

The commonly used alkylating agents are: *nitrogen mustard, cyclophosphamide, busulfan, chlorambucil,* and *melphalan*. With the exception of busulfan (an alkyl sulfonate), all the other agents are derivatives of nitrogen mustard (Fig. 3-6). Although modifications of this basic structure do not affect the mechanism of action, they do result in differences in absorption, site and rate of metabolism, and tissue affinity, which, in turn, determine the route of administration, rapidity of action, and side effects.

Nitrogen Mustard (Mechlorethamine Hydrochloride, HN_2, Mustargen)

Nitrogen mustard is prepared as a powder. Once reconstituted with water, it becomes very reactive and will undergo chemical transformation within a very short period of time. Consequently, it should be administered intravenously immediately or it will become inactivated. This should be done by injecting it into the tubing of an I.V. set that is already in place and which is running well; infiltration into the soft tissues may cause a severe tissue reaction, with erythema, ne-

Table 3-3 Cell-Cycle Nonspecific Agents

Class of Agent	Mechanism of Action
Alkylating Agents	Alkylation of DNA, RNA, and/or protein
Nitrogen mustard,	
Cytoxan, Busulfan,	
Chlorambucil, BCNU, CCNU	
Antibiotics	
Actinomycin D	Inhibits RNA polymerase
Adriamycin	Intercalates into DNA
Daunorubicin	Intercalates into DNA
Miscellaneous	
L-Asparaginase	Asparagine depletion
Prednisone	?
Procarbazine	Damages DNA
DTIC	?Alkylation

BASIC NITROGEN MUSTARD STRUCTURE

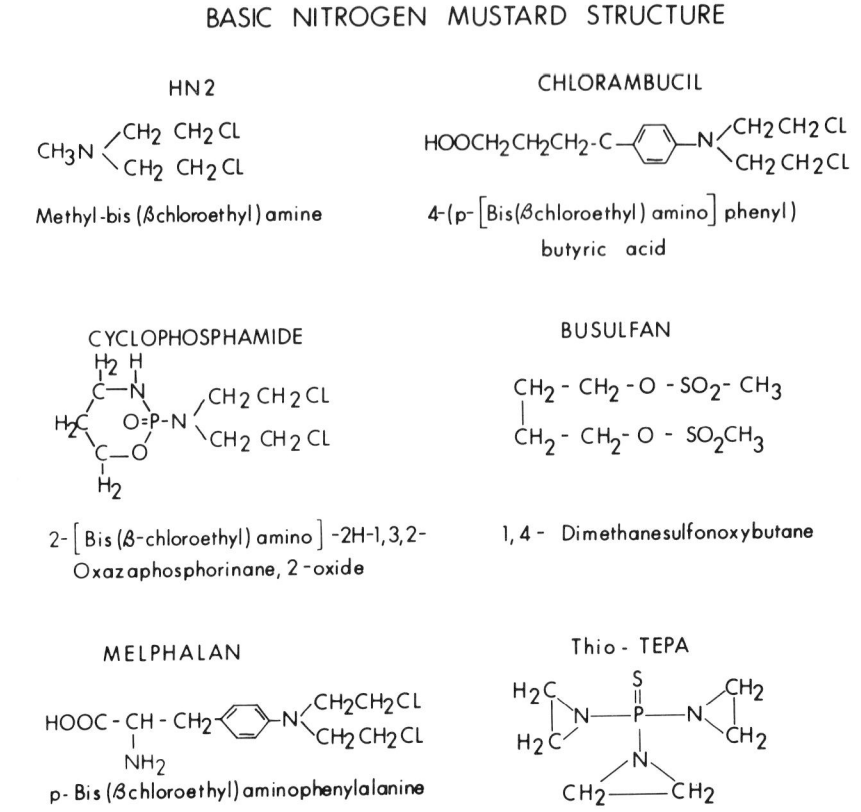

HN2
Methyl-bis (βchloroethyl) amine

CHLORAMBUCIL
4-(p-[Bis(βchloroethyl) amino] phenyl) butyric acid

CYCLOPHOSPHAMIDE
2-[Bis (β-chloroethyl) amino]-2H-1,3,2-Oxazaphosphorinane, 2-oxide

BUSULFAN
1,4- Dimethanesulfonoxybutane

MELPHALAN
p- Bis (βchloroethyl) aminophenylalanine

Thio-TEPA
Triethylene thiophosphoramide

Figure 3–6 Structural formulas of the alkylating agents. (Reprinted, by permission, from Greenwald, E. S.: Cancer Chemotherapy, Medical Examination Publishing Co.)

crosis, and sloughing of the skin. Indeed, the vesicant action of this compound is so pronounced that even spilling onto intact skin or the conjunctivae will cause severe reaction. Consequently, precautions such as the wearing of gloves and protective glasses should be observed during the reconstitution and withdrawal of the drug. All equipment used in this procedure should be either discarded immediately or rinsed with a solution containing equal volumes of 5 per cent thiosulfate and 5 per cent sodium bicarbonate for 45 minutes. If nitrogen mustard has been inadvertently extravasated into soft tissue, prompt infiltration of the area with sterile isotonic (1/6 molar) sodium thiosulfate and application of an ice compress for 6 to 12 hours may minimize the local reaction. Contact with skin or mucous membranes should be treated by irrigation with water for 15 minutes, followed by 2 per cent sodium thiosulfate solution.[74]

The earliest side effect noticeable by the patient will be nausea and vomiting. This can be controlled somewhat by prior administration of antiemetics and a sedative such as chloral hydrate. A more serious and potentially fatal complication is bone marrow suppression, with resultant leukopenia and thrombocytopenia. Other side effects include menstrual irregularities, toxic encephalopathy, and alopecia.

Once injected, nitrogen mustard has its primary effect within a few minutes, so care must be exercised in selecting the dosage. Because of this relative lack of control that the physician has over its action, nitrogen mustard has largely been supplanted by other alkylating agents that act more slowly and therefore can be controlled better. However, this agent still has an important place in the treatment of patients with *Hodgkin's disease* and *non-Hodgkin's lymphoma*. It is also used to treat *pleural malignancies* by direct intracavitary injection.

Cyclophosphamide (Cytoxan, Endoxan)

Cyclophosphamide is an N-phosphorylated cyclic derivative of nitrogen mustard (Fig. 3–6). The parent compound is inactive until oxidized by hepatic microsomal enzymes into active metabolites and, consequently, cyclophosphamide is effective when given by oral and intravenous routes, but not when injected directly into cavities.

Because of the inactivity of the cyclophosphamide molecule, it lacks the direct vesicant action of nitrogen mustard and does not cause irritation if spilled on the skin or extravasated during intravenous administration. Moreover, its slower rate of activity makes it easier to control than nitrogen mustard. However, in large doses it has equivalent tumoricidal activity and also equal side effects, particularly nausea and vomiting, bone marrow suppression, and alopecia.

A unique toxic sequel of the clinical use of cyclophosphamide is the development of hemorrhagic cystitis due to renal excretion of active metabolites in high concentrations;[81] black children appear to be affected by this complication over twice as frequently as whites. A large urine volume will dilute these metabolites and reduce the risk of bladder irritation; consequently, it is advisable to keep the patient well hydrated and for him to void frequently. Even in the absence of acute hemorrhagic cystitis, continued administration of the drug may result in hyperplastic and fibrotic changes affecting both the epithelial and muscular layers of the bladder, with eventual chronic cystitis. Carcinoma of the bladder has been reported in at least five patients after cyclophosphamide-induced hemorrhagic cystitis.[110]

In view of the general practice of keeping cyclophosphamide-treated patients well hydrated, it is important to consider that relatively high doses of this drug (greater than 50 mg/kg) may impair water excretion and lead to hyponatremia, weight gain, and inappropriately concentrated urine.[27] This may be a result of a direct effect of the active metabolite(s) on the distal renal tubule. The syndrome is usually self-limited.

Other side effects of cyclophosphamide include immunosuppression, sterility and testicular atrophy in males, amenorrhea and ovarian fibrosis in females, and fetal damage.[21] At very high dosage (120 mg/kg over a 4-day period) serious cardiac toxicity has been observed and death from diffuse hemorrhagic myocardial necrosis has occurred with a dosage of 240 mg/kg over 4 days.[15]

Cyclophosphamide is currently being used in protocols for *Hodgkin's disease, non-Hodgkin's lymphoma, rhabdomyosarcoma, Ewing's sarcoma, teratocarcinoma, acute lymphocytic leukemia,* and *neuroblastoma.*

Busulfan (Myleran)

Busulfan is a sulfonated alkylating agent (Fig. 3–6); it is usually administered by the oral route. When given in repeated doses, there is a gradually diminishing excretion in the urine and a progressive accumulation of the drug in the plasma, suggesting a slow elimination of the metabolic products.

The major toxic effect of busulfan is bone marrow suppression. There may be a lag period of 10 to 14 days before this becomes apparent and another lag period after the drug is discontinued before the blood count stops falling. This complicates the treatment of patients with this medication and may result in abrupt and occasionally irreversible drops in the neutrophil and platelet counts. Other side effects are seen mainly when the drug is administered for a prolonged period; these include hyperpigmentation, pulmonary fibrosis, ocular cataracts, and gynecomastia.

The major use of busulfan is in treatment of *chronic granulocytic leukemia*. Further details of its administration are discussed in Chapter Eight.

Chlorambucil (Leukeran)

Chlorambucil is an aromatic derivative of nitrogen mustard (Fig. 3–6) which can be administered orally. It is the slowest acting, least toxic, and most easily controllable of the alkylating agents. Although prolonged usage may result in marrow suppression, gastrointestinal symptoms, hepatotoxicity, and dermatitis, careful following of the patient and his relevant laboratory studies allows sufficient guidelines to avoid these toxic effects.

Since the major usage of this drug is in *chronic lymphocytic leukemia*, it is rarely used in children. However, it has also been used in treatment of *choriocarcinoma* and *testicular tumors*.

Melphalan (Alkeran, Phenylalanine Mustard, PAM)

This is a phenylalanine derivative of nitrogen mustard (Fig. 3–6), which can be given orally. It is used mainly in the treatment of *multiple myeloma*.

ANTIMETABOLITES

Antimetabolites are structural analogues of normal metabolites required for cell metabolism and growth; they interfere with these normal metabolic processes by being utilized to form an inappropriate end product or by inhibiting key enzymes.

In order to illustrate the mechanisms by which antimetabolites disrupt normal metabolic pathways, a brief review of folate and nucleic acid synthesis is given here.

The basic building blocks of DNA are deoxyribonucleotides derived from the purine (adenine, guanine) and pyrimidine (cytosine, thymine) bases. Certain antimetabolites interfere with the formation of these essential DNA components, whereas others actually incorporate themselves into the structure of the DNA molecule in place of the normal nucleotides and produce a functionally abnormal DNA.

An example of the manner in which antimetabolites can interfere with the synthesis of an essential nucleotide is afforded by the final step in the pathway of deoxythymidylate (dTMP) synthesis (Fig. 3–7). Deoxyuridylate (dUMP) is transformed to dTMP by the addition of a methyl group provided by methylene tetrahydrofolate (methylene-FH_4), a reaction catalyzed by the enzyme thymidylate synthetase. This reaction may be blocked either by inhibition of thymidylate synthetase or by inhibition of production of either of the substrates (dUMP or methylene-FH_4). As it turns out, *5-fluorouracil*, a pyrimidine analogue, inhibits thymidylate synthetase, whereas *methotrexate*, and other folate antagonists, can block the production of methylene-FH_4 by inhibiting the enzyme dihydrofolate reductase, which converts dihydrofolate to tetrahydrofolate. The final result in both

Cancer Chemotherapy

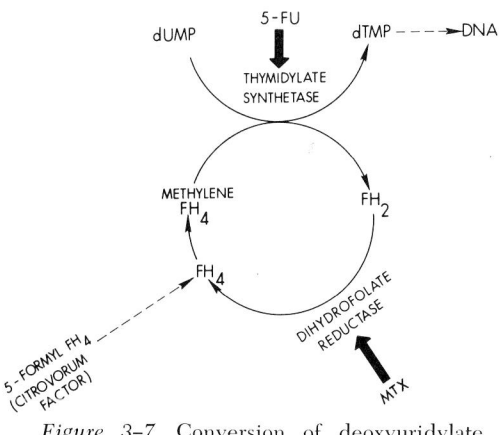

Figure 3-7 Conversion of deoxyuridylate (dUMP) to deoxythymidylate (dTMP) by transfer of a methyl group from methylene tetrahydrofolate (FH$_4$). This reaction can be blocked by methotrexate (MTX) or 5-fluorouracil (5-FU). The mechanism of citrovorum "rescue" of MTX-treated cells is also demonstrated.

instances is death of the cell due to depletion of dTMP.

Other clinically useful antimetabolites are *6-mercaptopurine* (6-MP), *6-thioguanine* (6-TG), *cytosine arabinoside*, and *5-azacytidine*. Both 6-MP and 6TG are purine analogues which incorporate themselves directly into the DNA molecular structure; 6-MP also blocks de novo purine biosynthesis and interconversions of purines. Cytosine arabinoside is a pyrimidine analogue whose modification is in the sugar moiety rather than in the pyrimidine base. It appears to work by inhibiting DNA polymerase. 5-Azacytidine is also a pyrimidine analogue.

Folate Antagonists— Methotrexate (Amethopterin)

Methotrexate is a folic acid analogue (Fig. 3-8) which forms a strong bond with the enzyme dihydrofolate reductase and thereby inhibits the synthesis of tetrahydrofolate, one of the active forms of the coenzyme. Since tetrahydrofolate is required as a donor of methyl groups for a number of important reactions, methotrexate inhibits a number of biochemical pathways, the most important of which are the de novo synthesis of purines and pyrimidines and specifically the synthesis of the pyrimidine deoxythymidylate (dTMP).

Deoxythymidylate (dTMP) is synthesized from its precursor deoxyuridylate (dUMP) by the transfer of a methyl group from methylene tetrahydrofolate (methylene-FH$_4$); the reaction is catalyzed by the enzyme thymidylate synthetase (Fig. 3-7). When formation of tetrahydrofolate (FH$_4$) is inhibited by methotrexate-induced blockage of dihydrofolate reductase, dTMP cannot be formed and is therefore unavailable for DNA synthesis. This results in the death of cells in the act of replicating DNA (S-phase of the cycle).

Methotrexate-treated cells can be "rescued" if a biologically active form of folic acid, 5-formyl tetrahydrofolic acid (citrovorum factor), is provided within minutes to hours after exposure to methotrexate. This agent bypasses the blockage of dihydrofolate reductase by providing tetrahydrofolate (FH$_4$) directly to the cells (Fig. 3-7). This phenomenon is of major importance both for prevention of deleterious side effects when an accidental overdosage of methotrexate is administered and for allowing treatment of tumors that are resistant to conventional doses of methotrexate, but sen-

Figure 3-8 Structural formulas of methotrexate and folic acid. (Reprinted by permission from New England Journal of Medicine 292: 1107, 1975.)

sitive to "toxic" doses of the drug. Methotrexate is thus the only cancer chemotherapeutic agent for which there is an antidote.

Toxicity appears to be related more closely to duration of drug exposure than to the peak blood level; thus the drug is more toxic when given in divided doses throughout the day or by slow continuous infusion than the same quantity given as a single dose.[39] Likewise, renal impairment will result in delayed excretion, prolonged higher blood levels, and greater toxicity.[82]

Methotrexate should never be administered before the BUN and creatinine levels are known. If these are abnormal, the dosage should be modified according to the following guidelines:[8]

BUN 20 to 30 mg/100 ml
or } Reduce dosage by 50 per cent
Creatinine 1.2 to 2.0 mg/100 ml

BUN > 30 mg/100 ml
or } Withhold methotrexate
Creatinine > 2.0 mg/100 ml

Acute Methotrexate Toxicity. Methotrexate toxicity may occur under both acute and chronic conditions of administration. The acute manifestations most often are first seen in the gastrointestinal tract; suppression of gut epithelial cell mitosis prevents replacement of sloughed cells and eventually leads to ulceration. Mouth ulcers, nausea, vomiting, anorexia, and diarrhea may result. The buccal ulcerations are characteristically shallow, painful, and white or yellow in color, with a red border.

Bone marrow injury usually manifests itself by neutropenia and thrombocytopenia, with these reaching a nadir one to three weeks after administration of the drug.

Acute pneumonitis may occur after oral, intravenous, or even intrathecal methotrexate administration. Pulmonary involvement is characteristically bilateral and interstitial and is accompanied by cyanosis, fever, nonproductive cough, and eosinophilia (in approximately half the patients).[52, 76, 102] Since infectious agents may also cause acute pneumonitis in patients receiving chemotherapy, an open lung biopsy is frequently necessary to establish a definitive diagnosis. Histologically, micronodular infiltrates composed of lymphocytes, plasma cells, histiocytes, eosinophils, and multinucleated giant cells, but no microorganisms, are seen with methotrexate pneumonia. Corticosteroid therapy may hasten clinical recovery,[102] although controlled studies have not been performed. Approximately 11 per cent of patients will die of the acute pulmonary disease,[102] while in some patients the pneumonitis may become chronic and produce marked interstitial fibrosis.

Other signs of acute toxicity include alopecia, perifolliculitis, brownish skin pigmentation, skin erythema, and inflammation of the vaginal, pleural, and bladder epithelium.

Chronic Methotrexate Toxicity. Continued methotrexate therapy for a number of years has been utilized for remission maintenance of acute lymphocytic leukemia. Patients receiving prolonged courses of methotrexate have developed interstitial pulmonary fibrosis,[76] hepatic fibrosis,[56, 76, 97] and osteoporosis.[86] These changes may develop quite insidiously; for example, most patients may be relatively asymptomatic during the development of hepatic toxicity. Hepatic damage can develop despite normal liver function tests and absence of hepatomegaly; BSP excretion tests and liver biopsy have been found to be the most reliable tests for detecting liver damage in these patients. Osteoporosis may go unrecognized until bone pain or fracture call attention to it.

Chronic intravenous infusions of methotrexate for maintenance therapy of acute lymphocytic leukemia have been associated with a progressive multifocal leukoencephalopathy; this occurs mainly in patients who have had prior central nervous system irradiation.[72, 73]

"High Dose" Methotrexate. In conventional dosage, methotrexate is useful in remission maintenance of *acute lymphocytic leukemia* as well as treatment of *choriocarcinoma*, *histiocytosis X*, and *Burkitt's lymphoma*. In higher dosage (greater than 1 gm/m² or 20 mg/kg) it has been used for treatment of *refractory acute lymphocytic leukemias*,[33] *lymphosarcoma*,[32] and *osteogenic sarcoma*,[85] as well as adjuvant therapy for occult *osteogenic sarcoma*.[59] The higher dosages can only be used if they are followed by citrovorum factor "rescue" to salvage normal cells.

The rationale for this form of therapy is based on the hypotheses that: (1) a very high concentration of methotrexate destroys cells by a mechanism different from that with conventional doses and results in preferential destruction of tumor cells; and (2) citrovorum factor may selectively rescue normal cells.

In addition to the toxic effects seen with conventional doses of methotrexate, high doses of methotrexate have also been associated with renal toxicity, apparently due to renal tubular damage resulting from precipitation of methotrexate.[42] This may be prevented, to some extent, by alkalinization and increased urine volume.

Intrathecal Methotrexate. Methotrexate is also administered intrathecally for treatment or prophylaxis of *central nervous system leukemia*. The usual dosage for this purpose is 12 mg/m² (maximum total dose = 15 mg);[24] this quantity has usually been diluted in preservative-free saline to a concentration of 1 mg/ml.

While this form of therapy is quite effective, it has, on occasion, been associated with significant neurotoxicity (Table 3–4), including meningeal irritation, seizures, encephalopathy, and paraplegia.[12, 45, 46] Less severe symptoms include headache, fever, vomiting, and CSF pleocytosis lasting two to five days. The frequency of these symptoms appears to be diminished when cranial irradiation is given concomitantly or Elliott's B solution (which has a chemical composition similar to that of cerebrospinal fluid) replaces saline as the diluent.[46] The basis for the more severe neurologic sequelae is not completely known, but may be related to prolonged high intrathecal concentrations of methotrexate; this is particularly true of patients with active CNS leukemia who have reduced egress of methotrexate from the cerebrospinal fluid.[12] Consequently, the *dosage of intrathecal methotrexate should be reduced when active CNS leukemia is present.*[45]

A significant increase in neurotoxicity has been reported in older patients and adolescents following intrathecal methotrexate. This may be the result of inappropriately high doses based on body surface area calculations (during late childhood and adolescence body weight and height increase more rapidly than brain size; consequently, doses based on body surface area are proportionately higher in relation to brain and CSF volume in these groups).[45]

Table 3–4 Signs and Symptoms of Neurotoxicity from Intrathecal Methotrexate[116]

COMMON (5–50 PER CENT)	UNCOMMON (<1 PER CENT)
Subacute meningeal irritation	Paraplegia
Stiff neck	Transient
Nausea and vomiting	Permanent
Headache	Seizures
Fever	Encephalopathy
Mild CSF pleocytosis	
Decreased opening pressure	

Systemic methotrexate toxicity can also result from intrathecal therapy, since the drug may be absorbed into the blood from the meninges. Therefore, systemic chemotherapy is usually discontinued when intrathecal methotrexate is given; in some institutions citrovorum factor is administered intravenously to counteract the systemic effects of methotrexate. Some groups have even noted arrest of neurologic deterioration after systemic treatment with citrovorum factor,[63] whereas others believe this relationship was fortuitous.[12]

Purine Analogues—
6-Mercaptopurine
(6-MP) (Purinethol),
6-Thioguanine (6-TG)
(Fig. 3-9)

Both 6-MP and 6-TG require conversion to their respective ribonucleotides for antitumor activity. In the ribonucleotide form, 6-MP appears to interfere with de novo purine synthesis as well as interconversions between the purines. However, the dominant component of its action appears to be related to its incorporation into DNA; 6-TG likewise appears to be incorporated into DNA.

6-MP is largely catabolized by the enzyme xanthine oxidase; inhibition of this enzyme by allopurinol (a drug used for management of hyperuricemia) prevents catabolism of 6-MP and consequently increased activity of this drug. *The daily dose of 6-MP should be reduced to 25 to 50 per cent of its usual level when allopurinol is being used concomitantly.* 6-TG is not catabolized by xanthine oxidase and, consequently, dosage reduction is not necessary when allopurinol is being used.

Since both of these drugs are readily absorbed by the gastrointestinal tract, they may be given by the oral route. Like the other antimetabolites, these drugs cause marrow suppression and gastrointestinal disorders (nausea, vomiting, anorexia). Less common toxicities are dermatitis, fever, hematuria, and crystalluria.[34]

Hepatotoxicity is not uncommon when patients are treated with 6-MP, especially when the dose exceeds 2 mg/kg/day;[34a, 97a] this complication may sometimes be avoided if the drug is withdrawn temporarily when oral lesions or severe leukopenia develop. Hepatotoxicity commonly manifests itself as cholestatic jaundice with elevated transaminase and alkaline phosphatase values; histologically a mixed pattern of parenchymal cell necrosis and intrahepatic cholestasis may be seen. The drug should be promptly discontinued at the first sight of hepatic dysfunction; in addition, subsequent reexposure to 6-MP may result in recurrence of liver damage.

Currently 6-MP is being utilized mainly for remission maintenance in *acute lymphocytic leukemia* and for treatment of *histiocytosis X*. 6-TG has been used in combination regimens for remission induction in *acute myeloid leukemia.*

Pyrimidine Analogues

Cytosine Arabinoside (Cytosar, Ara-C). Cytosine arabinoside is a nu-

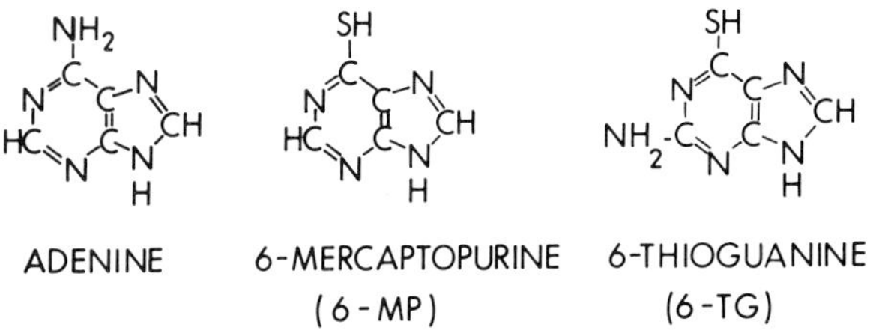

Figure 3-9 Structural formulas of adenine and its analogues 6-mercaptopurine (6-MP) and 6-thioguanine (6-TG).

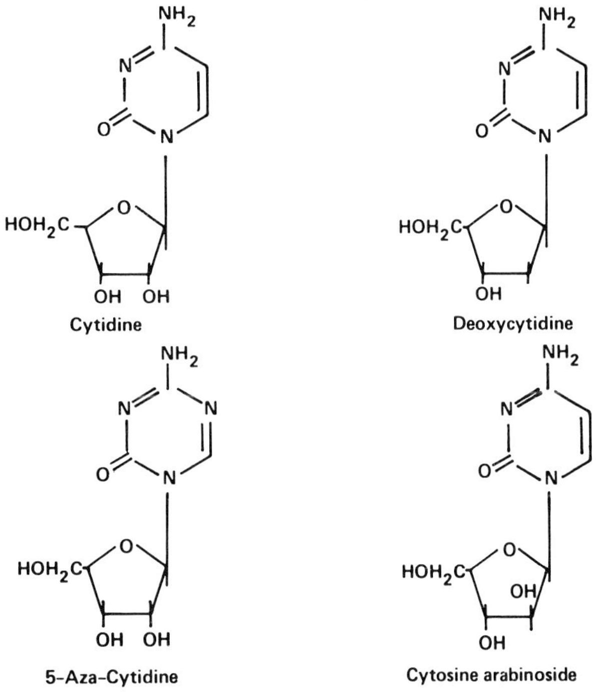

Figure 3–10 Structural formulas of cytidine and deoxycytidine and their analogues cytosine arabinoside and 5-azacytidine. (Reprinted, by permission from New England Journal of Medicine 292:1107, 1975.)

cleoside analogue which combines the pyrimidine base cytosine with the sugar arabinose (Fig. 3–10); it is unique in that its alteration resides in the sugar moiety of the molecule rather than in the pyrimidine base. As with most pyrimidine and purine analogues with antineoplastic activity, cytosine arabinoside requires phosphorylation to express this activity.

Cytosine arabinoside inhibits DNA polymerase and thereby blocks DNA replication; consequently, it exerts its effects primarily during the S-phase of the cell cycle. The drug is also incorporated into both DNA and RNA. Proliferating cells (hematopoietic, gastrointestinal, tumor) are the most severely affected. In addition to marrow suppression, marked megaloblastic changes can be induced in bone marrow precursor cells.

Cytosine arabinoside may be administered intravenously, subcutaneously, or intramuscularly; it has also been given intrathecally for treatment or prophylaxis of CNS leukemia. After a single rapid intravenous injection, the plasma half-life is less than 9 min and there is no measurable level after 15 to 60 min.[8] This is due to rapid deamination of the molecule by the enzyme pyrimidine nucleoside deaminase, which is found in leukocytes, liver, and kidney; 90 per cent of the dose is excreted within 24 hours as the deamination product.[8] Because of the rapid metabolic inactivation of this agent, higher blood levels can be maintained when it is given by slow continuous infusion over several hours than when given as a pulse dose.

Major side effects are nausea, vomiting, and bone marrow suppression (with megaloblastic changes). Other side effects are diarrhea, oral ulcerations, phlebitis, fever, abdominal pain, neuritis, rash, arthralgias, and alopecia. Because of the liver's role in detoxification of this agent, the dose should be reduced in the presence of hepatocellular dysfunction, particularly since the drug may cause further hepatic deterioration.

Cytosine arabinoside is a first-line drug for remission induction in *acute myelogenous leukemia.* It also has been used as a second-line drug for remission induction in *acute lymphocytic leukemia* (usually after the patient has relapsed and become refractory to vincristine/prednisone). Given intrathecally, cytosine arabinoside has been effective in the treatment of *meningeal leukemia.*

5-Azacytidine (Fig. 3-10). The main molecular consequences of this pyrimidine analogue are interference with the de novo synthesis of pyrimidine nucleotides and the formation of abnormal nucleic acids due to its incorporation. Although azacytidine shares certain metabolic reactions with cytosine arabinoside (including deamination by the same enzyme system), tumors resistant to cytosine arabinoside do not exhibit cross-resistance to azacytidine.

This agent may be administered subcutaneously or intravenously.[4] Side effects include nausea, vomiting, diarrhea, and prolonged marrow suppression. Clinical usefulness is mainly for treatment of *acute myelogenous leukemia* (AML); a 36 per cent response rate (with 20 per cent complete remissions) has been achieved in cases of AML which became refractory to other chemotherapeutic agents, and the median duration of remission in these patients was "encouragingly long."[109]

5-Fluorouracil (5-FU). 5-FU is an analogue of thymidine (5-methyluracil), one of the pyrimidine bases. Its primary effect appears to be the inhibition of thymidylate synthetase, the enzyme necessary to form deoxythymidylate (dTMP), and thereby the inhibition of DNA synthesis (Fig. 3-7).

5-FU is metabolized chiefly by the liver and is then excreted via the lungs as carbon dioxide; 10 to 30 per cent is excreted unchanged in the urine.

The major side effects are gastrointestinal and mouth ulcers, nausea, vomiting, diarrhea, and marrow toxicity. Alopecia, erythematous dermatitis, and reversible cerebellar ataxia are occasionally seen.

This agent is used mainly in the management of adult-type cancers (*carcinoma of the breast, gastrointestinal tract, cervix, and ovary*).

VINCA ALKALOIDS

The alkaloids *vincristine* and *vinblastine* are extracted from the periwinkle plant (*Vinca rosea* Linn). Although these two compounds differ only in methyl (vinblastine) or formyl

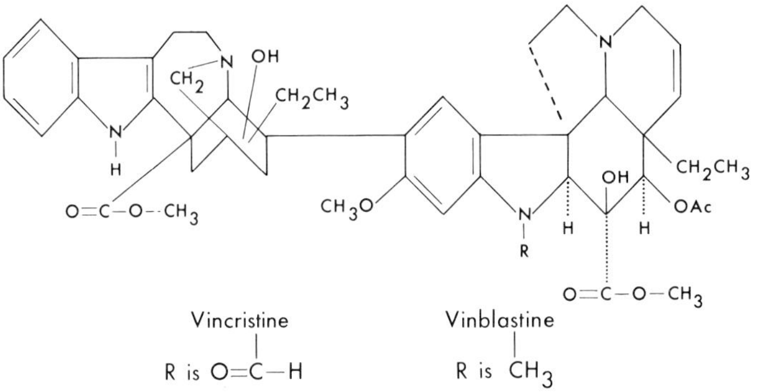

Figure 3-11 Structural formulas of the Vinca alkaloids. (From Cline, M. J., and Haskell, C. M.: Cancer Chemotherapy. 2nd Ed. Philadelphia, W. B. Saunders Co., 1975.)

(vincristine) side chains on a large parent molecule (Fig. 3–11), they have significantly different ranges of antitumor activity and side effects.

The mechanism of action of both these drugs appears to be related to binding of microtubular proteins; since these are essential contractile proteins of the mitotic spindle, arrest of mitosis at the metaphase stage results. Thus, these drugs are most effective against cells which are in mitosis (phase-specific).

Although these drugs can be given orally, absorption is unpredictable. Consequently, they are given intravenously with care to avoid extravasation, which can lead to local tissue necrosis.

Vincristine (Oncovin)

Vincristine is rapidly bound to tissues and has a short half-life in the serum. It is metabolized by the liver and excreted in the bile.

The principal toxic side effect of vincristine is neurotoxicity, possibly related to the role of microtubular protein in nerve tissues. Both peripheral neuropathic changes (mixed sensory and motor), autonomic nervous system toxicity (paralytic ileus, colicky abdominal pain, constipation), or cranial nerve palsies can occur. Generalized seizures may also occur in about 1 per cent of patients taking this drug.[60, 80] *Vincristine should be used with extreme caution in patients with a preexisting neuropathy, particularly variants of the Charcot-Marie-Tooth syndrome.*[114]

A majority of patients will lose deep tendon reflexes, and this should not be regarded as a sign of severe toxicity or as an indication to reduce or discontinue the drug.[116] However, numbness and paresthesias in the extremities, or distal motor weakness (demonstrable by inability to walk on the heels or extend the fingers or wrist) should be considered as early clues of significant neurotoxicity and an indication to stop therapy. Progression of this neuropathy may lead to wrist-drop, foot-drop (with a broad, slapping gait), or even quadriparesis. The prophylactic use of stool softeners and cathartics can be helpful in alleviating the bowel problems associated with vincristine.

Weiss and colleagues[116] have summarized a number of important generalizations about vincristine neurotoxicity:

1. The signs and symptoms of neuropathy are usually quite symmetrical. Strictly unilateral weakness, areflexia, or sensory changes generally are not consistent with a diagnosis of vincristine neurotoxicity.

2. In most cases there is a direct relationship between dose and toxicity, and a single inadvertent massive overdosage can produce serious neurologic impairment.

3. In patients with liver dysfunction, impaired hepatic inactivation of the drug may result in unusually severe neurotoxicity after routine doses.[95]

4. The manifestations of vincristine neuropathy are partially or completely reversible when the dosage is lowered or the drug is discontinued.

Other side effects include: inappropriate antidiuretic hormone secretion,[104] paroxysmal jaw pain, alopecia, and decreased spermatogenesis. Bone marrow suppression is not usually a serious problem unless very large doses are used.

Vincristine is useful as an induction agent for *acute lymphocytic leukemia*; it is also used as part of combination chemotherapy regimens for *rhabdomyosarcoma, neuroblastoma, Wilms' tumor, Ewing's sarcoma, teratocarcinoma*, and *lymphomas*.

Vinblastine (Velban)

Vinblastine produces a clinical spectrum of neurotoxicity similar to that of vincristine;[41, 116] however, unlike vincristine, it also produces severe bone marrow toxicity, which usually precedes neurotoxicity as the dose-limiting factor. Consequently, neurotoxicity is not usually a clinical problem. Nausea and vomiting may also occur.

Vinblastine has been used in the treatment of *Hodgkin's disease, non-Hodgkin's lymphoma,* and *histiocytosis X.*

ANTIBIOTICS

These drugs are produced by certain soil fungi. Their mechanism of action appears to result from the formation of stable complexes with DNA, with resultant inhibition of DNA replication or RNA transcription, or both. They are not specific for cell cycle or phase.

Drugs included in this classification are: *actinomycin D, Adriamycin, daunorubicin, bleomycin, mithramycin,* and *mitomycin C.* Most of the compounds are light-sensitive and must be protected from light to retain their activity.

Actinomycin D (Dactinomycin, Cosmegen) (Fig. 3-12)

Actinomycin D is the principal component of the mixture of actinomycin antibiotics produced by *Streptomyces parvullus.* When present in relatively low concentrations, actinomycin D binds to guanine residues in DNA and selectively inhibits the transcription of RNA by RNA polymerase. At higher concentrations, DNA synthesis is also inhibited.

There is an interesting synergistic interaction between actinomycin D and radiotherapy: patients receiving actinomycin D following radiotherapy have been noted to develop erythema and more extensive skin reactions in previously irradiated sites. In prospective studies it has been demonstrated that 500 to 600 rads are required to produce skin erythema, but in the presence of actinomycin D, as few as 100 rads will produce such erythema.[40] This may be because actinomycin D can inhibit repair of both sublethal and potentially lethal radiation damage to cells. It may thus be necessary to reduce the dosage of actinomycin D when radiotherapy has been used previously or is being used concomitantly.

Actinomycin D should be administered intravenously with care to avoid extravasation, which can result in local inflammation and necrosis of soft tissues. Other toxic effects include nausea and vomiting, diarrhea, proctitis, glossitis, alopecia, and bone marrow suppression. Because there appears to be a greater frequency of toxic effects (including death) in young infants, it has been suggested that this drug should be given to infants only over the age of 6 to 12 months.[83]

This agent is commonly used for

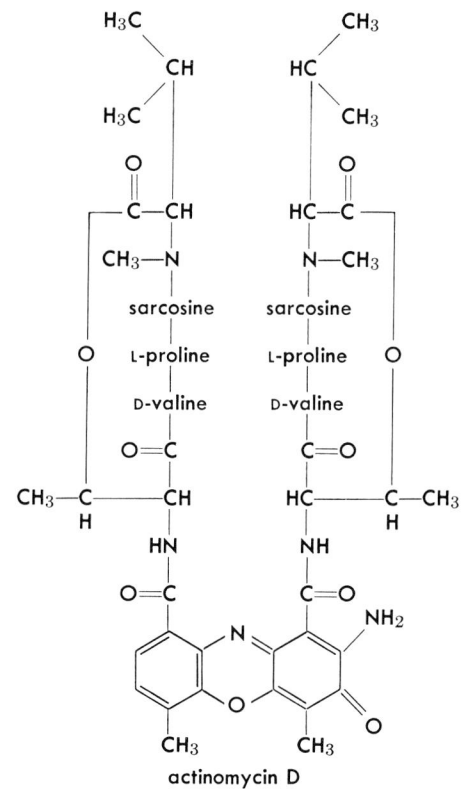

Figure 3-12 Structural formula of actinomycin D. (From West, E. S., Todd, W. R., Mason, H. S., and van Bruggen, J. T. [eds.]: Textbook of Biochemistry. 4th Ed. © 1966, The Macmillan Co., New York.)

treatment of *choriocarcinoma, Wilms' tumor,* and some *testicular tumors,* as well as being part of combination chemotherapy protocols for *rhabdomyosarcoma, Ewing's sarcoma,* and *teratocarcinoma.*

Doxorubicin (Adriamycin) and Daunorubicin (Daunomycin, Rubidomycin)

These agents are anthracycline antibiotics derived from *Streptomyces peucetius* var. *caesius* and differ only by a single OH group on carbon-14 (Fig. 3–13). They bind to DNA by intercalating between adjacent base pairs of the double helical structure;[111] this leads to uncoiling of the DNA helix and inhibition of DNA and RNA synthesis through template disordering and steric obstruction.[54]

Adriamycin is metabolized predominantly by the liver to adriamycinol and several aglycone derivatives; approximately half the drug is excreted intact in the bile, with another 30 per cent being excreted as conjugates.[5, 17] Impaired hepatic function can delay Adriamycin elimination and result in exaggerated clinical toxicity;[6] consequently, *modification of dosage is indicated if liver disease is present* (the dose should be reduced by 50 per cent if the bilirubin level is elevated and by 75 per cent if bilirubin is > 3 mg/dl).[24] By contrast, less than 6 per cent of the dose is excreted in the urine, and changes in renal function do not affect the pharmacokinetics of this agent.[6]

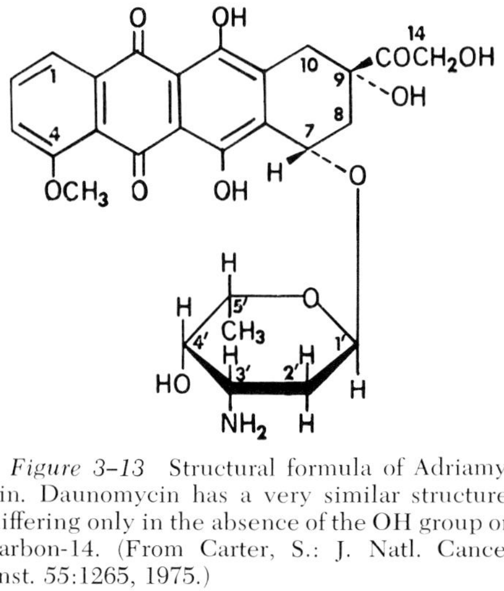

These drugs have similar pharmacologic characteristics and toxicities. Their major toxicity is bone marrow suppression, but they can also cause alopecia, stomatitis, vomiting, and tissue irritation and necrosis (if they extravasate during intravenous administration). Adriamycin skin ulcers develop insidiously and are much deeper than initially evident; superficial-appearing sloughs may thus progress to severe, deep loss (Fig. 3–14). Since these ulcers show no tendency toward spontaneous healing, it has been recommended that early treatment by either skin grafting or flap coverage be considered.[93] Adriamycin may also induce recall of a quiescent radiation reaction of the skin in a manner similar to that already described for actinomycin D.[19]

Drug induced stomatitis typically begins as a burning sensation with erythema of the oral mucosa, which may produce ulceration in 2 to 3 days, particularly in the sublingual and lateral tongue margins.

Cardiac toxicity is a unique side effect of these drugs; it may be manifested in two forms: (1) transient arrhythmias or nonspecific ECG changes early in the course of treatment, and (2) definitive cardiomyopathy with delayed, severe intractable congestive heart failure.

Careful monitoring of patients receiving Adriamycin or daunomycin with electrocardiograms (ECG) appears to have some usefulness in detecting early signs of cardiotoxicity. ECG abnormalities may be of two types:[49] (1) transient and unrelated to cardiac toxicity—these occur early in the course of treatment and include mild flattening of T waves sinus tachycardia, supraventricular tachy-

Figure 3–13 Structural formula of Adriamycin. Daunomycin has a very similar structure, differing only in the absence of the OH group on carbon-14. (From Carter, S.: J. Natl. Cancer Inst. 55:1265, 1975.)

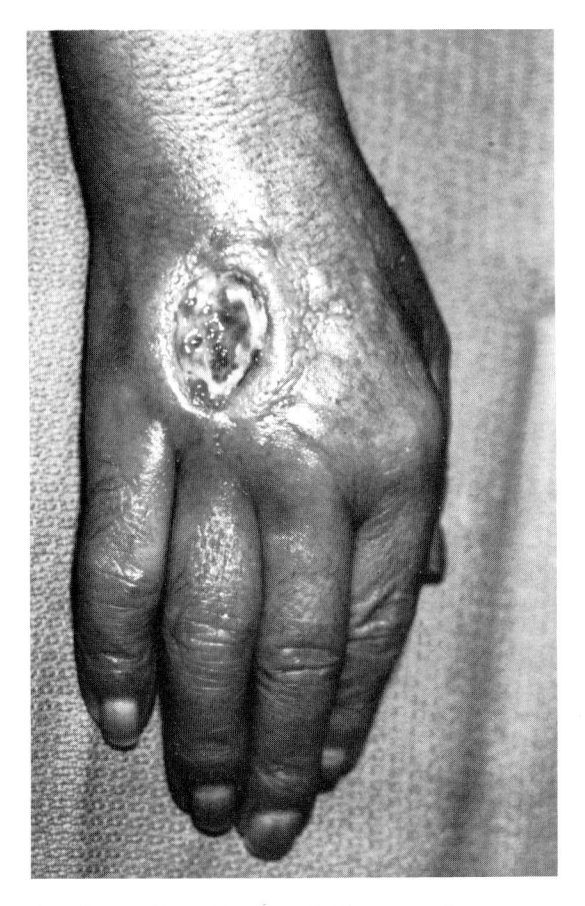

Figure 3–14 Ulcer of hand caused by infiltration of Adriamycin; lesion required removal of necrotic extensor tendons of middle two fingers. (From Rudolph, R., et al.: Cancer 38:1087, 1976.)

cardia, and premature ventricular contractions, or (2) late, irreversible changes which precede impending heart failure—these appear late in the course of treatment and consist of progressive flattening to inversion of T waves, decreased QRS voltage, and intraventricular conduction delay.

Friedman and associates[43a] studied physiologic and ultrastructural changes in the hearts of four cancer patients without previous heart disease who received Adriamycin. No cardiac abnormalities could be detected by serial x-ray films, ECGs, systolic time intervals, catheterization data, and radionuclide cardiac wall motion scans; cardiac damage could be detected only by percutaneous transjugular right ventricular endomyocardial biopsy. Early myocardial damage, including swollen cytoplasmic reticulum, myofibrillar degeneration, and fibrosis, was noted with cumulative doses as small as 180 mg/m.²

It is disappointing that cardiac function studies may not give early warning of congestive cardiomyopathy since early diagnosis of congestive heart failure appears to be essential for effective treatment of this complication. Treatment consists of prolonged administration (6 months or more in some cases) of digitalis and diuretics, a low-salt diet, and restriction of activities. Since these patients are extremely sensitive to digitalis, the total I.V. digitalizing dose (TDD) required is only 0.010 to 0.020 mg/kg digoxin or digitoxin; the recommended maintenance dose is 1/4 to 1/7 digoxin/TDD or 1/10 to 1/15 digitoxin/TDD.[49]

The mechanism by which Adriamycin and daunomycin produce cardiac toxicity is unclear. It may be related to: (1) structural similarities between these drugs and digitalis glycosides[21] or (2) suppression of DNA synthesis in the myocardium.[92] Pathologic changes consist of interstitial edema between myocardial fibers, destruction of myocardial cells, and disruption of sarcoplasm with or without vacuole formation;[26] these changes are nonspecific and have been described in other types of cardiomyopathy.

The development of cardiac toxicity is closely related to the *cumulative* doses of these drugs. The risk is minimal at *cumulative* doses of less than 550 mg/m² for Adriamycin[68] and 600 mg/m² for daunorubicin,[53] but exceeds 20 per cent for dosages above these levels.[13] Irradiation to the region of the heart, preexisting cardiac anomalies (arrhythmias, congenital or acquired heart disease), or concurrent cyclophosphamide therapy, appear to further increase the risks and *cumulative* dosages should be limited to 400 to 500 mg/m² in these instances.[49, 69, 85A]

Despite their close structural similarities, Adriamycin and daunorubicin differ markedly in their ranges of antitumor activity. Daunorubicin is useful primarily in the treatment of *acute leukemias*.[9, 115] However, Adriamycin has found use against a wide range of pediatric neoplasms, including *acute leukemias, Ewing's sarcoma, osteogenic sarcoma, non-Hodgkin's lymphomas, rhabdomyosarcoma, neuroblastoma*, and *teratocarcinoma*.[87]

Bleomycin (Blenoxane)

Bleomycin is a mixture of several polypeptide antibiotics produced by *Streptomyces verticillus;* it binds directly to DNA (thereby interfering with DNA replication as well as with RNA transcription) and can also produce single-stranded breaks in DNA.[44] There is also an inhibitory effect on progression of cells through the G_2 and M phases of the cell cycle.[2] Despite its effects on DNA synthesis, this agent has only minimal toxicity for rapidly proliferating normal tissues (e.g., bone marrow).

The clinical effects of bleomycin can be correlated with its propensity to localize in specific tissues, particularly lung, skin and a variety of malignant tumors; by contrast, hematopoietic tissue has a distinct lack of affinity for bleomycin.[78] This propensity for selective localization in malignant tissues has been utilized in nuclear medicine scanning techniques.

The major toxic effects of bleomycin are seen in the lungs. Pulmonary toxicity may be manifested initially by dyspnea, cough, low-grade fever, bibasilar rales, a bilateral interstitial infiltrate and hypoxemia. Pathologically this is characterized by interstitial edema, intraalveolar hyaline membrane formation, and hyperplasia of alveolar macrophages. In about 1 per cent of patients this may progress to marked interstitial pulmonary collagen deposition and fatal pulmonary fibrosis;[3, 14] the frequency of this dire complication appears to increase sharply at *cumulative* doses in excess of 400 mg and in patients over 70 years of age.[14] However, cases of pulmonary fibrosis have been reported at *total* doses of as little as 50 mg.[21] The appearance of dyspnea, rales, and an interstitial infiltrate in a patient being treated with bleomycin should prompt discontinuation of the drug as well as initiation of a vigorous diagnostic work-up to rule out other causes of interstitial pneumonia (see Chapter Seven). Although steroids have relieved symptoms and produced radiologic improvement in a few cases, their role in the treatment of this condition has not, as yet, been firmly established.

The second major (and unique) manifestation of bleomycin toxicity relates to the skin. These lesions begin to appear at *cumulative* doses of about 150 mg and begin with induration and erythema of the fingers and hands or in areas of previous radiotherapy. Considerable local pain and sensitivity to touch may limit the use of the fingers and desquamation and ulceration may result if the drug is not discontinued.

Other side effects of bleomycin include alopecia, nausea, fever, and rarely a fulminant, fatal reaction characterized by high fever, hypotension, and cardiorespiratory collapse. Bleomycin rarely causes bone marrow suppression, which makes it of great potential usefulness in combination chemotherapy.

Bleomycin is currently being used for treatment of *Hodgkin's disease, non-Hodgkin's lymphomas, testicular neoplasms,* and *squamous cell carcinoma of the head and neck.*[14, 119]

Mithramycin (Mithracin)
(Fig. 3–15)

Mithramycin is obtained from *Streptomyces caespitosus.*[88] It has been used in the treatment of embryonal cell carcinoma of the testis[65] and palliatively for treatment of hypercalcemia.[101] Initially severe toxicity was seen, including a severe hemorrhagic diathesis, fever, vomiting, skin eruptions, central nervous system reactions, stomatitis, hypocalcemia, and hepato-renal dysfunction.[65, 75] More recently a revised treatment protocol,[65] combined with very careful monitoring of liver function, coagulation parameters, and renal function has markedly reduced the incidence of these complications.

Mithramycin appears to exert its anti-hypercalcemic effects by virtue of inhibiting the rate and magnitude of osteoclastic bone resorption.[89] Its use should be considered in cases of severe hypercalcemia associated with skeletal metastases that fail to respond promptly to conventional therapy.

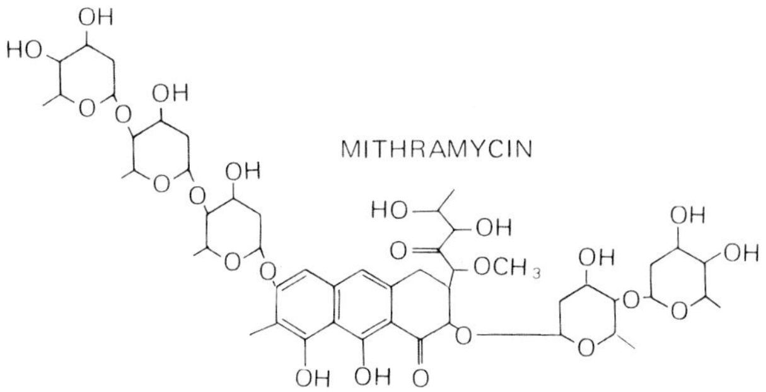

Figure 3–15 Structural formula of mithramycin. (From Krakoff, I. H.: CA 23:209, 1973.)

Miscellaneous Agents

L-*Asparaginase*

This enzyme, obtained from cultures of *Escherichia coli*, causes depletion of the amino acid L-asparagine by hydrolyzing it to L-aspartic acid and ammonia. Cells unable to produce their own supply of L-asparagine (e.g., acute lymphocytic leukemia cells) suffer impairment of protein synthesis and are unable to survive; organs with high protein synthesis rates, such as the liver and pancreas, are also adversely affected.

L-Asparaginase can be given by intramuscular or intravenous routes. It is not toxic to the bone marrow, gut, or hair follicles, but does have its own unique range of side effects. These include hypersensitivity reactions (urticaria, serum sickness, anaphylaxis), acute pancreatitis, hyperglycemia, liver dysfunction (fatty metamorphosis, elevated SGOT, alkaline phosphatase and bilirubin, and decreased albumin and fibrinogen), hypercalcemia, depression of coagulation factors, and central nervous system dysfunction.

Because of the risk of anaphylaxis, a physician should remain in attendance for at least 5 min after administration of the drug, and epinephrine, hydrocortisone, and Benadryl, as well as resuscitative equipment, should be readily available.

Pancreatitis occurs in as many as 16 per cent of children receiving L-asparaginase;[113] there is some evidence that the frequency of this complication may be dose-related, since it has rarely been a problem with doses below 200 I.U./kg/day[122] or 25,000 I.U./m²/day.[118] Serum amylase values should be regularly monitored while the patient is receiving L-asparaginase and for several weeks after it is discontinued, since pancreatitis may have a delayed onset.[113] Abdominal echography, as a monitor of pancreatic size, has been found to be helpful in the diagnosis of subclinical and early pancreatic injury and may permit prompt cessation of L-asparaginase therapy before more serious injury occurs.[94]

Approximately 25 to 50 per cent of patients receiving L-asparaginase will manifest a disorder in the level or quality of consciousness.[116] This encephalopathy, consisting of lethargy, somnolence, and confusion, usually begins within a day or so of therapy and clears rapidly after the end of treatment. Less commonly, an organic brain syndrome resembling alcoholic delirium tremens or Korsakoff's psychosis may develop 1 week or more after therapy and may last for several weeks. These neurologic dysfunctions are thought to relate to drug-induced metabolic abnormalities (excess L-aspartic acid and L-glutamic acid, and depleted L-asparagine and L-glutamine) and possibly also to drug-associated liver dysfunction.

L-Asparaginase has found its major usefulness for remission induction in *acute lymphocytic leukemia;* it has not been useful, however, for remission maintenance. This agent has also been used for treatment of *non-Hodgkin's lymphomas.*

Adrenal Corticosteroids

The mechanism of antitumor action of these agents remains unknown. Possible mechanisms may relate to the presence of corticosteroid receptor proteins within target cells[61] or to the accumulation of free fatty acids in the cytoplasm of sensitive cells, leading to direct nuclear damage.[107] Cortisol has a specific lytic effect on both normal and neoplastic lymphocytes, which may result from inhibition of glucose transport and subsequent decreased energy utilization.[106]

The site of action of glucocorticoids and other steroid hormones appears to be in the nucleus, and at the level of transcription. It is thought that the following sequence of events occurs when these hormones interact with target cells:[90] (1) binding of the steroid to its specific receptor and movement of this complex into the nucleus, (2) an action of the steroid-receptor complex on chromatin, possibly altering the synthesis of a substance involved in glucose uptake, and (3) as a consequence of impaired glucose metabolism, the inhibition of nucleic acid and protein biosynthesis, leading to cell lysis.

The corticosteroid agents used most frequently in cancer chemotherapy, because they induce minimal fluid retention, are prednisone and prednisolone. These agents are usually used in very large doses for a limited period of time in order to minimize the side effects of chronic steroid administration. Consequently their major use has been for induction of remission in diseases such as *acute lymphocytic leukemia, acute myelocytic leukemia, and malignant lymphomas* rather than for prolonged maintenance therapy.

Side effects include hyperglycemia, fluid and sodium retention, increased susceptibility to infection, psychotic reactions, and gastric irritation. Their relationship to peptic ulcer, previously a well accepted dogma, has recently been challenged.[25] Chronic administration may lead to truncal obesity, cushingoid facies, striae, osteoporosis, and hypertension.

Some of these deleterious effects can be ameliorated by placing the patient on a low-salt diet, with liberal administration of milk or antacids and careful observation for signs of infection.

In addition to their usefulness in treating acute leukemias and malignant lymphomas, steroids have also been found to be of value in treating symptoms in patients with cancer. Among these indications are *secondary hypercalcemia, cerebral edema, bone pain,* and *fever of malignancy.*

Nitrosoureas (BCNU, CCNU, Methyl-CCNU) (Fig. 3–16)

Nitrosoureas are a group of synthetic agents which appear to act through alkylation of nucleic acids and proteins plus carbamoylation of proteins;[23] they arrest cell-cycle progression in the G_2 phase.

These drugs can be given orally or intravenously. When given intravenously, their serum half-life is very short (less than 5 min for bischloronitrosourea or BCNU) owing to rapid tissue uptake and metabolism.[8, 21] They are primarily excreted in the urine. Because they are *lipid-soluble,* they are able to cross the blood-brain barrier easily, which makes them useful in the treatment of intracerebral lesions.

BCNU: 1,3-Bis(2-chloroethyl)-1-nitrosourea

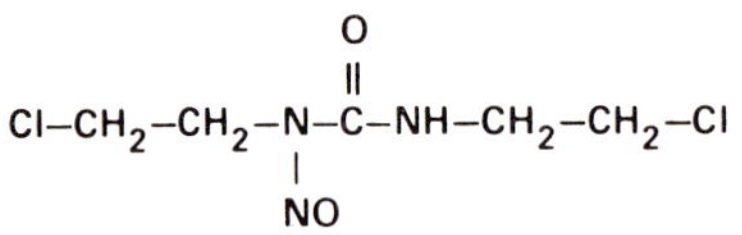

$$Cl-CH_2-CH_2-\underset{\underset{NO}{|}}{N}-\overset{\overset{O}{\|}}{C}-NH-CH_2-CH_2-Cl$$

CCNU: 1-(2-chloroethyl)-3-cyclohexyl-1-nitrosourea

$$Cl-CH_2-CH_2-\underset{\underset{NO}{|}}{N}-\overset{\overset{O}{\|}}{C}-NH-\bigcirc$$

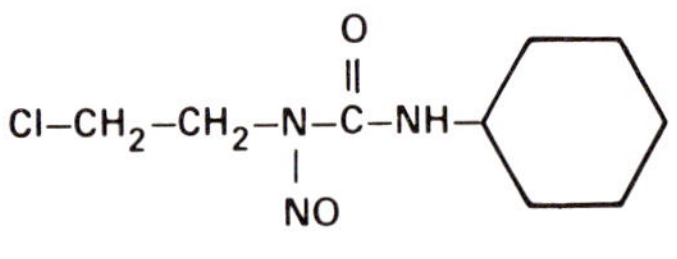

MeCCNU: 1-(2-Chloroethyl)-3-(4-methyl cyclohexyl)-1-nitrosourea

$$Cl-CH_2-CH_2-\underset{\underset{NO}{|}}{N}-\overset{\overset{O}{\|}}{C}-NH-\bigcirc-CH_3$$

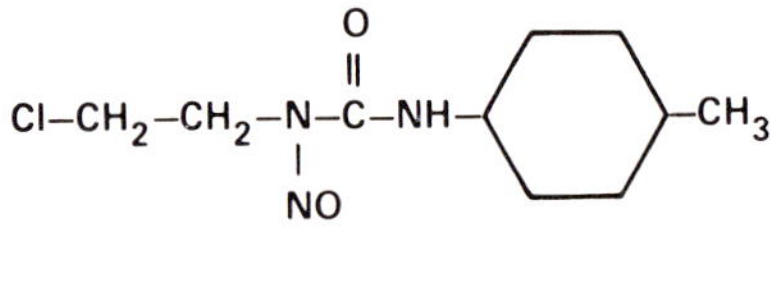

Figure 3–16 Structural formulas of the nitrosoureas. (From Oliverio, V. T., et al.: Cancer Treat. Rep. 60:703, 1976.)

Toxicity includes nausea, vomiting, venous irritation, and bone marrow suppression. The bone marrow suppressive effect of these drugs is of relatively later onset than that induced by other chemotherapeutic agents; blood counts reach their nadir on an average of 28 days after exposure to the drug (range 14 to 40 days).[30] This toxic effect on the marrow is dose-related, dose-limiting, and cumulative; the cumulative effects are manifested by lower nadirs at a given dose level, earlier appearance of nadirs, or longer durations of myelosuppression. These drugs may also produce kidney, liver, and lung toxicity.

The major clinical use of these agents has been in treatment of *brain tumors*[37] and *lymphomas*.[112, 120]

Procarbazine (Natulan, Matulane) (Fig. 3–17)

Procarbazine is a methylhydrazine derivative. Its mechanism of action appears to be mediated through the autooxidation of the methylhydrazine moiety with intracellular formation of hydrogen peroxide and subsequent damage to DNA.[10] It is nonspecific for cell-cycle phase.

The drug can be given orally or intravenously. Side effects include nausea and vomiting, bone marrow suppression, dermatitis, alopecia, postural hypotension, and central nervous system effects (euphoria, ataxia, nystagmus, paresthesias, Parkinsonism, depression, somnolence).

Since methylhydrazine is a weak monoamine oxidase inhibitor, foods with a high tyramine content (cheese, bananas) should be avoided. To minimize central nervous system depression, barbiturates, phenothiazines, narcotics, antihistamines, sedative antihypotensive drugs, and alcohol should not be given concomitantly. Likewise, sympathomimetic and tricyclic antidepressant drugs (e.g., imipramine) should be used with caution when the patient is receiving procarbazine.

Procarbazine is used for treatment of *non-Hodgkin's lymphoma* and as part of the MOPP protocol for *Hodgkin's disease*.[29]

Hydroxyurea (Hydrea)

Hydroxyurea is an inhibitor of ribonucleoside diphosphate reductase, an enzyme essential in DNA synthesis. It is specifically active during the S phase of the cell cycle. Being a small molecule, it is well absorbed from the gastrointestinal tract, reaching peak serum concentrations within 2 hours. Clearance from the serum is also rapid (by 6 hours) and excretion is mainly via the kidney.[70]

Toxicity includes bone marrow suppression and gastrointestinal symptoms. Uncommonly, skin reactions, alopecia, stomatitis, and neurologic problems may occur.[16]

This agent has been used in the treatment of busulfan-resistant *chronic granulocytic leukemia*, *melanoma*, and *advanced carcinoma of the ovary*.

Dimethyltriazeno Imidazolecarboxamide (DTIC) (Dacarbazine)

DTIC has a purine-like structure (Fig. 3–18), but has many of the biological characteristics of an alkylating agent[48] and is nonspecific for cell-cycle phase.[21] It is light-sensitive and must be stored in the dark.

Toxic signs include nausea and vomiting, as well as delayed bone marrow suppression. DTIC has been used

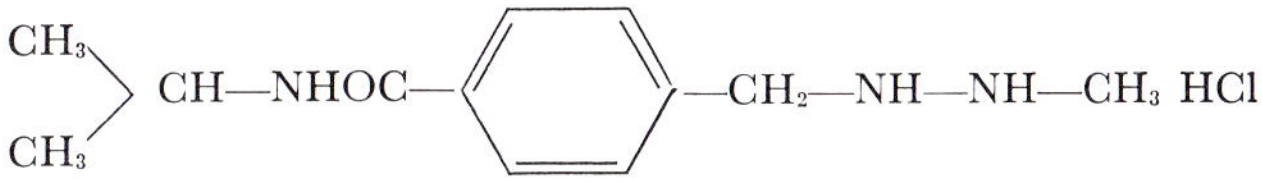

Figure 3–17 Structural formula of procarbazine. (From Billmeier, G. J., et al.: J. Pediatr. 75:892, 1969.)

DIC

Figure 3-18 Structural formula of imidazole carboxamide (DTIC). (From Cline, J. J., and Haskell, C. M.: Cancer Chemotherapy. 2nd Ed. Philadelphia, W. B. Saunders Co., 1975.)

in treatment of *melanoma*,[47] *lymphomas*,[43] and *soft tissue sarcomas*.[50]

Platinum Compounds

In 1965 Rosenberg and colleagues[91] reported that the discharge of an electric current from a platinum electrode through a nutrient broth containing *E. coli* produced platinum-containing compounds which inhibited replication of the bacteria. One of these compounds, cis-diaminodichloroplatinum (II) (DDP:NSC 119875), has been shown to be an effective antitumor agent as well.

Structurally, DDP is an inorganic complex formed by a central atom of platinum surrounded by chlorine and ammonia atoms in the cis position in the horizontal plane (Fig. 3-19). This chemical structure with its two labile chlorine atoms in the cis position is reminiscent of the mustard type bifunctional alkylating agents.

Some investigators feel that DDP exerts its antitumor effects by inhibiting cell division, and there is evidence that platinum coordination compounds bind to DNA and RNA.[71] Other authors hypothesize that the mechanism of action may involve enhancement of tumor antigenicity so that tumor cells become more susceptible to destruction by the immune system.

Although DDP and other platinum compounds are effective antitumor drugs, their effectiveness is limited by their toxicity, especially to the kidney. This nephrotoxic effect can be reduced by increasing the flow of urine through the patient's kidneys at the time the medication is administered.[71] Bone marrow suppression, nausea, and vomiting are also side effects of these drugs. Other toxic effects include tinnitus and high-frequency hearing loss.

DDP appears to be particularly effective against testicular tumors,[57] but it is still being tested for treatment of ovarian carcinoma, neuroblastoma, and a variety of other tumors.

REFERENCES

1. Adamson, R. H.: Metabolism of anticancer agents in man. Ann. N.Y. Acad. Sci. *179*: 432, 1971.
2. Barranco, S. C., and Humphrey, R. M.: The effects of bleomycin on survival and cell progression in Chinese hamster cells *in vitro*. Cancer Res. *31*:1218, 1971.
3. Bedrossian, C., Luna, M. A., Mackay, B., et al.: Ultrastructure of pulmonary bleomycin toxicity. Cancer 32:44, 1973.
4. Bellet, R. E., Mastrangelo, M. J., Engstrom, P. F., et al.: Clinical trial with subcutaneously administered 5-azacytidine

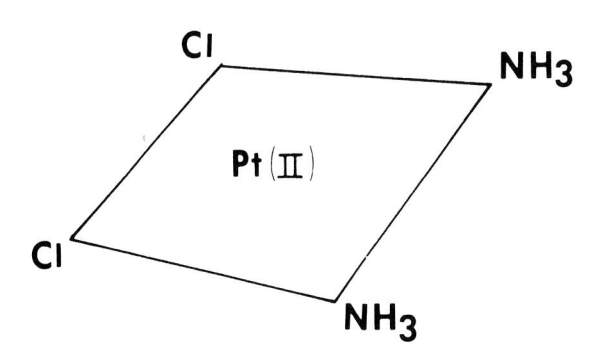

Figure 3-19 Structural formula of diaminodichloroplatinum. (From Higby, D. J., et al.: Cancer *33*:1219, 1974.)

(NSC-102816). Cancer Chemother. Rep., 58:217, 1974.
5. Benjamin, R. S., Riggs, C. E., Jr., and Bachur, N. R.: Pharmacokinetics and metabolism of Adriamycin in man. Clin. Pharmacol. Ther. *14*:592, 1973.
6. Benjamin, R. S., Wiernik, P. H., and Bachur, N. R.: Adriamycin chemotherapy—efficacy, safety and pharmacologic basis of an intermittent single high-dose schedule. Cancer *33*:19, 1974.
7. Berenson, M. P.: Recovery after inadvertent massive overdosage of vincristine (NSC-67574). Cancer Chemother. Rep. 55:525, 1971.
8. Bergevin, P. R., Tormey, D. C., and Blom, J.: Guide to the use of cancer chemotherapeutic agents. Mod. Treat. 9:185, 1972.
9. Bernard, J., Weil, M., Boiron, M., et al.: Acute promyelocytic leukemia: Results of treatment of daunorubicin. Blood *41*: 489, 1973.
10. Bernies, A., Kofler, M., Bollage, W., et al.: The degradation of DNA by new tumor inhibiting compounds: The intermediate formation of hydrogen peroxide. Experientia *19*:132, 1963.
11. Bertino, J. R., and Johns, D. G.: Folate antagonists. *In* Brodsky, I., and Kahn, S. B. (eds.): Cancer Chemotherapy Two: Twenty-Second Symposium. New York, Grune & Stratton, 1972.
12. Bleyer, W. A., Drake, J. C., and Chabner, B. A.: Neurotoxicity and elevated cerebrospinal fluid methotrexate concentration in meningeal leukemia. N. Engl. J. Med. 289:770, 1973.
13. Blum, R. H., and Carter, S. K.: Adriamycin: a new anticancer drug with significant clinical activity. Ann. Intern. Med. *80*: 249, 1974.
14. Blum, R. H., Carter, S. K., and Agre, K.: A clinical review of bleomycin—a new antineoplastic agent. Cancer *31*:903, 1973.
15. Buckner, C. O., Rudolph, R. H., Fefer, A., et al.: High-dose cyclophosphamide therapy for malignant disease: toxicity, tumor response and the effects of stored autologous marrow. Cancer 29:357, 1972.
16. Calabresi, P., and Parks, R. E.: Alkylating agents, antimetabolites, hormones, and other antiproliferative agents. *In* Goodman, L. S., and Gilman, A. (eds.): The Pharmacological Basis of Therapeutics. 4th Ed. New York, Macmillan Co., 1970.
17. Carter, S. K.: Adriamycin—a review. J. Natl. Cancer Inst. 55:1265, 1975.
18. Carter, S. K., and Soper, W. T.: Integration of chemotherapy into combined modality treatment of solid tumors. I. The overall strategy. Cancer Treatment Rev. *1*:1, 1974.
19. Cassady, J. R., Richter, M. P., Piro, A. J., and Jaffe, N.: Radiation-adriamycin interactions: preliminary clinical observations. Cancer 36:946, 1975.
20. Chabner, B. A., Drake, J. C., and Johns, D. G.: Deamination of 5-azacytidine by a human leukemia cell cytidine deaminase. Biochem. Pharmacol. 22:2763, 1973.
21. Chabner, B. A., Myers, C. E., Coleman, C. N., and Johns, D. G.: The clinical pharmacology of antineoplastic agents. N. Engl. J. Med. 292:1107, 1159, 1975.
22. Chabner, B. A., and Slavik, M.: Introduction: perspectives on high-dose methotrexate (NSC-740) therapy. Cancer Chemother. Rep. 6:1, 1975.
23. Cheng, C. J., Fujimura, S., Grunberger, D., and Weinstin, I. B.: Interaction of 1-(2-chlorethyl)-3-cyclohexyl-1-nitrosourea (NSC-79037) with nucleic acids and proteins *in vivo* and *in vitro*. Cancer Res. *32*:22, 1972.
24. Cline, M. J., and Haskell, C. M.: Cancer Chemotherapy. 2nd Ed. Philadelphia, W. B. Saunders Co., 1975.
25. Conn, H. O., and Blitzer, B. L.: Nonassociation of adrenocorticosteroid therapy and peptic ulcer. N. Engl. J. Med. 294:473, 1976.
26. Cortes, E. P., Lutman, G., Wanka, J., et al.: Adriamycin (NSC-123127) cardiotoxicity: a clinicopathologic correlation. Cancer Chemother. Rep. 6:215, 1975.
27. DeFronzo, R. A., Braine, H., Colvin, O. M., et al.: Water intoxication in man after cyclophosphamide therapy: time course and relation to drug activation. Ann. Intern. Med. 78:861, 1973.
28. DeVita, V. T., Jr., and Schein, P. S.: The use of drugs in combination for the treatment of cancer. N. Engl. J. Med. 288:998, 1973.
29. DeVita, V. T., Jr., Serpick, A. A., and Carbone, P. P.: Combination chemotherapy in the treatment of advanced Hodgkin's disease. Ann. Intern. Med. 73:881, 1970.
30. DeVita, V. T., Jr., Young, R. C., and Canellos, G. P.: Combination versus single agent chemotherapy: a review of the basis for selection of drug treatment of cancer. Cancer 35:98, 1975.
31. DeVita, V. T., Jr., Carbone, P. P., and Owens, A. H., Jr.: Clinical trials with BCNU. Cancer Res. 25:1876, 1965.
32. Djerassi, I.: High-dose methotrexate (NSC-740) and citrovorum factor (NSC-3590) rescue: background and rationale. Cancer Chemother. Rep. 6:3, 1975.

33. Djerassi, I., Farber, S., Abir, E., et al.: Continuous infusion of methotrexate in children with acute leukemia. Cancer 20:233, 1967.
34. Duttera, M. J., Carolla, R. L., Gallelli, J. F., et al.: Hematuria and crystalluria after high dose 6-mercaptopurine administration. N. Engl. J. Med. 287:292, 1972.
34a. Einhorn, M., and Davidsohn, I.: Hepatotoxicity of mercaptopurine. J.A.M.A. 188:802, 1964.
35. Elion, G. B., Singer, S., and Hitchings, G. H.: Antagonists of nucleic acid derivatives. VIII. Synergism in combinations of biochemically related antimetabolites. J. Biol. Chem. 208:477, 1954.
36. Fairley, K. F., Barrie, J. U., and Johnson, W.: Sterility and testicular atrophy related to cyclophosphamide therapy. Lancet 1:568, 1972.
37. Fewer, D., Wilson, C. B., Boldrey, E. B., and Enot, J. K.: Phase II study of 1-(2-choroethyl)-3-cholohexyl-1-nitrosourea (CCNU: NSC-79037) in the treatment of brain tumors. Cancer Chemother. Rep., 56:421, 1972.
38. Folkman, J.: Tumor angiogenesis: therapeutic implications. N. Engl. J. Med. 285:1182, 1971.
39. Frei, E., III: Effect of dose-schedule on response. In Holland, J. F., and Frei, E., III (eds.): Cancer Medicine. Philadelphia, Lea & Febiger, 1973.
40. Frei, E., III: The clinical use of actinomycin. Cancer Chemother. Rep. 58:49, 1974.
41. Frei, E., III, Franzino, A., Shnider, B. I., et al.: Clinical studies of vinblastine. Cancer Chemother. Rep. 12:125, 1961.
42. Frei, E., III, Jaffe, N., Tattersall, M. H. N., et al.: New approaches to cancer chemotherapy with methotrexate. N. Engl. J. Med. 292:846, 1975.
43. Frei, E., III, Luce, J. K., et al.: 5-(3,3-dimethyl-1-triazeno)-imidazole-4-carboxamide (NSC-45388) in the treatment of lymphoma. Cancer Chemother. Rep., 56:667, 1972.
44. Fujiwara, Y., and Kondo, T.: Strand-scission of HeLa cell deoxyribonucleic acid by bleomycin in vitro and in vivo. Biochem. Pharmacol. 22:323, 1973.
45. Gagliano, R. G., and Costanzi, J. J.: Paraplegia following intrathecal methotrexate. Report of a case and review of the literature. Cancer 37:1663, 1976.
43a. Friedman, M. A., Bozdech, M. J., Billingham, M., et al.: Adriamycin cardiotoxicity in humans: serial physiologic studies and endomyocardial biopsies. Clin. Res. 25:407A, 1977.
46. Geiser, C. F., Bishop, Y., Jaffe, N., et al.: Adverse effects of intrathecal methotrexate in children with acute leukemia in remission. Blood 45:189, 1975.
47. Gerner, R. E., Moore, G. E., and Didolklar, M. S.: Chemotherapy of disseminated malignant melanoma with dimethyl-triazeno imidazolecarboxamide and dactinomycin. Cancer 32:756, 1973.
48. Gerulath, A. H., and Loo, T. L.: Mechanism of action of 5-(3,3-dimethyl-1-triazeno)imidazole-4-carboxamide in mammalian cells in culture. Biochem. Pharmacol. 21:2335, 1972.
49. Gilladoga, A. C., Manuel, C., Tan, C. T. C., et al.: The cardiotoxicity of adriamycin and daunomycin in children. Cancer 37:1070, 1976.
50. Gottlieb, J. A., Bodey, G. P., et al.: An effective new 4-drug combination regimen (CY-VA-DIC) for metastatic sarcomas. Proc. Am. Ass. Cancer Res. Am. Soc. Clin. Oncol. 15:713 (abstr.), 1974.
51. Greene, H. S. N.: Heterologous transplantation of mammalian tumors. I. The transfer of rabbit tumor to alien species. J. Exp. Med. 73:461, 1941.
52. Gutin, P. H., Green, M. R., and Bleyer, W. A.: Methotrexate pneumonitis induced by intrathecal methotrexate therapy. Cancer 38:1529, 1976.
53. Halazun, J. F., Wagner, H. R., Gaeta, J. F., and Sinks, L. F.: Daunorubicin cardiac toxicity in children with acute lymphocytic leukemia. Cancer 33:545, 1974.
54. Hartmann, G., Goller, H., Koschel, K., et al.: Hemmung der DNA-abhängigen RNA und DNA-synthese durch Antibiotica. Biochem. Z. 341:125, 1964.
55. Henderson, E. S., and Samaha, R. J.: Evidence that drugs in multiple combinations have materially advanced the treatment of human malignancies. Cancer Res. 29:2272, 1969.
56. Hersch, E. M., Wong, V. G., Henderson, E. S., and Freireich, E. J.: Hepatotoxic effects of methotrexate. Cancer 19:600, 1966.
57. Higby, D. J., Wallace, H. J., Jr., Albert, D. J., and Holland, J. F.: Diaminodichloroplatinum: a phase I study showing responses in testicular and other tumors. Cancer 33:1219, 1974.
58. Holland, J. F., Scharlau, C., Gailani, S., et al.: Vincristine treatment of advanced cancer: a cooperative study of 392 cases. Cancer Res. 33:1258, 1973.
59. Jaffe, N., Frei, E., III, Traggis, D., et al.: Adjuvant methotrexate and citrovorum-factor treatment of osteogenic sarcoma. N. Engl. J. Med. 291:994, 1974.
60. Johnson, F. L., Bernstein, I. D., Hartmann, J. R., and Chard, R. L., Jr.: Seizures associated with vincristine sulfate therapy. J. Pediatr. 82:699, 1973.
61. Kaiser, N., Milholland, R. J., and Rosen, F.: Glucocorticoid receptors and mechanism of resistance in the cortisol-sensitive and -resistant lines of lymphosarcoma P1798. Cancer Res. 34:621, 1974.
62. Karon, M., Seiger, L., Leimbrock, S., et al.:

5-Azacytidine: a new active agent for the treatment of acute leukemia. Blood 42:359, 1973.
63. Kay, H. E. N., Knapton, P. J., O'Sullivan, J. P., et al.: Encephalopathy in acute leukemia associated with methotrexate therapy. Arch. Dis. Child. 47:344, 1972.
64. Kennedy, B. J.: Metabolic and toxic effects of mithramycin during tumor therapy. Am. J. Med. 49:494, 1970.
65. Kennedy, B. J.: Mithramycin therapy in testicular cancer. J. Urol. 107:429, 1972.
66. Lamerton, L. F.: Basic concepts of cell population kinetics. In Sartorelli, A. C., and Johns, D. G. (eds.): Antineoplastic and Immunosuppressive Agents. New York, Springer-Verlag, 1974.
67. Lawrence, H. J., Simone, J., and Aur, R. J. A.: Cyclophosphamide-induced hemorrhagic cystitis in children with leukemia. Cancer 36:1572, 1975.
68. Lefrak, E. A., Pitha, J., Rosenheim, S., and Gottlieb, J. A.: A clinicopathologic analysis of adriamycin cardiotoxicity. Cancer 32:302, 1973.
69. Lenaz, L., and Page, J. A.: Cardiotoxicity of adriamycin and related anthracyclines. Cancer Treat. Rev. 3:111, 1976.
70. Livingston, R. B., and Carter, S. L.: Single Agents in Cancer Chemotherapy. New York, Plenum Publishing Corp., 1970.
71. Marx, J. L.: Chemotherapy: renewed interest in platinum compounds. Science 192:774, 1976.
72. McIntosh, S., Klatskin, E., O'Brien, R. T., et al.: Chronic neurologic disturbance in childhood leukemia. Cancer 37:853, 1976.
73. Meadows, A. T., and Evans, A. E.: Effects of chemotherapy on the central nervous system. A study of parenteral methotrexate in long-term survivors of leukemia and lymphoma in childhood. Cancer 37:1079, 1976.
74. Drug Brochure: Trituration of Mustargen. West Point, Pa., Merck Sharpe & Dohme, Division of Merck & Co., Inc., March, 1974.
75. Monto, R. W., Talley, R. W., et al.: Observations on the mechanism of hemorrhagic toxicity in mithramycin (NSC-24559) therapy. Cancer Res. 29:697, 1969.
76. Nesbit, M., Krivit, W., Heyn, R., Sharp, H.: Acute and chronic effects of methotrexate on hepatic, pulmonary and skeletal systems. Cancer 37:1048, 1976.
77. Oettgen, H. F., Stephenson, P. A., Schwartz, M. K., et al.: Toxicity of E. coli L-asparaginase in man. Cancer 25:253, 1970.
78. Ohnuma, T., Holland, J. F., Masuda, H., et al.: Microbiological assay of bleomycin: inactivation, tissue distribution and clearance. Cancer 33:1230, 1974.

79. Oliverio, V. T.: Toxicology and pharmacology of the nitrosoureas. Cancer Chemother. Rep. 4:13, 1973.
80. Panoff, A.: Pathogenesis of epileptiform seizures in acute leukosis in childhood. Arch. Kinderheilk. 183:62, 1971.
81. Phillips, F. S., Sternberg, S. S., Cronin, A. P., and Vidal, P. M.: Cyclophosphamide and urinary bladder toxicity. Cancer Res. 21:1577, 1961.
82. Pitman, S. W., Parker, L. M., Tattersall, M. H. N., et al.: Clinical trial of high-dose methotrexate (NSC-740) with citrovorum factor (NSC-3590) toxocologic and therapeutic observations. Cancer Chemother. Rep. 6:43, 1975.
83. Pochedley, C.: Wilms' tumor. III. Special problems in therapy. N.Y. State J. Med. 71:1526, 1971.
84. Potter, V. R.: Sequential blocking of metabolic pathways in vivo. Proc. Soc. Exp. Biol. Med. 76:41, 1951.
85. Pratt, C. B., Roberts, D., Shanks, E., and Warmath, E. L.: Response, toxicity and pharmacokinetics of high-dose methotrexate (NSC-740) with citrovoroum factor (NSC-3590) rescue for children with osteosarcoma and other malignant tumors. Cancer Chemother. Rep. 6:13, 1975.
85a. Prout, M. N., Richards, M. J. S., Chung, K. J., et al.: Adriamycin cardiotoxicity in children. Case reports, literature review, and risk factors. Cancer 39:62, 1977.
86. Ragab, A. D., Frech, R. S., and Vietti, T. J.: Osteoporotic fractures secondary to methotrexate therapy of acute leukemia in remission. Cancer 25:580, 1970.
87. Ragab, A. D., Sutow, W. W., Komp, D. M., et al.: Adriamycin in the treatment of childhood solid tumors. A Southwest Oncology Group study. Cancer 36:1572, 1975.
88. Rao, K. V., Cullen, W. P., and Sobin, B. A.: New antibiotic with antitumor properties. Antibiot. Chemother. 12:182, 1962.
89. Robins, P. R., and Jowsey, J.: Effect of mithramycin on normal and abnormal bone turnover. J. Lab. Clin. Med. 52:576, 1973.
90. Rosen, F., and Milholland, R. J.: Mechanism of action of glucocorticoids. In Sartorelli, A. C., and Johns, D. G. (eds.): Antineoplastic and Immunosuppressive Agents. New York, Springer-Verlag, 1975.
91. Rosenberg, B., Van Camp, L., and Kriggs, T.: Inhibition of cell division in Escherichia coli by electrolysis products from a platinum electrode. Nature 205:698, 1965.
92. Rosenoff, S. H., Brooks, E., Bostick, F., et al.: Alterations of DNA synthesis in

cardiac tissue induced by adriamycin *in vivo*–relationship to fatal toxicity. Biochem. Pharmacol. 24:1898, 1975.
93. Rudolph, R., Stein, R. S., and Pattilo, R. A.: Skin ulcers due to adriamycin. Cancer 38:1087, 1976.
94. Samuels, B. I., Culbert, S. J., Okamura, J., and Sullivan, M. P.: Early detection of chemotherapy-related pancreatic enlargement in children using abdominal sonography. Cancer 38:1515, 1976.
95. Sandler, S. G., Tobin, W., and Henderson, E. S.: Vincristine-induced neuropathy: A clinical study of fifty leukemic patients. Neurology 19:367, 1969.
96. Sartorelli, A. C.: Some approaches to the therapeutic exploitation of metabolic sites of vulnerability of neoplastic cells. Cancer Res. 29:2292, 1969.
97. Sharp, H. L., White, J. G., and Krivit, W.: Methotrexate-induced liver injury. Proc. Am. Ass. Cancer Res. 18:60, 1967.
97a. Shorey, J., Schenker, S., Suki, W. N., et al.: Hepatotoxicity of mercaptopurine. Arch. Intern. Med. 122:54, 1968.
98. Skipper, H. E.: Cancer chemotherapy is many things. G. H. A. Clowes Memorial Lecture. Cancer Res. 31:1173, 1971.
99. Skipper, H. E., and Schnabel, F. M., Jr.: Quantitative and cytokinetic studies in experimental tumor models. *In* Holland, J. F., and Frei, E., III (eds.): Cancer Medicine. Philadelphia, Lea and Febiger, 1973.
100. Skipper, H. E., Schnabel, F. M., Jr., and Wilcox, W. S.: Experimental evaluation of potential anticancer agents. XII. On the criteria and kinetics associated with "curability" of experimental leukemia. Cancer Chemother. Rep. 35:1, 1964.
101. Slayton, R. B., Shnider, B. I., Elias, E., et al.: New approach to the treatment of hypercalcemia. The effect of short-term treatment with mithramycin. Clin. Pharmacol. Ther. 12:833, 1971.
102. Sostman, H. D., Matthay, R. A., Putman, C. E., and Smith, G. J. W.: Methotrexate-induced pneumonitis. Medicine 55:371, 1976.
103. Stephens, F. O.: "CRAB" care and cancer chemotherapy. Med. J. Aust. 2:41, 1976.
104. Suskind, R. M., Brusilow, S. W., and Zehr, J.: Syndrome of inappropriate secretion of antidiuretic hormone produced by vincristine toxicity (with bioassay of ADH level). J. Pediatr. 81:90, 1972.
105. Sutow, W. W., and Valeriote, F.: General aspects of chemotherapy. *In* Sutow, W. W., Vietti, T. J., and Fernbach, D. J. (eds.): Clinical Pediatric Oncology. St. Louis, C. V. Mosby, 1973.
106. Talley, R. W.: Corticosteroids. *In* Holland, J. F., and Frei, E., III (eds.): Cancer Medicine. Philadelphia, Lea and Febiger, 1973.

107. Turnell, R. W., and Burton, A. F.: Studies on the mechanism of resistance to lymphocytolysis induced by corticosteroids. Cancer Res. 34:39, 1974.
108. Valeriote, F., and Vietti, T. J.: Cellular kinetics and conceptual basis of chemotherapy. *In* Sutow, W. W., Vietti, T. J., and Fernbach, D. J. (eds.): Clinical Pediatric Oncology. St. Louis C. V. Mosby, 1973.
109. Von Hoff, D. D., Slavik, M., and Muggia, F. M.: 5-Azacytidine. A new anti-cancer drug with effectiveness in acute myelogenous leukemia. Ann. Int. Med. 85:237, 1976.
110. Wall, R. L., and Clausen, K. P.: Carcinoma of the urinary bladder in patients receiving cyclophosphamide. N. Engl. J. Med. 293:271, 1975.
111. Waring, M.: Variation of the supercoils in closed circular DNA by binding of antibiotics and drugs: evidence for molecular models involving intercalation. J. Mol. Biol. 54:247, 1970.
112. Wasserman, T. H., Slavik, M., and Carter, S. K.: Review of CCNU in clinical cancer therapy. Cancer Treat. Rev. 1:131, 1974.
113. Weetman, R. M., and Baehner, R. L.: Latent onset of clinical pancreatitis in children receiving L-asparaginase therapy. Cancer 37:780, 1974.
114. Weiden, P. L., and Wright, S. E.: Vincristine neurotoxicity. N. Engl. J. Med. 286:1369, 1972.
115. Weil, M., Glidewell, O. J., Jacquillar, C., et al.: Daunorubicin in the therapy of acute granulocytic leukemia. Cancer Res. 33:921, 1973.
116. Weiss, H. D., Walker, M. D., and Wiernik, P. H.: Neurotoxicity of commonly used antineoplastic agents. N. Engl. J. Med. 291:75, 127, 1974.
117. Whitcomb, M. E., Schwartz, M. I., and Tormey, D. C.: Methotrexate pneumonitis: case report and review of the literature. Thorax 27:636, 1972.
118. Whitecar, J. P., Jr., Bodey, G. P., Harris, J. E., and Freireich, E. J.: L-asparaginase. N. Engl. J. Med. 282:732, 1970.
119. Yagoda, A., Mukherji, B., Young, C., et al.: Bleomycin, an antitumor antibiotic. Clinical experience in 274 patients. Ann. Intern. Med. 77:861, 1972.
120. Young, R. C., DeVita, V. T., Jr., Serpick, A. A., and Cannelos, G. P.: Treatment of advanced Hodgkin's disease with (1,3 bis (2-chloroethyl)-1-nitrosourea) (BCNU). N. Engl. J. Med. 285:475, 1971.
121. Zimmerman, A. M., Padilla, G. M., and Cameron, I. L.: Drugs and the Cell Cycle. New York, Academic Press, 1973.
122. Zubrod, C. G.: The clinical toxicities of L-asparaginase in treatment of leukemia and lymphoma. Pediatrics 45:555, 1970.
123. Zubrod, C. G.: The basis for progress in chemotherapy. Cancer 23:202, 1973.

Chapter Four

RADIOTHERAPY

William N. Brand

The common characteristic of the various electromagnetic emissions used in radiotherapy is their ability to ionize atoms. Ionization of an atom occurs when a packet of electromagnetic radiant energy collides with an orbital electron and knocks it out of position. Electrons displaced in such a fashion expend their energy by ionizing other atoms. This energy may be transferred through a chain of chemical reactions, eventually producing damage to biologically important molecules (Fig. 4–1). Such macromolecular damage is not brought about directly by ionization but is mediated through the formation of free radicals (i.e., atoms or molecules containing unpaired electrons), which are highly reactive. Since cells consist primarily of water (70 to 90 per cent), most biological damage results from the formation of hydrogen (H·) and hydroxyl (OH·) free radicals.

Ionizing radiations may be of two types: electromagnetic (x-rays and gamma rays) and particulate (neutrons, alpha particles, and beta particles). By convention the term "x-ray" refers to ionizing electromagnetic irradiation produced by a man-made generator (the x-ray machine), whereas "gamma rays" refer to a similar form of energy produced by the disintegration of the nucleus of radioactive atoms (e.g., ^{60}cobalt). X-rays are produced by the acceleration of particles (usually electrons); when these particles strike a target (usually tungsten) their energy is absorbed, and heat and electromagnetic radiations are produced.

The units of x-ray or gamma-ray exposure are the *roentgen (R)*, a measurement of ionization in air, and the radiation absorbed dose *(rad)*, a representation of the quantity of radiation actually absorbed in tissue. A dose of one rad represents the amount of radiation that deposits 100 ergs per gram of irradiated tissue.

Cellular Effects of Ionizing Radiation

The critical target in cell death is the nucleus. DNA and RNA may be damaged by ionizing radiation in several different ways: (1) damage to nucleotide bases (particularly the pyrimidine bases, cytosine, thymine, and uracil), (2) single strand breaks, and (3) double helix strand breaks. This may be manifested by chromosome destruction, mitotic delay, mutation, and cell cycle changes. As a result of this damage to the nucleic acids, reproductive function is seriously compromised. Metabolic functions of the irradiated cell

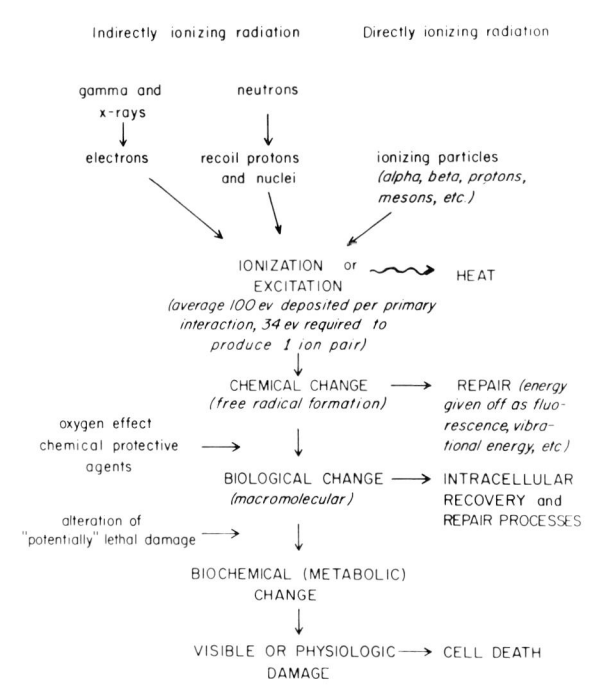

```
Indirectly ionizing radiation        Directly ionizing radiation

    gamma and              neutrons
     x-rays                   ↓
       ↓          recoil protons      ionizing particles
    electrons    and nuclei           (alpha, beta, protons,
                                      mesons, etc.)
           ↘         ↓          ↙
              IONIZATION or  ⤳  HEAT
              EXCITATION
           (average 100 ev deposited per primary
            interaction, 34 ev required to
                produce 1 ion pair)
                      ↓
                CHEMICAL CHANGE  →  REPAIR (energy
                (free radical formation)   given off as fluo-
  oxygen effect       ↓                    rescence, vibra-
  chemical protective →                    tional energy, etc)
  agents
                BIOLOGICAL CHANGE  →  INTRACELLULAR
                (macromolecular)       RECOVERY and
  alteration of                        REPAIR PROCESSES
  "potentially" lethal damage →
                      ↓
                BIOCHEMICAL (METABOLIC)
                     CHANGE
                      ↓
                VISIBLE OR PHYSIOLOGIC → CELL DEATH
                     DAMAGE
```

Figure 4–1 Development of radiation injury in cells. (From Little, J. B., and Williams, J. R.: *In* Lee, D. H. K. (ed.): Handbook of Physiology, Section 9, Reaction to Environmental Agents. Bethesda, Md., American Physiological Society, 1977.)

are also altered following irradiation and this may be reflected by alterations in membrane permeability, protein synthesis, and enzyme configuration.

Because the major effect of irradiation is on the nucleic acids, parenchymal tissues that normally undergo frequent renewal by mitotic division (e.g., bone marrow, germ cells) are the most radiosensitive, whereas those that normally renew very slowly or not at all are relatively radioresistant. Intermediate in radiosensitivity are the small "intraparenchymal" blood vessels, damage to which may mediate the acute destruction of the relatively radioresistant parenchymal tissues.[4]

Ionizing radiations produce either sublethal or lethal damage to cells. Sublethal injury is associated with repair and recovery, whereas lethal injury is manifested by failure to successfully replicate genetic material and the inability to undergo mitosis. If the number of tumor cells lethally irradiated exceeds the tumor's ability to repopulate with viable cells, there will be clinically observable tumor shrinkage. If the amount of ionizing radiation given is sufficient to reduce the surviving cell fraction to some minimal critical number, the tumor may be eradicated. Repopulation also occurs in normal tissue and it is this repopulation, coupled with repair of sublethal damage, that permits the successful administration of ionizing radiation to a tumor-bearing volume that includes critical amounts of normal tissue.

Figure 4–2 illustrates a typical cell survival curve in response to irradiation. The initial portion of the curve, the so-called "shoulder," represents the ability of the irradiated cells to accumulate and repair sublethal damage. The second, steeper (linear) portion of the curve illustrates the fairly constant lethality with increasing dose to a homogeneously sensitive population of cells. The final portion of the curve shows a break from the homogenous sensitivity, which implies some form of protection from ionizing radiation (usually anoxia). In general, the

Figure 4-2 Typical cell survival curve. That portion defined as *a* shows the summated effect of repair of sublethal injury and repopulation. Curve *b* shows exponential kill of cells of a homogenous population associated with higher doses. Curve *c* illustrates the effect of anoxia on the surviving population.

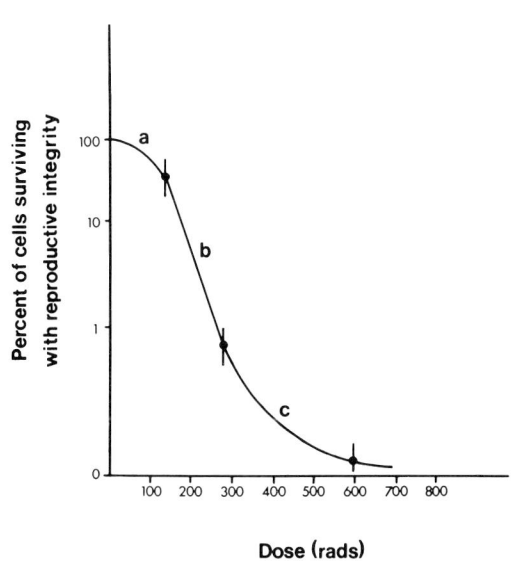

more resistant the cells are to radiation effects, the broader the shoulder and the less steep the slope will be.

It is reasonable to assume that almost any tumor can be destroyed by irradiation if the dose delivered is sufficiently high. Unfortunately, the dosage required for 100 per cent eradication of many tumors may be associated with an unacceptable amount of destruction of normal tissue. This point illustrates the limitations of the term "radiosensitivity" which should perhaps be considered to be a reflection of the tolerance of the normal tissues within the irradiated volume to the dose selected. The radiation therapist must, therefore, define a critical or dose-limiting organ or tissue within the volume to be irradiated. For example, if both lungs contain multiple metastatic deposits of tumor, the radiation tolerance of the pulmonary parenchyma determines the "radiosensitivity" or "radioresistance" of the tumor. If, in this example, the tumors in the lungs were metastatic from an orbital rhabdomyosarcoma, the primary site might be controlled by irradiation alone (a radiation-induced cataract will certainly follow, yet we judge this to be an acceptable complication for the chance of cure of the child); however, the metastatic pulmonary lesions could not be eradicated by radiotherapy without also destroying pulmonary function. For most patients radiotherapy results in sequelae to normal tissues that lie somewhere between the simple complication of a radiation cataract and fatal radiation pneumonitis.

RELATIONSHIP OF DOSE AND VOLUME

The larger the cancer, the higher the dose required for eradication. Several factors account for this phenomenon:

1. On a statistical basis alone, the number of viable tumor cells remaining after a given dose of radiotherapy is greater for a large tumor than for a small tumor.

2. Large tumors generally have a poorer vascular supply than do small tumors; consequently, a higher proportion of cells will be hypoxic and less sensitive to radiotherapy.

3. The growth fraction (i.e., proportion of cells actively dividing) is smaller in a large tumor than it is in a small tumor (see discussion of Gompertzian kinetics in Chapter Three).

In general, total doses used in pediatric oncology tend to cluster in three broad ranges: (1) 1000 to 2000 rads (acute lymphoblastic leukemia, histocytosis X, pulmonary irradiation in Wilms' tumor); (2) 2000 to 4000 rads (Wilms' tumor, neuroblastoma, Hodgkin's disease, non-Hodgkin's lymphoma); (3) 4000 to 6000 rads (retinoblastoma, brain tumors, soft tissue sarcomas, and Ewing's sarcoma). In any curative attempt, full cancericidal doses should be delivered with the first irradiation. Inadequate dosage can so alter subsequent radiation response that a cancer that was initially radiocurable can be rendered radioincurable. This alteration of the radiation response can be attributed to several factors:

1. Selection of a radioresistant population by destroying the more radiosensitive cells.
2. Radiation-produced mutations may lead to production of a more resistant cell type.
3. Changes in the tumor bed. After irradiation, subendothelial connective tissues proliferate in blood vessels, with subsequent narrowing of the vascular lumen. This results in a decrease in oxygen availability, which may compromise the effect of radiotherapy (since ionization of oxygen may play an important role in the cytocidal effect of radiation).

FRACTIONATION

When a given dose of irradiation is divided into several daily increments (*fractionation*), the biological effect is usually less than if the treatment had been given in a single dose. This decreased response with daily fractionation appears to be related to cell recovery occurring between the increments and to the capability of cells not lethally damaged to adapt to radiation-induced alterations of the surrounding tissue. In general, normal cells have a greater and faster capacity than tumor cells to repair this damage;[29] consequently, after each treatment the normal tissue cells will recover more completely than the tumor cells from the effects of the radiotherapy. This relationship between timing and dose of radiotherapy (the *time-dose relationship*) makes it mandatory that the dose or irradiation should be stated with the corresponding time period over which the dose was delivered. A complete expression of treatment should include total dose, number of fractions, and elapsed time in calendar days.

Typically, radiation treatments are given in five fractions per week (some radiation therapists prefer four to six fractions per week). The usual total weekly dose varies between 750 and 1000 rads, depending on the volume and tissue included in the beam and the general condition of the child. In some instances, however, particularly when rapid palliation is the aim of treatment, a single high increment dose (600 to 1000 rads) may be employed. While such a high dose of radiation has no place in curative efforts, delivering 1000 rads to as much as one half of the child's body may bring about dramatic relief from pain or pressure caused by large tumor masses. It is estimated that this dose of radiation will kill more than 95 per cent of the cells in a tumor mass. We have used this technique in several children with disseminated rhabdomyosarcoma and neuroblastoma who were refractory to drug therapy when conventional radiation fractionation was deemed inappropriate.

NORMAL TISSUE TOLERANCE AND DAMAGE

Injuries to normal tissues following radiation therapy may be divided roughly into acute and chronic effects. Acute effects are usually seen during the course of (or immediately following) therapy, whereas late effects may develop at times varying from several months to as late as 5 to 10 years following therapy.

In general, the acute effects reflect the cellular dose-survival characteristics of the tissue and physiologic phenomena resulting from cell killing (e.g., altered proliferation kinetics such as repopulation and recruitment). Normal tissues typically involved in acute radiation reactions include the bone marrow, gastrointestinal tract, skin, oropharynx, and bladder. Bone marrow depression, mucositis, hair loss, and gastrointestinal upset are ultimately the result of failure to maintain the integrity of the proliferative compartments of the corresponding cell-renewal systems.

Late damage to various critical organs can result from: (1) loss of parenchymal cells; (2) injury to the fine vasculature; (3) dysfunction of fibrocytes; or (4) a combination of the above. Histologically a gradual disappearance in both the number of cells in the vascular compartment of the organ and in the functioning of parenchymal cells is observed. Injury in many of these organs appears to be due to damage to the capillary network and small arterioles, as well as primary loss of functional cells.

SYSTEMIC EFFECTS OF RADIOTHERAPY

RADIATION SICKNESS

Radiation sickness is manifested clinically by headache, anorexia, nausea, and vomiting. It is thought to be related to absorption of breakdown products of the irradiated tissues and, consequently, the incidence and severity are related to the volume of tissue treated and the daily dose. Radiation sickness is more apt to occur when the abdomen is included within the treatment field; in contrast, large daily doses may be administered to the head and neck and to the extremities without producing this complication. Radiation sickness can be prevented or minimized, in most instances, by adjusting the treatment technique (i.e., reduction in the daily dosage or in the volume of tissue treated). Antiemetic drugs may also be useful in controlling symptoms. It is important to recognize that the symptoms of radiation sickness are short-lived, usually disappearing within 48 hours after the last dose of radiation; consequently, persistence of these symptoms for a period of greater than 48 hours after the conclusion of treatment requires a careful search for some other etiology.

BONE MARROW SUPPRESSION

Rapid fall in the white count and platelet count may occur as a result of irradiation to large portions of the red marrow. When the trunk is irradiated, blood counts should be followed carefully (at least two to three times per week). Usually these values begin to decrease during the second week of treatment and reach their nadir during the third and fourth weeks. Treatment should be interrupted if the absolute neutrophil count decreases below 600/mm^3 or the total white count falls below 2000/mm^3.[13]

The degree of bone marrow suppression can be related to the volume of functional bone marrow within the field of irradiation and the dosage of radiation applied. In the adult over 20 years of age, 25 to 40 per cent of the functional marrow is in the spine, 15 to 40 per cent in the pelvis, and 10 to 30 per cent in the sternum and ribs;[1] in children these proportions may be lower because of active marrow in the long bones.

SKIN AND MUCOUS MEMBRANE REACTIONS

Skin and mucous membrane reactions may develop following radiotherapy to many areas of the body. The initial skin reaction may be erythematous and this may be followed by desquamation or a moist "radioepidermitis" consisting of denuded dermis covered by a thin layer of fibrin. In the absence of secondary infection these lesions usually are painless. Bronzing and scaling of the epidermis may follow. Desquamation reactions may be treated with mild lubricating ointments. Powders containing heavy metals should be avoided during treatments, since they may augment the radiation effects. Heavily perfumed soaps, lotions, and underarm deodorants also should not be applied to irradiated areas. If the desquamation is moist in character, the area should be kept clean and excessive crust removed by soaking. Local antibiotics should be applied if the area becomes infected. After the healing of a moderately severe reaction, the skin may appear grossly normal but it is never biologically normal. Injuries or infections may cause reactions limited to the treated volume; for instance, erythema may reappear following systemic treatment with actinomycin D. When the radiation dosage has been high enough to cause vascular damage, an "x-ray burn" characterized by local necrosis may result.

The initial reaction of a mucous membrane to irradiation also is erythema; this may gradually progress to a mucositis characterized by a white glistening membrane overlying the surface. Histologically this is an accumulation of desquamated cells, leukocytes, and fibrin associated with destruction and desquamation of the superficial layers of the epithelium. Local anesthetics can alleviate symptoms in the mouth, pharynx, and esophagus.

LOCAL EFFECTS OF RADIOTHERAPY

Head

In almost every instance, when the skull is irradiated, epilation will result. Hair regrows except in those rare circumstances when a part of the scalp has received a dose considerably in excess of 6000 rads. Except for bony lesions of the skull, the head is usually irradiated only in prophylactic treatment of acute lymphoblastic leukemia (2000 to 2400 rads) and in the treatment of primary malignant tumors of the brain (4000 to 6000 rads). The only CNS effect of the lower dose level has been the observation that some children receiving prophylactic irradiation for leukemia experience a transient period of somnolence following completion of the treatment. No late effects on pituitary or hypothalamic function have been observed and no alteration in intellect is apparent.

The treatment of primary brain tumors involves a limited volume in a sensitive portion of the brain (tumor about the third ventricle) or the entire brain (medulloblastoma). In these instances it is frequently difficult to separate the acute effects of ionizing radiation from those of the trauma associated with the growth of the tumor and neurosurgical procedures. Late effects other than necrosis from excessive dose are not well defined. The recent report by Richards and associates[23] suggests that irradiation in the region of the pituitary-hypothalamic area results in deficiencies, particularly of growth hormone. The oldest child studied was eight at the time of irradiation. All received doses in the range of 4000 to 5000 rads. The mechanism is not entirely clear since it has also been observed that children with Cushing's disease may resume growth following pituitary-hypothalamic irradiation with similar doses. In general, these doses are employed in the treatment of astrocytomas, third ventricular tumors, ependymomas, and medulloblastomas. No clear-cut evidence of impaired intellectual function has been found in treated survivors.

Not infrequently, the ear is included in the treatment of malignant brain tumors and serous otitis may develop, as well as an external otitis secondary to desquamation in the external canal. Doses of 4000 to 6000 rads have no known effect on the acoustic nerve; however, loss of high tone discrimination may result following irradiation.

Defects can develop in the teeth as a result of suppression or qualitative alteration of saliva when the salivary glands are included within the field of irradiation. The most frequent changes are multiple, superficial defects usually affecting the crowns of the teeth. Consequently, the patient should be followed closely by an oral surgeon/dentist and maintain a good oral hygiene program.

ORBIT

The orbit and its contents may be included in the beam at any of the three dose levels. In the case of leukemic infiltrates along the optic nerve or choroid, doses of about 2000 rads have been employed. In the case of retinoblastoma, doses of 3500 to 4500 rads are generally recommended, and for rhabdomyosarcoma of the orbit, primary treatment with 5000 to 6000 rads is used. It is well known that the lens is one of the most sensitive of normal tissues. When the lens is subjected to any of the three dose levels, a radiation cataract can be expected to develop. The time for development of a cataract may be measured in years and is dose-dependent. In the higher dose ranges, the retina itself may be threatened, as well as the cornea, if care if not taken to avoid high doses on the surface. Retinal and vitreous hemorrhages are frequently encountered complications in the dose range of 4000 to 6000 rads. If the lacrimal gland has been treated at the higher dose level, production of tears may diminish and the surface of the eye will be prone to chronic irritation. Fortunately, the availability of artificial tears has limited this problem.

Depending upon the age of the child, the irradiated facial bones about the orbit may show some growth deformity. In general, however, other facial bones are rarely included except in cases of metastatic disease or when smaller doses are employed, as for histiocytosis X. An exception to this is the rare primary Ewing's tumor of the mandible.

CHEST

The doses employed in treatment of tumors that arise in the lung, mediastinum, or thoracic cage are usually in the range of 1000 to 2000 or 2000 to 4000 rads. Some degree of radiation pneumonitis can be expected in all children who receive a dose of 2000 rads to both lungs. Severe, possibly fatal, respiratory insufficiency may develop if more than 75 per cent of the pulmonary tissues have received this dose. However, fatal radiation pneumonitis may occur even with doses below 2000 rads, particularly if the patient has received prior therapy with actinomycin D.[3]

Radiation pneumonitis may present as two clinical entities: (1) an acute exudative pneumonitis which occurs 1 to 2 months after treatment; or (2) interstitial fibrosis appearing several months to several years after treatment.

Radiation pneumonitis may be asymptomatic, associated with a dry, hacking cough and mild exertional dyspnea, or it may progress to severe respiratory distress, spiking temperature, and cor pulmonale. Steroids are probably best reserved for the patient with moderately severe dyspnea and should not be used if only asymptomatic radiologic findings are present. Once steroids are instituted, they must be tapered slowly, as rapid cessation frequently results in a rebound of symptoms and pulmonary infiltrates.

In practice, both lungs are irradiated in the combined treatment of metastatic Wilms' tumor to a dose of 1200 to 1500 rads. A small part of lung tissue may be treated with a higher dose if a nodule persists following the initial whole lung treatment. The clinical sequelae will be minimal.

Thoracic neuroblastoma is usually treated with doses of 2000 to 3500 rads to a field that includes a limited volume of lung. No significant pulmonary sequelae are expected. In the very young child treated in this manner, significant skeletal and muscle deformities may occur.

In the treatment of Hodgkin's disease (Stages I, II, and III) a large field mantle technique with lung shielding and doses of 4000 rads are employed. In children and adults with large mediastinal masses, we have favored initial treatment with chemotherapy to reduce the mediastinal mass so that greater amounts of lung can be shielded.

Radiation-induced heart disease is most commonly manifested as acute pericarditis and less commonly as myocarditis. Pericarditis, if it develops, usually occurs within a year after completion of therapy. It is manifested by pleuritic chest pain, a pericardial friction rub, ECG abnormalities, and enlargement of the cardiac silhouette on x-ray. We have seen cases in which children who received 3000 to 4000 rads to the aorta have developed aortic hypoplasia coincident with the margins of the irradiated volume. Others have observed similar changes in the abdominal aorta and other large arteries.

Of greater importance with large midline fields is the spinal cord tolerance, which varies with dose, fractionation, and length of cord irradiated. In general, doses of 4000 rads or less given in daily fractionation over 1 month are not likely to cause clinically evident spinal cord damage. Radiation myelitis occurs in two clinical forms: transient and progressive. The transient form is reversible and complete recovery is possible; symptoms include numbness or hyperesthesia in the limbs. One form of this is *Lhermitte's syndrome*, which consists of electrical paresthesiae in the upper and lower extremities induced by anterior flexion of the head. There are no demonstrable neurologic defects and the condition gradually disappears over the subsequent three to four months. Progressive myelitis, on the other hand, is not reversible and is clinically manifested by a weakness or paralysis of muscles. Once the neurologic signs and symptoms have become severe, they rarely disappear and may progress to partial cord transection.

ABDOMEN

Doses employed in treatment of the localized forms of both Wilms' tumor and neuroblastoma are similar and range from 2000 rads in the very young to 3500 rads in older children. In the usual case, the flank is irradiated. All or part of other organs may of necessity be included in the volume irradiated. These include liver, large and small bowel, stomach, spleen, adrenal glands, and large arteries.

Fortunately, there are only a few situations where whole abdominal irradiation is necessary in childhood (Stage III dysgerminoma, Wilms' tumor with gross contamination, and non-Hodgkin's lymphoma confined to the abdomen). Generally, weekly doses in the range of 600 to 800 rads are tolerated depending on the general condition of the child, and a total dose of 2000 to 3000 rads is given with appropriate shielding of liver and kidney as mentioned above. Para-aortic and iliac lymph node irradiation as employed in the treatment of Hodgkin's disease at doses of about 4000 rads is usually well tolerated. The major sequela will be hematopoietic depression from inclusion of a large portion of the pelvic bone marrow.

Radiation of vertebral bodies results in early epiphyseal closure and growth arrest (for doses in excess of 2000 rads).[18] Children are especially sensitive to irradiation of the vertebral column when under 6 years of age and at the time of the adolescent growth spurt.[22] Consequently, the treatment portals should extend across the entire body of the relevant vertebrae in order to avoid scoliosis. Although the eventual height that the patient will reach is somewhat shorter than if he were untreated, stature is not severely affected, since normally only 2 to 4 vertebrae are in the treatment field.

We have seen three children given doses of irradiation to the renal bed following nephrectomy for Wilms' tumor in whom the right colon appeared hypoplastic years after irradiation. There are other instances of apparent hypoplasia of that portion of the abdominal aorta included in the field.

Radiation Nephritis

The symptoms of acute radiation nephritis usually appear within 6 months of irradiation with doses in the range of 2000 rads over three to five weeks;[16] they include lassitude, headache, dyspnea, vomiting, nocturia, and peripheral edema. Severe hypertension may also be present. Laboratory findings include proteinuria, hyposthenuria, azotemia, and a normochromic, normocytic anemia. Chronic radiation nephritis usually becomes manifest about 18 months or later after radiotherapy. The clinical course consists of slowly progressive anemia, hypertension, and impairment of renal function. Such patients may eventually succumb to the effects of chronic uremia, malignant hypertension, or congestive heart failure. This late phase of radiation nephropathy is primarily contingent upon the severity of the sclerosis of the small and medium arteries.[28] This late stage may seemingly arise de novo after several years of well-being in which the patient was asymptomatic.

Radiation Hepatitis

Doses to the whole of the liver should not exceed 2500 rads, and these should be modified downwards if given in association with a recent partial hepatectomy or adjuvant chemotherapy. After doses of between 3500 to 4000 rads, nearly half the patients will show radiation damage, and with doses of over 4000 rads, 75 per cent will develop radiation hepatitis.[11] The presenting symptoms of radiation hepatitis are usually an insidious enlargement of the liver with ascites appearing 2 to 6 weeks following radiotherapy. Jaundice is not usually observed initially but may develop later on. Elevated serum alkaline phosphatase levels appear to correlate well with the degree of functional injury. Levels of the other hepatic enzymes (e.g., SGOT, LDH) may also be increased. The pathologic picture of this acute phase is characterized by hepatic cell necrosis, centrilobular vein thrombosis, and connective tissue proliferation within the lumen of the small efferent veins. Owing to the remarkable ability of the liver parenchyma to regenerate, a major portion of the liver can be severely compromised without hepatic failure developing. Thus, 4000 to 5000 rads may be delivered over several weeks to a large segment of the liver without producing severe functional impairment;[26] however, severe structural damage may occur. Hepatic fibrosis may be a later sequela of the structural damage occurring following acute irradiation injury to the liver.

Radiation Enteritis

Intestinal injury ("radiation enteritis") may follow whole abdominal radiation in childhood. The symptoms of this complication include vomiting, diarrhea, malabsorption, and inability to tolerate oral fluid; partial or complete bowel obstruction may be an occasional late sequela. Histologic appearance of the bowel at the time of delayed radiation injury shows severe villus blunting, lymphatic dilatation, and moderately dense inflammatory infiltrate.[7] A fractionated low-residue, low-fat diet which is free of gluten and protein derived from cow's milk appears to be useful in managing this complication.[7]

Pelvis

Except for the rare case of leukemic involvement of the ovary and early stage dysgerminoma, the pelvis is rarely treated with doses in the lower ranges. More typically, doses of 3000 to 5000 rads are employed and the sequelae will be discussed for that range. Tumors encountered in childhood include soft tissue sarcomas, malignant sacrococcygeal teratomas, and Ewing's sarcoma.

The bladder mucosa tolerates significant doses of radiation except in combination with cyclophosphamide, when acute cystitis may result in severe hemorrhage.

The germ cells of both male and female gonads, on the other hand, are very sensitive to radiation, and permanent sterility will probably occur after fractionated doses of 1000 to 1200 rads.[28] The interstitial (Leydig) cells of the testis are less sensitive to radiation and, consequently, testosterone production and the development of secondary sexual characteristics are not affected. The ovary is more sensitive to radiation than the testis, and doses as low as 200 rads may produce appreciable cellular death.[30] The granulosa cells are also relatively radiosensitive and, consequently, the production of estrogen and the development of secondary female characteristics are likely to be adversely affected by the radiotherapy dosages used for treatment of most pelvic tumors.

When the large intestine is irradiated, watery diarrhea and intermittent cramping may develop. When the rectum is included in the irradiated volume, rectal discomfort or tenesmus with mucus or blood in the stool may develop.

In treating sarcomas of the vagina, bladder, and prostate, care should be taken to avoid as much of the pelvic bony structure as possible. Some of the worst deformities result from irradiation of the bony pelvis in infancy. In addition, as much bone marrow as possible should be spared by careful attention to this detail. In the case of Ewing's sarcoma, however, usually a very large volume encompassing the primary bony site and most of the pelvic organs is necessary. Since these children are usually over eight years of age, the bony sequelae will not be as prominent, but marrow reserve may be impaired and limit the use of chemotherapy.

Extremities

Tumors arising primarily from the extremities (Ewing's sarcoma and soft tissue sarcomas) generally require doses of 4000 to 6000 rads over 4 to 6 weeks for eradication. The higher doses are usually given to only a part of the extremity after an initial 4000 to 5000 rads is delivered to the whole of the bone, as in the case of Ewing's sarcoma, or to the muscle compartment, as in the case of soft tissue sarcoma. Two points are important in treating extremities. The skin of an extremity (particularly in a small child) does not have the same tolerance to irradiation as does the skin over the trunk of the body, and a severe moist desquamation may be observed in the skin of an extremity at doses of only one half to two thirds that expected for the same complication on the trunk. Second, with doses of about 4500 rads, the soft tissues distal to the part of the extremity irradiated may undergo atrophy and contracture from a lack of sufficient blood flow through the vasculo-connective tissue irradiated proximally. This can best be avoided by sparing, if possible, a strip of normal soft tissue in the irradiated volume after a dose of 4000 rads. A poorly functioning limb following irradiation is not an acceptable sequela, since preservation of good function is the sole purpose in irradiating malignant tumors of the extremity. Both bone and muscle will suffer some degree of atrophy with the doses employed. The bone changes may be without clinical consequences until the bones are stressed; however, once complications develop (e.g., pathologic fracture, osteomyelitis), they may be difficult to treat. Consequently, prevention of stress to these areas needs to be emphasized.

INTERACTION BETWEEN RADIATION THERAPY AND CANCER CHEMOTHERAPY

It is rare indeed when a child treated with radiation is not also receiving concomitant chemotherapy. Since both modalities of treatment may compete for critical normal tissue tolerance, it is imperative that the collaborating radiation therapist and chemotherapist clearly define the intent and limitations of each modality as it relates to cure and identify the demands on normal tissue anticipated from each modality. During treatment, careful monitoring of bone marrow reserve and gastrointestinal toxicity, as well as of pulmonary, cardiac, renal, hepatic, and urinary tract manifestations of the combined therapies, is mandatory.

Certain antitumor drugs, particularly the antineoplastic antibiotics actinomycin D, Adriamycin, and bleomycin appear to be broad-spectrum augmentors of radiation injury.[19, 20] With the exception of the brain and eye, all other organs may show enhanced injury when these agents are used in combination with radiotherapy. As a result of this sensitization, the total effect of the drug and radiation together is greater than the sum of the expected number of cells killed from radiation alone and from the drug alone. This augmentation effect occurs not only when the drug is given concurrently with radiation, but can also occur as a "recall" phenomenon when the drug is administered at a later date after radiation. This is most prominent in the skin, where a reactivation of the erythematous and sometimes desquamating reaction may occur within the radiation field.

A second class of drug-radiation interaction appears to involve agents which are themselves toxic to normal tissues. Thus, agents that have specific critical organ toxicity when used alone are highly dangerous when used in combination with radiation doses that also injure the organ. Examples of this are the enhanced toxicity of Adriamycin with radiation on the heart, methotrexate with radiation on the brain, and cyclophosphamide with radiation on the bladder.

The augmentation of radiation dose damage by cancer chemotherapeutic agents is a serious problem in a wide range of tissues necessitating accurate knowledge of the dose-effect factor and appropriate modification of the radiation treatment.

LATE EFFECTS OF IRRADIATION

The long-term effects of radiotherapy may be subtle, requiring the passage of months, if not years, to become manifest. They include aberrations of growth and development, impairment of the functional capacity of various organs, oncogenesis, and gonadal effects with varying degrees of infertility and genetic consequences.[6]

Li and Stone[15] have reported that half of the long-term survivors of childhood cancer in their series had some major defect attributable to their therapy, and many of these defects related to the deleterious effects of irradiation on growing skeletal and muscular tissues.

The risk of tumor development following irradiation appears to follow a linear dose-response pattern. Examples of malignancies developing following radiation exposure include: (1) leukemia—1 to 2 cases per 10^6 persons per year per rad (atomic bomb irradiation),[24] (2) thyroid cancer—2.5 cases per 10^6 persons per year per rad (following irradiation to the neck and chest),[9] (3) bone tumors—4 cases per 10^6 persons per year per rad (following internally absorbed radium in radium dial workers).[8] Li and associates recently reviewed the late effects in 414 long-term survivors of childhood cancer and found a 12 per cent cumulative probability of a second cancer within 20 years after initial diagnosis. Most of the second malignancies were soft tissue and bone sarcomas arising in previously irradiated tissues.

REFERENCES

1. Atkinson, H. R.: Bone marrow distribution as a factor in estimating radiation to the blood-forming organs. A survey of present knowledge. J. Coll. Radiol. Aust. 6:149, 1962.
2. Bloomer, W. D., and Hellman, S.: Normal tissue responses to radiation therapy. N. Engl. J. Med. 293:80, 1975.
3. Braun, S. R., Dolico, G. A., Olson, C. E., and Caldwell, W.: Low-dose radiation pneumonitis. Cancer 35:1322, 1975.
4. Casarett, G. W.: Similarities and contrasts between radiation and time pathology. In Strehler, B. (ed.): Advances in Gerotological Research. Vol. 1. New York, Academic Press, 1964.
5. Committee for Radiation Oncology Studies: Normal tissue tolerance and damage. Cancer 37:2046, 1976.
6. D'Angio, G. J.: The late consequences of successful cancer treatment given children and adolescents. Radiology 114:145, 1975.
7. Donaldson, S. S., Jundt, S., Ricour, C., et al.: Radiation enteritis in children. A retrospective review, clinicopathologic correlation, and dietary management. Cancer 35:1167, 1975.
8. Hasterlik, R. J., Finkel, A. J., and Miller, C. E.: The late effects of radium deposition in man. Radiation Standards. Part II. 87th Congress of the United States, second session, pp. 943–946, 1963.
9. Hempelmann, L. H., Pifer, J. W., Burke, G. J., et al.: Neoplasms in persons treated with x-rays in infancy for thymic enlargement—A report of the third follow-up survey. J. Natl. Cancer Inst. 38:317, 1967.
10. Hendee, W. R.: Medical Radiation Physics. Chicago, Year Book Medical Publishers, 1970.
11. Ingold, J. A., Reed, G. B., Kaplan, H. S., and Bagshaw, M. A.: Radiation hepatitis. Am. J. Roentgenol. 93:200, 1965.
12. Johns, H. E.: The Physics of Radiology. Springfield, Ill., Charles C Thomas, 1969.
13. Kligerman, M. M.: Principles of radiation therapy. In Holland, J. F., and Frei, E., III (eds.): Cancer Medicine. Philadelphia, Lea & Febiger, 1973.
14. Li, F. P., Cassady, J. R., and Jaffe, N.: Risk of second tumors in survivors of childhood cancer. Cancer 35:1230, 1975.
15. Li, F. P., and Stone, R.: Survivors of childhood cancer. Ann. Int. Med. 84:551, 1976.
16. Luxton, R. W., and Kunkler, P. B.: Radiation nephritis. Acta Radiol. 2:169, 1962.
17. Moss, W. T., Brand, W. N., and Battifora, H.: Radiation Oncology. 4th Ed. St. Louis, C. V. Mosby Co., 1973.
18. Parker, R. G., and Berry, H. C.: Late effects of therapeutic irradiation in the skeleton and bone marrow. Cancer 37:1162, 1976.
19. Phillips, T. L., and Fu, K. K.: Quantification of combined radiation therapy and chemotherapy effects on critical normal tissues. Cancer 37:1186, 1976.
20. Phillips, T. L., Wharam, M. D., and Margolis, L. W.: Modification of radiation injury to normal tissues by chemotherapeutic agents. Cancer 35:1678, 1975.
21. Pizzarello, D. J., and Witcofski, R. L.: Medical Radiation Biology. Philadelphia, Lea & Febiger, 1972.
22. Probert, J. C., and Parker, B. R.: The effects of radiation therapy on bone growth. Radiology 114:155, 1975.
23. Richards, G. E., Wara, W. M., Grumbach, M. M., Kaplan, S. L., Sheline, G. E., and Conte, F. A.: Delayed onset of hypopituitarism: sequelae of therapeutic irradiation of central nervous system, eye, and middle ear tumors. J. Pediatr. 89:553, 1976.
24. Rubin, P., and Casarett, G. W.: Clinical Radiation Pathology. Philadelphia, W. B. Saunders Co., 1968.

25. Rubin, P., Landman, S., Mayer, E., et al.: Bone marrow regeneration and extension after extended field irradiation in Hodgkin's disease. Cancer 32:699, 1973.
26. Seydel, H. G.: The risk of tumor induction in man following medical irradiation for malignant neoplasm. Cancer 35:1641, 1975.
27. United Nations Scientific Committee on the Effects of Atomic Radiation: Ionizing Radiation—Levels and Effects. New York, United Nations, 1972.
28. White, D. C.: The histopathologic basis for function decrements in late radiation injury in diverse organs. Cancer 37:1126, 1976.
29. Withers, H. R.: Capacity for repair in cells of normal and malignant tissues. *In* Time and Dose Relationships in Radiation Biology as Applied to Radiotherapy. Upton, N.Y., Brookhaven National Laboratory, Associated Universities, Inc., 1970.
30. Zuckerman, S.: The sensitivity of the gonads to radiation. Clin. Radiol. 16:1, 1965.

Chapter Five

TUMOR IMMUNOLOGY AND IMMUNOTHERAPY

The fundamental thesis of tumor immunology is that cells undergoing neoplastic change acquire new antigens (*tumor-specific antigens*), which the immune system can identify as "foreign", and as a consequence, humoral and cell-mediated immune responses are elicited, which may result in tumor rejection. According to this concept, clinical cancer develops when the immune system is intrinsically defective, when the growing tumor fails to elicit an appropriate immunologic response, or when the rejection reaction is overwhelmed by the tumor or its products. The goal of immunotherapy is to tip the immunologic balance in the host's favor.

TUMOR ANTIGENS

The majority of animal tumors and all tumors that have been properly evaluated in man manifest antigens which are recognizable as foreign by the immune system.[46a] In experimental systems "new" antigens are found in all tumors induced by chemical carcinogens, oncogenic viruses, or foreign bodies; they may also be found, to a lesser extent, in some "spontaneous" tumors.[75] These tumor-associated antigens have been demonstrated within the cell nucleus, in the cytoplasm, on the cell membrane, or as extracellular products.

Chemically, tumor antigens appear to be very similar to histocompatibility (HLA) antigens; that is, they are probably glycoproteins with molecular weights of approximately 50,000. Some of these antigens (*oncofetal antigens*) appear to be similar to embryonic or fetal antigens; these may reappear as a result of derepression during malignant transformation of genetic information normally repressed in adult cells. The best-characterized oncofetal antigens are *carcinoembryonic antigen* (CEA) and *alpha-fetoprotein* (AFP). These are discussed in Chapter 2.

Chemical carcinogens and physical agents (e.g., ionizing radiation) generally induce tumor-specific antigens that are unique for each tumor; tumors induced by oncogenic viruses, on the other hand, have tumor-specific transplantation antigens that are specific for all tumors induced by the same virus regardless of the morphology or biology of the tumor. These virus-induced antigens are of two major types: (1) structural viral antigens regularly detectable in RNA virus-induced tumors that continually shed virus from the cell membrane; and (2) newly formed antigens not present either in the normal cells prior to neoplastic transformation or in the viral particles.[105, 107, 120]

A number of human tumors have been shown to be antigenic; among these are Burkitt's lymphoma, melanoma, neuroblastoma, lymphoreticular tumors, carcinomas of the breast, colon, and bladder, and soft tissue sarcomas.

Clinical evidence of immune responses to tumor antigens in humans may be summarized as follows.

1. Certain human tumors manifest local accumulations of lymphocytes, and there is a positive correlation between the relative intensity of lymphoid cell accumulation and the length of survival.[6, 19, 65, 71]

2. Some cancer patients have demonstrable delayed hypersensitivity skin tests to extracts of the membranes of their own tumors as well as to extracts of homologous tumors of the same type; these responses show some correlation with the clinical course.[26, 52]

3. Spontaneous remission has been reported in more than 130 human tumors; over half of these tumors were neuroblastomas, choriocarcinomas, renal adenocarcinomas, and malignant melanomas, tumor types for which immunologic responses of the host to the tumor have been demonstrated.[24, 98]

4. Lymphocytes from cancer patients are often reactive in vitro to their own tumor cells as well as to tumor cells cultured from other patients with the same type of neoplasm; this phenomenon occurs whether the patients are in remission or have actively growing tumors.[45] However, no specific in vitro reactivity to tumor cells is seen with lymphocytes from patients with other forms of cancer or from healthy subjects.[45]

THE IMMUNE SYSTEM AND CANCER

Adaptive immunity in humans is subserved by the cells of the lymphoid system. These cells arise from the primitive pluripotent cells located in the bone marrow;[1, 61, 114, 120] they then migrate to lymphoid organs where, under appropriate inductive influences, they differentiate into functional, immunologically competent lymphocytes (Fig. 5–1). Two distinct populations of circulating lymphocytes have been well characterized (Table 5–1): (1) those that are processed by the thymus gland (*T-lymphocytes*) and take part in cellular immune reactions (delayed hypersensitivity, allograft rejection, and graft-versus-host reactions); and (2) those that are independent of the thymus (*B-lymphocytes*) and act as precursors for the cells that synthesize the various circulating immunoglobulins. A third subpopulation, known as "null" cells, lacks recognizable characteristics of both T- and B-cells; these cells proba-

Table 5–1 Characteristics of T- and B-Lymphocytes

	SITE OF MATURATION	IMMUNOLOGIC FUNCTION	MARKERS
T-cell	Thymus	Delayed hypersensitivity Homograft rejection	Sheep erythrocyte receptors Human T-lymphocyte antigens (HTLA) Terminal deoxynucleotidyl transferase
B-cell	Bone Marrow	Antibody formation	Surface immunoglobulins Receptors for C'3 components and IgG

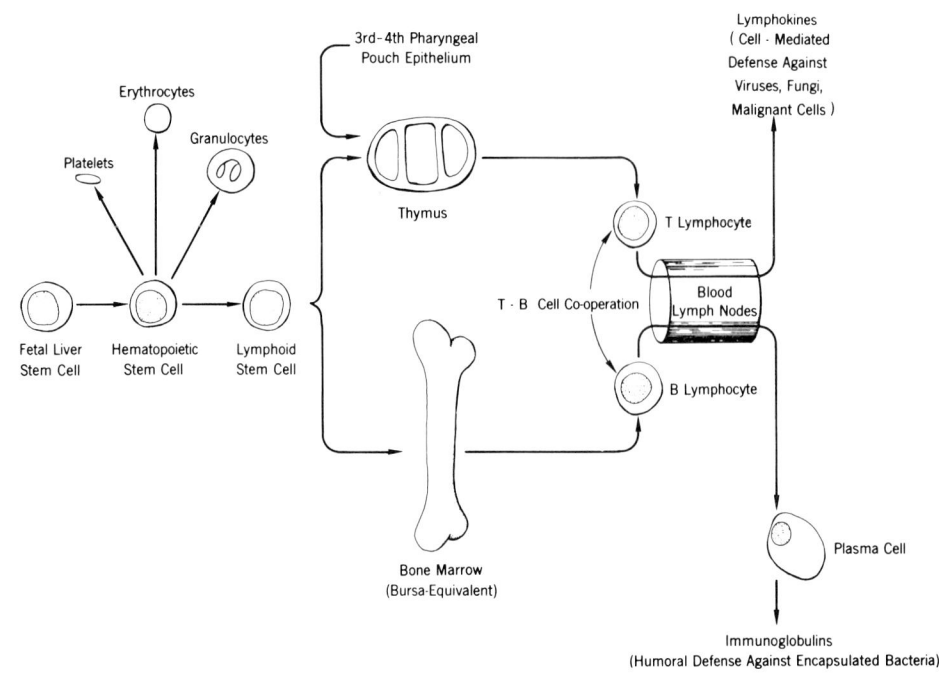

Figure 5-1 Pathways of differentiation of human lymphocytes. (From Kersey, J. H., Gajl-Peczalska, K. J., and Nesbit, M. E.: J. Pediatr. 84:789, 1974.)

bly represent a heterogeneous group consisting of hematopoietic stem cells, precursors to T- and B-cells, and other lymphocytes of unknown function. A unique class of lymphocytes, not yet fully characterized, is the "natural killer" or K-cell variant.

T-Cells

T-cells arise from a subpopulation of lymphocytes in the bone marrow that is committed to T-cell differentiation (*prothymocytes*). After migrating to the thymus, these cells are "processed" by the thymic microenvironment. This processing, which may involve thymic hormones (*thymosin, thymopoietin,* and possibly others), results in the induction of a set of characteristic markers whereby T-cells may be identified.[36, 37, 61, 104] While in the thymus these cells are known as *thymocytes.* The cells then enter the peripheral circulation, where certain of their markers are lost whereas other markers may be newly acquired.

The major markers for identification of T-cells are a *surface receptor for sheep erythrocytes, a surface human T-lymphocyte antigen (HTLA),* and an enzyme, *terminal deoxynucleotidyl transferase (TdT).*

The *surface receptor for sheep erythrocytes* is present on T-cells during their residence in the thymus and in the circulation.[56, 125] These cells can be identified by their ability to bind sheep erythrocytes (E) in a "rosette-like" configuration (Fig. 5-2); thymocytes form these rosettes at both 4°C and 37°C, whereas the more mature peripheral blood T-cells form rosettes only at 4°C.[7] Using such techniques, it has been demonstrated that 50 to 78 percent of peripheral blood lymphocytes in normal adults are E-rosette forming cells.

Human T-lymphocyte antigen (HTLA) is detected by using anti-

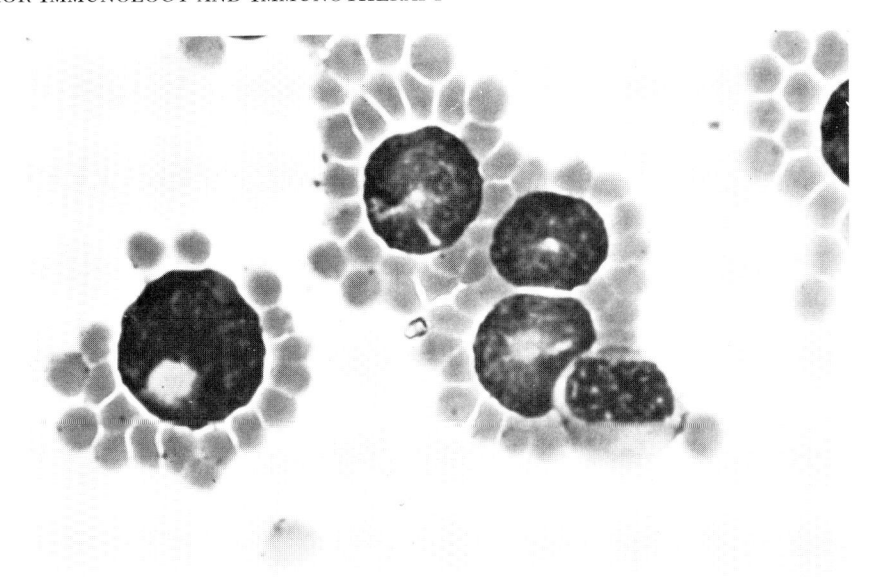

Figure 5–2 Lymphoblasts from a T-cell leukemia showing "rosette" formation with sheep erythrocytes. (Courtesy of Dr. John Quinn.)

serum produced in various animal species against human thymocytes; approximately 50 to 70 per cent of adult human peripheral blood lymphocytes carry this marker.[59] Another surface marker, the *human-thymus leukemia associated antigen* (H-Thy-L) has been demonstrated in extracts of normal thymocytes, but not in peripheral T-lymphocytes.[32]

Terminal deoxynucleotidyl transferase (TdT) is an enzyme which has the unique property of polymerizing polydeoxynucleotides onto a primer in the absence of a template. It has been detected in highest concentrations in thymocytes, but it completely disappears before the final maturation of the T-cell to a circulating lymphocyte.[32, 64, 74]

Cell-Mediated Responses to Tumor. T-lymphocytes play a major role in cellular immunity against fungal, viral, and certain bacterial pathogens; they are also the cells which mediate the delayed hypersensitivity reaction. Functional tests have indicated that T cells are subdivided into *helper cells* (which assist in B-cell function), *suppressor cells* (which regulate the immune response), and *cytotoxic T cells* (which recognize and destroy tumors and allografts in the absence of specific antibody). In experimental systems, T-cells have demonstrated the ability to kill tumor cells both in vivo[5] and in vitro.[8] Activation of T-cells starts a sequence of events which includes cell replication, the emergence of "killer" cells that directly attack "foreign" cells, and the production of lymphokines, which chemically mediate inflammation, macrophage localization, and macrophage activation.

From studies with animal models, it appears that effective immune responses to tumor-specific antigens are similar to any cellular immune response to a weak histocompatibility transplantation antigen.[120] After initial processing there is recognition of the new tumor membrane antigens by interaction with cell surface recognition receptors of long-lived T-lymphocytes. This interaction then triggers proliferation of a clone of cells specifically directed against tumor cells; as these T-lymphocytes undergo blastic transformation, they may release cytotoxic chemical mediators directly or activate macrophages to release these substances.

B-Cells

B-lymphocytes are independent of the thymus and (in humans) may be derived from the bone marrow. In avian species the precursors of B-cells must pass through a gut-associated lymphoid organ (the bursa of Fabricius) before acquiring the characteristics of B-cells. In man, although an equivalent to this organ is presumed to exist, it has not been identified as yet.

B-lymphocytes are identifiable by the presence of *surface immunoglobulins* as well as *surface receptors for heat-aggregated gamma globulin and complement components*. These cells are the precursors of the plasma cells, which synthesize immunoglobulins for humoral immune responses.

Humoral Responses to Tumor. Antitumor antibodies may act by several different mechanisms: (1) direct cytotoxicity—mediated by binding to the tumor cell surface with resultant complement fixation and cell lysis; (2) binding to the surface of lymphocytes or monocytes (*cytophilic antibody*) and "arming" them to become specifically cytotoxic; (3) combining with circulating tumor antigen released from the surface of tumor cells and causing this "blocking factor" to be cleared from the system.

Tumor-specific antibodies have been demonstrated against most common human solid tumors.[108] Some patients who have experienced removal or regression of neuroblastoma, soft tissue sarcomas, and melanoma have circulating antibody that is cytotoxic in vitro for these tumors; this antibody frequently decreases strikingly or disappears at the time of tumor recurrence.[67, 82, 102, 124] Such studies suggest that circulating antibody may be an effective factor in controlling micrometastases when bulk tumor has been removed, but may be overwhelmed when a large source of circulating tumor antigens is present.

K-Cells

Natural killer or K-cells were first described in mice as a unique class of cells manifesting cytotoxic activity to Moloney leukemia. These cells lack both T- and B-cell surface markers. They are found most commonly in the spleen, but small numbers are also found in lymph nodes and bone marrow; they do not occur in the thymus. The cytotoxicity of K-cells appears to be antibody-dependent and involves binding of the Fc portion of the antibody molecule to the surface of the K-cell. Apparently surface receptors for the Fc portion of the antibody molecule are present on the surface of the K-cell; similar (but not necessarily identical) Fc receptors are carried by monocytes and macrophages (for cytophilic antibody), granulocytes, and mast cells (for IgE).

THE EFFECTS OF CANCER ON THE IMMUNE SYSTEM

The presence of a growing tumor interferes with immunologic function in at least two general ways. First, there is a nonspecific and generalized suppression of immunocompetence and second, there is a tumor-specific immunologic deficiency related to the release of "blocking factors" by the growing tumor. In general, the extent of immunosuppression correlates with the stage of the disease and the level of tumor cell burden in the host. Any therapeutic maneuver which reduces tumor bulk may reverse both the nonspecific and specific immunosuppression and alter the immune balance in the patient's favor. Thus, any therapeutic endeavor that reduces the tumor-cell burden is a form of "immunotherapy."

Suppression of Generalized Immunocompetence

Immunodeficiency associated with progressive tumor growth and correlated directly with the size of the tumor burden has been demonstrated

Table 5-2 Tumor-Associated Immunosuppression

DISEASE	MAJOR DEFECT
Hodgkin's disease	Cell-mediated immunity and other T-lymphocyte functions[2, 13, 123]
Chronic lymphocytic leukemia	Reduced immunoglobulin levels and impaired antibody synthesis[15]
Acute leukemia	Cell-mediated immunity[48]
Solid tumors	Cell-mediated immunity[56] Inflammatory response[20, 55]

in Hodgkin's disease, non-Hodgkin's lymphoma, chronic lymphocytic leukemia, chronic myelocytic leukemia, acute lymphocytic leukemia, acute myelocytic leukemia, and various solid tumors (Table 5–2). Such generalized immunosuppression may be mediated by (1) factors released into the serum by the tumor that impair lymphocyte function, (2) stress, (3) nutritional deficiency, (4) the continuing action of carcinogens and oncogenic viruses, (5) intercurrent illnesses, (6) genetic factors, and (7) age (immunologic responses are especially poor during early infancy and old age).

Suppression of Tumor-Specific Immunity—"Blocking Factors"

Studies have shown that a growing neoplasm constantly releases soluble tumor-associated antigens into the bloodstream where they can circulate as free tumor antigen[57] or as "immune complexes" composed of a small fragment of tumor antigen bound to a tumor-specific antibody molecule.[106] Such immune complexes are detectable in the bloodstream of more than one third of cancer patients and in the glomeruli of patients with leukemia and various forms of lymphoma.[117]

These "blocking factors" have been demonstrated to block the lymphocyte-mediated destruction of tumor cells in vitro[41, 44, 45] and it may be both logical and consistent with available evidence to postulate that either blocking factor–like complexes or free tumor antigen fragments behave in vivo by the same mechanisms that govern in vitro activity—i.e., by either blocking specific lymphocyte recognition of tumor cells or triggering the lymphocytes ineffectively in sites remote from the tumor mass.[108] These mechanisms may act first regionally, on draining lymph nodes, and then, as the tumor evolves, systemically.

CANCER IN THE IMMUNOLOGICALLY DERANGED HOST—THE IMMUNOLOGIC SURVEILLANCE HYPOTHESIS

The immunologic surveillance hypothesis proposes that the immune system constantly monitors the body for the appearance of "foreign" tumor cells[9, 10] and that clinical cancer arises when this host control system against neoplasia breaks down. One of the major corollaries of this hypothesis is that there should be a major increase in the incidence of neoplasms in the immunologically deranged host. In humans there are at least four circumstances in which immunodeficiency or immunologic abnormalities are associated with an increased incidence of malignancy: (1) primary immunodeficiency diseases, (2) immunosuppressive chemotherapy, (3) autoimmune diseases, and (4) aging.

It is tempting, therefore, to speculate that the high incidence of malignancy in immunologically deranged individuals is related to defective immunosurveillance. However, in that event one would expect that the relative frequency of the various types of tumors seen in such individuals would be similar to that for the general population; for example, acute lymphoblastic leukemia, central nervous system tumors, and neuroblastoma should be the predominant malignancies seen in immunologically defective children. This however, does not turn out to be the case. For instance, when the types of tumors which develop in children with primary immunodeficiency diseases were compared with those of the general United States population, a much higher proportion of lymphoreticular solid tumors was found in the former group. Whereas lymphoreticular tumors constituted only 8 per cent of all malignancies in the general childhood population, they accounted for 67 per cent of the tumors in the immunodeficient children[60, 62] (Table 5-3). Likewise, patients receiving immunosuppressive medications following organ transplant have a relatively increased incidence of lymphoreticular malignancy.

Although most cases of malignant lymphoma reported in immunologically deranged patients have been classified as "reticulum cell sarcoma," some authors believe that many of these tumors represent a distinctive histologic entity. The tumors contain a monotonous proliferation of cells resembling phytohemagglutinin-stimulated peripheral lymphocytes in culture or the paracortical cells of antigen-stimulated lymph nodes;[72] such cells have been termed "immunoblasts" and the tumors "immunoblastic sarcomas." The anatomic distribution of these lymphoproliferative tumors is also distinctive; in transplant patients 46 per cent involve the central nervous system and in 33 per cent the lesion is confined to these areas,[72] as compared to a 0.4 to 1.5 per cent involvement of the central nervous system by malignant lymphomas arising in nontransplant patients.

The relatively high incidence of lymphoreticular malignancy seen in immunologically defective individuals suggests the possibility that a damaged lymphoid system may be more prone to develop malignant transformation than a normal one, particularly in the face of chronic antigenic stimulation (possibly by oncogenic viruses).

Primary Immunodeficiency Diseases. In 1974 Kersey and associates[62] reported for the Immunodeficiency–Cancer Registry that a total of

Table 5-3 A Comparison of the Forms of Cancer Seen in the General Pediatric Population With Those Seen in Children With Immunodeficiency Diseases[60]

TUMOR TYPE	RELATIVE MORTALITY RATES (PER CENT)	
	General Pediatric Population	Children With Immunodeficiency Diseases
Leukemia (all types)	48	25
Central nervous system	16	4
Lymphoreticular ("reticulum cell sarcoma," lymphosarcoma, etc.)	8	67
Bone	4	2
Other	24	2

60 children under 15 years of age were known to have died of cancer. These included:

Severe combined immunodeficiency	9 cases
X-linked immunodeficiency	4 cases
Wiskott-Aldrich syndrome	14 cases
Ataxia-telangiectasia	29 cases
Variable (late-onset) immunodeficiency	3 cases
IgA deficiency	1 case

They estimated the mortality rate for cancer in children with primary immunodeficiency to be 0.8 per 100 per year; this is approximately 100 times the mortality rate for cancer in the general childhood population (0.007 per 100 per year).[78]

SEVERE COMBINED IMMUNODEFICIENCY DISEASE (SCID). SCID represents the most extreme form of functional deficiency of both T- and B-lymphocytes; patients with this disorder lack both humoral (B-cell) and cellular (T-cell) immune responses. They are unable to produce circulating antibody in response to antigenic stimuli and have very low immunoglobulin levels; they are also profoundly lymphopenic and cannot mount in vivo or in vitro cellular immune reactions. As a result of their severe immunologic defect, these patients are very susceptible to infections with fungi, viruses, protozoa, and bacteria of low pathogenicity.

SCID is a heterogeneous entity with a variable inheritance pattern (autosomal recessive, sex-linked, and sporadic) and some patients are deficient in the enzymes adenosine deaminase and nucleoside phosphorylase.

The incidence of malignancy in SCID has been estimated at 2 per cent.[60] Particularly noteworthy is the high incidence of lymphoreticular malignancies (leukemia, lymphosarcoma, Hodgkin's disease) in the first 2 years of life, a period during which solid lymphoid malignancies are virtually unknown in immunologically normal children.

INFANTILE X-LINKED AGAMMAGLOBULINEMIA (BRUTON TYPE). This appears to be a disorder of B-cells. Patients so afflicted have low serum immunoglobulin levels and lack humoral immunity, but have normal cellular immune responses. They suffer mainly from infections with encapsulated pyogenic organisms (pneumococcus, *H. influenzae*, streptococcus, meningococcus, and *Pseudomonas aeruginosa*).

The estimated risk of malignancy in patients with Bruton's disease is 6 per cent; lymphoreticular malignancies and leukemia are the most common tumor types.[60]

DIGEORGE SYNDROME. This results from embryonic maldevelopment of the derivatives of pharyngeal pouches III and IV, among which are the thymus and parathyroid glands. Patients have deficiency of T-lymphocyte–mediated cellular immunity and have a high incidence of viral and fungal infections. There have been no reported cases of malignancy.[60]

COMMON VARIABLE IMMUNODEFICIENCY. This heterogeneous group of disorders is loosely defined by the fact that the immunologic deficiency develops after a period of apparently normal immunologic function. They may have hypogammaglobulinemia or dysgammaglobulinemia plus evidence of defective cellular immunity.

The incidence of malignancy in this group is approximately 8 per cent.[60] Although lymphoreticular malignancies are the predominant types of cancer in this group, 29 per cent are nonlymphoid (nearly half of these are gastric carcinoma).

ATAXIA-TELANGIECTASIA. This autosomal recessive multisystem disease is characterized by cerebellar ataxia, dilated ocular and cutaneous vessels (telangiectasia), recurrent sinopulmonary infections, defects in both humoral and cellular immunity, and a

10 per cent incidence of malignancy.[60, 69, 120] Most of the neoplasms involve lymphoid tissues, but cases of gastrointestinal, central nervous system, skin, and ovarian malignancy have also been reported.[60, 120] Since very little lymphoid tissue is present in ataxia-telangiectasia, hilar or mediastinal lymphadenopathy seldom accompanies pulmonary infections; hence the appearance of adenopathy is highly suggestive of lymphoma in these patients.[103]

It has been estimated that heterozygotes for this disorder constitute 1 per cent of the normal population; for such individuals under age 45, the risk of dying from a malignant neoplasm is estimated to be 5 times the risk for the general population.[115] There appears, in particular, to be a predisposition to develop leukemia, lymphoma, and ovarian, biliary, and gastric carcinomas.[115]

WISKOTT-ALDRICH SYNDROME. This X-linked recessive disorder is characterized by the triad of eczema, thrombocytopenia, and recurrent infections with all classes of organisms. Both humoral and cellular immunity are affected; serum IgM levels are very low, while IgG and IgA levels may be normal. Antibody responses to polysaccharide antigens are particularly defective, and it has been postulated that the basic defect in Wiskott-Aldrich syndrome is in recognition or processing of antigen.

Nearly 10 per cent of children with this syndrome die with malignancy.[103] Of these, the vast majority have a malignant reticuloendotheliosis, primarily involving the lymphoid tissues of the body, but with frequent involvement of the gastrointestinal tract, liver, kidneys, adrenals, and brain.

SELECTIVE IgA DEFICIENCY. This is a relatively common disorder, occurring in from 1:700 to 1:3500 individuals in the general population;[31] affected individuals may be asymptomatic or suffer from sinopulmonary and gastrointestinal infections.

The incidence of malignancy has not, as yet, been determined; however, several patients have been reported with gastrointestinal and pulmonary carcinomas.[60]

Patients Receiving Immunosuppressive Therapy. Iatrogenic alterations of immunity which develop during treatment of a number of diseases are also associated with an increased incidence of malignancy. These include: (a) organ transplant recipients, (b) patients with nonmalignant diseases treated with immunosuppressive agents, and (c) patients with malignancy treated with cancer chemotherapy.

ORGAN TRANSPLANT RECIPIENTS. Malignancies have been encountered in three groups of organ homograft recipients: (1) patients in whom a cancer arises de novo at some time after transplantation, (2) those in whom a cancer was accidentally transmitted with the transplant, (3) those with tumors present before the transplantation.

Patients With De Novo Cancers Arising After Organ Homograft. There is a 5 to 6 per cent incidence of de novo malignant neoplasms in immunosuppressed organ homograft recipients; this frequency is approximately 100 times greater than that observed in the same age range in the general population.[88] Most of these cancers occurred in young adults (average age, 38 years; range, 8 to 70 years) and the average time of appearance of the tumors is 28 months after transplantation.[87]

The cancers seen in this group are of two major types, epithelial (67 per cent) and mesenchymal (33 per cent); of the former group the most common sites are skin, lip, and cervix uteri, whereas the most common mesenchymal tumors are various types of solid lymphoma.[87, 100] It is of interest to note that, although the incidence of "reticulum cell sarcoma" (a solid lymphoreticular malignancy) is 700 times greater in women receiving renal transplants than in the general female population, the incidence of breast cancer (the most common neoplasm of women) is not increased in the transplant group; this again indicates a striking relationship between impaired immunity and lymphoreticular neoplasia that is not wholly compatible with the theory of immune surveillance.

Patients With Transplanted Cancers. Penn[87] has described a group of 46 patients with renal or cardiac transplants from donors who had cancer at the time of donation or who showed evidence of malignancy some months afterwards (renal transplant donors). Although the transplanted organs appeared to be grossly free of tumor, in two patients the kidney and adjacent structures were involved by cancer, and in 10 other patients there was, in addition, evidence of distant spread of the neoplasm. At least six of these patients have died of the transplanted tumor and one patient died of complications relating to the tumor; immunosuppression was discontinued in the remaining three patients, and the cancers apparently underwent rejection and disappeared.

Although it is rarely possible to successfully transplant a malignant tumor from one human to another healthy person, these results show that chronic immunosuppressive therapy makes it possible for the transferred malignant cells to become established in the transplanted organ, invade the surrounding tissues, and metastasize widely.

Patients With Cancer Present Before Transplantation. Of this group of patients, 69 per cent of the transplants were performed specifically for treatment of cancer of the kidneys, liver, or other organs; in the other 31 per cent of patients the cancers were incidental to a renal transplant procedure (i.e., they involved skin, thyroid, testis, bladder, and other organs).[88] At the time of transplantation all neoplasms appeared to be localized and there was hope of obtaining a "cure." Virtually all patients received immunosuppressive therapy with azathioprine and prednisone, as well as other agents. Of the 101 patients, 38 per cent developed recurrent or metastatic tumors within an average period of 12 months following transplantation; it is not possible, however, to determine whether this figure represents an increased incidence caused by the chronic immunosuppressive therapy or merely reflects the natural history of the neoplasms.

PATIENTS WITH NONMALIGNANT DISEASES. Chronic immunosuppressive therapy for treatment of psoriasis, chronic renal disease, rheumatoid arthritis, systemic lupus, dermatomyositis, chronic cold agglutinin disease, and ulcerative colitis has been associated with the development of malignancy, particularly leukemia and lymphoma.[87] Although the development of malignancy in the patients with underlying autoimmune disease may reflect an innate propensity of these patients to cancer,[12, 34, 97, 122] conditions such as psoriasis are not usually associated with cancer unless treated with immunosuppressive agents or arsenic. Consequently, Penn's report of malignancy in 22 psoriasis patients treated with methotrexate or aminopterin suggests that the immunosuppression caused by these drugs may be a factor in oncogenesis.[87]

PATIENTS WITH MALIGNANT DISEASES. With the possible exception of mithramycin, the major cytotoxic drugs presently used in cancer chemotherapy are capable of suppressing both humoral and cell-mediated immunity.[94] It is thus possible that the chemotherapy used for treating a malignancy may depress cellular immunity and favor further growth and dissemination of the neoplasm or adversely affect whatever balance is present between sensitized lymphocytes, which tend to destroy malignant cells, and blocking factors, which tend to protect them; moreover, suppression of "immune surveillance" may also lead to the development of a second or third malignancy. In this regard, it has been well established that patients with cancer are prone to develop a second malignancy;[68, 80] in survivors of childhood cancer, for instance, the 20-year cumulative probability of a second cancer is 12 per cent.[68]

The role of cancer chemotherapy in the development of malignancy is probably complex and may involve potentiation of environmental carcinogens, permitting growth of oncogenic viruses, and direct oncogenic effects in addition to immunosuppression.

Patients With Autoimmune Diseases. There appears to be an increased incidence of malignancy in certain patients with autoimmune diseases, particularly dermatomyositis; the incidence of malignancy associated with this condition is approximately 13 to 15 per cent.[97, 122] In patients with dermatomyositis the sites most frequently involved by malignancy are stomach, breast, lung, ovary, reticuloendothelial system, colon, and rectum.[122]

Canoso and Cohen reported an 11.4 per cent incidence of malignancy in a series of 70 patients with systemic lupus erythematosus followed for a median interval of 6½ years,[12] and considered their results strongly suggestive of a link between lupus and malignancy. Of the eight cases of cancer seen in their series, five were epithelial carcinomas of the cervix; six of these eight patients had been treated with immunosuppressive therapy.

Although Oleinick found no increased frequency of death from lymphoreticular malignancies in lupus patients,[85] other authors have described an increased incidence of autoimmune phenomena in patients with malignant lymphomas and other malignancies; these can precede or follow the appearance of the tumors and have been shown to involve most types of autoimmune diseases and most types of lymphoid malignancy.[28, 47, 58, 76]

Aging. Malignancies among the general population have their greatest incidence beyond the age of 40 years; likewise, aged experimental animals have a greater propensity to accept transplants of malignant cells.[9, 39, 42, 70] These phenomena may be related to the deterioration of immunologic responsiveness, particularly cellular immunity, which occurs with aging. Immunologic senescence may not be the only explanation for the relationship between cancer and aging, however. It is also possible that this phenomenon may be a reflection of the duration of exposure to spontaneous or environmental carcinogenic stimuli or a result of age-related changes in endocrine function.

IMMUNOTHERAPY

The ultimate goal of immunotherapy is immunization of the patient against his own tumor. From a large number of studies in experimental animals, as well as some experience with human cancer, it is now possible to define some of the conditions necessary for successful treatment by immunologic stimulation.

1. The patient must be immunologically competent.
2. The tumor must have strong antigenicity.
3. The tumor burden must be relatively small — in experimental animals, host defenses are capable of destroying small numbers of tumor cells (10^6 to 10^7), but the presence of 10^8 (one hundred million) or more tumor cells almost always results in unrelenting tumor progression.[81] Since a neoplasm only 1 cm in diameter contains approximately 10^9 (1 billion) tumor cells (more than enough to overwhelm immunologic defenses), reduction of tumor burden by surgery, radiotherapy, or chemotherapy, or a combined

approach, is necessary before immunotherapy can be expected to eradicate the neoplasm.

TYPES OF IMMUNOTHERAPY

Immunotherapy may be classified into three categories: active, passive, and adoptive (Table 5–4). *Active immunotherapy* attempts to increase the host's intrinsic response to the tumor, *passive immunotherapy* involves the transfer of serum containing antitumor antibodies, and *adoptive immunotherapy* attempts a transfer of immunologically competent cells or information that will be adopted by the host as his or her own.

Active Immunotherapy

Active immunotherapy attempts to stimulate the host's intrinsic immunity to tumor antigens. This may be achieved by the use of nonspecific adjuvant agents, which cause an increase in the general level of immunocompetence, or by the use of tumor-specific stimuli, such as tumor cells or tumor antigens.

Nonspecific Agents. Adjuvants such as bacille Calmette Guérin (BCG), *Corynebacterium parvum* (*C. parvum*), levamisole, and polynucleotides appear to mediate their effects through a nonspecific and extremely complex activation of macrophages, B-lymphocytes, and T-lymphocytes. As a result, the reticuloendothelial system is stimulated to produce an immune response to a variety of antigens, including tumor antigens.[4, 21, 27]

BACILLE CALMETTE GUÉRIN. BCG is an attenuated strain of *Mycobacterium bovis* used as a vaccine against tuberculosis. In cancer treatment trials, it is usually administered by scarification or intradermal inoculation. Despite its attenuated state, it is still a viable organism, which may cause problems in an immunosuppressed host; thus, granulomatous hepatitis and pneumonitis, as well as other systemic reactions, have been reported.[4, 112] The methanol extraction residue (MER) of BCG circumvents the hazards associated with the administration of live BCG and has few known (and largely minor) clinical side effects. Studies using this agent for nonspecific immunotherapy are currently in progress.

The most extensive trials of live BCG have been in the treatment of malignant melanoma and the acute leukemias. Indeed, the most dramatic evidence of antitumor activity by immunotherapy in humans is seen in the regression of primary or metastatic cutaneous melanoma tumors after intralesional injection of BCG.[25] Local recurrences of melanoma have been treated by intralesional inoculation of BCG, with a reported regression rate of 90 per cent of the injected nodules.[84] However, only 17 per cent of uninjected adjacent nodules regressed and little effect was seen on visceral metastases, suggesting that there was not an effective system response.[25, 76, 84] In a more recent study, patients receiving adjuvant BCG therapy after surgical removal of a primary melanoma had half the incidence of metastatic disease after a 2-year interval that a control group treated by surgery alone had.[23] The results thus far, therefore, appear to suggest that immunologic adjuvant therapy with BCG is effective primarily when BCG is in direct contact with the tumor and when the

Table 5–4 Forms of Immunotherapy

1. Active: stimulation of host's intrinisic immunity to tumor antigens
   a. Nonspecific: adjuvants such as BCG, *C. parvum*, polynucleotides
   b. Specific: injection of killed autologous or allogeneic tumor cells
2. Passive: transfer of immune serum
3. Adoptive: transfer of immune cells or immunologic information
   a. Lymphocyte transfusions
   b. Transfer factor
   c. Immune RNA
   d. Thymosin

tumor mass is small. Preliminary trials also indicate that combining BCG with chemotherapy might beneficially affect survival in melanoma patients.

The results of treatment of the acute leukemias by BCG immunotherapy will be presented in Chapter Eight.

CORYNEBACTERIUM PARVUM. *Corynebacterium parvum* is an anaerobic bacterium. When given intravenously or intraperitoneally to mice, it causes intense reticuloendothelial system stimulation, with particular augmentation of macrophage function.[14, 86] B-cell function is also increased, but paradoxically, T-cell function may be temporarily depressed;[50, 101] Cheng and coworkers[14] found decreased T-cell function in humans as well following administration of *C. parvum*, but Israël and Edelstein,[54] in contrast, have found increased T-cell function and augmented immunologic competence. Thus, the patient may resist opportunistic infections and, possibly, second malignancies as a result of immunotherapy.

FUTURE POTENTIAL OF NONSPECIFIC IMMUNOTHERAPY. In summary, the potentialities of immunotherapy with adjuvant agents are still being defined. Studies with experimental animals have demonstrated the necessity for the appropriate timing, dosage, and route of administration of these agents; much work is currently in progress to determine the appropriate parameters for treating various human malignancies.

Specific Agents. Active immunotherapy may be made more specific by the injection of live or killed autologous or allogeneic tumor cells, sometimes altered by the addition of haptens or by treatment with neuraminidase to make them more antigenic.[79] Living tumor cells, when administered intradermally in numbers that are insufficient to cause a progression in tumor growth, generally are the most effective immunogens;[81] the possibility that living autologous tumor cells could result in tumor growth at the inoculation site has inhibited the use of such vaccines in humans, however. Since patients with cancer may have a weakened immune capacity, only frequent immunization with highly antigenic cells may prove adequate to improve immune function sufficiently to alter the course of the disease.

Passive Immunotherapy

The use of serum from donors sensitized against tumor cells has not been very successful.[70, 79] Serum from patients in remission from cancer has been injected into patients with active cancer of the same type, but with transient, if any, effects.[79] In addition, there is evidence that serum from cancer patients may actually enhance tumor growth, possibly because of the presence of blocking factors. The injection of live tumor cells (and perhaps even killed ones) into normal individuals in order to develop immune sera raises serious ethical questions and has been rarely used in humans.

Adoptive Immunotherapy

Adoptive immunotherapy attempts to confer immunity on an unresponsive recipient by transferring immunoreactive cells or immunologic information from a donor who is reactive against a given antigen. In human cancer therapy the donor may be a normal person who has become sensitized to a tumor antigen or a "cured" cancer patient. Such maneuvers are potentially useful but again raise moral and ethical problems. Immunization of normal persons with tumor material (even killed tumor cells) may involve contamination by the causative agent (perhaps viral); likewise, removal of lymphoid cells from the "cured" patient may conceivably upset a delicate immunologic balance and permit relapse of tumor in these patients. Furthermore, graft-versus-host disease may develop as a complication of lymphocyte transfusion if the host is immunosuppressed while rejection of transfused lymphocytes will occur if the host is immunocompetent.

Some of the problems complicating the transfer of intact lymphocytes might be obviated by substituting leukocyte extracts (e.g., transfer factor and immune RNA) for the living cell.

Transfer factor appears to transfer cell-mediated immunity exclusively without transferring the ability to make antibodies.[75, 79] It has been used successfully in the treatment of nontumorous conditions such as mucocutaneous candidiasis and some cases of Wiskott-Aldrich disease.[29] There has been much less success so far in treating tumors. Because transfer factor appears to be species-specific, the only available source for this substance for cancer immunotherapy is from patients in long-term remission or from family members whose lymphocytes are cytotoxic against the tumor cells in vitro.

Immune RNA is extracted from lymphocytes or macrophages which have been sensitized to certain viruses, tumor cells, or transplantation antigens; it is capable of transferring immunologic reactivity against these antigens to nonsensitized hosts. Unlike transfer factor, immune RNA is not species-specific. Therefore, material effective against human tumors could be prepared from the macrophages or lymphocytes from animals specifically immunized with the target tumor;[118] however, huge amounts of RNA appear to be necessary to transfer the ability to overcome a large tumor cell burden.[3]

Thymosin is a hormone produced in the thymus gland which stimulates T-cells. It may be useful in restoring or conferring normal maturation of T-cells in the cancer-bearing host when aging or stress have produced thymic involution.

REFERENCES

1. Abdou, N. I., and Abdou, N. L.: Bone marrow: the bursa equivalent in man? Science 175:446, 1972.
2. Aisenberg, A. C.: Immunologic status of Hodgkin's disease. Cancer 19:385, 1966.
3. Alexander, P., and Hall, J. G.: The role of immunoblasts in host resistance and immunotherapy of primary sarcomata. Adv. Cancer Res. 12:1, 1970.
4. Bast, R. C., Jr., Zbar, B., Borsos, T., and Rapp, H. J.: BCG and cancer. N. Engl. J. Med. 290:1413, 1458, 1974.
5. Bernstein, I. W.: Immunologic defenses against cancer. J. Pediatr. 83:906, 1973.
6. Black, M. M., Opler, S. R., and Speer, F. D.: Microscopic structure of gastric carcinomas and their regional lymph nodes in relation to survival. Surg. Gynec. Obstet. 98:725, 1954.
7. Borella, L., and Sen, L.: E receptors on blasts from untreated acute lymphocytic leukemia (ALL): comparison of temperature dependence of E rosettes formed by normal and leukemic lymphoid cells. J. Immunol. 114:187, 1975.
8. Brunner, K. T., and Cerottini, J. C.: Cytotoxic lymphocytes as effector cells of cell-mediated immunity. In Amos, B. (ed.): Progress in Immunology. New York, Academic Press, 1971.
9. Burnet, F. M.: The concept of immunological surveillance. Progr. Exp. Tumour Res. 13:1, 1970.
10. Burnet, F. M.: Immunological surveillance in neoplasia. Transplant. Rev. 7:4, 1971.
11. Canellos, G. P., DeVita, V. T., Arseneau, J. C., et al.: Carcinogenesis by cancer chemotherapeutic agents—second malignancies complicating Hodgkin's disease in remission. Rec. Results Cancer Res. 49:108, 1974.
12. Canoso, J. J., and Cohen, A. S.: Malignancy in a series of 70 patients with systemic lupus erythematosus. Arthritis Rheum. 17:383, 1974.
13. Chase, M. W.: Delayed-type hypersensitivity and the immunology of Hodgkin's disease, with a parallel examination of sarcoidosis. Cancer Res. 26:1097, 1966.
14. Cheng, V. T., Suit, H. D., Wang, C. C., and Cummings, C.: Nonspecific immunotherapy by *Corynebacterium parvum*. Phase I toxicity study in 12 patients with advanced cancer. Cancer 37:1687, 1976.
15. Cone, L., and Uhr, J. W.: Immunological deficiency disorders associated with chronic lymphocytic leukemia and multiple myeloma. J. Clin. Invest. 43:2241, 1964.
16. Cooper, M. D., Peterson, R. D. A., South, M. A., et al.: The functions of the thymus

system and the bursa system in the chicken. J. Exp. Med. *123*:75, 1966.
17. Dickler, H. B., and Kunkel, H.: Interaction of aggregated γ-globulin with B lymphocytes. J. Exp. Med. *136*:191, 1972.
18. Dimitrov, N. V., Andre, S., Elioponlos, G., et al.: Effect of *Corynebacterium parvum* on bone marrow cell cultures. American Society of Hematology, Seventeenth Annual Meeting (Abstr. 203), 1974.
19. Dixon, F. J., and Moore, R. A.: Testicular tumors; a clinico-pathological study. Cancer *6*:427, 1953.
20. Dizon, Q. S., and Southam, C. M.: Abnormal cellular response to skin abrasions in cancer patients. Cancer *16*:1288, 1963.
21. Editorial: Immunostimulation. Lancet *2*: 349, 1976.
22. Eilber, F. R., and Morton, D. L.: Impaired immunological reactivity and recurrence following cancer surgery. Cancer *25*:362, 1970.
23. Eilber, F. R., Morton, D. L., Holmes, E. C., et al.: Adjuvant immunotherapy with BCG in treatment of regional-lymph node metastases from malignant melanoma. N. Engl. J. Med. *294*:237, 1976.
24. Everson, T. C., and Cole, W. H.: Spontaneous Regression of Cancer. Philadelphia, W. B. Saunders Co., 1966.
25. Fahey, J. L., Brosman, S., Ossorio, R. C., et al.: Immunotherapy and human tumor immunology. Ann. Intern. Med. *84*:454, 1976.
26. Fass, L., Heberman, R. B., and Ziegler, J.: Delayed cutaneous hypersensitivity reactions to autologous extracts of Burkitt-lymphoma cells. N. Engl. J. Med. *282*: 776, 1970.
27. Freund, J.: The mode of action of immunologic adjuvants. Adv. Tuberc. Res. *7*: 130, 1956.
28. Fudenberg, H. H.: Genetically determined immune deficiency as a predisposing cause of "autoimmunity" and lymphoid neoplasia. Am. J. Med. *51*:295, 1971.
29. Fudenberg, H. H., Levin, A. S., Spitler, L. E., et al.: The therapeutic uses of transfer factor. Hosp. Pract. *9*:95, 1974.
30. Gatti, R. A., and Good, R. A.: Occurrence of malignancy in immunodeficiency diseases—a literature review. Cancer *28*:89, 1971.
31. Gatti, R. A.: Immunodeficiency disease. *In* Practice of Medicine. New York, Harper & Row, Publishers, 1972.
32. Gelfand, E. W., and Chechik, B. E.: Unmasking the heterogeneity of acute lymphoblastic leukemia. N. Engl. J. Med. *294*:275, 1976.
33. Glade, P. R., Zaldivar, N. M., Mayer, L., and Cahill, L. T.: The role of cellular immunity in neoplasia. Pediatr. Res. *10*:517, 1976.
34. Goldenberg, G. J., Paraskevas, F., and Israels, L. G.: Lymphocyte and plasma cell neoplasms associated with autoimmune diseases. Semin. Arthritis Rheum. *1*:174, 1971.
35. Goldman, J. M., and Th'ng, K. H.: Phagocytic function of leukocytes from patients with acute myeloid and chronic granulocytic leukaemia. Brit. J. Haematol. *25*: 299, 1973.
36. Goldstein, A. L., Slater, F. D., and White, A.: Preparation, assay, and partial purification of a thymic lymphocytopoietic factor (thymosin). Proc. Natl. Acad. Sci. U.S.A. *56*:1010, 1966.
37. Goldstein, G., Scheid, M. P., Hammerling, U., et al.: Isolation of a polypeptide that has lymphocyte differentiating properties and is probably represented universally in living cells. Proc. Natl. Acad. Sci. U.S.A. *72*:11, 1975.
38. Good, R. A., Biggar, W. D., and Park, B.: Immunodeficiency in man. *In* Amos, B. (ed.): Progress in Immunology. New York, Academic Press, 1971.
39. Good, R. A.: Relations between immunity and malignancy. Proc. Natl. Acad. Sci. U.S.A. *69*:1026, 1972.
40. Gutterman, J. U., Mavligit, O., Gottlieb, J. A., et al.: Chemoimmunotherapy of disseminated malignant melanoma with dimethyltriazeno imidazole carboxomide and Bacille Calmette Guérin. N. Engl. J. Med. *291*:592, 1974.
41. Halliday, W. J.: Blocking effect of serum from tumor-bearing animals on macrophage migration inhibition with tumor antigens. J. Immunol. *106*:855, 1971.
42. Hanna, M. G., Jr., Nettesheim, P., and Snodgrass, M. J.: Decreasing immune competence and development of reticulum cell sarcomas in lymphatic tissue of aged mice. J. Natl. Cancer Inst. *46*:809, 1971.
43. Harris, J., Sengar, D., Stewart, T., and Hyslop, D.: The effect of immunosuppressive chemotherapy on immune function in patients with malignant disease. Cancer *37*:1058, 1976.
44. Hellström, I., Hellström, K. E., Evans, C. A., et al.: Serum-mediated protection of neoplastic cells from inhibition by lymphocytes immune to their tumor-specific antigens. Proc. Natl. Acad. Sci. U.S.A. *62*:362, 1969.
45. Hellström, I., Hellström, K. E., Bill, A. H., et al.: Studies on cellular immunity to human neuroblastoma cells. Int. J. Cancer *6*:172, 1970.
46. Hellström, I., Hellström, K. E., Sjögren, H. O., et al.: Serum factors in tumor-free patients cancelling the blocking of cell-mediated immunity. Int. J. Cancer *8*:185, 1971.
46a. Hellström, K. E., and Hellström, I.: Lymphocyte mediated cytotoxicity and

blocking serum activity to tumor antigens. Adv. Immunol. *18*:209, 1974.
47. Hersh, E. M., Gutterman, J. U., and Mavligit, G. M.: Cancer and host defense mechanisms. Pathiobiol. Ann. *5*:133, 1975.
48. Hersh, E. M., Whitecar, J. P., Jr., McCredie, K. B., et al.: Chemotherapy, immunocompetence, immunosuppression, and prognosis in acute leukemia. N. Engl. J. Med. *285*:1211, 1971.
49. Hoover, R., and Fraumeni, J. F., Jr.: Risk of cancer in renal-transplant recipients. Lancet *2*:55, 1973.
50. Howard, J. G., Christie, G. H., and Scott, M. T.: Biological effects of *Corynebacterium parvum* IV Adjuvant and inhibitory activities on B lymphocytes. Cell. Immunol. *7*:290, 1973.
51. Hoyer, J. R., Cooper, M. C., Gabrielsen, A. E., et al.: Lymphopenic forms of congenital immunologic deficiency diseases. Medicine *47*:201, 1968.
52. Hughes, L. E., and Lytten, B.: Antigenic properties of human tumors: delayed cutaneous hypersensitivity reactions. Brit. Med. J. *1*:209, 1964.
53. Humphrey, L. J.: Tumor immunity in man. J. Surg. Res. *10*:493, 1970.
54. Israël, L., and Edelstein, R.: Nonspecific immunostimulation with *Corynebacterium parvum* in human cancer. In M. D. Anderson Hospital and Tumor Institute: Immunological Aspects of Neoplasia. Baltimore, Williams & Wilkins, 1975.
55. Johnson, M. W., Maibach, H. I., and Salmon, S. E.: Skin reactivity in patients with cancer. N. Engl. J. Med. *284*:1255, 1971.
56. Jondal, M., Holm. G., and Wigzell, H.: Surface markers on human T and B lymphocytes. J. Exp. Med. *136*:207, 1972.
57. Jose, D. G., and Seshadri, R.: Circulating immune complexes in human neuroblastoma: direct assay and role in blocking specific cellular immunity. Int. J. Cancer *13*:824, 1974.
58. Joseph, R. R., Tourtellotte, C. D., Barry, W. E., et al.: Prolonged immunological disorder terminating in hematological malignancy: a human analogue of animal disease? Ann. Intern. Med. *72*:699, 1970.
59. Kersey, J., Sabad, A., Gajl-Peczaleska, K., et al.: Acute lymphoblastic leukemic cells with T (thymus-derived) lymphocyte markers. Science *182*:1355, 1973.
60. Kersey, J. H., Spector, B. D., and Good, R. A.: Primary immunodeficiency diseases and cancer: The immunodeficiency-cancer registry. Int. J. Cancer *12*:333, 1973.
61. Kersey, J., Kazimiera, J. G.-P., and Nesbit, M. E.: The lymphoid system: abnormalities in immunodeficiency and malignancy. J. Pediatr. *84*:789, 1974.
62. Kersey, J. H., Spector, B. D., and Good, R. A.: Cancer in children with primary immunodeficiency diseases. J. Pediatr. *84*:263, 1974.
63. Klein, G.: Tumor antigens. Ann. Rev. Microbiol. *20*:223, 1966.
64. Kung, P. C., Gottlieb, P. D., and Baltimore, D.: Terminal deoxynucleotidyl transferase: serological studies and radioimmunoassay. J. Biol. Chem. *251*:2399, 1976.
65. Lauder, I., and Aherne, W.: The significance of lymphocytic infiltration in neuroblastoma. Brit. J. Cancer *26*:321, 1972.
66. Levin, A. G., McDonough, E. F., Miller, D. G., and Southam, C. M.: Delayed hypersensitivity response to DNFB in sick and healthy persons. Ann. N.Y. Acad. Sci. *120*:400, 1964.
67. Lewis, M. G., Ikonopisov, R. L., Nairn, R. C., et al.: Tumor-specific antibodies in human melanoma and their relationship to the extent of the disease. Brit. Med. J. *3*:547, 1969.
68. Li, F. P., Cassady, J. R., and Jaffe, N.: Risk of second tumors in survivors of childhood cancer. Cancer *35*:1230, 1975.
69. Louis-Bar, D.: Sur un syndrome progressif comprenant des télangiectases capillaires cutanées et conjonctivales symétriques à disposition naevoïde et des troubles cérébelleux. Confin. Neurol. *4*:32, 1941.
70. Marchelonis, J.: Immunology and Cancer. In Pascal, R. R., Silva, F., and King, D. W. (eds.): Cancer Biology. 1. Induction, Regulation, Immunology, and Therapy. New York, Stratton Intercontinental Medical Book Corporation, 1976.
71. Martin, R. F., and Beckwith, J. B.: Lymphoid infiltrates in neuroblastomas: their occurrence and prognostic significance. J. Pediatr. Surg. *3*:161, 1968.
72. Matas, A. J., Hertel, B. F., Rosai, J., et al.: Post-transplant malignant lymphoma. Amer. J. Med. *61*:716, 1976.
73. McBride, R. A.: Graft versus host reaction in lymphoid proliferation. Cancer Res. *26*:1135, 1966.
74. McCaffrey, R., Harrison, T. A., Parkman, R., et al.: Terminal deoxynucleotidyl transferase activity in human leukemic cells and in normal human thymocytes. N. Engl. J. Med. *292*:775, 1975.
75. McKhann, C. F., and Yarlott, M. A., Jr.: Tumor immunology. CA *25*:187, 1975.
76. Miller, D. G.: The association of immune disease and malignant lymphoma. Ann. Intern. Med. *66*:507, 1967.
77. Miller, J. F. A. P.: T-cell regulation of immune responsiveness. Ann. N.Y. Acad. Sci. *249*:9, 1975.

78. Miller, R. W.: Fifty-two forms of childhood cancer: United States mortality experience, 1960–1966. J. Pediatr. 75:685, 1969.
79. Mitchell, M. S.: An introduction to tumor immunology and immunotherapy. Gynec. Oncol. 4:1, 1976.
80. Moertel, C. G., Dockerty, M. B., and Baggenstoss, A. H.: Multiple primary malignant neoplasms. I. Introduction and presentation of data. Cancer 14:221, 1961.
81. Morton, D. L., Eilber, F. R., Joseph, W. L., et al.: Immunological factors in human sarcomas and melanomas. A rational basis for immunotherapy. Ann. Surg. 172:740, 1970.
82. Morton, D. L.: Immunological studies with human neoplasms. J. Reticuloendothel. Soc. 10:137, 1971.
83. Morton, D. L.: Immunotherapy of cancer. Cancer 30:1647, 1972.
84. Morton, D. L. Eilber, F. R., Holmes, E. C., et al.: BCG immunotherapy of malignant melanoma: summary of a seven-year experience. Ann. Surg. 180:635, 1974.
85. Oleinick, A.: Leukemia or lymphoma occurring subsequent to autoimmune disease. Blood 29:144, 1967.
86. O'Neill, G. J., Henderson, D. C., and White, R. G.: The role of anaerobic Corynebacterium on specific and nonspecific immunological reactions. I. Effect of particle clearance and humoral and cell-mediated immunological responses. Immunology 24:977, 1973.
87. Penn, I.: Occurrence of cancer in immune deficiencies. Cancer 34:858, 1974.
88. Penn, I.: Second malignant neoplasms associated with immunosuppressive medications. Cancer 37:1024, 1976.
89. Penn, I., and Starzl, T. E.: Malignant tumors arising de novo in immunosuppressed organ transplant recipients. Transplantation 14:407, 1972.
90. Pisano, J. C., DiLuzio, N. R., and Salky, N. K.: Absence of macrophage humoral recognition factor(s) in patients with carcinoma. J. Lab. Clin. Med. 76:141, 1970.
91. Raff, M.: Surface antigenic markers for distinguishing T and B lymphocytes in mice. Transplant. Rev. 6:52, 1971.
92. Ross, G. D., Polley, M. J., Rabellino, E. M., and Grey, H. M.: Two different complement receptors on human lymphocytes. One specific for C3b and one specific for C3b inactivator-cleaved C3b. J. Exp. Med. 138:798, 1973.
93. Sample, W. F., Gertner, H. R., and Chretien, P. B.: Inhibition of phytohemagglutinin-induced in-vitro lymphocyte transformation by serum from patients with carcinoma. J. Natl. Cancer Inst. 46:1291, 1971.
94. Santos, G. W.: Immunosuppressive drugs. I. Fed. Proc. 26:907, 1967.
95. Schoenberg, B. S., Greenberg, R. A., and Eisenberg, H.: Occurrence of certain multiple primary cancers in females. J. Natl. Cancer Inst. 43:15, 1969.
96. Schottenfeld, D., Berg, J. W., and Vitsky, B.: Incidence of multiple primary cancers. II. Index cancers arising in the stomach and lower digestive system. J. Natl. Cancer Inst. 43:77, 1969.
97. Schuermann, H.: Maligne Tumoren bei Dermatomyositis und progressiver Sklerodermie. Arch Dermat. Syph. 192:575, 1951.
98. Schwartz, A. D., Dadash-Zadeh, M., Lee, H., and Swaney, J. J.: Spontaneous regression of disseminated neuroblastoma. J. Pediatr. 85:760, 1974.
99. Schwartz, R. S.: Immunoregulation, oncogenic viruses, and malignant lymphomas. Lancet 1:1266, 1972.
100. Schwartz, R. S.: Another look at immunologic surveillance. N. Engl. J. Med. 293:181, 1975.
101. Scott, M. T.: Biological effects of the adjuvant Corynebacterium parvum. I. Inhibition of PHA, mixed lymphocyte and GVH reactivity. Cell. Immunol. 5:459, 1972.
102. Selvaraj, R. J., McRipley, R. J., and Sbarra, A. J.: The metabolic activities of leukocytes from lymphoproliferative and myeloproliferative disorders during phagocytosis. Cancer Res. 27:2287, 1967.
103. Shackleford, G. D., and McAlister, W. H.: Primary immunodeficiency diseases and malignancy. Am. J. Roentgenol. 123:144, 1975.
104. Silverstone, A. E., Cantor, H., Goldstein, G., and Baltimore, D.: Terminal deoxynucleotidyl transferase is found in prothymocytes. J. Exp. Med. 144:543, 1976.
105. Sjögren, H. O., and Bansal, S. C.: Antigens in virally induced tumors. In Amos, B. (ed.): Progress in Immunology. New York, Academic Press, 1971.
106. Sjögren, H. O., Hellström, I., Bansal, S. C., et al.: Suggestive evidence that the "blocking antibodies" of tumor-bearing individuals may be antigen-antibody complexes. Proc. Natl. Acad. Sci. U.S.A. 68:1372, 1971.
107. Smith, R. T.: Tumor-specific immune mechanisms. N. Engl. J. Med. 278:1207, 1268, 1326, 1968.
108. Smith, R. T.: Possibilities and problems of immunologic intervention in cancer. N. Engl. J. Med. 287:439, 1972.
109. Smith, R. W., Terry, W. D., and Sell, K. W.: An antigenic marker for human thymic lymphocytes. J. Immunol. 110:884, 1973.
110. Solowey, A. C., and Rapoport, F. T.: Immunologic responses in cancer pa-

tients. Surg. Gynecol. Obstet. *121*:756, 1965.
111. Southam, C. M., and Moore, A. E.: Induced immunity to cancer cell homografts in man. Ann. N.Y. Acad. Sci. *73*:635, 1958.
112. Sparks, F. C., Silverstein, M. J., Hunt, J. S., et al.: Complications of BCG immunotherapy in patients with cancer. N. Engl. J. Med. *289*:827, 1973.
113. Starzl, T. E., Penn, I., Putnam, C. W., et al.: Iatrogenic alterations of immunologic surveillance in man and their influence on malignancy. Transplant. Res. *7*:112, 1971.
114. Stutman, O., and Good, R. A.: Immunocompetence of embryonic hemopoietic cells after traffic to thymus. Transplant. Proc. *3*:923, 1975.
115. Swift, M., Sholman, L., Perry, M., and Chase, C.: Malignant neoplasms in the families of patients with ataxia-telangiectasia. Cancer Res. *36*:209, 1976.
116. Teller, M. N.: Interrelationships among aging, community, and cancer. *In* Sigel, M., and Good, R. A. (eds.): Tolerance, Autoimmunity and Aging. Springfield, Ill., Charles C Thomas, 1972.
117. Theofilopoulos, A. N., Wilson, C. B., and Dixon, F. J.: The Raji cell radioimmune assay for detecting immune complexes in human sera. J. Clin. Invest. *57*:169, 1976.
118. Thor, D. E., and Dray, S.: The cell migration-inhibition correlate of delayed hypersensitivity. Conversion of human nonsensitive lymph node cells to sensitive cells with an RNA extract. J. Immunol. *101*:469, 1968.
119. Tornyos, K.: Phagocytic activity of cells of the inflammatory exudate in human leukemia. Cancer Res. *27*:1756, 1967.
120. Waldmann, T. A., Strober, W., and Blaese, R. M.: Immunodeficiency disease and malignancy: various immunological deficiencies of man and the role of immune processes in the control of malignant disease. Ann. Intern. Med. *77*:605, 1972.
121. Ward, P. A., and Berenberg, J. L.: Defective regulation of inflammatory mediators in Hodgkin's disease. N. Engl. J. Med. *290*:76, 1974.
122. Williams, R. C., Jr.: Dermatomyositis and malignancy: a review of the literature. Ann. Intern. Med. *50*:1174, 1959.
123. Winkelstein, A., Mikulla, J. M., Sartiano, G. P., and Ellis, L. D.: Cellular immunity in Hodgkin's disease: comparison of cutaneous reactivity and lymphoproliferative responses to phytohemagglutinin. Cancer *34*:549, 1974.
124. Wood, W. C., and Morton, D. L.: Microcytotoxicity test: detection in sarcoma patients of antibody cytotoxic to human sarcoma cells. Science *170*:1318, 1970.
125. Wybran, J., Carr, M. D., and Fudenberg, H. H.: The human rosette-forming cell as a marker of a population of thymus-derived cells. J. Clin. Invest. *51*:2537, 1972.
126. Yoneda, M., and Bollum, F. J.: Deoxynucleotide-polymerizing enzymes of calf thymus gland. I. Large scale purification of terminal and replicative deoxynucleotidyl transferase. J. Biol. Chem. *240*:3385, 1965.

Chapter Six

PSYCHOLOGICAL AND SOCIAL SUPPORT OF THE PATIENT AND FAMILY

Julia M. Cotter and Allen D. Schwartz

The diagnosis of any serious illness, especially one that is potentially fatal, has a tremendous impact on the child and his family. The procedures to which the child is subjected, the effects of treatment, and the uncertainty of the future place a great stress upon the child and those close to him. The ability of the child and his family to cope with this stress and to handle the problems throughout the course of treatment depend in large part upon the strengths and abilities to function which they had prior to the diagnosis. Families who already have good internal supports, such as good parent-child and marital relations, emotional stability, and individual ego strengths, and strong external supports, such as support from extended family members and satisfactory work roles and social roles, will be more capable of coping with stress than those without such supports. Even members of the healthiest family system, however, will have every aspect of their family life—including their interpersonal relationships, economic stability, and religious beliefs—placed under stress when confronted with the impact of a potentially fatal illness. Other major factors affecting a family's ability to cope are its relationship with medical and allied medical personnel, and the degree to which its nonmedical needs are met. Each stage of the illness has its own special stresses and requires understanding in order that those involved in care might adequately support the family.

THE INITIAL DIAGNOSIS

When the patient and family are referred to a "specialist" the parents usually have some suspicion that their child has a serious illness. Thus, they already have some degree of anxiety prior to meeting the new physician. This may be expressed as anger directed toward the referring physician for what the parents mistakenly believe to be his inability to make the correct diagnosis, or his delay in making the diagnosis. Once the diagnosis of a malignant disease is confirmed the manner in which the information is presented to both patient and parents is of crucial importance. It is usually best to tell the parents together. Most physicians have advocated a realistic and honest approach. Parents and other members of the family or close friends whom parents wish to include in knowing the diagnosis need to be told the same information. A lengthy conference with the physician is necessary to explain the nature of the illness and the treatment that is to follow. It is reassuring to parents to be told from the outset what they can expect in terms of therapy, side effects, and prognosis. Generally this must be repeated several times in order for parents to be able to emotionally and intellectually digest all of the new information. If parents are given a realistic and honest picture, the usual reaction is one of shock and anticipatory grief. Generally there is not a high level of denial since the words "leukemia" and "cancer" are well enough known that most people are readily aware of their implications. Parents often find that the prognosis may be better than they initially expected, for some believe that once such a diagnosis is made, the child may never leave the hospital. They may sometimes feel anger toward the physician who tells them the diagnosis. As a result they are often in a situation where they can not express their anger for fear of offending the very person upon whom they are now dependent. It is not unusual for parents to relate that they experienced such a reaction later during the course of the child's illness, and they are often surprised when discussing their feelings with other parents to find that this reaction is not unique to them or abnormal.

Several emotional issues are raised at the time of diagnosis. The parents are concerned about the etiology of the illness. They often feel guilty and may believe that they are in some way to blame for their child's illness. They wonder if the disorder was caused by a deficient diet, hereditary factors, or by some accident or trauma at birth or during the child's life. Whatever form it takes, the questions they are asking are "Am I to blame?," and "Could this have been prevented?" Many parents desire to fix the blame, even upon themselves, in an attempt to master or control a situation; that is, if there is a reasonable explanation for why their child has the disease, such as some past event over which they had control, maybe there is an answer over which they may also have control. Parents often feel guilty that they did not recognize illness earlier. Many times the child had complained of being tired or of having aches and pains which the parents had ignored or had not taken seriously. If the parents had previously taken the child to a physician who assured them that all was well, a great deal of anger might be directed toward the physician. There is often fear that a delay in the diagnosis either on their part or the part of their doctor has made a difference regarding the outcome. Parents need the opportunity to ventilate their feelings and be given reassurance that they were in no way responsible for the disease. They often have a great deal of dependency upon their physician, and need to hear these reassurances repeatedly.

Another major concern of the parents is what the child should be told about his illness and how he will react emotionally. They also want to know what to tell others, such as siblings, friends, and teachers. Parents generally will rely on the physician's advice on how to handle these situations.

Depending upon the child's age and his ability to understand, a realistic approach usually appears to be best. A great deal has been published regarding the child's ability to intellectually grasp information about his illness and the concept of death. In general, children above the age of 6 years are well able to comprehend that they are "sick" and have some ability to conceptualize death. Thus, most children 6 years of age and older, and some younger, more mature children need to know that their illness has a name and what that name is. All children need to be given reasons for the treatment and uncomfortable procedures they must undergo. Otherwise, treatment may be interpreted as a punishment. For many children, especially those between 6 and 11 years of age, the procedures and side effects of therapy will produce more anxiety than the illness itself. Most children 11 years of age and older express fears of the illness itself and its prognostic implications. Like their parents, their initial reaction is one of grief and shock, many of them having heard about the illness before. In an initial conference it is important to ask the adolescent what the word "leukemia" (or whatever the diagnosis might be) means to him. One 15 year old boy began crying as soon as the physician stated the word "leukemia." When asked what the word meant to him, he said "People die from it. A boy in my class had leukemia and he died two years ago." Such youngsters need reassurance about the benefits of treatment, and must know what to expect, but a very optimistic view can be presented. The physician can be realistic and optimistic at the same time. The physician usually is only fooling himself if he believes that he can keep the knowledge of the diagnosis from the teenager. Denying to the adolescent that a serious illness exists often denies him the opportunities to express his fears and concerns to his parents and physician. If he feels that the truth is being kept from him, he may believe little else of what factual information is given to him. Particularly for the adolescent, it is important that a private relationship be established with the physician that does not involve the parents. Thus, the youngster knows that he will be told information directly and not through parents, and that he has the opportunity to ask questions and express concerns directly to the physician without upsetting his parents. However, the physician should avoid keeping secrets between the parents and child, and open communication within the family should be encouraged.

REMISSION

After the initial diagnosis, parents and older children anxiously await being told that the disease is in remission or "under control." Until this time, there is a natural tendency for parents to move closer toward their child and become more protective. Once the child's condition is in remission, much tension is alleviated in most families. Whereas the initial task had been to have the family accept the diagnosis and therapy, the task is now for the patient and family to return to as normal a life as is possible, albeit a life that has in many ways been changed by the disease. The child and family must now begin to incorporate the diagnosis and treatment into their lifestyle. In most instances children can quickly return to school and resume their normal activities. The treatment and its side effects must now be dealt with, and problems such as hair loss and the other effects of therapy now assume major importance. During this stage, the parents and older children will often seek information about the illness that initially they were unable to ask about or did not wish to hear.

The emotionally stable patient and family will usually be able to adapt and cope with the illness and the uncertainty it brings and resume previous social, family, and work roles. Those with a history of prior difficulties in coping often have a resurgence of their previous problems. For example, if there was a tendency before the illness occurred for the parents to overprotect the child, the diagnosis of the illness will reenforce and strengthen this behavior pattern, which will continue even during the time the child's illness is under complete medical control. This may be manifested, for example, by the child's sleeping with the parents. If, prior to the illness, there were marital or parent-child disturbances, the impact of the illness may deepen them further. If a parent or child had previous episodes of depression, anxiety, or psychosomatic complaints, these problems often become more severe.

Paradoxically, the medical advances made in the treatment of many childhood malignancies have created new problems, because the uncertainty of the outcome has now increased. Illnesses that were uniformly lethal can now often be cured, but no physician can ever be certain which child will survive. The unknown is often more difficult for some to face than the certainty of death. It is therefore important that the physician be available to the family to answer their questions and to offer reassurance throughout the course of care, even when the child has no obvious evidence of illness and may have reached the point where he is no longer receiving chemotherapy. The long-term psychological effects from having been treated for and cured of a potentially fatal illness such as cancer are now being evaluated in a number of medical centers. Such studies may lead to future changes in our present approach and management of children and their families, just as our new understanding of the long-term organic effects of therapy is now influencing present treatment regimens.

RECURRENCE OF DISEASE

When the illness recurs, a crisis situation is again created. Family members usually understand the meaning and prognostic implications of a relapse. The family and child generally react with feelings of shock and grief, and the fears and feelings of anguish present at the initial diagnosis are often reactivated. In many instances, the grief at relapse is even more intense than that experienced during the initial diagnosis, because the hope for cure has been lessened. Again, the parents and older children may attempt to master the situation by searching for reasons or meanings. They may again become angry at the physician because he was unable to control the disease. The child often feels anger and frustration because of the reinstitution of therapy and procedures that he thought he might not have to experience again. The physician must now realistically explain the present situation to the parents and child, allow them to express their fears and concerns, and again help them with the emotional tasks of facing an uncertain future.

THE DYING CHILD

The stage is often reached when treatment can no longer effectively control the disease and there is little more that can be offered medically except palliative therapy. When the disease has been of chronic nature, parents have in many ways prepared for this stage of the illness. At this point, the family must accept the fact that the child will probably die. The process which helps parents prepare for this has been called "anticipatory mourning," and has been defined by Futterman and Hoffman[4] as "a set of processes that are directly related to the awareness of the impending loss, to its emotional impact and to the adaptive mechanisms whereby emotional attachment to the child is relinquished over time." Family members begin to recognize the inevitability of death and consequently begin to feel the emotional impact of the impending loss.

Several conflicting tasks are now faced by the parents at this time. They must support their child emotionally and maintain a normal relationship, but they must also begin to separate emotionally from the child. They must focus on their child's immediate emotional and physical needs but must also look to the future and to their own needs and those of other family members. Parents seldom lose all hope as long as their child is alive. The conflicts created by such a burden often produce anxiety in the parents, who feel they are walking on an "emotional tightrope," as they continually try to find some balance between retaining hope and facing loss.

During this period, family members need the opportunity to ventilate and share their feelings. They need to know that it is normal to be anxious or depressed, to cry, and to openly express their feelings. Many parents will welcome the opportunity to discuss their past experiences with their child and to repeatedly discuss and relive the history of their child's illness. This is an effort to integrate this tragedy into their lives. In our experience, if parents are allowed the opportunity to express themselves, they will, with proper guidance, use the process of anticipatory mourning to accept death. They now begin to realistically face the impending death of their child and a future without him, while still hoping for a "miracle." Parents may one day acknowledge that their child is dying and the next day talk about "If he should make it." In situations in which the terminal stage is prolonged, parents often need to maintain hope in order to continue their relationship with their child. At this point, some families may decide to care for the child at home. If families are emotionally prepared to care for their child, and are aware of what to expect, home care to the terminal patient can, in selected instances, be a positive and healthy experience.

The child's ability to recognize and accept the fact that he has a terminal illness depends upon his age, his personality, and the degree to which others support him. Most children under 5 years of age fear a separation from parents and other loved ones rather than death itself. They generally view death as a sleep or a restriction of activity, and need reassurance that they will not be left alone.

Children 5 to 10 years of age may view death in a more personified manner, such as becoming an angel or going to heaven. They are often more fearful of the treatment procedures than of death itself. During this time of life children often express their feelings and fears symbolically, through games or pictures, or by talking about a grandparent or a pet who died.

Example: Elizabeth, a 7 year old girl with leukemia, was playing with toy soldiers. She had lined them up on the social worker's desk when she accidentally knocked one to the floor. She gasped and said "He's dead." She then asked the social worker whether the man could be put back on the table. The worker asked what she thought. Elizabeth said "No, he's dead," and put the soldier aside. She was asked where the soldier was. Elizabeth replied, "He's in heaven with his grandfather." This then led to a discussion of her perception of heaven and who lived there. At no time did she talk about her own fate. The child was told nothing by the worker of what she was actually discussing. It would have been traumatic to Elizabeth if it had been pointed out to her that she was talking about herself. If she had been ready to discuss such matters, she would have made the connection herself.

Dr. Kübler-Ross, in her book *Questions and Answers On Death and Dying*, has stated that "No patient should be told that he is dying. I do not encourage people to force patients to face their own death when they are not ready for it. Patients should be told that they are seriously ill. When they are ready to bring up the issue of death and dying, we should answer them, we should listen to them, we should hear their questions, but you do not go around telling patients they are dying and depriving them of a glimpse of hope that they may need in order to live until they die."[11] Thus, one must be available to discuss with the child what he wants to discuss, but the pace must be set by the child. One 8 year old girl asked her physician what would happen if the drugs didn't work. Instead of answering, the physician asked if she were worred about that. The girl replied "Yes, because I don't want to lose my hair again." Clearly, the child was not asking about death, but a misinterpretation of her question might have brought up a premature discussion which the child was not emotionally prepared to handle.

The issue of discussing death is particularly relevant to adolescents who, in many cases, seek direct information. Adolescents are well able to conceptualize death. Like adults, they understand that death is permanent. Adolescents need not be told that they are dying, but must be given the opportunity to discuss the questions they have. Frequently adolescents are depressed, which obviously is a normal reaction under the circumstances. It is often painful for staff members to work with the dying adolescent for a number of reasons. Adolescence is normally a time when one is absorbed with plans for the future, school, and dating, and is often associated with the happiest times of life. Physicians, nurses, and other personnel can easily identify with adolescents and young adults, but they may make the staff feel uncomfortable because the patients know they are dying.

Example: Charles, a 15 year old boy with acute lymphocytic leukemia, was an intelligent, articulate young man. He was very well liked by peers and adults, including hospital staff, because of his friendly, warm personality. Throughout the course of his illness, Charles presented an almost casual attitude regarding his illness. When he became seriously ill, he continued to maintain this facade. He joked about his illness and always spoke about returning home from the hospital. As his illness became progressively worse, he began to verbalize his fears of dying. It eventually became very difficult for both family members and staff to listen to Charles' expressions of his fears, particularly because it contrasted sharply with his previous denial and "happy" personality. Eventually the family members were able to discuss with the staff the emotional problems that Charles was expressing and how they might respond to his needs. Consequently, Charles' feelings were met with openness, and he was able to receive the support and comfort he needed by both family and staff during the terminal phase of his illness.

In summary, some of the general concepts for meeting the emotional needs of patients and families during the terminal stage of illness are as follows:

1. Support the family's strengths and the relationship between the family and the patient.

2. Allow the family and child to set the pace in dealing with the issue of dying; be gently realistic without pushing towards acceptance of the realities of the situation.

3. Allow anger to be expressed. Give both the patient and the family as much control over the situation as is possible and do not interpret outbursts as a personal attack upon you.

4. Do not discourage expressions of grief. To be upset is normal and grieving is a means of coping.

5. Allow the patient and family to have hope.

AFTER THE CHILD DIES

After the child dies, the family will go through a process of mourning that may last for several months. Families should know this ahead of time and can be helped to prepare for this period. If parents know that they will feel depressed, dream about their child, become upset during certain times of the year, such as the anniversary of the child's death, his birthday, the Christmas season, or other times which are normally associated with celebrating or joy, they will at least understand that their reactions are normal. Depression is only abnormal if it persists intensely for an extended period of time and interferes with the person's ability to resume the normal tasks of life. Some families may experience a sense of relief that their ordeal and that of the child is finally over. It is helpful if parents have an opportunity to discuss such feelings, for the relief they may experience following their child's death may often result in new feelings of guilt. It is very important for parents to feel that they can contact the physician after the child's death. Often they will have questions that they were emotionally unable to ask before the child's death, and now wish to discuss. Some follow-up support should be available to the family by the physician, social worker, or other health care personnel who have been involved with the family during their ordeal until the family is again functioning well.

STAFF REACTIONS

The death of a child is always tragic and normally evokes painful feelings in everyone. Like parents, medical and allied medical personnel may also experience shock, anger, and anguish at the impending death of a child. These feelings cannot be avoided and can sometimes be made use of to foster emotional growth, but they must not be allowed to interfere with the care delivered to the patient and family.

The responsibility of caring for a child with a catastrophic illness may present particular problems to the primary physician and house staff, who have been taught that the goal of medical treatment is to cure the child. Their inability to do this may be interpreted as a failure of professional expectations. If treatment does not cure, the physician may feel guilty and angry at what is perceived as failure and inadequacy. Physicians may also become upset because of the various uncomfortable, but necessary, procedures they must perform on the child. They often ask themselves when treatment should be stopped on a child who is dying. One must constantly weigh the quality of life given the child against the possible chances of achieving another meaningful remission.

Occasionally the family may make excessive demands on the physician's time and emotional resources. While the physician may be aware that the anger sometimes expressed by the family is not really directed at him (or her), he must realize that their constant need for reassurances is a manifestation of their anxiety. The pressures of time and the responsibilities to other patients may sometimes make it difficult for him to give the time he feels the patient and family deserve.

Schowalter[15] pointed out that the response of the physician handling the dying child may take the form of "emotional overinvolvement or callous withdrawal," both reactions being harmful to the physician, the patient, and the family. He noted the difficulty house officers had in spending time with the dying child, and their tendency to underestimate the child's level of awareness of his illness and medical conditions. These reactions, of course are not unique to physicians; other members of the health care team often respond in a similar manner. Often a sign of "protective isolation" on the door of the hospital room of a child in effect protects the doctor and staff more than the patient, for it gives them an excuse for not continually entering the room to be faced with the family and child. When the child is in the terminal stage of illness we have found it is valuable for all of those persons involved in the care to meet together to discuss both the medical and emotional needs of the patient and family, and to express their own needs and feelings about the impending death of the child. For several reasons, the deaths of some children may be more difficult to face than others, especially if a staff member has developed a closeness to a particular patient and family, has a child of the same age, or in some way identifies with the patient or family. It is not desirable to become emotionally immune to death, but rather to be able to come to an acceptance of death, to give emotional support and comfort to others when needed, and to allow staff members to experience and express their own emotions.

SELECTED READING

1. Ablin, A. R., Bengir, C. M., Stein, R. C., et al.: A conference with the family of a leukemic child. Amer. J. Dis. Child. 122:362, 1971.
2. Easson, W. M.: The family of the dying child. Pediatr. Clin. N. Am. 19:1157, 1972.
3. Fischoff, J., and O'Brien, N.: After the child dies. J. Pediatr. 88:140, 1976.
4. Futterman, E., and Hoffman, I.: Crisis and adaptation in the families of fatally ill children. In Anthony, J., and Koupernik, C. (eds.): The Child in His Family: The Impact of Disease and Illness. Vol. 2. New York, John Wiley and Sons, Inc., 1973.
5. Gould, R. K., and Rothenberg, M. B.: The chronically ill child facing death—How can the pediatrician help? Clin. Pediatr. 12:447, 1973.
6. Karon, M., and Vernick, J.: An approach to the emotional support of fatally ill children. Clin. Pediatr. 7:274, 1968.
7. Kirkpatrick, J., Hoffman, I., and Futterman, E. H.: Dilemma of trust: Relationship between medical care givers and parents of fatally ill children. Pediatrics 54:169, 1974.
8. Knapp, V., and Hansen, H.: Helping the parents of children with leukemia. Social Work 18:70, 1973.
9. Koch, C. R., Hermann, J., and Donaldson, M. H.: Supportive care of the child with cancer and his family. Sem. Oncol. 1:81, 1974.
10. Koocher, G. P.: Talking with children about death. Amer. J. Orthopsychiat. 44:404, 1974.
11. Kübler-Ross, E.: Questions and Answers on Death and Dying. New York, Macmillan Co., 1974.
12. Lascari, A., and Stehbens, J. A.: The reactions of families to childhood leukemia. Clin. Pediatr. 12:210, 1973.
13. Petrillo, M., and Singer, S.: Emotional care of hospitalized children. Philadelphia, J. B. Lippincott Co., 1972.
14. Schoenberg, B., Carr, A. C., Peretz, D., et al.: Loss and Grief: Psychological Management in Medical Practice. New York, Columbia University Press, 1970.
15. Schowalter, J. E.: Death and the pediatric house officer. J. Pediatr. 76:706, 1970.
16. Schulman, J. L.: Coping with Tragedy: Successfully Facing the Problems of a Seriously Ill Child. Chicago, Follett Publishing Co., 1976.
17. Spinetta, J. J., and Maloney, L. J.: Death anxiety in the outpatient leukemic child. Pediatrics 56:1034, 1975.
18. Townes, B. D., Wold, D. A., and Holmes, T. H.: Parental adjustment to childhood leukemia. J. Psychosomatic Res. 18:9, 1974.
19. van Eys, J.: Supportive care for the child with cancer. Pediatr. Clin. N. Am. 23:215, 1976.

Chapter Seven

ONCOLOGIC EMERGENCIES

The primary plan for care of a patient with a newly diagnosed malignancy is non-oncologic in nature. At this juncture the major responsibility of the medical staff caring for the child is to stabilize his general condition and to recognize life-threatening complications rather than to be concerned with searching the literature for the latest treatment modality for the neoplasm. Only on rare occasions is it necessary to perform surgery or to start specific chemotherapy or radiotherapy on the day of admission. Instead, attention should be paid to detection of anemia, occult infection, a bleeding diathesis, metabolic abnormalities, or symptoms arising from pressure on a vital organ. It does the patient little good to receive the most up-to-date cancer treatment or be transferred to a comprehensive treatment center if causes of potential serious morbidity or mortality are overlooked by the primary physician until their effects are irreversible.

Once the patient has received specific antitumor therapy, complications may arise from the therapy (e.g., bone marrow suppression) or from recurrence of the tumor and it is the responsibility of the physician following the patient to recognize and treat these promptly and appropriately.

This chapter discusses some of the major emergency situations which may arise in the child with a neoplastic disease. All of the conditions described are treatable and potentially reversible if recognized and treated correctly—and all of them are associated with dire consequences if the diagnosis is delayed or missed.

METABOLIC EMERGENCIES

HYPERURICEMIA

Hyperuricemia is the most frequent cause of acute renal failure in patients with leukemia; it may also be a significant problem in patients with lymphosarcoma and other solid tumors. Since this problem frequently complicates the patient's course at the time of diagnosis or shortly after the initiation of therapy, failure to recognize and treat it appropriately may seriously compromise the patient's ultimate prognosis.

In humans uric acid is the final product in the degradative metabolism of purines, which are vital building blocks of DNA and RNA. At a blood pH of 7.4, uric acid exists largely in solution as the monovalent salt, sodium urate; however, at a urinary pH of 5, uric acid is very insoluble and tends to precipitate as crystals. These uric acid crystals may obstruct the renal tubules and produce oliguric renal failure.

Hyperuricemia in neoplastic disease usually reflects excessive uric acid production secondary to an increased nucleic acid turnover by the mass of abnormal cells. Following cytotoxic therapy, neoplastic cells become necrotic and present more DNA and RNA to be catabolized, thereby leading to a further increase in uric acid levels. Antecedent renal disease or obstructive uropathy may accentuate this tendency by interfering with uric acid excretion. Other factors which increase the likelihood of uric acid nephropathy are: a persistently low urinary pH and prolonged dehydration.

The clinical manifestations of hyperuricemia are usually related to renal insufficiency and consist of lethargy, nausea, or vomiting; uric acid calculi may produce hematuria, renal colic, and oliguria or anuria. Uric acid crystals may be visible in the urinary sediment. Extreme hyperuricemia may produce a neurologic syndrome consisting of anorexia, nausea, persistent vomiting, extreme lethargy, weakness, coma, and convulsions.[42] Gouty arthritis is rare in hyperuricemic patients with acute leukemia because of a lack of polymorphonuclear cells to mediate the inflammatory joint changes; however, patients with chronic leukemia or solid tumors may have gouty symptoms.

Treatment of Hyperuricemia

Treatment of hyperuricemia consists of measures to (1) decrease uric acid production, (2) promote uric acid solubility in the urine, and (3) reduce uric acid concentration in the urine (Table 7–1). These measures should be instituted in every case of acute leukemia and lymphosarcoma prior to initiating specific chemotherapy (regardless of the initial uric acid level), particularly in patients with high leukocyte counts and massive organ enlargement due to tumor involvement.

Uric acid production may be decreased by the drug allopurinol (4 hydroxypyrazolo-[3,4-d] pyrimidine), a competitive inhibitor of the enzyme xanthine oxidase which catalyzes the final steps in the degradation of purines to uric acid, according to the sequence at the bottom of the page.

The most frequent side effect seen with allopurinol therapy is a maculopapular skin rash; exfoliative, urticarial, and purpuric lesions as well as erythema multiforme (Stevens-Johnson syndrome) have also been reported. Patients receiving ampicillin appear to be especially prone to develop skin eruptions when taking allopurinol concurrently.[8] It is considered prudent to discontinue allo-

Table 7–1 Treatment of Hyperuricemia

Allopurinol*	100 mg P.O. TID (for children > 6 y.o.) 50 mg P.O. TID (for children < 6 y.o.)
Fluid (D5 ¼S)	3000 ml/m² daily
NaHCO₃	35–45 mEq/m² daily (to maintain urine pH 7.0–7.5)

*The dose of allopurinol should be reduced if renal failure is present (see text)

$$purine \longrightarrow hypoxanthine \xrightarrow{xanthine\ oxidase} xanthine \xrightarrow{xanthine\ oxidase} uric\ acid$$

with allopurinol inhibiting the xanthine oxidase steps

purinol therapy at the first appearance of a skin rash, because sometimes the skin eruption is followed by a more severe hypersensitivity reaction. Less common side effects of allopurinol include rare cases of vasculitis, renal failure, and peripheral neuritis. It is important to remember that the purine analogue 6-mercaptopurine (6MP) requires xanthine oxidase for its metabolic breakdown; consequently, *undue toxicity may result from 6MP unless its dose is reduced to 25 per cent of the usual dose when allopurinol is used concomitantly.*

Since allopurinol and its metabolites are excreted only by the kidney, accumulation of the drug can occur in renal failure. The dose of allopurinol, therefore, should be reduced under these conditions. With a creatinine clearance of 10 to 20 ml/min, the dosage should be reduced by one third; when the creatinine clearance is less than 10 ml/min, the daily dosage should not exceed one third the usual dose. With extreme renal impairment (creatinine clearance less than 3 ml/min), the interval between doses may also need to be lengthened.

An adequate urine output is essential for treating hyperuricemia, and the patient may require intravenous supplementation to maintain the desired urine flow of 100 ml/m²/hour.[35] This can be given in the form of D5 ¼S with added sodium bicarbonate to alkalinize the urine (desired pH, 7.0 to 7.5). Acetazolamide (Diamox) may also be used to alkalinize the urine. Furosemide (Lasix) should be avoided, since it tends to produce an acid urine.

If the patient is anuric or oliguric, an attempt at osmotic diuresis with mannitol (25 g/m² intravenously over 15 min.) has been recommended following insertion of ureteral catheters (if urate sludge is seen blocking the ureters at cystoscopy).[35] If an increase in urine output does not occur, the patient should be treated for acute renal failure by appropriate fluid and protein restriction and the uric acid removed by peritoneal dialysis or hemodialysis.[16]

HYPERCALCEMIA

Normally the serum calcium level is maintained within a narrow range (9 to 11 mg/dl or 4.5 to 5.5 mEq/liter) by means of a dynamic equilibrium between gastrointestinal intake, bone accretion and resorption, and loss from the body. Hypercalcemia may occur in cancer patients as a result of direct bone resorption by osteolytic bone metastases or through stimulation of osteoclasts by humoral mediators (parathormone, parathormone-like substances, osteoclast activating factor, vitamin D and its metabolites, or prostaglandins).

The clinical effects of hypercalcemia are multiple and may involve a number of organ systems. Meyers divides them into five categories:[27] (1) neurologic—drowsiness, lethargy, confusion, coma, muscular weakness, abnormalities in the deep tendon reflexes; (2) gastrointestinal—anorexia, nausea, vomiting, constipation; (3) renal—polydypsia, polyuria, albuminuria, hyposthenuria, failure; (4) cardiac—tachycardia, bradycardia, arrhythmia, decreased QT interval, failure; (5) miscellaneous—potassium depletion, alkalosis.

In patients with mild hypercalcemia (12 to 13 mg/dl), treatment should be aimed at hydration and restoration of electrolyte balance; a low calcium diet should also be provided. If these simple measures do not suffice, serum calcium values may be lowered by oral phosphates or glucocorticoids.[38]

Severe hypercalcemia (above 15 mg/dl) is a medical emergency requiring immediate and vigorous therapy. Such patients may present with a catastrophic syndrome characterized by abdominal pain, intractable vomiting, profound weakness, severe dehydration, and rapid deterioration of renal function, progressing to coma and death. Isotonic saline should be given intravenously in order to reverse dehydration and promote calcium excretion. Since the saline should be given at a rate sufficient to induce a brisk diuresis, careful cardiovascular monitoring is required; furosemide (1 mg/kg as a bolus injection every 6 to 8 hours as needed) may also be employed.[38] The addition of a nonresorbable anion, such as sulfate, will further facilitate calcium excretion,[10, 31] but may result in fluid overload and secondary electrolyte imbalance (hypernatremia, hypokalemia).[21] Mithramycin, an antitumor antibiotic, given at a dose of 25 µg/kg intravenously has been demonstrated to lower serum calcium and may be useful in patients with skeletal metastases who fail to respond promptly to conventional therapy;[43] however, it has bone marrow suppressive effects and is still considered to be under investigation. Should the above measures fail, calcium may be removed by peritoneal dialysis or hemodialysis against solutions low in calcium.

When calcium is lowered to normal or near-normal levels, oral phosphate is useful for chronic use; treatment directed at eliminating or reducing the tumor will also be effective in preventing recurrence of hypercalcemia. Since inactivity promotes resorption of calcium from bone, it is important to avoid prolonged immobilization.

HYPOCALCEMIA

Hypocalcemia has been found in 10 per cent of leukemic children, generally in the advanced stages.[23] This complication may also arise immediately following initial therapy of acute lymphocytic leukemia, when phosphate is released by destroyed lymphoblasts (whose content of organic and inorganic phosphorus is relatively high). The symptoms include disturbances in consciousness, convulsions, carpopedal spasms, and hallucinations.

Treatment consists of intravenous administration of 10 per cent calcium gluconate, preferably under ECG monitoring.

SPINAL CORD COMPRESSION

Spinal cord compression may result from malignant disease in the epidural space or collapse of a vertebral body; early recognition of the threat to spinal cord integrity and prompt, effective therapy are necessary to minimize the possibility of irreversible paraplegia.

Clinical Findings

The clinical signs of neurologic dysfunction resulting from extradural spinal tumor may be divided into three categories based on the location of the lesion:[3] (1) compression of the *spinal cord* itself (above T_{10}); (2) compression of the *conus medullaris* (T_{10} to L_2); (3) compression of the *cauda equina* (below L_2) (Table 7–2).

Pain in the back is almost invariably the initial symptom of *spinal cord compression*. This may start as a vague backache, but root compression then causes pain along the distribution of the affected nerve; cervical or lumbar lesions produce pain radiating down the arm or leg whereas thoracic lesions have a girdle-like effect.[9] Such pain, usually increasing in intensity and constancy, and aggravated by sneezing, coughing, or straining, may be the sole complaint for a period varying from a few days to many months. The acute phase of the illness is then heralded by: (1) further disorders of sensation (prickling, numbness, loss of feeling, or coldness in the legs as well as impaired sensation to pinprick, light touch, temperature, and vibration), (2) progressive symmetric muscle weakness, (3) abnormal reflexes (increased deep tendon reflexes, ankle clonus, and positive Babinski sign), and (4) bladder and bowel disturbances. Sphincter control is usually the last

Table 7-2 Clinical Localization of Intraspinal Metastatic Lesions

	SPINAL CORD	CONUS MEDULLARIS	CAUDA EQUINA
Vertebral level	Above T_{10}	T_{10}–L_2	Below L_2
Motor impairment	Symmetric; may progress rapidly to profound weakness	Symmetric; mild to moderate weakness	Asymmetric; rarely severe
Tendon reflexes	Increased	Increased knee jerk; decreased ankle jerk	Asymmetric; depressed
Plantar response	Abnormal	May be abnormal	Normal
Sensory abnormalities	Symmetric; level common	Symmetric; saddle distribution	Asymmetric; dermatomal
Sphincter disturbances	Late	Early	Late; may be absent

(From Baten, M., and Vannucci, R. C.: J. Pediatr. 90:207, 1977.)

function to be affected and has the most ominous prognosis. If these symptoms are not evaluated and treated appropriately, a fulminating loss of cord function culminating in irreversible paraplegia will ensue.

Involvement of the *conus medullaris* may also produce weakness, but muscle tone is often normal and the deep tendon reflexes may demonstrate a mixed pattern of increased knee and depressed ankle jerks. Sensory abnormalities to pinprick characteristically involve the perineal or posterior thigh regions. Sphincter disturbances are common.

When the *cauda equina* is involved, there may be normal or mild loss of strength in a lower extremity along with an ipsilateral reduction of deep tendon reflexes. Plantar reflexes are flexor. Sphincter disturbances occur in approximately half the patients.

Radiologic Findings

The possibility of spinal cord compression should also be considered whenever a posterior mediastinal mass is evident on chest x-ray, large abnormal retroperitoneal lymph nodes are present on lymphangiogram, or a paraspinal mass is seen. Other radiologic signs which may suggest the presence of, and help localize, a cord-compressing lesion include collapse of a vertebral body or pedicle erosion. Vertebral lesions adjacent to, or directly overlying, the sites of epidural lymphoma may be demonstrable radiologically in over half of lymphoma patients with cord compression; in other patients, in whom vertebral lesions are not seen on x-ray, lymphomatous invasion may be found in excised laminae.

Since lumbar puncture may hasten the progression of a partial disability to complete paraplegia, it is usually done with facilities for intervention available and is followed by myelography without withdrawal of the needle. Indeed, myelography is the definitive procedure for demonstration of intraspinal metastatic disease. The demonstration of a filling defect by lumbar myelography is usually adequate to confirm the presence and location of the lower limits of an extradural mass. If there is an intraspinal block with total obstruction to flow of contrast material, cisternal myelography may then be performed to define the cephalad limit of tumor and to determine if multiple lesions are present at different levels (Fig. 7-1). The contrast medium may then be left in situ to follow the response to therapy.

Treatment of Spinal Cord Compression

Although there is universal agreement that spinal cord compression is a medical emergency requiring immediate treatment, the proper management of this condition remains con-

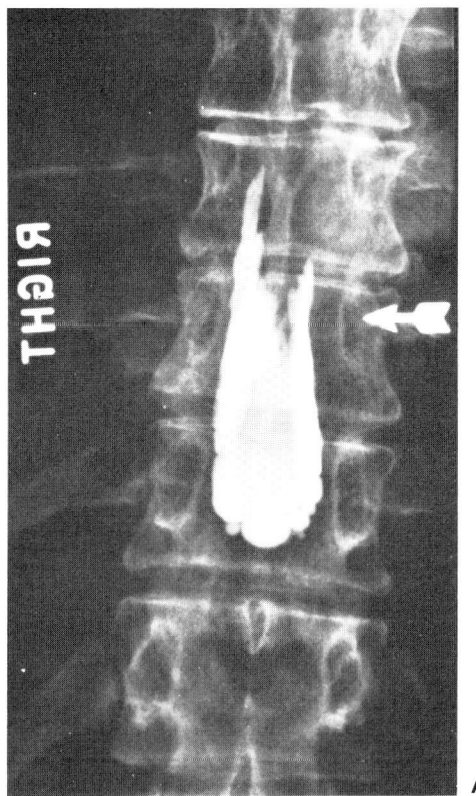

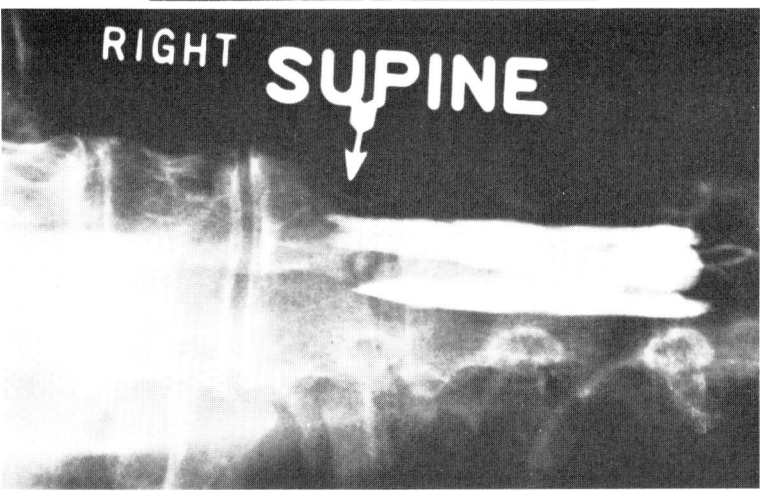

Figure 7-1 Lumbar (A) and cisternal (B) myelogram in a Hodgkin's disease patient with epidural spinal cord compression showing complete block. Patient presented with a 1 month history of back pain and 24 hours of rapidly progressive neurological signs. (From Somasundaram, M., and Posner, J. B.: Neurological complications of Hodgkin's disease. *In* Lacher, M. J. [ed.]: Hodgkin's Disease. New York, John Wiley & Sons 1976.)

troversial. The major alternative approaches are laminectomy, radiotherapy, or a combination of these. Chemotherapy and steroids may be used as adjuvant modalities; for example, dexamethasone (Decadron) may be given parenterally (0.05 mg/kg q6h) as soon as the diagnosis of cord compression is confirmed to help reduce the edema produced by the tumor.

Laminectomy is indicated in patients with severe neurologic defect or rapid progression of symptoms and signs over a 24-hour period;[32, 44] in addition to decompression, it provides a tissue diagnosis. Surgery should then be followed by irradiation (which can be delivered so as to avoid the recent midline surgical incision). Laminectomy with partial tumor removal is designed to provide immediate relief of pressure, whereas postoperative irradiation should effect complete permanent decompression (for radiosensitive tumors). Attempts to completely remove all tumor tissue surgically often carry the risk of compromising the blood supply of the spinal cord, especially the epidural arteries (when the tumor extends anteriorly).[32]

Radiotherapy, without preceding laminectomy, is particularly effective in relieving cord compression due to lymphoma and should also be considered for patients with widely separated lesions, those who are poor surgical risks, and those whose signs are slowly progressive and not very severe. However, the therapeutic response should be followed by frequent neurologic examinations and follow-up myelograms; if there is an inadequate response, laminectomy should be performed.

The conventional radiotherapeutic approach is to give small initial increments of dosage and to continue treatment over a period of 2 to 4 weeks. This is designed to avoid early pressure increase due to tumor swelling and edema, with subsequent aggravation of the neurologic defect. Some authors,[28, 39, 40, 44] however, believe that the risk of early tumor edema has been exaggerated and have utilized initial high doses of irradiation with the feeling that the rapid tumor shrinkage should more than compensate for radiation-induced tumor swelling.

If the patient has received prior irradiation to the area for vertebral involvement or a previous cord compression episode, the therapist must carefully consider the limit of the spinal cord's tolerance to irradiation — inadvertent overlap of treatment fields may result in radiation-induced transverse myelitis. The threshold value for symptomatic radiation myelopathy is about 3500 rads over 3 weeks or 4000 rads over 4 weeks and is time-dependent (relatively larger absorbed doses are tolerated if extended over a longer period).[2, 6, 13] However, individual susceptibilities may vary.

SUPERIOR VENA CAVA SYNDROME

Major factors contributing to the vulnerability of the superior vena cava (SVC) to compression are the thinness of its wall, its low intravascular pressure, and its anatomic position. Being locked tightly into a compartment of the right anterior superior mediastinum in intimate proximity to the right main stem bronchus, the SVC is completely encircled by chains of lymph nodes which drain all structures of the right thoracic cavity and the lower part of the left thoracic cavity.

In approximately 97 per cent of instances, the SVC syndrome is secondary to malignant disease,[25] usually lymphoproliferative disease in children or bronchogenic carcinoma in adults. Benign causes include thyroid goiter, fibrosing mediastinitis, tuberculosis, and aortic aneurysms.

Obstruction of the SVC may be manifested by (1) dilatation of the collateral veins of the chest wall and neck, (2) edema and plethora of the face, neck, and upper part of the torso,

(3) respiratory distress, (4) suffusion and edema of the conjunctiva (with or without proptosis), and (5) "wet brain" syndrome (drowsiness, stupor, unconsciousness, and seizures).

Lokich and Goodman point out that *"the major pitfalls in management of the SVC syndrome relate to overzealous efforts to establish the site of obstruction and to determine a specific histopathologic diagnosis."*[25] Such procedures as venography, venous pressure manometry, lung scan, bronchoscopy, mediastinal exploration, and upper extremity venous injections may lead to life-threatening respiratory obstruction, aspiration, and hemorrhage. Since SVC syndrome is recognizable by clinical criteria, many of these diagnostic procedures are not necessary and may produce complications; likewise, intravenous injections in the upper extremity are contraindicated because of the risk of thrombosis, phlebitis, and poor drug distribution. Consequently *all intravenous infusions should be administered through the veins of the lower extremities.*

If the SVC obstruction has been only slowly progressive or the clinical manifestations are mild, surgical biopsy of the region may be pursued directly by cervical mediastinal exploration.[25] Otherwise diagnosis should be deferred until therapeutic maneuvers permit relief of obstruction, for manipulation of the tissues around the SVC may lead to respiratory compromise or massive hemorrhage as a consequence of dilated collateral veins and edematous tissue. If surgical biopsy is deemed necessary to establish a tissue diagnosis under these circumstances, search should be made for abnormal superficial lymph nodes or other accessible tissue (e.g., bone marrow).

Treatment of SVC Syndrome

Radiation therapy is considered the primary therapeutic modality.[15, 25] Rapid high-dose irradiation has been shown to give symptomatic relief within 72 hours without compromising the patient's condition by so-called "radiation edema."[15, 39, 40] The treatment consists of 400 rads to midplane for 3 days, then slowing the rate to 150 to 180 rads/day until a total dose of 3000/5000 rads has been given (depending on the pathology of the tumor and the general condition of the patient).[15] The use of nitrogen mustard concomitantly with radiotherapy does not appear to confer additional benefits;[24] however, the combined use of hydrocortisone with radiotherapy may be of benefit to children with non-Hodgkin's lymphoma.[14]

For instances where the SVC syndrome is caused by lymphoma (Hodgkin's or non-Hodgkin's), chemotherapy may be as effective as radiation. Intravenous nitrogen mustard (0.4 mg/kg) (Fig. 7–2) or cyclophosphamide (30 mg/kg) along with judicious diuretic therapy may be used.[11] For non-Hodgkin's lymphoma, intravenous hydrocortisone (8 mg/kg) given in the first 24 hours, may produce dramatic regression (particularly when combined with radiotherapy); an oral steroid may be substituted thereafter as the clinical condition improves.[14] Chemotherapy may also be utilized when the mediastinum has already received the maximum tolerated dosage of radiotherapy.

Rapid response to therapy may result in hyperuricemia and uric acid nephropathy; thus, adequate hydration, alkalinization of the urine, and use of allopurinol should be provided when there is a large volume of tumor.

PAIN

When the patient with cancer complains of pain, any of a number of mechanisms may be responsible. These include (1) compression of a nerve root, trunk, plexus, or the spinal

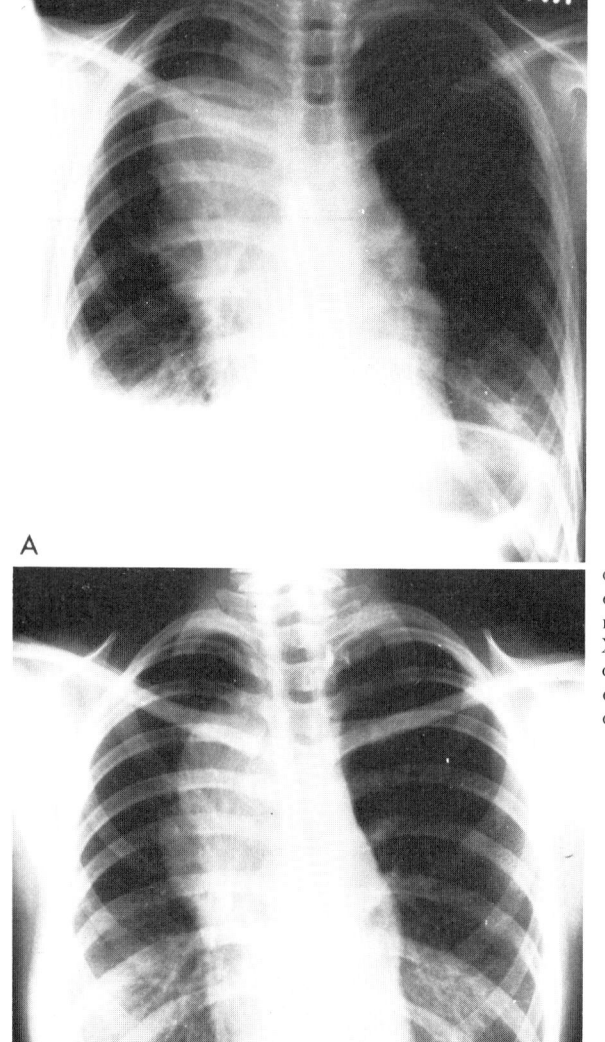

Figure 7-2 Superior vena cava syndrome in a patient with Hodgkin's disease. *A*, Large mediastinal mass and right pleural effusion are evident. *B*, X-ray taken 36 hours after patient received nitrogen mustard; the mass has decreased in size and the effusion has cleared.

cord by tumor or an adjacent bone fracture, (2) perivascular or perineural lymphangitis (with irritation of the sensory nerve endings) secondary to infiltration of a blood vessel or nerve by tumor cells, (3) partial or complete occlusion of blood vessels with secondary venous engorgement and/or arterial ischemia, (4) infiltration and tumefaction in tissues tightly enclosed by fascia, periosteum, or other pain-sensitive structures, (5) necrosis, infection, and inflammation of pain-sensitive structures, or (6) obstruction of a hollow viscus.

Since pain is a subjective emotional experience, the patient's perception of it may vary considerably, depending on his emotional state. Thus, in the presence of cancer, emotional factors such as fear, apprehension, anxiety, and depression may accentuate painful stimuli. Likewise, the physician's approach to the patient's complaints may have a profound effect on the success of treatment; it is therefore necessary to approach the patient with an attitude of concern and confidence.

Treatment of Pain

Initially all complaints of pain should be viewed as indicative of an underlying pathologic mechanism, and primary therapeutic efforts should be directed toward eliminating the cause rather than suppressing the symptoms. In most instances this involves surgical, chemotherapeutic, or radiotherapeutic elimination of the tumor. Even in cases beyond hope of cure, appropriate palliative antitumor therapy may provide effective relief of pain. Infection also is a common cause of pain in cancer patients and should be treated by appropriate measures.

When the tumor can no longer be treated definitively, the symptomatic relief of pain becomes a major priority. This usually involves the administration of systemic analgesics, but neurosurgical techniques are sometimes required when the pain becomes uncontrollable with other measures. Generally the least potent analgesic capable of producing adequate relief should be used, but there should be no hesitation about using potent narcotic agents if they are required.

Non-narcotic Analgesics. Aspirin remains the agent of choice for single-drug oral non-narcotic analgesia;[29, 30] however, the combination of aspirin with codeine, oxycodone, or pentazocine appears to produce significantly greater pain relief than aspirin alone.[30] On the other hand, the commonly used combination of aspirin, phenacetin, and caffeine (APC) is no more effective than aspirin alone for pain relief and can produce significant renal damage owing to papillary necrosis and interstitial nephritis.[1, 5]

Despite its analgesic effectiveness and relatively low cost, aspirin is not always the best choice for analgesia because it may produce significant side effects, including gastrointestinal ulceration and hemorrhage, hypersensitivity reactions, and certain asthmatic conditions.[9a] A major side effect of aspirin is interference with platelet aggregation through inhibition of ADP release from platelet granules. This will prolong the bleeding time even in normal individuals and may cause significant accentuation of a mild or moderate hemorrhagic diathesis. Thus, *aspirin is absolutely contraindicated in any patient with thrombocytopenia, deficiency of any of the plasma coagulation factors, or any other condition compromising the hemostatic mechanism.*

Acetaminophen (Tylenol) is probably the analgesic of choice for mild pain when aspirin is contraindicated. Although lacking the anti-inflammatory action of aspirin, it is an effective analgesic and antipyretic and does not cause gastritis or functional platelet defects.[9a, 37]

Propoxyphene (Darvon), ethoheptazine (Zactane), and promaxine (Sparine) appear to be significantly inferior to aspirin in analgesic effectiveness.[29, 30]

Narcotic Analgesics. Codeine is probably the most commonly used oral narcotic analgesic for mild to moderate pain. Its effectiveness is enhanced when used in conjunction with aspirin, but it may be used alone in cases where aspirin is contraindicated. Meperidine (Demerol) is also used frequently for moderate to severe pain. Its oral absorption is somewhat variable, but it is tolerated well by children and is convenient for ambulatory use. When pain is severe, either parenteral meperidine or morphine can be used.

Most patients given a morphine-like drug for relief or pain, especially in a hospital, are able to discontinue its use without difficulty even when they have developed a mild degree of dependence; only a small percentage become compulsive abusers.[9a] Consequently, *the fear of producing drug addiction should never prevent the administration of morphine or other potent narcotics to a patient with a terminal malignancy.*

Unfortunately many physicians tend to order (and nurses to administer) suboptimal dosages of narcotic agents because they overestimate the duration of action of the drug or underestimate the dosage requirement necessary to produce adequate analgesia; undertreatment may actually encourage craving for the drug to alleviate pain, which can be misinterpreted as addiction.[26] Thus, in order to achieve the maximum benefit from narcotic analgesics it is probably best to offer them at regular intervals that are shorter than the average duration of pain relief (Table 7–3) rather than make their administration dependent on the patient's complaint of pain.[7]

Side effects which legitimately should limit the dosage or frequency, or both, of administration of a narcotic drug include: oversedation, mood alteration, respiratory depression, nausea, vomiting, constipation, and urinary retention.

Neurosurgical Procedures for Palliation of Pain. When pain can no longer be controlled by other means, neurosurgical interruption of pain impulses may offer the patient considerable comfort for the remaining portion of his lifespan. Neurosurgical intervention should be undertaken while the patient's condition is good enough to tolerate general anesthesia and his anticipated survival is sufficiently long (at least 3 months or more) to justify the discomfort of the postoperative pain and limitation of activity.[34]

PERIPHERAL NERVE BLOCK. Pain due to regional involvement can often be alleviated effectively by a *peripheral nerve block* produced by injection of xylocaine or neurolytic drugs, such as absolute alcohol or phenol. Although such relief is usually temporary (lasting from 1 to 6 hours with xylocaine to 6 months with alcohol or phenol), it is frequently useful in determining if permanent destruction of the nerve(s) will provide significant relief.

RHIZOTOMY. Dorsal rhizotomy involves the destruction of the dorsal nerve route through which practically all spinal sensory flow into the central nervous system is channeled. This technique is appropriate for segmental somatic pain when it arises in an area where loss of all sensory modalities will not constitute a disability. Thus, it may be a good choice for treatment of pain of the thoracic or abdominal

Table 7–3 Time of Onset and Duration of Action of Narcotic Analgesics[9a]

Drug	Route of Administration	Onset of Peak Effect (min)	Duration of Action (hr)
Codeine	P.O., S.C., I.M.	15–30	4–6
Meperidine	P.O., S.C.	40–60	2–4
	I.M.	30–50	2–4
Morphine	S.C.	50–90	Up to 7
	I.M.	30–60	Up to 7
	I.V.	20	Up to 7

dermatomes; however, it must be recognized that useful pain symptoms which can give early warning of an inflamed hollow viscus (gallbladder, appendix) may be abolished. Sensory rhizotomy for pain in an extremity is effective in selected cases[45] but may result in a useless limb lacking proprioceptive discrimination. Chemical rhizotomy using intrathecal injections of absolute alcohol or phenol in glycerol appears to be useful for treatment of pain mediated by the lumbar and sacral routes,[33] but a potential hazard of this technique is impairment of bladder innervation and subsequent bladder flaccidity.

SUBARACHNOID SALINE INJECTION. Subarachnoid injection of superchilled saline solution ("saline slush") has been used for relief of pain in patients in whom neurosurgery is contraindicated or in those who have not gained relief from neurosurgical procedures.[4] Because the initial instillation of cold saline is painful, this procedure must be performed under general anesthesia. Unfortunately, this technique does not seem to relieve pain as reliably in neoplastic disease as it does in certain non-neoplastic conditions, and multiple irrigations are sometimes necessary.[34] The simplicity of this technique, as well as its relative lack of interference with bladder or bowel function, makes it useful in some cases, however.

Other Pain Relief Procedures. *Cordotomy* entails interruption of the spinothalamic tract. This may be performed surgically by an incision into the anterolateral quadrant of the spinal cord, contralateral to the site of pain. *Percutaneous cordotomy* is a new technique whereby a needle is stereotactically inserted between the C_{1-2} interspace to the anterolateral quadrant of the spinal cord and a thermal lesion of the spinothalamic tract is made with radiofrequency waves conducted through the needle.

Intracerebral surgery for pain relief is usually the procedure of last resort. Bilateral nonspecific destruction of large amounts of frontal white matter may produce significant personality deterioration. More selective techniques such as *frontal leucotomy* or *frontothalamic section* may be less destructive to personality and serve to alter the emotional reaction to pain even if the pain is still perceived. Furthermore, surgery of the frontal lobes does not produce sensory loss or motor and sphincter dysfunction. *Thalamotomy* may also be of value in relieving pain without producing personality deterioration; pain appears to be alleviated in these instances by altering structures at the level at which pain is consciously perceived.[46]

ANEMIA

Anemia is a frequent finding in the child with malignancy; it may be present at the time of initial presentation or may develop during the course of therapy. The etiology of anemia in the pediatric oncology population may reflect any of the multiple causes of anemia in the general pediatric population. However, severe anemia is almost always due to: (1) hypoproduction of erythrocytes secondary to suppression of the normal bone marrow elements by malignant infiltrates, chemotherapy, or radiotherapy, or (2) loss of whole blood through hemorrhage.

The acute leukemias are the pediatric malignancies that most commonly produce anemia through bone marrow infiltration; the solid tumors of childhood, particularly lymphoma and neuroblastoma, also may involve the bone marrow. When anemia develops under these circumstances it is frequently accompanied by *leukoerythroblastic changes* (i.e., nucleated red blood cells and immature granulocytes) on the peripheral smear; the peripheral blood may also contain teardrop-shaped red blood cells, poikilocytes and circulating blast cells.

Chemotherapy and radiotherapy produce anemia by damaging the rapidly dividing precursor cells of the bone marrow, which are ultimately destined to provide mature cells to replace senescent erythrocytes. Since the life span of the mature red cell (120 days) is much longer than that of neutrophils or platelets, the hemoglobin level is less rapidly and significantly affected than are the neutrophil and platelet counts. Consequently, significant anemia is rarely seen when pulse chemotherapy is used. However, if the drugs are administered on a daily basis or if large intermittent doses are given before bone marrow recovery is complete, severe anemia may develop.

Another frequent cause of anemia in the child with malignancy is the so-called *anemia of chronic disease*. This state is characterized by a modest acceleration in red cell destruction and a failure of the bone marrow to compensate for this with adequate production. Generally, the anemia is mild to moderate (hemoglobin rarely falls below 9 g/dl) and is accompanied by only a modest increase in the reticulocyte count. Although the serum iron level and the iron binding capacity are low, the marrow iron stores are increased due to defective utilization of iron for erythropoiesis. The anemia of chronic disease will not respond to iron therapy or to other hematinics, but will usually resolve when the malignancy has been treated adequately.

MANAGEMENT OF ANEMIA

Hypoproduction Anemia

When anemia is due to bone marrow failure, the initial treatment is replacement of red cell mass. *Packed red cells* are preferred to whole blood for this purpose in order to minimize the volume load on the cardiovascular system. It is important to recognize that the anemia has probably developed gradually over a period of time and the patient has compensated for it by increasing the plasma volume, thereby putting an added strain on the heart. Too rapid replacement of blood under these conditions may precipitate or aggravate congestive heart failure. Consequently, clinical judgment is required in order to prevent cardiac decompensation. A good general rule to follow is to replace the red cells at a rate approximate to that at which the anemia developed.

When the anemia is not too severe and the patient shows no sign of cardiovascular stress, packed red cells may be given at a rate of 10 cc/kg over a period of 3 to 4 hours with continuous monitoring for signs of tachypnea, tachycardia, or other signs of heart failure. When the patient is severely anemic (hemoglobin less than 5 g/dl) or appears to be on the verge of congestive heart failure, the packed cells should be given at a slower rate (3 cc/kg over 3 to 4 hours); this may be repeated every 8 hours until the patient's condition has stabilized. Occasionally a modified exchange transfusion, with removal of a volume of whole blood equal to the volume of packed cells transfused, may also be useful. The general goal of transfusion therapy is to raise the patient's hemoglobin level to above 10 g/dl.

Hemorrhagic Anemia

When the anemia is due to acute hemorrhage, the patient is depleted of plasma volume as well as red cell mass. Under these circumstances, the agent of choice is *whole blood*. This should be given at a rate commensurate with the rate of hemorrhage. Thus, a patient with a very acute voluminous hemorrhage should be transfused aggressively while a patient whose anemia is due to a chronic or occult hemorrhage may be transfused more slowly or may even be managed with oral iron therapy.

Other Red Cell Preparations

One complication of transfusion therapy, particularly when multiple transfusions have been administered, is the development of antibodies to leukocyte and platelet antigens. This may be manifested clinically by febrile reactions or chills during, or within three hours after, transfusion of whole blood or packed red cells. The development of these antibodies to tissue (HL-A) antigens will also cause difficulties should a bone marrow transplantation be performed. It is therefore desirable, if transplantation is a possible consideration, to transfuse the patient with red blood cell products from which most leukocytes and platelets have been removed. Among the products which have been developed for this purpose are: (1) *leukocyte-poor packed red blood cells*, and (2) *frozen red blood cells*.

Leukocyte-poor packed red blood cells are prepared by separating the leukocytes and platelets from whole blood by means of inverted centrifugation or serial batch washings using the IBM Cell Processor. *Frozen red cells* are prepared by freezing blood in the presence of glycerol, which is a cryoprotective compound. When the blood is thawed for transfusion, the glycerol is removed by washing and the red cells are reconstituted with saline. The extensive washing procedure used to prepare this product removes blood group antibodies, plasma proteins, plasma electrolytes, leukocytes platelets and some, if not all, of the hepatitis virus

NEUTROPENIA

When serious neutropenia arises in pediatric oncology patients, it is usually the result of the replacement of the normal bone marrow elements by malignant infiltrates or suppression of the bone marrow by cytotoxic chemotherapy.

Neutropenia arising from myelosuppressive chemotherapy usually is most severe from 8 to 16 days after drug administration; for the majority of these agents the marrow effect is transient and is completely reversible. The nitrosoureas are unique among cytotoxic agents in that they are usually associated with a longer delay in marrow suppression (nadir around day 28) and may produce cumulative marrow toxicity.

In clinical practice the best estimation of the adequacy of the body's production of neutrophils is the Absolute Neutrophil Count (ANC). This is calculated by multiplying the total white cell count by the percentage of band cells and polymorphonuclear neutrophils (PMN's) in the differential count. This calculation is essential in following children with compromised bone marrow function because the total white cell count may be misleading. Consider two patients, both of whom have a total white cell count of 5000/mm.^{3} The first has the following differential count: 45 per cent polymorphs, 5 per cent bands, 40 per cent lymphocytes, 5 per cent monocytes, and 5 per cent esoinophils (ANC = 5000 × 50 per cent = 2500/mm^3). The second has 4 per cent polymorphs, 1 per cent bands, 80 per cent lymphocytes, 10 per cent monocytes, and 5 per cent eosinophils (ANC = 5000 × 5 per cent = 250/mm^3). It is apparent that although both these patients have the same total white count (5000/mm^3), the first patient has a much more ample supply of neutrophils than does the second.

As shown in Figure 7–3, the risk of the infection is maximal when the ANC is below 100/mm,^{3} and nearly all episodes of bacteremia and disseminated fungal infection occur in patients with ANC below 500/mm^3.[57] The frequency of infection then decreases sharply with increasing ANC and reaches a plateau at 1000/mm.^{3}

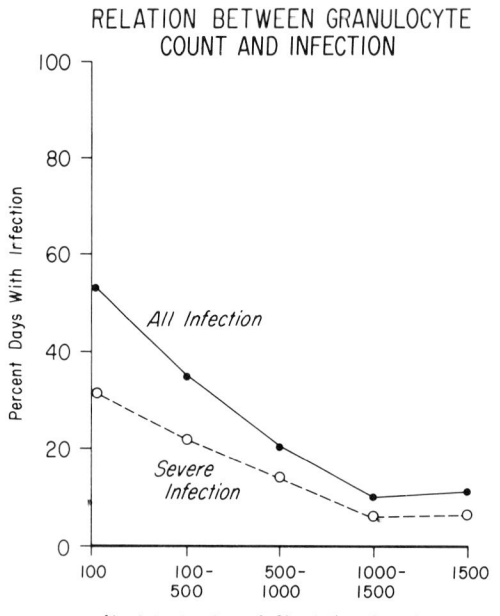

Figure 7-3 Relationship of absolute neutrophil count to risk of infection. (From Bodey, G. P.: Infections in patients with cancer. *In* Holland, J. F., and Frei, E., III: Cancer Medicine. Philadelphia, Lea & Febiger, 1973.)

MANAGEMENT OF NEUTROPENIA

Since the half-life of the circulating neutrophils is approximately 7 hours, transfusion therapy is not useful in maintaining an adequate neutrophil count in the severely neutropenic patient. It is essential, however, to diagnose early and treat aggressively any infectious complications that may arise.

When fever, signs of inflammation, or any other indications of occult infection appear in a patient with ANC < 500/mm,³ all orifices and other potential sites of infection should be cultured and broad-spectrum antibiotic coverage initiated—this is discussed further in the section entitled Infectious Complications.

When documented sepsis, meningitis, or other serious infection develops in the severely neutropenic patient, granulocyte transfusion therapy may be useful in supplementing antibiotic therapy until the patient's bone marrow recovers. Granulocytes may be obtained from patients with chronic granulocytic leukemia or from normal donors using cell separation or filtration leukapheresis techniques. In most instances, efforts are now made to use histocompatibility testing to identify HL-A compatible donor-recipient pairs. In general, only patients with ANC < 200/mm,³ documented infection, and an anticipated delay in recovery of bone marrow function should be considered for granulocyte transfusion. In order to be maximally effective, the transfusion should be given daily for a period of at least 5 to 10 days.

HEMORRHAGE

Effective hemostasis requires adequate numbers of functional platelets, adequate levels of plasma coagulation proteins, and vascular integrity. In the patient with cancer a potentially fatal hemorrhagic diathesis may develop as a result of compromise of any or all of these mechanisms either by the malignancy itself, by complications of the malignancy, or by therapeutic maneuvers directed against the malignancy.

PLATELET ABNORMALITIES

Hemorrhagic problems related to platelets are usually due to a reduction in the number of circulating platelets (thrombocytopenia); this may be the result of either of two things: inadequate production or accelerated destruction (Table 7-4).

Table 7-4 Mechanisms of Thrombocytopenia

1. Inadequate production
    Bone marrow infiltration by the malignancy
    Bone marrow suppression by chemotherapy
2. Accelerated destruction
    Consumption coagulopathy
    Sepsis
    Autoimmune
    Splenic sequestration ("hypersplenism")

The intensity of the hemorrhagic diathesis is usually directly related to the degree of thrombocytopenia. The earliest indication of a platelet problem is frequently some form of mucocutaneous bleeding (petechiae, purpura, excessive bleeding from puncture sites, epistaxis). This does not usually occur spontaneously until the platelet count is below 20,000 to 30,000/mm,[3] and the risk that severe spontaneous internal bleeding will occur does not usually develop until the platelet count is less than 10,000/mm.[3] When the platelet count is below 1000/mm[3] the daily risk of major bleeding is of the order of 30 per cent.[18]

Occasionally a hemorrhagic problem may be produced or accentuated by functional impairment of the platelets. This may occur as the result of certain drugs (e.g. aspirin) or as an intrinsic defect of platelets seen in association with certain hematologic malignancies (preleukemia, acute myelogenous leukemia, myelomonocytic leukemia, juvenile chronic myelogenous leukemia). Ancillary events, such as trauma, surgery, hypertension, sepsis, or severe sunburn, may also result in major hemorrhage even when the platelet count is at a relatively "safe" level (i.e., above 30,000 to 50,000/mm[3]). Postpubertal females may develop severe hemorrhage at the time of normal menses—such patients should be placed on suppression estrogen therapy (e.g., oral contraceptives). The general principles of management of the thrombocytopenic patient are shown in Table 7-5.

Table 7-5 Management of the Thrombocytopenic Patient

1. Appropriate therapy for underlying illness
2. Platelet transfusion (if platelet count <20,000/mm[3] and thrombocytopenia is due to underproduction of platelets)
3. Avoid aspirin
4. Avoid intramuscular injections and deep venipunctures
5. Suppressive estrogen therapy (for postpubertal females)

Thrombocytopenia Due to Platelet Hypoproduction

An early step in the evaluation of the patient with thrombocytopenia is examination of the bone marrow. If the marrow is diffusely infiltrated by leukemic cells (or metastatic solid tumor), then thrombocytopenia is a reflection of decreased platelet production. Such patients will not be capable of normal platelet production until the tumor population is significantly reduced or eradicated. Thrombocytopenia secondary to chemotherapy-induced marrow suppression presents the picture of a bone marrow panhypoplasia. Peripheral blood counts begin to fall by 4 to 14 days after the drug is administered, with the nadir reached somewhere between days 8 and 16.

The treatment of thrombocytopenia, when it is due to hypoproduction (regardless of the etiology), is transfusion with platelet concentrates. In some centers platelet transfusions are given "prophylactically" when the platelet count is less than 20,000 to 30,000/mm,[3] whereas in others, platelet transfusion is reserved for the times when active bleeding is present.

One *unit* of platelets is considered to be the number of platelets derived from one unit of whole blood (approximately 1 to 1.5 × 10[11] platelets);[18] the expected increase in the patient's platelet count following a transfusion of platelet concentrate can be expressed as follows: 10[11] platelets (1 unit) will raise the platelet count by 12,000/mm[3] per square meter of body surface area. Thus, in order to raise the platelet count to a reasonably safe level (50,000 to 60,000/mm[3]), the patient should be transfused with 4 to 5 units of platelets per square meter of body surface.

In a normal individual platelets have a lifespan of 10 days. However, for patients with neoplastic disease, particularly those with splenomegaly, fever, infection, platelet antibodies, or gross bleeding, the survival time is considerably shorter. Thus, platelet transfusions are usually required every 3 to 5 days until the patient's bone marrow recovers.

Several recent modifications have added to the effectiveness of platelet transfusion. The use of HLA-compatible donors has resulted in significantly better survival of transfused platelets and thereby reduced the frequency of transfusions. The technique of platelet plasmapheresis has enabled physicians to obtain multiple platelet units from the same donor, which reduces the risk of hepatitis exposure and volume overload.

Thrombocytopenia Due to Accelerated Platelet Destruction

If the marrow aspirate appears to be of normal cellularity and adequate numbers of megakaryocytes are evident, it is unlikely that inadequate production is the mechanism for the thrombocytopenia. In this situation, the thrombocytopenia may be the result of accelerated destruction secondary to a consumption coagulopathy, septicemia, an autoimmune reaction, or splenic sequestration.

Disseminated Intravascular Coagulation (Consumption Coagulopathy). Disseminated intravascular coagulation may occur if widespread inappropriate activation of the clotting system leads to intravascular fibrin formation. This may be produced via three mechanisms: (1) damage to vascular endothelium with exposure of collagen, leading to activation of Factor XII and platelet aggregation, (2) introduction of thrombogenic substances into the circulation, and (3) decreased levels of inhibitors of coagulation or blockade of the reticuloendothelial system so that activated clotting factors are not cleared from the circulation.

Patients with intravascular coagulation develop a consumption coagulopathy whereby "labile" coagulation factors are consumed faster than they can be produced and their levels are therefore reduced; prominent among these are *factors II, V, and VIII, fibrinogen,* and *platelets.* Thus, the patient will have, in addition to thrombocytopenia, a prolonged partial thromboplastin time, a prolonged prothrombin time, and a reduced fibrinogen level. Since the fibrinolytic mechanism is also activated, elevated levels of fibrin monomer and fibrin degradation products appear in the plasma.

Among the multitude of causes of disseminated intravascular coagulation in patients with malignancies are *release of thromboplastin-like material by the tumor itself* (seen in neuroblastoma, acute promyelocytic leukemia, acute myelomonocytic leukemia), *hemorrhagic pancreatitis, infection, intravascular hemolysis, hypoxia, acidosis,* and *tissue injury.*

The key to clinical management of intravascular coagulation is the effective removal of the underlying condition(s) which triggered the coagulation process. This may involve vigorous efforts at control of infection, acidosis, hypoxia, and hypotension, or removal of tumor tissue. Once this has been accomplished, the platelets and coagulation factors should return to adequate hemostatic levels within 12 to 24 hours; however, if the defects are severe and the patient is either actively bleeding or at risk of having serious bleeding, careful replacement of platelets and clotting factors by transfusion of platelet concentrates or fresh frozen plasma (10 ml/kg) may be utilized. Heparin is no longer commonly used for treatment of disseminated intravascular coagulation since it may aggravate the bleeding diathesis. This form of therapy may play a role, however, in patients with prominent thrombotic manifestations (e.g., gangrenous fingers and toes, renal vein thrombosis), patients with acute promyelocytic leukemia, and those patients with an unresectable tumor which appears to be releasing thromboplastin-like material.

Septicemia. It is likely that multiple mechanisms may produce thrombocytopenia in the septic patient; among these are direct effects of the microorganism or its toxins on platelets, diffuse vascular damage which may trigger intravascular coagulation, or sequestration of platelets by an activated reticuloendothelial system. It is thus not surprising that a variety of changes in the hemostatic mechanism may accompany septicemia; the most frequent of these is thrombocytopenia which may occur either with or without evidence of concomitant disseminated intravascular coagulation.[12]

The pattern of coagulation changes appears to correlate well with the patient's blood pressure—i.e., those patients who have normal blood pressure may have thrombocytopenia, but tend to have elevated levels of factor V, factor VIII, and fibrinogen, whereas those with hypotension ("septic shock") are virtually all thrombocytopenic and have accompanying disseminated intravascular coagulation (low levels of factor V, factor VIII, and fibrinogen, plus elevated levels of fibrin split products) (Table 7-6).

Splenic Sequestration. Thrombocytopenia may be associated with splenomegaly of virtually any cause; the mechanism appears to be increased pooling of platelets in the spleen. In children with cancer, the likely causes of such splenomegaly are (1) infiltration of the spleen by tumor cells, (2) portal hypertension secondary to malignant hepatic involvement, hepatic vein thrombosis, or cirrhosis, and (3) splenic vein obstruction or thrombosis.

Thrombocytopenia due to hypersplenism is frequently associated with neutropenia and anemia as well, since leukocytes and erythrocytes are also trapped in the enlarged spleen. In these situations, the bone marrow shows generalized hyperplasia of normal marrow constituents.

Thrombocytopenia secondary to hypersplenism tends to be moderate in degree (usually $\geq$ 30,000 to 50,000/mm^3) and is rarely associated with clinical bleeding manifestations. Removal of the spleen in conditions of hypersplenism is thus necessitated by anemia and increased transfusion requirements rather than by hemorrhagic symptoms. Although splenectomy will usually bring the blood counts back to normal, the operation should only be performed if its benefits counterbalance the risks of surgery and the increased susceptibility of the postsplenectomy patient to overwhelming sepsis.

Autoimmune Thrombocytopenia. Thrombocytopenia secondary to immune destruction of platelets is usually a diagnosis of exclusion, since it is frequently difficult to demonstrate antiplatelet antibodies by in vitro

Table 7-6 Summary of the Relations Between Blood Pressure and Coagulation Data in Children with Septicemia[12]

Blood Pressure	Platelets	"Consumption Factors"*	"Vitamin K Factors"†	Fibrinolysis Euglobulin Lysis Time	Fibrinolytic Split Products
Normal	Normal or reduced	Normal or increased	Normal or reduced	Normal	Absent
Reduced	Reduced	Reduced	Normal or reduced	Normal	Present

*Factors II, V, and VIII, and fibrinogen.
†Factors II, VII, IX, and X.
(Reprinted, by permission, from the New England Journal of Medicine, Vol. 279, p. 854, 1968.)

techniques. Thus the diagnosis is dependent upon the demonstration of (1) a morphologically normal bone marrow with abundant megakaryocytes, (2) shortened platelet survival, (3) a normal coagulation profile, and (4) absence of other known causes of thrombocytopenia (infection, drugs, splenomegaly).

Of the malignancies seen in childhood, lymphoma (especially Hodgkin's disease) is the most likely to be associated with this condition, and in some cases thrombocytopenia may be the sole clinical manifestation of active disease. The most satisfactory treatment of this complication is to control the underlying lymphoma—steroids are often ineffective in raising the platelet count until this occurs.[17] In one series splenectomy corrected the thrombocytopenia in 9 of 10 cases and uncovered occult splenic lymphoma in 5 cases.[17]

ABNORMALITIES OF COAGULATION FACTORS

Liver Disease

The liver synthesizes all of the major clotting factors except factor VIII. When the liver is damaged by malignant infiltrates, chemotherapy, radiotherapy, viral hepatitis, or other processes, there may be reduced synthesis of these clotting factors, with a resultant prolongation of the partial thromboplastin time and prothrombin time. The platelet count, on the other hand, is usually within normal limits unless there is an associated consumption coagulopathy (this sometimes occurs in liver disease because of failure of the reticuloendothelial component of the liver to clear activated clotting factors from the circulation).

The fact that the factor VIII and platelet levels are normal in patients with liver disease but low in patients with intravascular coagulation provides a useful means of discriminating between these two disorders (Table 7–7).

Treatment consists of transfusion with fresh plasma or fresh-frozen plasma (10 ml/kg).

Vitamin K Deficiency

The vitamin K–dependent factors are II, VII, IX, and X. Deficiency of these factors may develop if the patient becomes depleted of vitamin K because of dietary inadequacy, prolonged gut "sterilization," hepatic insufficiency, malabsorption, or biliary obstruction. This condition may be differentiated from the coagulopathy of liver disease by the normal levels of

Table 7–7 Laboratory Studies Useful in Differentiating the Common Coagulation Abnormalities in Cancer Patients

	BONE MARROW DISEASE	DISSEMINATED INTRAVASCULAR COAGULATION	LIVER DISEASE	VITAMIN K DEFICIENCY
Platelet count	Decreased	Decreased	Normal or decreased	Normal
Factor II	Normal	Decreased	Decreased	Decreased
Factor V	Normal	Decreased	Decreased	Normal
Factor VIII	Normal	Decreased	Normal	Normal
Fibrinogen	Normal	Decreased	Decreased	Normal
Fibrin monomer	Normal	Increased	Normal or increased	Normal
RBC morphology (peripheral blood)	Normal, may have teardrop RBCs and nucleated RBCs	Helmet cells, fragmented RBCs	Target cells	Normal

factor V and fibrinogen and from disseminated intravascular coagulation by the normal factor V, factor VIII, and platelet levels (Table 7–7).

In the event of severe hemorrhage, the patient may be treated with fresh plasma, fresh-frozen plasma (10 ml/kg), or fresh whole blood (20 ml/kg). However, in less urgent situations, treatment with vitamin K preparations will usually restore hemostatic effectiveness within 12 to 24 hours.

INFECTIOUS COMPLICATIONS

Infection is a major source of morbidity and mortality in cancer patients; it is the cause of death in about 60 to 80 per cent of patients with leukemia and lymphoma[56, 71, 74, 99, 100, 102, 108, 110, 130] and 40 per cent of patients with solid tumors.[100, 104]

Regardless of the underlying type of neoplasm, the development of infection can be related to one or more of the following defense mechanisms having been compromised: (1) mechanical barriers, (2) neutrophilic phagocytes, (3) cell-mediated and humoral immunity, and (4) the spleen.

Mechanical Barriers. In order for an organism to cause infection, it must first breach the mechanical barrier imposed by the skin and mucous membranes of the nasopharyngeal, pulmonary, gastrointestinal, and genitourinary tracts. The child with cancer is especially susceptible to factors that interrupt the integrity of these tissues; among these factors are decubitus ulcers, cutaneous tumor growth, necrotizing enteropathy, surgical incisions, intravenous lines, and skin necrosis secondary to infiltration of certain antitumor drugs.

Infection is also liable to occur when drainage of an area is blocked by an obstructive lesion. Thus, pneumonia may develop distal to a bronchial lesion, pyelonephritis behind a lesion obstructing a ureter, and purulent sinusitis behind a lesion blocking the drainage of the sinus. The offending microorganisms in these situations are usually the native flora of the region (e.g., gram-negative bacilli in urinary tract and gastrointestinal tract lesions, anaerobic bacteria in sinus lesions).

Neutrophilic Phagocytes. Once an infectious organism has breached the mechanical barrier of the skin or mucous membranes, it is the role of the neutrophilic phagocytes to prevent local consolidation and widespread dissemination of the infection. The lethality of infection in most cancer patients is directly attributable to a quantitative defect in circulating neutrophils. Neutropenia is seen most frequently in patients with acute leukemia, but may also occur as a result of myelosuppressive chemotherapy or marrow involvement by metastatic tumor.

Cell-Mediated and Humoral Immunity. The malignancies most commonly associated with a primary impairment of immunologic function are the lymphomas. Because of defects in T-cell and monocyte function, Hodgkin's disease patients in particular are unduly susceptible to facultative intracellular parasites, such as fungi, the tubercle bacillus, *Brucella*, and *Listeria monocytogenes*.

Patients with leukemia also appear to have impaired immunologic function, even before they are given chemotherapy; this may be manifested by defective cell-mediated immunity[98] and low levels of immunoglobulins.[107] Although not all leukemic patients manifest these defects initially, those who do seem to have a relatively poorer prognosis[98, 107, 108] than those with normal values. Similar deficiencies in host defense mechanisms may also be found in patients with other tumors, particularly when they have advanced disease.

Immunodeficiency may also be a result of treatment with antineoplastic chemotherapeutic agents which impair T- and B-cell function. In addition, corticosteroids interfere with the inflammatory response by decreasing capillary permeability, stabilizing lysosomal membranes and interfering with migration of leukocytes. Patients receiving chemotherapeutic agents and corticosteroids, consequently, have a high incidence of bacterial, fungal, viral, and protozoal infections. In some series,[139a] as many as 16 per cent of deaths in leukemic patients occur while the patient is in complete remission and are attributable to nonbacterial infections, mainly *Pneumocystis carinii*, Herpes viruses, cytomegalovirus, and pathogenic fungi. These infections are not usually related to neutropenia and are more likely the result of immunosuppression.

After the discontinuation of immunosuppressive chemotherapy, both lymphocyte and immunoglobulin levels return to normal within several months.[65] In fact, there may be such a sudden burst of proliferation and differentiation of immunocompetent cells that the marrow lymphocyte count may be in excess of 40 per cent and may mistakenly lead to the diagnosis of leukemic relapse.[65]

The Spleen. The only malignancy for which splenectomy is a routine part of management is Hodgkin's disease; recently some patients with acute and chronic myelogenous leukemia have also been splenectomized.

Splenectomized patients have an increased propensity for overwhelming infections with gram-positive organisms, particularly the pneumococcus. In one series of splenectomized Hodgkin's disease patients, there was a 10 per cent incidence of gram-positive septicemia and/or meningitis; the mortality rate of these patients was in excess of 50 per cent.[74]

Preventive Measures

General. Because of their increased susceptibility to infection, special precautions should be observed in the care of children with malignant diseases, particularly at times when they are severely neutropenic. Especially important is the preservation of the integrity of the skin and mucous membranes as mechanical barriers. This involves special attention to skin cleanliness and dental hygiene. The risk of anorectal complications may be reduced by minimizing or avoiding procedures such as digital examinations, rectal temperature readings, and enemas, which traumatize the rectal mucosa.

Indwelling scalp vein needles, venous catheters, and hyperalimentation lines have a high frequency of bacterial contamination (35 to 90 per cent),[56, 76, 81] which increases with the period of time they are left in place. The best way to prevent infections resulting from intravenous therapy is to use the intravenous route only when absolutely necessary and to limit the use of any site to as brief a period as possible (preferably less than 48 to 72 hours). Small butterfly-type needles are preferable to indwelling plastic catheters because of a lower rate of phlebitis and septicemia associated with them.[125] The site of injection should be cleaned thoroughly with an antiseptic scrub and covered with an antibiotic ointment and a sterile gauze. If sepsis related to intravenous therapy develops despite these precautions, replacement of all the involved apparatus is imperative.

Careful observation for signs of cutaneous, periodontal, perianal, urinary tract, and respiratory tract infections should be continuously maintained. When fever of unknown origin is present or when the patient shows signs of an active infection, modification or discontinuation of antineoplastic chemotherapy is indicated.

Children with malignant diseases should avoid exposure to individuals with contagious illnesses such as varicella, shingles, measles, influenza, pyoderma, and so forth. *Inoculation with a live virus preparation (polio, rubeola, mumps, smallpox, influenza, rubella) is absolutely contraindicated in patients with neoplastic diseases; killed virus vaccines may be administered, however.*

The vigilance with which cancer patients should be isolated from normal individuals is to a large extent determined by the degree of impairment of host defense mechanisms. When significant neutropenia is present (ANC < 500/mm^3), the patient should probably not attend school or be exposed to crowds; in the event of severe neutropenia (ANC < 100/mm^3), reverse isolation is probably merited. At some institutions, protected environments have been devised to minimize exposure to all organisms, both exogenous and endogenous (see below).

Protected Environment. The compromised host is susceptible to infection both by endogenous and environmental agents; consequently, prophylactic programs have been designed that have endeavored to eradicate the patient's own skin, gastrointestinal, and oropharyngeal flora as well as to isolate him from exposure to nosocomial organisms.

The two major types of patient isolation units which have undergone extensive study are the Life Island and the laminar air flow room. The Life Island consists of a bed enclosed in a plastic tent[59] supplied by air passed through high-efficiency filters capable of removing 99.99 per cent of all viable organisms. The laminar air flow room combines high-efficiency air filtration with air flowing in a horizontal fashion at 90 ft/min to prevent particles from settling (laminar air flow); since the entrance door is located "downstream" from the patient, any outside air will be caught in the laminar flow and filtered before it reaches the patient (Fig. 7–4). Personnel entering these areas wear sterile caps, masks, gloves, gowns, and boots. The patients are served "sterile" food,[144] and all equip-

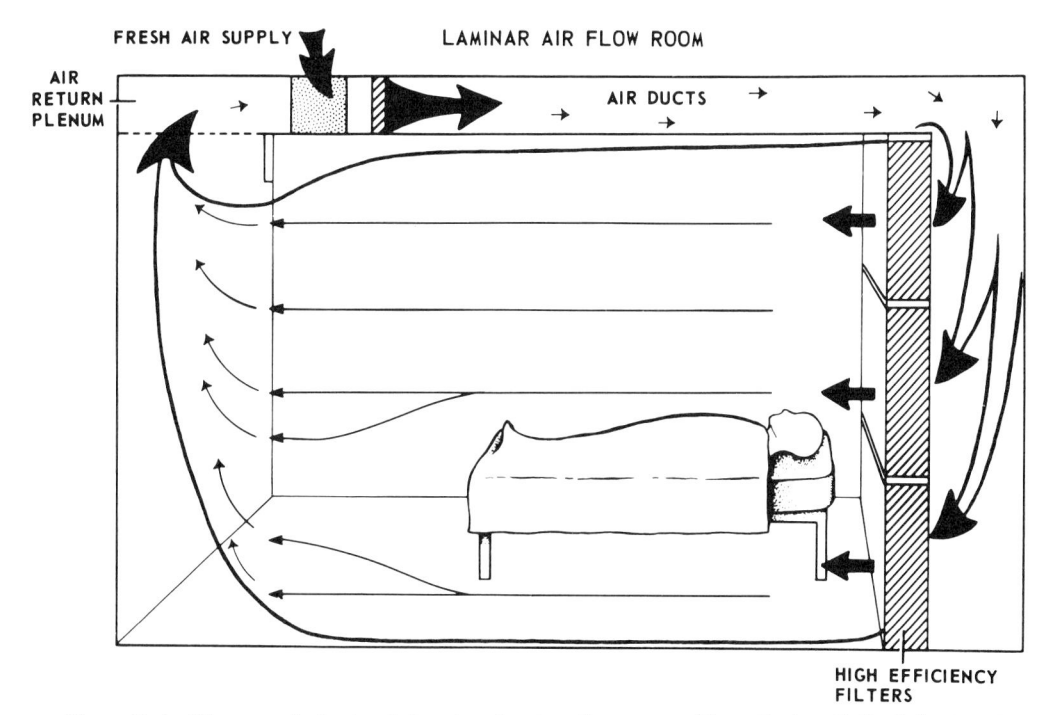

Figure 7–4 Diagram of air circulation in a laminar flow room. (From Bodey, G. P.: Infections in patients with cancer. *In* Holland, J. F., and Frei, E., III: Cancer Medicine. Philadelphia, Lea & Febiger, 1973.)

ment used in the room has also been sterilized. These protected environments reduce microbial contamination by 60-fold (Life Island) to 600-fold (laminar flow room);[55] 70 per cent (Life Island) to 90 per cent (laminar flow room) of the air samples are sterile.

In order to eliminate endogenous flora, topical and nonabsorbable oral antibiotics are administered and the patients are bathed frequently with germicidal soap solutions. Despite these efforts, persistence of endogenous flora remains a major problem. Thus, bacterial pathogens and fungi persist in the throats of 25 per cent of patients,[61] and fungi persist in the stools of over half the patients. Potentially pathogenic organisms also persist in the groin and the perianal areas of some patients.[63]

In one study, patients placed within an isolation unit and given prophylactic oral nonabsorbable antibiotics had half as many severe infections as a corresponding control group; whereas approximately 25 per cent of the control patients died of infection, none in the study group succumbed to infection.[111] The use of prophylactic antibiotics alone without the isolation unit did not significantly reduce the incidence or mortality rate of infections. Despite the ability of the protected environment/prophylactic antibiotic regimen to prevent infectious complications and improve short-term survival, there was no significant improvement in remission rates or long-term survival in patients so treated.[111] However, these maneuvers conceivably may allow an increased number of patients to live a sufficient time to receive an adequate trial of cancer chemotherapy or to receive more intensive chemotherapy regimens. Further studies are necessary before it can be determined whether the benefits of the protected environment justify the emotional burden placed on the child, the family, and the medical staff, and the significantly higher cost entailed.

Prophylaxis of Varicella. In normal children, varicella (chickenpox), is usually a benign cutaneous disease with a mortality rate of 0.12 to 0.4 per cent.[69] However, in children with acute leukemia or with neoplasms who are being treated with chemotherapeutic agents or corticosteroids, varicella can be a source of significant morbidity and mortality. In one recent series,[86] 32 per cent of patients who contracted varicella while receiving anticancer therapy had visceral dissemination, and 7 per cent died. Each of these deaths was associated with varicella pneumonia.

Because varicella is associated with such problems in children with neoplastic diseases, and because of its highly contagious nature, attempts have been made to protect these children from the effects of the virus. The initial attempts involved the use of gamma globulin and specific zoster immune globulin (ZIG), which can ameliorate[133] or prevent[68] varicella in normal children. However, gamma globulin appears not to have any modifying effect on varicella in children with neoplastic disease,[86,89] and ZIG, while ameliorating the effects of the illness,[68,105] does not appear to prevent it in children who are not previously immune.[90]

Zoster immune plasma (ZIP) obtained from adults 2 to 6 weeks after recovery from herpes zoster is currently the agent of choice for prophylaxis of varicella in children with neoplastic disorders. It appears to prevent the appearance of clinical varicella in over 70 per cent of patients and ameliorates the disease considerably in the others.[89,121]

In order to be maximally effective, ZIG or ZIP should be administered within 72 hours of exposure, since, after this period of time, the virus has already penetrated the cells and is not accessible to circulating antibody.[110] Cessation of anticancer therapy prior to the onset of lesions also appears to lessen the risk of severe disseminated disease.[86]

Tuberculosis Prophylaxis. All newly diagnosed cancer patients should be skin tested for tuberculosis and treated with isoniazid for 12 to 18 months if the skin test is positive and (1) the patient has leukemia or lymphoma or (2) the patient is to be treated with immunosuppressive agents or corticosteroids. It should be borne in mind that patients with leukemia and lymphoma (particularly Hodgkin's disease) are frequently anergic to skin testing, and consequently a negative skin test cannot be regarded as ruling out completely occult tuberculosis, particularly if there are suspicious lesions on chest x-ray.

INFECTION-RELATED SYNDROMES IN CANCER PATIENTS

Fever of Obscure Origin

Episodes of fever are always a cause of concern in cancer patients. Although certain malignancies (especially leukemias, lymphomas, and Wilms' tumor) can cause pyrexia, the possibility of infection as the basis for the temperature elevation must always be considered. Unfortunately neither the character nor the severity of the fever is of any help in determining whether the cause is the malignancy itself or an associated infection. In general, apart perhaps from newly diagnosed Hodgkin's disease, it is safest to suspect prolonged unexplained fever as being due to occult infection.

Episodes of fever are due to infection in 50 per cent of lymphoma patients, 60 per cent of leukemia patients, and 80 per cent of solid tumor patients.[64, 67] Over 90 per cent of these infections are caused by bacteria or fungi,[110] the lungs, skin, and gastrointestinal tract being the most common sites of infection.

Fever is particularly difficult to evaluate in neutropenic patients because the lack of an appropriate inflammatory response may prevent the classic clinical signs and symptoms from appearing. To add to the difficulty, these infections may disseminate rapidly and have a fatal outcome if not treated promptly. Some clues as to the nature of the underlying illness may be derived from certain helpful signs and symptoms (Table 7–8), but generally a painstaking physical examination must be performed and screening laboratory tests

Table 7–8 Signs and Symptoms Useful in Evaluating Unexplained Fever in Cancer Patients

SIGNS/SYMPTOMS	NATURE OF INFECTION	PROBABLE ORGANISM
Dysphagia	Esophagitis	*Candida*, Herpes simplex
Colicky pain, diarrhea	Enteritis	*Salmonella*
Painful defecation	Perianal cellulitis	Gram-negative bacteria, anaerobic bacteria
White retinal exudates	Fungemia	*Candida*
Oral lesions	Thrush, oral ulcers	*Candida*, Herpes simplex, gram-negative bacteria
Ecthyma gangrenosum	Septicemia	*Pseudomonas*
Vesicular cutaneous lesions (localized)	Shingles	Varicella-zoster
Vesicular cutaneous lesions (generalized)	Chickenpox	Varicella-zoster
Generalized lymphadenopathy	Lymphadenitis	*Toxoplasma*, Cytomegalovirus, EB virus
Indwelling urinary catheter	Urinary tract infection	Gram-negative bacteria
Hyperalimentation line	Bacteremia, fungemia	Various bacteria and fungi (especially *Candida*)
Tachypnea (without rales)	Interstitial pneumonitis	Gram-negative bacteria, fungi viruses, protozoa

obtained. These tests include: chest x-ray, urinalysis, blood, urine, and throat cultures, and lumbar puncture. Serologic tests for cytomegalovirus, infectious mononucleosis, toxoplasmosis, and histoplasmosis may also be helpful. Bone marrow aspiration and culture are useful in diagnosing disseminated histoplasmosis and tuberculosis as well as other bacterial and fungal infections. When the patient manifests tachypnea which is disproportionate to the degree of fever, measurement of arterial PO_2 may provide an early clue to interstitial pneumonitis even before changes are manifest on the chest film.

In many instances the child with a malignancy and fever of unknown origin is acutely ill, and it is undesirable to delay therapy until the result of the above studies pinpoint the etiology of the fever. Consequently, broad-spectrum antibiotic therapy is initiated immediately after cultures have been obtained. The selection of appropriate antibiotic therapy is influenced not only by the likely offending organism, but also by the degree of impairment of the host's defense mechanisms. If adequate circulating neutrophils are present, a combination of gentamicin with methicillin (or cephalosporin) will provide sufficient broad-spectrum coverage; carbenicillin should be added if significant neutropenia is present[48, 62, 110] (Table 7-9). Methicillin is preferred over cephalosporin for use with gentamincin because combined cephalothin-gentamicin therapy is associated with a high incidence of primary renal tubule damage in severely ill patients with malignant disease.[127]

If the cultures remain negative but the patient becomes afebrile within 72 to 96 hours, the antibiotics should be continued for a full 7 to 10 day course (Fig. 7-5), since early discontinuance may result in relapse of infection and death.[132] If the cultures remain negative but fever does not respond to the antibiotic regimen, then the antibiotics should be discontinued and the patient reevaluated.[81] In particular, an extensive search for fungi should be made, since approximately 20 per cent of patients with protracted fever that is unresponsive to antibiotics turn out to have fungal infection.[132] Most of these fungal infections are not recognized premortem; since sputum and blood cultures are usually negative or inconclusive, a definite diagnosis can usually only be made by demonstrating hyphae in tissue section of liver, bone marrow, lung, and other organs.[120] Some authors feel that a trial of amphotericin B may be indicated if the patient has been on steroids and has pneumonia or prolonged fever (> 21 days) unresponsive to antibiotic therapy.[120] However, since toxicity is frequent and a prolonged course of therapy is often required before a response is seen, empiric amphotericin B therapy is rarely utilized.

Recently the combination of trimethoprim-sulfamethoxazole (Bactrim) has been reported to be effective against 54 per cent of the infections occurring in a group of cancer patients who had failed to respond to prior antibiotic therapy.[94] This may reflect

Table 7-9 A Broad-Spectrum Antibiotic Regimen for Cancer Patients with Unexplained Fever[53, 75]

	PEDIATRIC DOSE	ADULT DOSE	
Carbenicillin	80 mg/kg q4h	5 g q4h	I.V. over 20–30 min
Gentamicin	1–1.7 mg/kg q8h	80 mg q8h	I.V. over 60 min
Methicillin	50–100 mg/kg q6h	3–4 g q6h	I.V. over 30–60 min

There should be an interval of at least 1 hour between the infusion of carbenicillin and gentamicin.[147]

Gentamicin dose may need reduction for patients with impaired renal function.

ONCOLOGIC EMERGENCIES

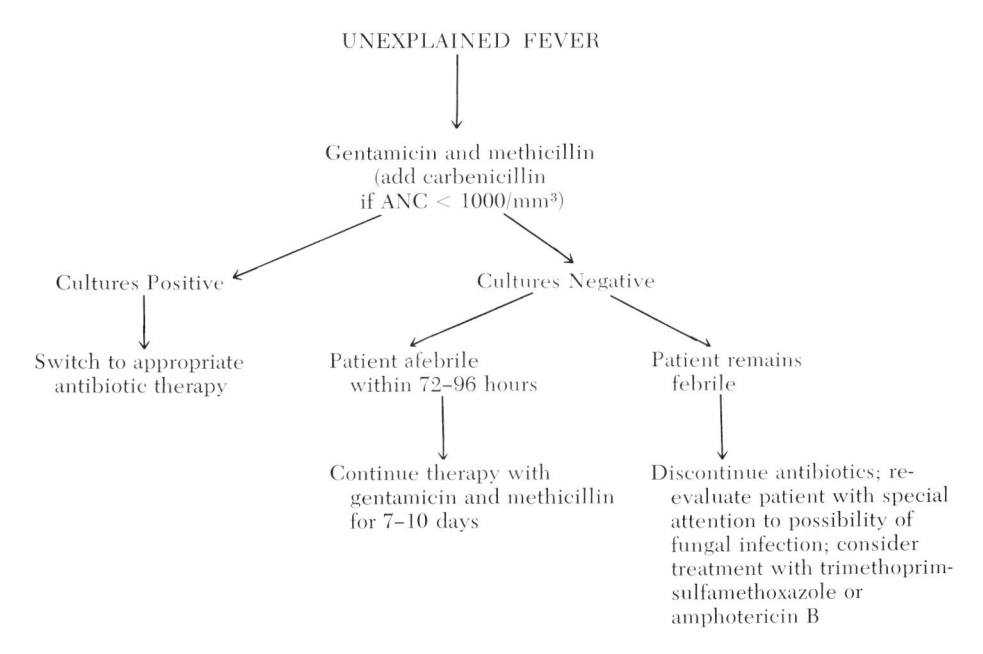

```
                    UNEXPLAINED FEVER
                            |
                            v
              Gentamicin and methicillin
                 (add carbenicillin
                 if ANC < 1000/mm³)
              /                    \
   Cultures Positive          Cultures Negative
         |                    /              \
         v                   v                v
  Switch to appropriate   Patient afebrile    Patient remains
  antibiotic therapy      within 72–96 hours  febrile
                              |                   |
                              v                   v
                     Continue therapy with    Discontinue antibiotics; re-
                     gentamicin and methicillin  evaluate patient with special
                     for 7–10 days            attention to possibility of
                                              fungal infection; consider
                                              treatment with trimethoprim-
                                              sulfamethoxazole or
                                              amphotericin B
```

Figure 7–5 Approach to fever in patients with malignancy.

the sensitivity of non-bacterial (e.g., *Toxoplasma, Pneumocystis carinii*) infections, as well as those due to bacteria, to this combination.

Once a specific organism has been identified as the cause of fever, therapy should then be guided by in vitro sensitivities; ideally in neutropenic patients the drugs used should be bactericidal rather than bacteriostatic. The combination of gentamicin and carbenicillin is particularly effective against *Pseudomonas* species in the neutropenic patient. However, this combination should not be used to treat any other known gram-negative infections because carbenicillin has only marginal activity against *Klebsiella* and *Serratia* species and partially inactivates the more effective agent, gentamicin.[62] Furthermore, carbenicillin is relatively irritating to veins and is expensive. Consequently, it should be discontinued after three or four days if *Pseudomonas* is not cultured and the patient is well.

Tables 7–10 and 7–11 list the com-

Table 7–10 Bacterial Infections in Cancer Patients

Organism	Drug(s) of Choice
Gram-positive cocci	
Pneumococcus	Penicillin G
Streptococcus	Penicillin G
Enterococcus	Penicillin G and streptomycin
Staphylococcus aureus	Methicillin
Gram-positive bacilli	
Clostridia	Penicillin G
Listeria monocytogenes	Erythromycin and tetracycline
Gram-negative bacilli	
Pseudomonas aeruginosa	Gentamicin (ANC > 1000/mm³) Carbenicillin and gentamicin (ANC < 1000/mm³)
Escherichia coli	Ampicillin
Salmonella	Chloramphenicol
Klebsiella pneumoniae	Gentamicin
Proteus mirabilis	Ampicillin
Proteus species	Kanamycin
Serratia marcescans	Gentamicin
Mima-Herellea	Tetracycline
Bacteroides	Tetracycline
HIGHER BACTERIA	
Nocardia	Sulfonamide-ampicillin
Mycoplasma	
tuberculosis	Isoniazid-streptomycin

Table 7-11 Non-Bacterial Infections in Cancer Patients

Organism	Drug(s) of Choice
Fungi	
Aspergillus	Amphotericin B
Candida	Amphotericin B
Coccidioides	Amphotericin B
Cryptococcus	Amphotericin B
Histoplasma	Amphotericin B
Sporotrichum	Amphotericin B
Phycomycetes	Amphotericin B
Viruses	
Cytomegalovirus	
Herpes simplex	Iododeoxyuridine (IUDR)
Varicella-zoster	Adenine arabinoside°
Protozoa	
Toxoplasma	Pyrimethamine-sulfadiazine
Pneumocystis carinii	Trimethoprim-sulfamethoxazole

°Based on one randomized, controlled crossover study.[146]

mon organisms seen in cancer patients and the drugs most frequently used to treat them. These recommendations must be regarded as subject to modification as sensitivities change and newer drugs are developed.

Septicemia

The impact of antibiotic therapy has resulted in a marked alteration in the spectrum of bacterial infections occurring in cancer patients. Prior to the introduction of penicillin, *Pneumococcus* and *Streptococcus* were the predominant agents involved in fatal infections of cancer patients. Penicillin-resistant *Staphylococcus aureus* then became the predominant organism, accounting for 30 per cent of all fatal infections in patients with acute leukemia;[96] since the introduction of methicillin in the early 1960's, the incidence of fatal *Staphylococcus* infections of leukemia patients has dropped to less than 5 per cent.[56]

Infections caused by gram-negative bacilli are now the most serious threat in neutropenic or immunosuppressed patients, accounting for approximately 85 per cent of episodes of septicemia in cancer patients.[56] The majority of these infections are caused by *Escherichia coli*, *Klebsiella* species, and *Pseudomonas aeruginosa*; however, *Staphylococcus aureus*, and *Streptococcus* as well as other relatively nonpathogenic organisms, such as *Serratia marcescens*, *Bacteroides*, *Salmonella*, *Bacillus cereus*, *Listeria monocytogenes*, and *Clostridia*, have also been associated with serious infections in these patients. Indeed *any organism consistently cultured from a leukemic or immunosuppressed cancer patient should be regarded as clinically significant and the patient treated accordingly.*

The most common sites of gram-negative infection are the oropharynx, lungs, gastrointestinal tract, skin, and urinary tract. All of these may lead to septicemia if the patient is severely neutropenic and cannot localize the infection.

Pseudomonas sepsis may be accompanied by characteristic peripheral lesions known as *ecthyma gangrenosum*. The classical lesions are ulcerations with ecchymotic and gangrenous centers and bright red borders (Fig. 7-6); however, variants of echthyma gangrenosum such as erythematous elevated indurated nodules with fluctuation, vesicles, small papules, and cellulitis have also accompanied *Pseudomonas* sepsis. These lesions all appear to stem from *Pseudomonas*-induced vasculitis followed by hemorrhagic necrosis.[129] Although *Pseudomonas* is the most common cause of necrotizing dermal plaques in the compromised host, other agents, such as *Aspergillus*, *Mucor*, *Cryptococcus*, *Aeromonas hydrophilia*, and the agent of phaeohyphomycosis have also occasionally produced a similar picture.[128] Skin biopsy and cultures are therefore sometimes necessary for a definitive diagnosis.

Candida sepsis also is associated with a characteristic lesion—*Candida endophthalmitis*. The patient may complain of ocular difficulties, includ-

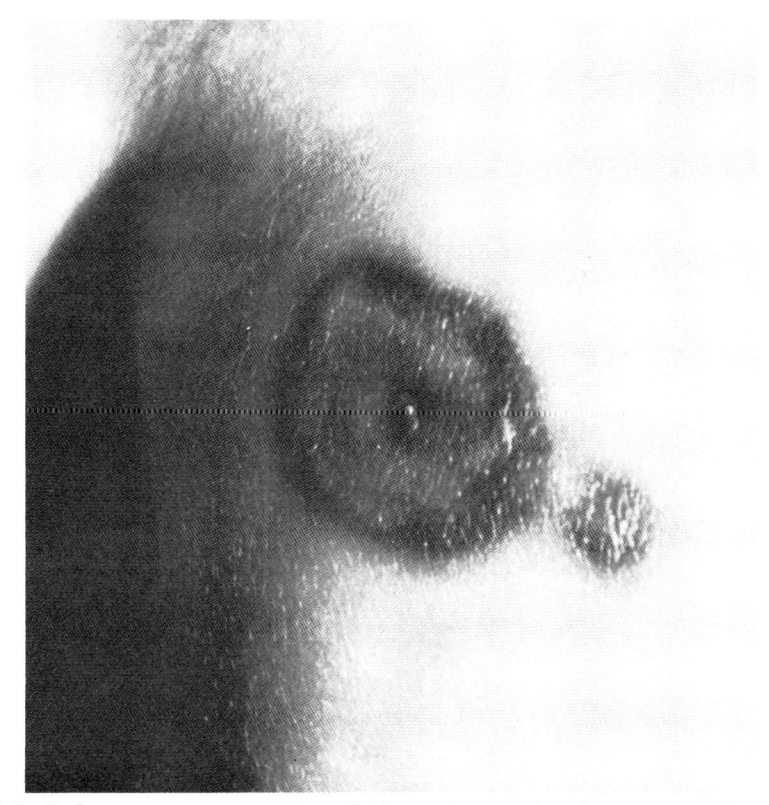

Figure 7-6 Ecthyma gangrenosum. (From Chilcote, R. R., and Baehner, R. L.: Pediatr. Ann. 3:71, 1974.)

ing photophobia, conjunctivitis, and blurred vision; these are accompanied by characteristic multiple white, fluffy, raised lesions on the retina (Fig. 7-7).[83, 114] If not treated, *Candida* endophthalmitis causes severe visual impairment or blindness, and subsequent enucleation of the eye may be required.[114]

Table 7-12 lists the syndromes accompanying some of the common viral, fungal, and protozoal infections seen in patients with compromised host defenses.

Pulmonary Infections

Pneumonia may be caused by a wide spectrum of biologic agents, including bacteria, fungi, viruses, and protozoa (Table 7-13). Because of the broad spectrum of etiologic agents to be considered, as well as the difficulty in isolating many of these organisms from the sputum, it is frequently necessary to obtain pulmonary tissue by means of a needle or open-lung biopsy. Closed needle biopsy has an 85 per cent yield, a 30 per cent incidence of complications (mainly pneumothorax), and a 0.5 per cent mortality; open-lung biopsy has a 95 per cent yield, a 6 per cent morbidity rate, and a 1.5 per cent mortality rate.[101] Obtaining an adequate pulmonary sample is important for diagnostic, prognostic, and therapeutic purposes, since 70 per cent of patients in whom a treatable basis for pneumonitis is found eventually recover, compared with only 25 per cent of those with no specific diagnosis.[93] Biopsy specimens should be cultured for bacteria and fungi and stained with gram-stain, hematoxylin and eosin,

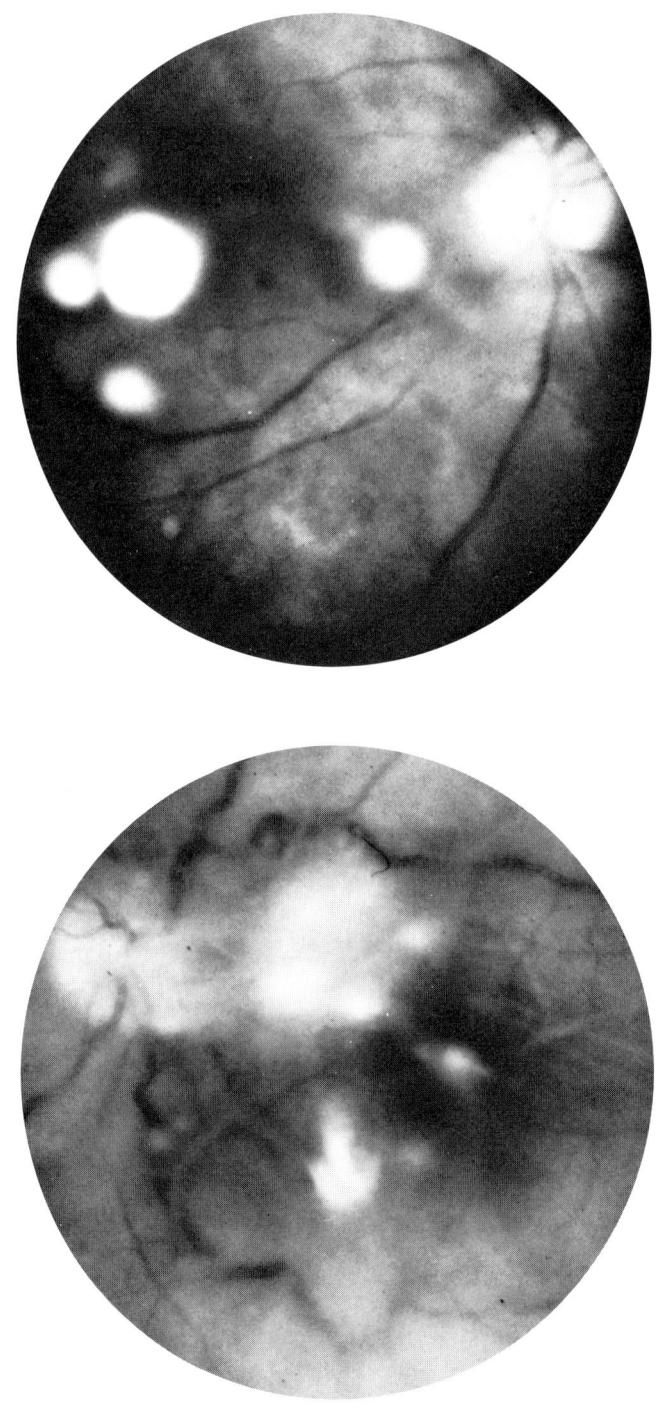

Figure 7-7 Candida endophthalmitis (Reprinted from Weinstein, A. J., et al.: Arch. Intern. Med. *132*:749, 1973.)

ONCOLOGIC EMERGENCIES

Table 7-12

SYNDROMES ACCOMPANYING VIRAL INFECTIONS	SYNDROMES ACCOMPANYING FUNGAL INFECTIONS

CYTOMEGALOVIRUS[47, 49, 78, 95]
  Viremia*
  Virus excretion (urine, throat)*
  Fever
  Fever with rash
  Hepatitis
  Atypical lymphocytes in peripheral blood
  Pneumonitis
  Chorioretinitis
 	
HERPES SIMPLEX[50, 113, 122]
  Large chronic necrotic ulcers of lips, nose, eyelids
  Generalized mucocutaneous vesicular eruption
  Esophagitis
  Necrotizing tracheobronchitis
  Bronchopneumonia
  Encephalopathy
 	
VARICELLA-ZOSTER[69, 86, 126]
  Shingles (localized zoster)
  Chickenpox
  Pneumonitis
  Disseminated zoster
  Encephalitis
  Hepatitis
	MONILIA (CANDIDA)[83, 84, 88]
	  Fungemia
	  Endophthalmitis
	  Mucositis
	  Esophagitis
	ASPERGILLUS[119, 128]
	  Fever
	  Pulmonary infiltrates
	  Abscesses of brain, heart, liver, and/or GI tract
	  Sinus infections
	HISTOPLASMA[77]
	  Fever
	  Hepatosplenomegaly
	  Variable chest x-ray findings
	PHYCOMYCOSIS (Mucor) (Rhizopus)[52, 118]
	  Rhinocerebral infection
	  Cavitary pneumonia
	  Renal vein thrombosis
	  Fever
	
	SYNDROMES ACCOMPANYING PROTOZOAL INFECTIONS
	
	TOXOPLASMA[70, 85, 117, 141]
	  Fever
	  Lymphadenopathy
	  Central nervous system disease
	  Hepatosplenomegaly
	  Pneumonitis
	  Chorioretinitis
	PNEUMOCYSTIS CARINII[143]
	  Interstitial pneumonitis

*The presence of viremia or excretion of virus is not a useful means of determining active CMV, since most of these patients are asymptomatic.[78] Fourfold rises in antibody titer may represent dissemination of CMV, however.[95]

---

and Gomori's methenamine silver technique (which will identify *Pneumocystis carinii*).

In patients with acute leukemia and lymphoma, the differential diagnosis of interstitial pneumonitis should also include involvement by the primary neoplastic process. Thus, of 44 patients with primary lymphoma, 50 per cent had a lymphomatous interstitial infiltrate in the lung.[93] Occasionally lung biopsy will reveal both neoplastic cells and an infectious agent.

The majority of pneumonias in cancer patients are caused by bacteria, particularly *gram-negative* organisms; this is especially true of pneumonias appearing early in the patient's course (before prolonged hospitalization, administration of broad-spectrum antibiotics, or steroid therapy). The gram-negative pneumonias, in particular, are associated with low-grade aspiration and are consequently frequently predominantly distributed in the

Table 7-13 Infectious Agents Associated with Interstitial Pneumonitis in Cancer Patients

Gram-negative bacteria
  (*Pseudomonas, Klebsiella*)
Fungi (*Candida, Aspergillus, Nocardia,*
  phycomycosis agents)
Viruses (cytomegalovirus, varicella, measles)
Protozoa (*Toxoplasma, Pneumocystis carinii*)

lower lobes. If the patient is neutropenic, pneumonia may be difficult to diagnose initially because of a lack of physical findings, sputum production, or x-ray changes. The presence of fever and tachypnea in such a patient should raise the suspicion of pneumonia, and frequently a repeat x-ray 48 to 72 hours later may show evidence of a pneumonic process. When x-ray changes are present in the neutropenic patient with gram-negative pneumonia, the usual pattern is an alveolar infiltrate; however, some cases of gram-negative pneumonia have a mixed alveolar and interstitial pattern (Fig. 7–8) which may cause them to be mistaken for fungal, viral, or protozoal infections.[151] As gram-negative pneumonias are usually necrotizing in nature, they usually progress rapidly to produce cavitation, sputum production, and extensive pulmonary involvement. *Pseudomonas*, the commonest cause of gram-negative pneumonia, produces a diffuse bronchopneumonia with nodular infiltrates and small areas of radiolucency (microabscesses), usually involving the lower lobes and sparing the apices.[56]

Tuberculosis should be considered in the differential diagnosis of pulmonary infections, particularly in leukemia and lymphoma patients, and those patients being treated with corticosteroids. The chest x-ray usually shows apical involvement, but cavitation or a miliary pattern may also be present. Since many of these patients are anergic to studies of delayed hypersensitivity, a negative tuberculin reaction should not be considered significant evidence against the possibility of a tuberculous process.

When pneumonia develops in oncology patients after prolonged hospitalization, antibiotic therapy, or corticosteroid therapy, fungal agents are frequently responsible. The most common offenders are *Candida*,

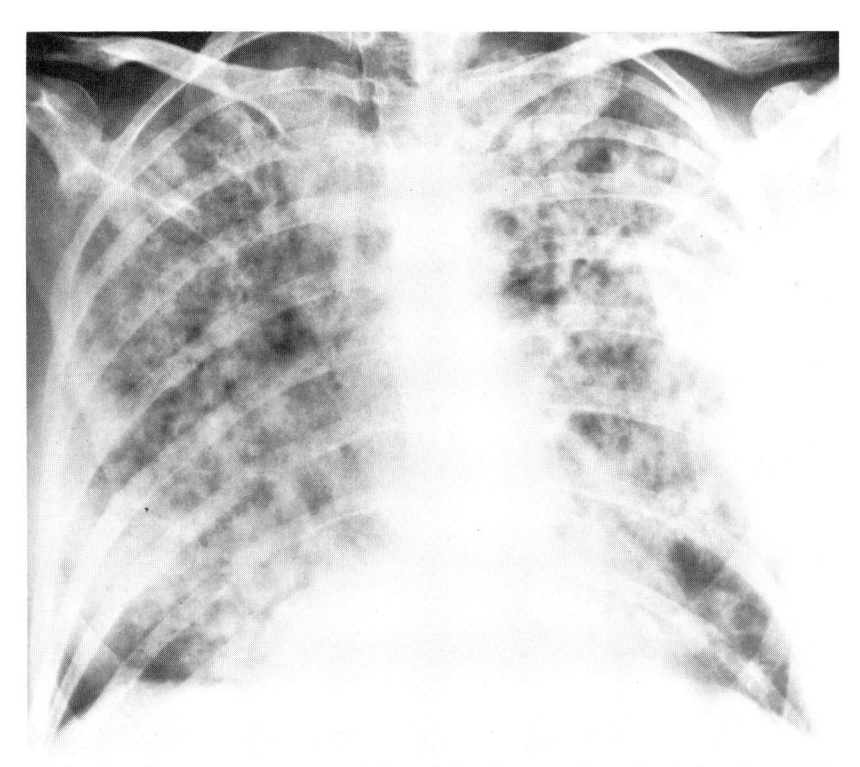

Figure 7–8 Pseudomonas pneumonia: bilateral involvement by mixed alveolar and interstitial infiltrate. (From Zorzona, J., et al.: Am. J. Roentgenol. *127*:989, 1976.)

ONCOLOGIC EMERGENCIES

Aspergillus, and the agents of phycomycosis, all of which may produce necrotizing bronchopneumonia, miliary abscesses, hemorrhagic pulmonary infarction, cavitation, interstitial infiltrates, empyema, or pleural effusion. Histoplasmosis and coccidioidomycosis may produce pulmonary lesions which mimic tuberculosis.

Viral pneumonia may be caused by *cytomegalovirus, varicella,* and *measles*. Although more ubiquitous agents (e.g., rhinoviruses, adenoviruses) may also cause pneumonia, the pneumonia they produce is neither more frequent nor more severe in cancer patients than in the general population.[72, 110] Clinical manifestations may include tachypnea, dyspnea, cyanosis, fine, moist rales, and interstitial pulmonary infiltrate on chest x-ray. These pneumonias may progress rapidly and terminate fatally.

Pneumocystis carinii and *Toxoplasma gondii* are protozoan agents which can cause pneumonia in compromised hosts. Pneumonia is practically the only manifestation of *Pneumocystis* infection, but toxoplasmosis is associated with fever, lymphadenopathy, hepatosplenomegaly, and central nervous system involvement in addition to pulmonary infiltrates. *Pneumocystis* is the most common cause of interstitial pneumonitis in patients with leukemia and lymphoma.[91] Its usual clinical signs are fever, a dry, nonproductive cough, tachypnea, and progressive cyanosis; auscultatory findings are minimal and rales are not usually audible. Chest x-ray shows interstitial granular haziness of the perihilar areas initially; this usually progresses to generalized irregular patches of consolidation. Diagnosis is complicated by the fact that the organisms are not usually evident in the sputum and cannot be cultured from the blood. Transthoracic needle aspiration or needle or open biopsy of the lung may be necessary to demonstrate the organisms; these samples should be processed with Gomori's methenamine silver technique, which will identify *Pneumocystis carinii* as cystic structures with an outer double-layered wall containing 2 to 8 internal bodies (Fig. 7–9).

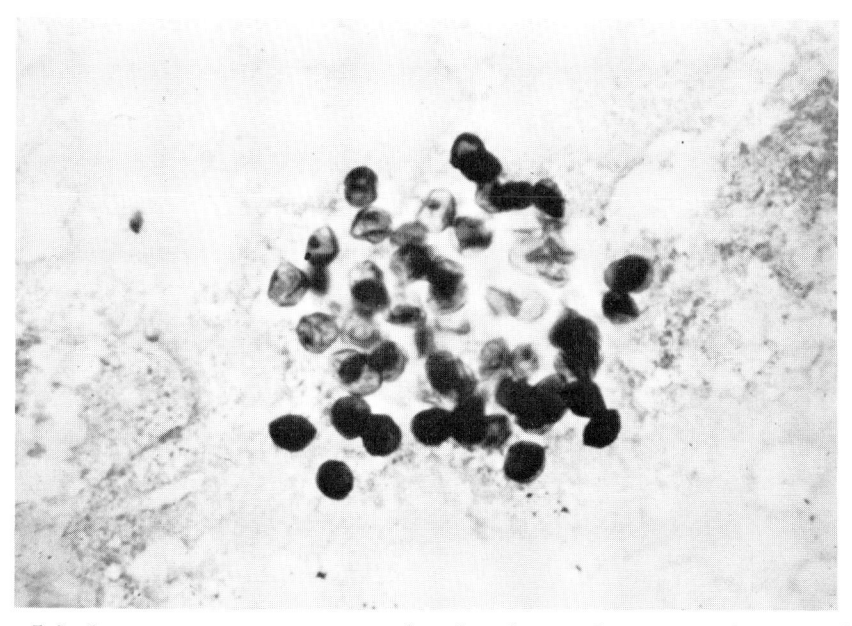

Figure 7–9 *Pneumocystis carinii* organisms from lung biopsy of a patient with interstitial pneumonia (methanamine silver technique).

Pneumocystis carinii has in the past been treated with pentamidine isethionate.[80] This treatment has resulted in 63 to 78 per cent cure rate if treatment is maintained for at least nine days,[102, 143] but has adverse side effects in nearly half the patients receiving it; these include impaired renal function, liver dysfunction, injection-site reactions, hypotension, hypoglycemia, and severe allergic manifestations. More recently, the combination of trimethoprim-sulfamethoxazole* (Bactrim) has been found to equal pentamidine in effectiveness (79 per cent recovery rate) and to have fewer side effects.[102] The efficacy of trimethoprim and sulfonamide appears to derive from the synergistic effect on folate metabolism. Trimethoprim inhibits dihydrofolate reductase by competing with dihydrofolate, whereas sulfonamide inhibits dihydrofolate synthesis by competing with paraminobenzoic acid.

Since *P. carinii* pneumonia is such an important cause of morbidity and mortality in pediatric oncology patients, it would be highly desirable to try to minimize its occurrence. An encouraging recent development in this regard is the demonstration by Hughes and co-workers[103] that trimethoprim-sulfamethoxazole was effective in preventing the development of *P. carinii* pneumonia in a group of 80 children considered to be at high risk for its development (versus a 21 per cent incidence in a placebo-treated group).

Central Nervous System Infections

Listeria monocytogenes and *Cryptococcus* are common CNS pathogens in cancer patients. Meningitis caused by these organisms is often associated with few clinical manifestations. Headaches, visual defects, and mild abnormalities of the sensorium are common symptoms; fever and nuchal rigidity are more likely to be seen with *Listeria* meningitis than with cryptococcal infection. *Listeria* is one of the few gram-positive organisms that are rod-shaped, and consequently isolation of a gram-positive bacillus from the CSF or blood of a patient with cancer should immediately call this diagnosis to mind even if the laboratory mistakenly reports it as a diphtheroid contaminant. *Cryptococcus* is seen almost exclusively in patients with leukemia or lymphoma;[73] it provokes a lymphocytic CSF response and can be identified by India ink negative staining (Fig. 7–10).

Brain abscesses in cancer patients are most commonly associated with gram-negative and anaerobic bacteria, particularly if the patient is neutropenic or has had head and neck surgery.[81] Staphylococcal and gram-negative meningitis also are more common in patients who have had surgery for head and neck tumors. Fungal brain abscesses may be due to *Aspergillus*, Phycomycetes, or *Nocardia*, and these patients usually have pulmonary infiltrates as well.[73]

Encephalitis is frequently viral in nature (Herpes simplex, measles, or varicella–zoster). However, the possibility of toxoplasmosis should also be considered in the differential diagnosis of any CNS disorder in an oncology patient, particularly since it is a treatable illness.[141] Three major patterns of neurologic involvement have been seen with toxoplasmosis: (1) diffuse encephalopathy with or without seizures; (2) meningoencephalitis; (3) singular or multiple progressive mass lesions.[141] Diagnosis is made by means of the Sabin-Feldman dye test, IgM fluorescent antibody test, or complement fixation test.

Progressive multifocal leukoencephelopathy is seen most commonly in patients with leukemia and lymphoma. Its exact etiology remains unconfirmed, but a viral etiology of at least some cases is probable. The condition

---

*Daily drug dosages: trimethoprim (20 mg/kg); sulfamethoxazole (100 mg/kg). The drugs may be given orally or parenterally.

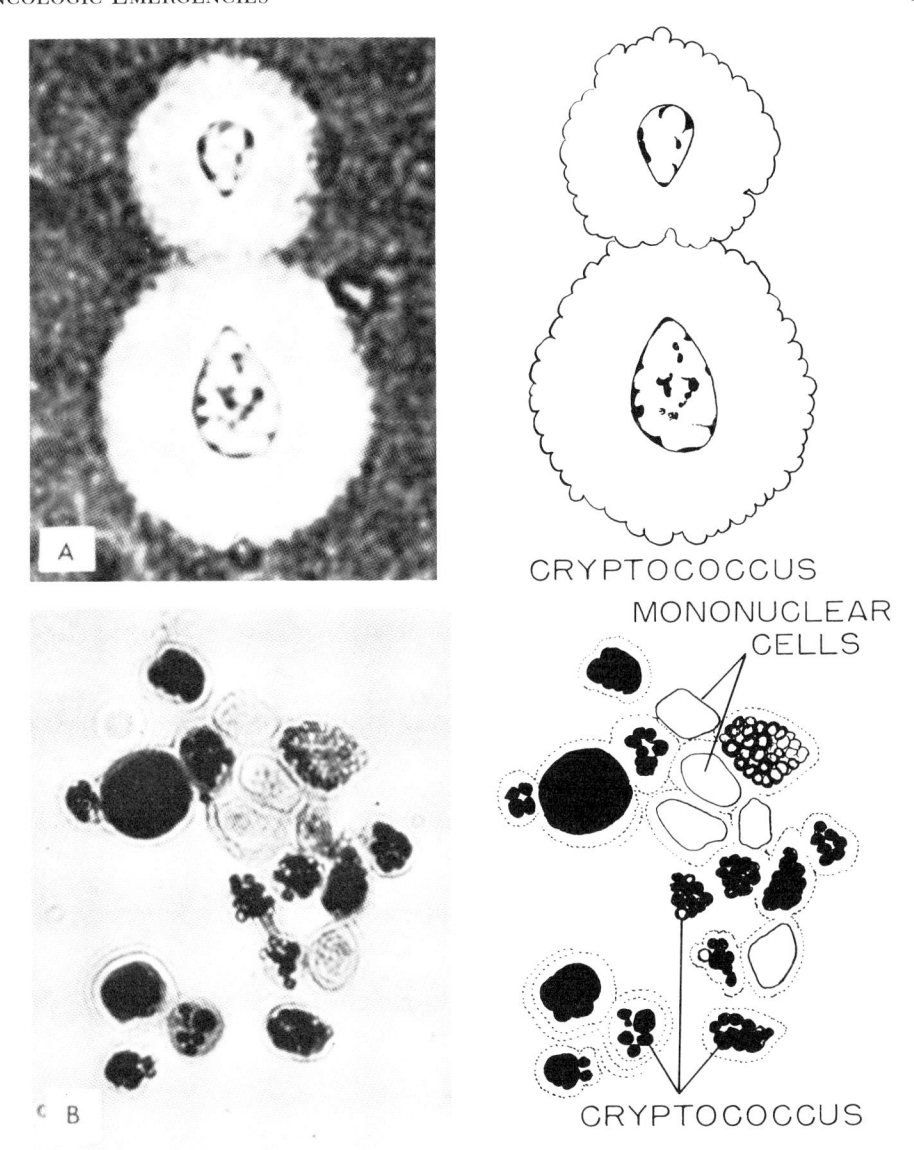

Figure 7–10 Cryptococcus neoformans. A, Indian ink preparation shows large capsule which excludes india ink from two organisms which have just budded. B, Gram stain showing gram-positive internal structures and large gram-negative capsules. Some of the organisms are budding. Mononuclear cells are also present. (From Armstrong, D., and Chmel, H.: Infectious complications of Hodgkin's disease. *In* Lacher, M. J. [ed.]: Hodgkin's Disease. New York, John Wiley & Sons, 1976.)

is characterized by insidious onset of nonspecific mental changes (disorientation, decreased mental acuity, emotional lability, visual field defects, blindness, dysarthria, and sensory loss). There is usually a relentless progression of symptoms, with death occurring within 3 to 4 months. On postmortem examination, the brain shows the following pathologic findings: multiple areas of demyelination in the cerebral hemispheres, cerebellum, and brain stem, bizarre giant hyperplastic astrocytes, and inclusions within the nuclei of oligodendrocytes.

Oropharyngeal and Esophageal Infections

Herpes Simplex. Oral ulcerations observed in patients with myeloproliferative and lymphomatous disorders are frequently the result of infection with Herpes simplex and must be distinguished from those associated with certain chemotherapeutic agents (e.g., methotrexate). Viral cultures of the lesions may be helpful in this regard. Herpes simplex may also cause large necrotic ulcers on the face, especially about the lips, nose, and eyelids; these lesions usually begin as small papulovesicular eruptions which become necrotic and slowly enlarge peripherally for several weeks before healing commences.[122] The frequent topical application of 0.5 per cent idoxuridine ointment may be beneficial in healing these lesions.[50, 122] Local irradiation has also proved useful, especially in promoting healing of oral lesions.[50]

Candidiasis. *Candida* infection of the oral mucous membranes (thrush) or esophagus is most frequently seen in patients with hematologic malignancies, especially if they have been treated with steroids or broad-spectrum antibiotics. The oral lesions appear as white or greyish-white plaques surrounded by an erythematous halo and are sometimes difficult to distinguish from the necrotic lesions seen with methotrexate toxicity.

Esophageal lesions are characterized by dysphagia, intense retrosternal or epigastric pain, and abnormal sensations in the throat.[112] Barium swallow frequently demonstrates impaired esophageal motility, narrowing, a cobblestone epithelium, erosions, and/or ulcerations (Fig. 7–11). If untreated, the mycelia may enter the systemic circulation through ruptured esophageal vessels and disseminate to other organs, leading to the death of the patient.

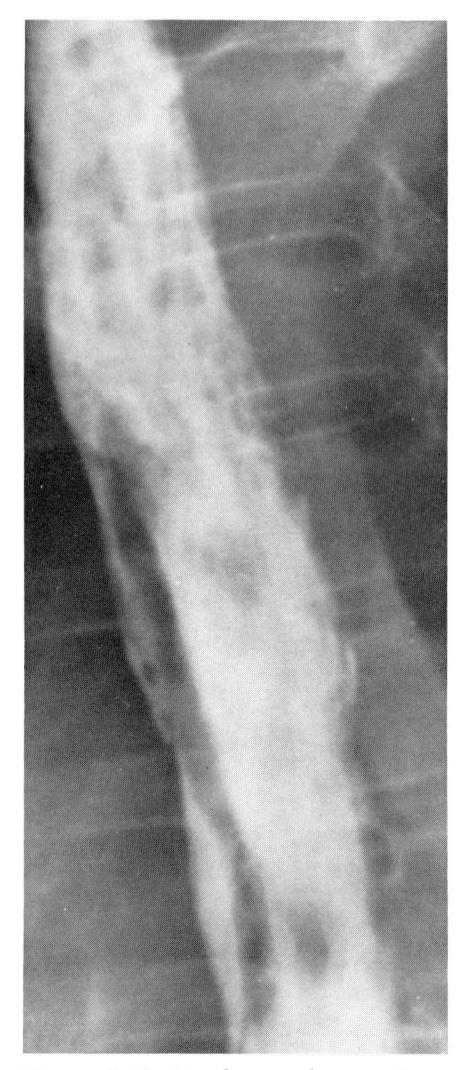

Figure 7–11 Monilia esophagitis. Barium swallow demonstrates defects of various sizes and shapes producing an irregular cobblestone pattern. (From Lewicki, A. M., and Moore, J. P.: Amer. J. Roentogenol. *125*:218, 1975.)

Oral and esophageal moniliasis are usually treated with oral mycostatin. When the patient does not respond to this treatment, other causes of dysphagia such as Herpes and other viruses, chemotherapy (especially methotrexate and Adriamycin), radiotherapy, esophageal malignancy, and gastric reflux should be ruled out before subjecting the patient to amphotericin B treatment for presumed resistant moniliasis.[113]

Anorectal Infections

The rectum should be considered a possible site of infection in all febrile neutropenic patients, especially those with hematologic malignancies; perianal complications are especially frequent in patients with acute monocytic leukemia and acute myelomonocytic leukemia.[136] Sometimes these infections are iatrogenically induced by irritation of the perianal region.

Presenting features of anorectal infections include indurated, tender red areas, fluctuant ischiorectal abscesses, fistulas with edematous sentinel piles, and thrombosed infected ulcerated hemorrhoids. Early diagnosis is sometimes difficult, however, because impaired hosts often produce only a slight inflammatory response.

When the above features are present or if the patient complains of perianal pain, broad-spectrum antibiotic therapy should be instituted (gram-negative and anaerobic bacteria are the most frequent offending organisms); warm compresses or sitz baths, stool softeners, and analgesics are also useful. Surgical treatment should be avoided in the severely neutropenic patient, since incision into the involved area may result in extensive propagation, with subsequent necrosis of the entire buttock; an obvious fluctuant abscess should be drained, however.[137] Thrombocytopenia should be corrected before any drainage procedures are initiated in order to avoid intractable hemorrhage.

When patients with active leukemia show perianal pathology, leukemic infiltrates may be present and low-dose radiation therapy to the perianal area is indicated.[137] Radiotherapy can also be given to patients who have thrombosed external hemorrhoids with induration around the base. The dosage used is 300 to 400 rads over 1 to 3 days.

Infections Caused by Anaerobic Bacteria

Anaerobic bacterial infections occur most frequently in situations where tumors obstruct the bronchi or interrupt the integrity of the oral, gastrointestinal, or genitourinary tract. Most intraabdominal, pelvic, and anorectal infections in pediatric oncology patients are caused by anaerobes; *Bacteroides* species and anaerobic streptococci are the organisms most commonly found.

Treatment of these infections requires adequate drainage, removal of necrotic tissue, and appropriate antibiotic therapy. Penicillin G and streptomycin are effective for treating infection with anaerobic streptococci and tetracycline is active against *Bacteroides*. Clindamycin and chloramphenicol also have an excellent spectrum against anaerobes.[130]

REFERENCES

1. Abel, J. A.: Analgesic nephropathy. Clin. Pharmacol. Ther. *12*:583, 1971.
2. Atkins, H. L., and Tretter, R.: Radiation myelopathy: Time-dose considerations. Acta Radiol. *5*:79, 1966.
3. Baten, M., and Vannucci, R. C.: Intraspinal metastatic disease in childhood cancer. J. Pediatr. *90*:207, 1977.
4. Battista, A. F.: Subarachnoid cold saline wash for pain relief. Arch. Surg. *103*:672, 1971.
5. Beaver, W. T., Mild analgesics: A review of their clinical pharmacology. Part II. Am. J. Med. Sci. *251*:576, 1966.
6. Boden, G.: Radiation myelitis of the brain stem. J. Faculty Radiol. *2*:79, 1950.
7. Bonica, J. J.: The total management of the patient with chronic pain. Drug Ther. *3*:33, 1973.
8. Boston Collaborative Drug Surveillance Program: Excess of ampicillin rashes associated with allopurinal or hyperuricemia. N. Engl. J. Med. *286*:505, 1972.
9. Botterell, E. H., and FitzGerald, G. W.: Spinal cord compression produced by extradural malignant tumors: Early recognition, treatment, and results. Can. Med. Assoc. J. *80*:791, 1959.
9a. Catalano, R. B.: The medical approach to management of pain caused by cancer. Semin. Oncol. *2*:379, 1975.
10. Chakmakjian, Z. H., Bethune, J. E., et al.:

Sodium sulfate treatment of hypercalcemia. N. Engl. J. Med. 275:862, 1966.
11. Cline, M. J., and Haskell, C. M.: Cancer Chemotherapy. 2nd Ed. Philadelphia, W. B. Saunders, 1975.
12. Corrigan, J. J., Jr., Ray, W. L., and May, N.: Changes in the blood coagulation system associated with septicemia. N. Engl. J. Med. 279:851, 1968.
13. Coy, P., Baker, S., and Dolman, C. L.: Progressive myelopathy due to radiation. Can. Med. Assoc. J. 100:1129, 1969.
14. D'Angio, G. J., Mitus, A., and Evans, A. E.: The superior mediastinal syndrome in children with cancer. Amer. J. Roentgenol. 93:537, 1965.
15. Davenport, D., Ferree, C., Blake, D., and Raben, M.: Response of superior vena cava syndrome to radiation therapy. Cancer 38:1577, 1976.
16. Deger, G. E., and Wagoner, R. D.: Peritoneal dialysis in acute uric acid nephropathy. Mayo Clin. Proc. 47:189, 1972.
17. Fink, K., and Al-Mondhiry, H.: Idiopathic thrombocytopenic purpura in lymphoma. Cancer 37:1999, 1976.
18. Freireich, E. J., Shively, J. A., and DeJongh, D. S.: Platelet replacement. In Neoplasia in Childhood. A collection of papers presented at the Twelfth Annual Clinical Conference on Cancer, 1967, at the University of Texas M. D. Anderson Hospital and Tumor Institute. Chicago, Year Book Medical Publishers, Inc., 1969.
19. Friedman, M., Kim, T. H., and Panahon, A. M.: Spinal cord compression in malignant lymphoma. Treatment and results. Cancer 37:1485, 1976.
20. Haddad, P., Thaell, J. F., Kiely, J. M., et al.: Lymphoma of the spinal extradural space. Cancer 38:1862, 1976.
21. Heckman, B. A., and Walsh, J. H.: Hypernatremia complicating sodium sulfate therapy for hypercalcemic crisis. N. Engl. J. Med. 276:1082, 1967.
22. Khan, F. R., Glicksman, A. S., Chu, F. C. H., and Nickson, J. J.: Treatment by radiotherapy of spinal cord compression due to extradural metastases. Radiology 89:495, 1967.
23. Jaffe, N., Kim, B. S., and Vawter, G. F.: Hypocalcemia—A complication of childhood leukemia. Cancer 29:392, 1972.
24. Levitt, S. H., Jones, T. K., Kilpatrick, S. J., and Bogardus, C. R.: Treatment of malignant superior vena caval obstruction. A randomized study. Cancer 24:447, 1969.
25. Lokich, J. J., and Goodman, R.: Superior vena cava syndrome. Clinical management. J.A.M.A. 231:58, 1975.
26. Marks, R. M., and Sachar, E. J.: Undertreatment of medical inpatients with narcotic analgesics. Ann. Intern. Med. 78:173, 1973.
27. Meyers, W. P. L.: Hypercalcemia in neoplastic disease. Arch. Surg. 80:308, 1960.
28. Millburn, L., Hibbs, G. G., and Hendrickson, F. R.: Treatment of spinal compression from metastatic carcinoma. Cancer 21:447, 1968.
29. Moertel, C. G., Ahlmann, D. L., Taylor, W. F., et al.: A comparative evaluation of marketed analgesic drugs. N. Engl. J. Med. 286:813, 1972.
30. Moertel, C. G., Ahlmann, D. L., Taylor, W. F., et al.: Relief of pain by oral medications. J.A.M.A. 229:55, 1974.
31. Muggia, F. M., and Heinemann, H. O.: Hypercalcemia associated with neoplastic disease. Ann. Intern. Med. 73:281, 1970.
32. Mullins, G. M., Flynn, J. P. G., El-Mahdi, A. M., et al.: Malignant lymphoma of the spinal epidural space. Ann. Intern. Med. 74:416, 1971.
33. Nathan, P. W.: Treatment of intractable pain by chemical rhizotomy with phenol solutions. In Gillingham, F. J. (ed.): Neurosurgery. Philadelphia, J. B. Lippincott Co., 1970.
34. Nelson, K. M., Bourke, R. S.: Neurosurgical management of pain. In Holland, J. F., and Frei, E., III (eds.): Cancer Medicine. Philadelphia, Lea & Febiger, 1973.
35. Perry, M. C., Hoagland, H. C., and Wagoner, R. D.: Uric acid nephropathy. J.A.M.A. 236:961, 1976.
36. Rastegar, A., and Thier, S. O.: The physiologic approach to hyperuricemia. N. Engl. J. Med. 286:470, 1972.
37. Reuter, S., and Montgomery, W. W.: Aspirin vs. acetaminophen after tonsillectomy. Arch. Otolaryn. 80:214, 1964.
38. Root, A. W., and Harrison, H. E.: Recent advances in calcium metabolism. II. Disorders of calcium homeostasis. J. Pediatr. 88:177, 1976.
39. Rubin, P., Green, J., Holzwasser, G., et al.: Superior vena caval syndrome. Slow low dose versus rapid high dose schedules. Radiology 81:388, 1963.
40. Rubin, P., Poulter, C. A., and Miller, G.: Spinal cord decompression of epidural lymphomas by rapid high doses of irradiation alone. Radiol. Clin. North Am. 6:106, 1968.
41. Scholz, D. A., Purnell, D. C., Goldsmith, R. S., et al.: Hypercalcemia and cancer. CA 25:27, 1975.
42. Sinks, L. F., Newton, W. A., Jr., Nagi, N. A., and Stevenson, T. D.: A syndrome associated with extreme hyperuricemia in leukemia. J. Pediatr. 68:578, 1966.
43. Stapleton, F. B., Lukert, B. P., and Linshaw, M. A.: Treatment of hypercalcemia

associated with osseous metastases. J. Pediatr. 89:1029, 1976.
44. Tefft, M., Mitus, A., and Schulz, M. D.: Initial high dose irradiation for metastases causing spinal cord compression in children. Amer. J. Roentgenol. 106:385, 1969.
45. White, J. C.: Posterior rhizotomy: A possible substitute for cordotomy in otherwise intractable neuralgias of the trunk and extremities of nonmalignant origin. Clin. Neurosurg. 13:20, 1966.
46. White, J. C., and Sweet, W. H.: Pain and the Neurosurgeon. Springfield, Ill., Charles C Thomas, 1959.

INFECTIOUS COMPLICATIONS

47. Abdallah, P. S., Mark, J. B. D., and Merigan, T. C.: Diagnosis of cytomegalovirus pneumonia in compromised hosts. Amer. J. Med. 61:326, 1976.
48. Armstrong, D.: Life-threatening infections in cancer patients. Cancer 23:138, 1973.
49. Armstrong, D., Haghbin, M., Balakrishnan, S. L., and Murphy, M. L.: Asymptomatic cytomegalovirus infection in children with leukemia. Am. J. Dis. Child. 122:404, 1971.
50. Aston, D. L., Cohen, A., and Spindler, M. A.: Herpes virus hominis infection in patients with myeloproliferative and lymphoproliferative disorders. Brit. Med. J. 4:462, 1972.
51. Baker, R. D.: Pulmonary mucormycosis. Am. J. Path. 32:287, 1956.
52. Bennett, J. E.: Chemotherapy of systemic mycoses. N. Engl. J. Med. 290:30, 320, 1974.
53. Bloomfield, C. D., and Kennedy, B. J.: Cephalothin, carbenicillin, and gentamicin combination therapy for febrile patients with acute non-lymphocytic leukemia. Cancer 34:431, 1974.
54. Bodey, G. P.: Fungal infections complicating acute leukemia. J. Chron. Dis. 19:667, 1966.
55. Bodey, G. P.: Studies of a patient laminar air flow facility. Proceedings of the 1969 ISA Annual Conference and Exhibit, October, 1969, Houston, Texas. Instrument Society of America, Publication #69-655, 1969, pp. 1–7.
56. Bodey, G. P.: Infections in patients with cancer. In Holland, J. F., and Frei, E., III (eds.): Cancer Medicine. Philadelphia, Lea & Febiger, 1973.
57. Bodey, G. P., Buckley, M., Sathe, Y. S., and Freireich, E. J.: Quantitative relationships between circulating leukocytes and infection in patients with acute leukemia. Ann. Intern. Med. 64:328, 1966.
58. Bodey, G. P., Freireich, E. J., and Frei, E., III: Studies of patients in a laminar air flow unit. Cancer 24:972, 1969.
59. Bodey, G. P., Hart, J., Freireich, E. J., and Frei, E., III: Studies of a patient isolator unit and prophylactic antibiotics in cancer chemotherapy. Cancer 22:1018, 1968.
60. Bodey, G. P., and Rodriguez, V.: Advances in the management of *Pseudomonas aeruginosa* infections in cancer patients. Eur. J. Cancer 9:435, 1973.
61. Bodey, G. P., and Rodriguez, V.: Infections in cancer patients on a protected environment-prophylactic antibiotic program. Am. J. Med. 59:497, 1975.
62. Bodey, G. P., Rodriguez, V., and Luce, J. K.: Carbenicillin therapy of gram-negative bacilli infections. Am. J. Med. Sci. 257:408, 1969.
63. Bodey, G. P., Watson, P., Cooper, C., and Freireich, E. J.: Protected environment units for the cancer patient. CA 21:215, 1971.
64. Boggs, D. R., and Frei, E., III: Clinical studies of fever and infection in cancer. Cancer 13:1240, 1960.
65. Borella, L., Green, A. A., and Webster, R. G.: Immunologic rebound after cessation of long-term chemotherapy in acute leukemia. Blood 40:42, 1972.
66. Borella, L., and Webster, R. G.: The immunosuppressive effects of long-term combination chemotherapy in children with acute leukemia in remission. Cancer Res. 31:420, 1971.
67. Browder, A. A., Huff, J. W., and Petersdorf, R. G.: The significance of fever in neoplastic disease. Ann. Intern. Med. 55:932, 1961.
68. Brunell, P. A., Ross, A., Miller, L. H., and Kuo, B.: Prevention of varicella by zoster immune globulin. N. Engl. J. Med. 280:1191, 1969.
69. Bullowa, J. G. M., and Wishik, S. M.: Complications of varicella. Am. J. Dis. Child. 49:923, 1935.
70. Carey, R. M., Kimball, A. C., Armstrong, D., and Lieberman, P. H.: Toxoplasmosis: Clinical experiences in a cancer hospital. Am. J. Med. 54:30, 1973.
71. Casazza, A. R., Duvall, C. P., Carbone, P. P.: Infection in lymphoma: Histology, treatment and duration in relation to incidence and survival. J.A.M.A. 197:710, 1966.
72. Chambers, R.: Progress Report for 1971. NCI Leukemia Service Virus Surveillance Contract. Bethesda, Md., National Cancer Institutes, 1971.
73. Chernik, N. L., Armstrong, D., and Posner, J. B.: Central nervous system infections in patients with cancer. Medicine 52:563, 1973.
74. Chilcote, R. R., Baehner, R. L., Hammond,

D., et al.: Septicemia and meningitis in children splenectomized for Hodgkin's disease. N. Engl. J. Med. 295:798, 1976.
75. Chilcote, R. R., and Baehner, R. L.: Infection in childhood cancer: Experience in management of infection in acute leukemia. In Pochedly, C. (ed.): Clinical Management of Cancer in Children. Acton, Mass., Publishing Sciences Group, Inc., 1975.
76. Collins, R. N., Braun, P. A., Zinner, S. H., and Kass, E. H.: Risk of local and systemic infection with polyethylene intravenous catheters. N. Engl. J. Med. 279:340, 1968.
77. Cox, F., and Hughes, W. T.: Disseminated histoplasmosis and childhood leukemia. Cancer 33:1127, 1974.
78. Cox, F., and Hughes, W. T.: Cytomegaloviremia in children with acute lymphocytic leukemia. J. Pediatr. 87:190, 1975.
79. Curry, C. R., and Quie, P. G.: Fungal septicemia in patients receiving parenteral hyperalimentation. N. Engl. J. Med. 285:1221, 1971.
80. De Vita, V. T., Emmer, M., Levine, A., Jacobs, B., and Berard, C.: *Pneumocystis carinii* pneumonia. N. Engl. J. Med. 280:287, 1969.
81. Dilworth, J. A., and Mandell, G. L.: Infections in patients with cancer. Semin. Oncol. 2:349, 1975.
82. Editorial: Fever in malignant disease. Brit. Med. J. 1:591, 1974.
83. Edwards, J. E., Jr., Foos, R. Y., Montgomerie, J. Z., and Guze, L.: Ocular manifestations of *Candida* septicemia. Review of 76 cases of hematogenous *Candida* endophthalmitis. Medicine 53: 47, 1974.
84. Eras, P., Goldstein, M. J., and Sherlock, P.: *Candida* infection of the gastrointestinal tract. Medicine 51:367, 1972.
85. Feldman, H. A.: Toxoplasmosis. N. Engl. J. Med. 279:1370, 1968.
86. Feldman, S., Hughes, W. T., and Daniel, C. B.: Varicella in children with cancer: Seventy-seven cases. Pediatrics 56:388, 1975.
87. Feldman, S., Webster, R. G., and Sugg, M.: Influenza in children and young adults with cancer. 20 cases. Cancer 39:350, 1977.
88. Fishman, L. S., Griffin, J. R., et al.: Hematogenous *Candida* endophthalmitis: A complication of candidemia. N. Engl. J. Med. 286:675, 1972.
89. Geiser, C. F., Bishop, Y., Meyers, M., Jaffe, N., and Yankee, R.: Prophylaxis of varicella in children with neoplastic disease: Comparative results with zoster immune plasma and gamma globulin. Cancer 35:1027, 1975.
90. Gershon, A. A., Steinberg, S., and Brunell, P. A.: Zoster immune globulin. A further assessment. N. Engl. J. Med. 290:243, 1974.
91. Goodell, B., Jacobs, J. B., Powell, R. D., and De Vita, V. T.: Pneumocystis carinii: The spectrum of diffuse interstitial pneumonia in patients with neoplastic diseases. Ann. Intern. Med. 72:337, 1970.
92. Gordon, J. E.: Chickenpox: An epidemiological review. Am. J. Med. Sci. 244:132, 1962.
93. Greenman, R. L., Goodall, P. T., and King, D.: Lung biopsy in immunocompromised hosts. Am. J. Med. 59:488, 1975.
94. Grose, W. E., Bodey, G. P., and Rodriguez, V.: Sulfamethoxazole-trimethoprim for infections in cancer patients. J.A.M.A. 237:352, 1977.
95. Henson, D., Siegel, S. E., Fuccillo, D. A., et al.: Cytomegalovirus infections during acute childhood leukemia. J. Infect. Dis. 126:469, 1972.
96. Hersh, E. M., Bodey, G. P., Nies, B. A., and Freireich, E. J.: Causes of death in acute leukemia: A ten-year study of 414 patients from 1954–1963. J.A.M.A. 193:105, 1965.
97. Hersh, E. M., and Freireich, E. J.: Host defense mechanisms and their modification by cancer chemotherapy. In H. Busch (ed.): Methods in Cancer Research. Vol. 4. New York, Academic Press, 1968.
98. Hersh, E. M., Whitecar, J. P., Jr., McCredie, K. B., et al.: Chemotherapy, immunocompetence, immunosuppression, and prognosis in acute leukemia. N. Engl. J. Med. 285:1211, 1971.
99. Hughes, W. T.: Fatal infections in childhood leukemia. Amer. J. Dis. Child. 122:283, 1971.
100. Hughes, W. T.: Infection problems in childhood cancer. Proceedings of the Seventh National Cancer Conference. Philadelphia, J. B. Lippincott, 1973.
101. Hughes, R. L., Bogdonoff, M. L., Faber, L. P., et al.: Lung biopsy in the acutely ill—when and how? Chest 62:484, 1972.
102. Hughes, W. T., Feldman, S., and Chaudhary, S.: Comparison of trimethoprim-sulfamethoxazole (TMP-SMZ) and pentamidine (PNT) in the treatment of *Pneumocystis carinii* (PCP) pneumonitis. Pediatr. Res. 10:399, 1976.
103. Hughes, W. T., Kuhns, S., et al.: Successful chemoprophylaxis for *Pneumocystis carinii* pneumonitis. Pediatr. Res. 11: 501, 1977.
104. Inagki, J., Rodriguez, V., and Bodey, G. P.: Causes of death in cancer patients. Cancer 33:568, 1974.
105. Judelsohn, R. G., Meyers, J. D., Ellis, R. J.,

105. and Thomas, E. K.: Efficacy of zoster immune globulin. Pediatrics 53:476, 1974.
106. Kass, E. H., and Schneiderman, L. J.: Entry of bacteria into the urinary tracts of patients with inlying catheters. N. Engl. J. Med. 256:556, 1957.
107. Khalifa, A. S., Take, H., Cejka, J., and Zuelzer, W. M.: Immunoglobulins in acute leukemia in children. J. Pediatr. 85:788, 1974.
108. Kiran, O., and Gross, S.: The G-immunoglobulins in acute leukemia in children; hematologic and immunologic relationship. Blood 33:198, 1969.
109. Levine, A. S., Graw, R. G., Jr., and Young, R. C.: Management of infection in patients with leukemia and lymphoma: Current concepts and experimental approaches. Semin. Hematol. 9:141, 1972.
110. Levine, A. S., Schimpff, S. C., Graw, R. C., Jr., and Young, R. C.: Hematologic malignancies and other marrow failure states: Progress in the management of complicating infections. Semin. Hematol. 11:141, 1974.
111. Levine, A. S., Siegel, S. E., Schreiber, A. D., Hauser, J., Preisler, H., Goldstein, I. M., Seidler, F., Simon, R., Perry, S., Bennett, J. E., and Henderson, E. S.: Protected environments and prophylactic antibiotics—a prospective controlled study of their utility in the therapy of acute leukemia. N. Engl. J. Med. 288:477, 1973.
112. Lewicki, A. M., and Moore, J. P.: Esophageal moniliasis. A review of common and less frequent characteristics. Am. J. Roentgenol. 125:218, 1975.
113. Lightdale, C. J., Wolf, D. J., Marcucci, R. A., and Salyer, W. R.: Herpetic esophagitis in patients with cancer: Antemortem diagnosis by brush cytology. Cancer 39:223, 1977.
114. Lou, P., Kazdan, J., Bannatyne, R. M., and Cheung, R.: Successful treatment of Candida endophthalmitis with a synergistic combination of amphotericin B and rifampin. Am. J. Ophthalmol. 83:12, 1977.
115. Louria, D. B., et al.: Listerosis complicating malignant disease. A new association. Ann. Intern. Med. 67:261, 1967.
116. Lowenbraun, S., Young, V., Kenton, D., and Serpick, A. A.: Infection from intravenous "scalp-vein" needle in a susceptible population. J.A.M.A. 212:451, 1970.
117. Lunde, M. N., Gelderman, A. H., Hayes, S. L., et al.: Serologic diagnosis of active toxoplasmosis complicating malignant diseases: Usefulness of IgM antibodies and gel-diffusion. Cancer 25:637, 1970.
118. Meyer, R. D., Rosen, P., and Armstrong, D.: Phycomycosis complicating leukemia and lymphoma. Ann. Intern. Med. 77:871, 1972.
119. Meyer, R. D., Young, L. S., Armstrong, D., and Yu, B.: Aspergillosis complicating neoplastic disease. Am. J. Med. 54:6, 1973.
120. Mirsky, H. S., and Cuttner, J.: Fungal infection in acute leukemia. Cancer 30:348, 172.
121. Movasagghi, M.: The prevention and treatment of varicella-zoster infection in patients at high risk. Clin. Pediatr. (Phila.) 12:299, 1973.
122. Muller, S. A., Herrmann, E. C., Jr., and Winkelmann, R. K.: Herpes simplex infections in hematologic malignancies. Am. J. Med. 52:102, 1972.
123. Ogra, P. L., Sinks, L. F., and Karzon, D. T.: Poliovirus antibody response in patients with acute leukemia. J. Pediatr. 79:444, 1971.
124. Orfanakis, M. G., Wilcox, H. G., and Smith, C. B.: In vitro studies of the combined effects of ampicillin and sulfonamides on Nocardia asteroides and results of therapy in four patients. Antimicrob. Agents Chemother. 1:215, 1972.
125. Peter, G., Lloyd-Still, J. D., and Lovejoy, F. H., Jr.: Local infection and bacteremia from scalp vein needles and polyethylene catheters in children. J. Pediatr. 80:78, 1972.
126. Pinkel, D.: Chickenpox and leukemia. J. Pediatr. 58:729, 1961.
127. Plager, J. E.: Association of renal injury with combined cephalothin-gentamicin therapy among patients severely ill with malignant disease. Cancer 37:1937, 1976.
128. Prystowsky, S. D., Vogelstein, B., Ethinger, D. S., et al.: Invasive aspergillosis. N. Engl. J. Med. 295:655, 1976.
129. Reed, R. K., Larter, W. E., Sieber, O. F., Jr., et al.: Peripheral nodular lesions in Pseudomonas sepsis: The importance of incision and drainage. J. Pediatr. 88:977, 1976.
130. Ries, K., and Kaye, D.: Bacterial and fungal infections. In Sutnick, A. I., and Engstrom, P. L. F. (eds.): Oncologic Medicine: Clinical Topics and Practical Management. Baltimore, University Park Press, 1976.
131. Robinson, H. J.: Adrenal steroids and resistance to infection. Antibiot. Chemother. 7:199, 1960.
132. Rodriguez, V., Burgess, M., and Bodey, G. P.: Management of fever of unknown origin in patients with neoplasms and neutropenia. Cancer 32:1007, 1973.
133. Ross, A. H.: Modification of chicken pox in family contacts by administration of gamma globulin. N. Engl. J. Med. 267:369, 1962.
134. Ryan, J. A., Jr., Abel, R. M., Abbott, W. M.,

et al.: Catheter complications in total parenteral nutrition: A prospective study of 200 consecutive patients. N. Engl. J. Med. 290:757, 1974.
135. Schimpff, S. C., Satterlee, W., Young, V. M., et al.: Empiric therapy with carbenicillin and gentamicin for febrile patients with cancer and granulocytopenia. N. Engl. J. Med. 284:1061, 1971.
136. Schimpff, S. C., Wiernik, P. H., and Block, J. G.: Rectal abscesses in cancer patients. Lancet 2:844, 1972.
137. Sehdev, M. K., Dowling, M. D., Jr., Seal, S. H., and Stearns, M. W., Jr.: Perianal and anorectal complications in leukemia. Cancer 31:149, 1973.
138. Sickles, E. A., Young, V. M., Greene, W. H., et al.: Pneumonia in acute leukemia. Ann. Intern Med. 79:528, 1973.
139. Sidransky, H., and Pearl, M. A.: Pulmonary fungus infections associated with steroid and antibiotic therapy. Dis. Chest. 39:630, 1961.
139a. Simone, J. V., Holland, E., and Johnson, W.: Fatalities during remission of childhood leukemia. Blood 39:759, 1972.
140. Sinkovics, J. G., Smith, J. P.: Septicemia with *Bacteroides* in patients with malignant disease. Cancer 25:663, 1970.
141. Townsend, J. J., Wolinsky, J. S., Baringer, J. R., and Johnson, P. C.: Acquired toxoplasmosis. A neglected cause of treatable nervous system disease. Arch. Neurol. 32:335, 1975.
142. Vietti, T. J., and Ragab, A. H.: Complications and total care of a child with acute leukemia. Cancer 35:1007, 1975.
143. Walzer, P. D., Perl, D. P., Krogstad, D. J., et al.: *Pneumocystis carinii* pneumonia in the United States. Epidemiologic, diagnostic, and clinical features. Ann. Intern. Med. 80:83, 1974.
144. Watson, P., and Bodey, G. P.: Sterile food service for patients in protected environments. J. Am. Diet. Assoc. 56:515, 1970.
145. Weinstein, L., and Chang, T.: The chemotherapy of viral infections. N. Engl. J. Med. 289:725, 1973.
146. Whitley, R. J., Ch'ien, L. T., Dolin, R., et al.: Adenine arabinoside therapy of herpes zoster in the immunosuppressed. NIAID collaborative antiviral study. N. Engl. J. Med. 294:1193, 1976.
147. Winters, R. E., Chow, A. W., Hecht, R. H., and Hewitt, W. L.: Combined use of gentamicin and carbenicillin. Ann. Intern. Med. 75:925, 1971.
148. Wollman, M. R., Young, L. S., Armstrong, D., and Haghbin, M.: Anti-*Pseudomonas* heat-stable opsonins in acute lymphoblastic leukemia in children. J. Pediatr. 86:376, 1975.
149. Young, L. S., Armstrong, D., Blevins, A., and Lieberman, P.: *Nocardia asteroides* infection complicating neoplastic disease. Am. J. Med. 50:356, 1971.
150. Young, R. C., Bennett, J. E., Vogel, C. L., Carbone, P. P., and De Vita, V. T.: Aspergillosis: The spectrum of the disease in 98 patients. Medicine 49:147, 1970.
151. Zorzona, J., Goldman, A. M., Wallace, S., et al.: Radiologic features of gram-negative pneumonias in the neutropenic patient. Am. J. Roentgenol. 127:989, 1976.

Chapter Eight

THE LEUKEMIAS

The leukemias are a diverse group of diseases which have in common an apparently unrestrained proliferation (or accumulation) of white blood cells in the absence of a demonstrable stimulus. Without treatment, these diseases have a high mortality rate, mainly as a consequence of bone marrow failure.

Although the term leukemia ("white blood") is sometimes considered to be synonymous with a high peripheral blood leukocyte count, some patients may have a normal or low leukocyte count. The presentation of such patients may be termed *subleukemic* if primitive (blast) cells are evident in the peripheral blood and *aleukemic* if there are no blast cells in the peripheral blood. The term *preleukemic* refers to individuals with unexplained anemia, neutropenia, or thrombocytopenia who have bone marrow findings suggestive, but not diagnostic, of leukemia initially, but then develop frank leukemia, usually after a prolonged or "smoldering" course. The diagnosis of preleukemia is a retrospective one, often made months or years after hematologic abnormalities are first noted.

Traditionally, leukemias have been classified morphologically by the predominant cell line involved *(lymphocytic, myelocytic, monocytic, undifferentiated)* or temporally by the survival time of the untreated patient *(acute* versus *chronic)*. Prior to the use of chemotherapy, survival time usually reflected the severity of the maturation defect; leukemias characterized by a predominance of primitive (blast) cells tended to run an *acute*, fulminant course, whereas those characterized predominantly by mature cells tended to run a protracted or *chronic* course. Recent advances in the treatment of some of the more undifferentiated leukemias have resulted in significant prolongation of life and, consequently, patients with some forms of "acute" leukemia may now run a relatively "chronic" course. However, the old terminology persists and today the term *acute leukemia* refers to a condition characterized by a high proportion of blast cells, whereas *chronic leukemia* is one with predominantly mature cells.

Epidemiology

Age

Age patterns differ greatly from one type of leukemia to another. Approximately 95 per cent of the leukemias seen in childhood are of the acute variants (Fig. 8–1). *Acute lymphocytic*

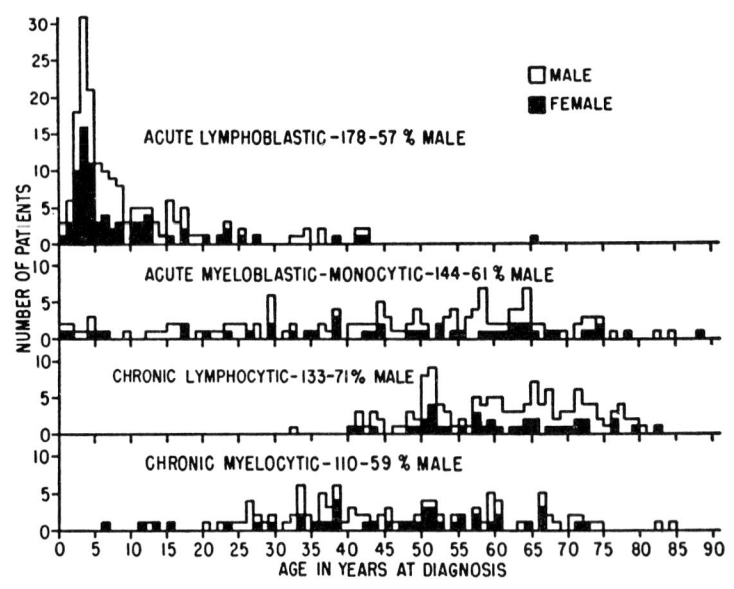

Figure 8–1 Age and sex of 565 patients with leukemia. (From Boggs, D. R., et al.: Medicine 41:163, 1962.)

leukemia (ALL) shows a peak in incidence in the 3 to 5 year age group (approximately 40 per cent of childhood leukemia cases occur during these peak years) and is not often seen in adults. *Acute myelocytic leukemia* (AML) and its variants, on the other hand, show no childhood peak and constitute the vast majority of acute leukemia cases in adults. *Chronic granulocytic leukemia* is unusual in very young children, occurring more commonly in persons of middle age or older. *Chronic lymphocytic leukemia* occurs extremely rarely, if ever, in children, but is a common form of leukemia in persons over the age of 50 years.

Sex

In most series there is a higher proportion of boys than girls with acute leukemia. This seems to become evident after the first year of life and becomes most prominent for children of ages 6 to 15, of whom approximately two thirds of patients are boys. The male excess in this age group appears to be significantly greater for myelogenous and undifferentiated forms than it is for the lymphocytic form.[96]

Race

In the past all forms of leukemia were found more commonly in whites than nonwhites,[115] but the difference has tended to diminish in recent years.[97] Nonetheless, a recent U.S. survey found the incidence of leukemia to be almost twice as high in white children as in black children (4.2/100,000/yr. vs. 2.4/100,000/yr.).[347a] Likewise, until recently nonwhites did not manifest the ALL peak in the 3 to 5 year age group.[97] These differences have been attributed to environmental rather than genetic factors.

Time-Space Clustering of Leukemia

In the past decades several apparent "epidemics" of acute leukemia have been reported. The most celebrated was the occurrence in Niles, Illinois, of eight cases of acute leukemia over a 3-year period in children who shared a close geographic proximity.[141] However, reports have also come from Georgia,[84] London,[317] and New Zealand.[129] The significance of these reports remains unclear since they may merely reflect coincidence or ex post facto setting of geographic and temporal boundaries. A more recent study, which attempted to find evidence of clustering by allowing for a long latent period between exposure to a presumed leukemogenic agent and clinical onset of the disease, has found only slight evidence of clustering, and this was considered to be attributable to chance.[296]

There has been no consistent correlation of leukemia frequency with month of birth[138, 299, 317] or month of onset of clinical symptoms.[138, 184]

Familial Incidence of Leukemia

A question that concerns all parents of leukemic children is whether there is a risk that their other children might develop the disease. Several studies have demonstrated that siblings of leukemic children do have a higher incidence of leukemia, the relative risk being 2.3 to 4 times that of the general pediatric population.[77a, 213] Nonetheless, the actual chance that a sibling will develop leukemia is still relatively remote (1:720 to 1:1000), and parents should be reassured in this regard.

Gunz and associates[128a] surveyed the families of 909 patients with leukemia of all types and found an increased incidence among both first-degree relatives (2.8 to 3 times expected) and more distant ones (2.3 times expected). Thus, between 1 in 12 and 1 in 13 patients with leukemia had one or more relatives with leukemia and 1 in 48 had a first-degree relative with leukemia; concordant disease (same cell type) occurred in more than half of such families. Both increased familial tendency and the likelihood for concordant cell type were most marked for chronic lymphocytic leukemia, less marked for acute leukemia, and probably absent for chronic granulocytic leukemia.

Gunz's group also collated data on 22 families with multiple cases of leukemia;[128a] among the 90 cases of leukemia in these families, 61 per cent were acute leukemia, 35.6 per cent were chronic lymphocytic leukemia, and 3.3 per cent were chronic granulocytic leukemia. Eleven families were entirely concordant for acute leukemia and seven for chronic lymphocytic leukemia.

Patients with Very High Risk of Developing Leukemia

Leukemia, like cancer in general, is not an entirely random event; some individuals appear to be at unusually high risk for developing it. These include: *identical twins of children with acute leukemia, children with congenital disorders characterized by chromosomal anomalies* (Bloom's, Fanconi's, and Down's syndromes), *patients receiving therapeutic irradiation* for ankylosing spondylitis and polycythemia vera, and *atomic bomb survivors* (Table 8–1).

Identical Twins of Children with Acute Leukemia. No other malignancy of childhood or adulthood demonstrates the extraordinary risk of monozygotic twin concordance seen in childhood acute leukemia. However, the risk varies considerably, depending on the age at which the first twin develops clinical disease. If this occurs within the first year of life, the other twin will almost invariably also develop leukemia. Up to the age of 5 years the likelihood that the second twin will develop leukemia is in the range of 10 to 20 per cent; the leukemia is of a similar morphologic type (usually lymphoblastic) and also occurs at a young age. The risk then decreases with increasing age, so that by the time twins are 6 to 7 years of age or older, the risk for the second twin

Table 8-1 Groups at Exceptionally High Risk of Leukemia[213]

Group	Approximate Risk	Time Interval
Identical twin of child with leukemia	1 in 5	Weeks or months
Radiation-treated polycythemia vera	1 in 6	10–15 years
Bloom's syndrome	1 in 8	<30 years of age
Hiroshima survivors (within 1000 meters of hypocenter)	1 in 60	12 years
Down's syndrome	1 in 95	<10 years of age
Radiation treated patients with ankylosing spondylitis	1 in 270	15 years
Sib of child with leukemia	1 in 720	10 years
U.S. Caucasian children	1 in 2880	10 years

approaches that of the general population.

The search for an explanation for this extremely high concordance rate is complicated by the fact that these children are not only identical for genetic endowment, but also for intrauterine and early postnatal experiences;[85] moreover, they frequently share a common circulatory system during intrauterine life, which could facilitate passage of leukemic cells from one twin to the other.[63] Thus, if leukemic transformation occurred in one twin while the placental vessels were united, it is almost inevitable that the other twin would be colonized by the leukemic clone. Concordant leukemia in monozygotic twins may, therefore, represent only one occurrence of leukemia, not two.

Patients with Congenital Chromosomal Abnormalities. Bloom's syndrome and Fanconi's constitutional aplastic anemia are characterized by genetically induced chromosome fragility leading to an increase in chromosomal breaks when cells are cultured in vitro. Bloom's syndrome is also accompanied by short stature and photosensitive telangiectasia of the face (Fig. 8–2). When leukemia develops in this condition, it is usually of the acute myelogenous type. Fanconi's anemia is also associated with short stature, as well as congenital anomalies (hyperpigmentation of the skin, renal anomalies, skeletal anomalies, mental retardation). Patients with Fanconi's anemia commonly develop acute monocytic or myelomonocytic leukemia.[96]

Patients with Down's syndrome (trisomy 21) have an incidence of acute leukemia that is greater than 15 times that of the general population.[214] Rosner and Lee,[260] in their review of the world literature, found 276 recorded cases of Down's syndrome and leukemia (47 in newborns, 227 in children less than 20 years of age and 2 in adults). Of the 227 children, 31 per cent

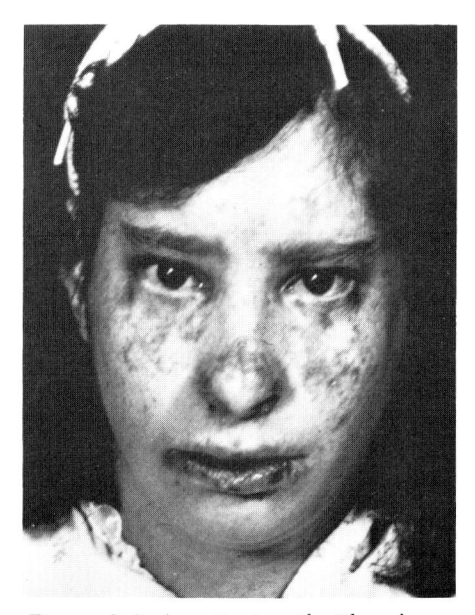

Figure 8–2 A patient with Bloom's syndrome. (From Bloom, D., et al.: J. Pediatr. 68:103, 1966.)

had AML and 69 per cent had ALL; among the 47 newborns, 58 per cent had AML and 42 per cent had ALL.

ETIOLOGY

The etiology of the leukemias is very likely multifactorial, involving a complex interaction between the host and various environmental agents. Among the environmental factors which have been implicated in the development of acute leukemia are: (1) ionizing irradiation, (2) chemical carcinogens, and (3) infectious agents (primarily viral).

Ionizing Irradiation

Evidence documenting the role of irradiation has come from studies of individuals who have received *diagnostic, therapeutic*, and *atomic bomb irradiation*.

Children who were exposed to diagnostic irradiation while in utero have been reported in some studies to have a higher incidence of leukemia,[302] particularly when they had been exposed in the first trimester. The development of leukemia in these patients appears to be nonrandom in that the higher risk appears to be confined to a subgroup with other identifiable high-risk factors (allergic diathesis, early childhood viral disease). The etiologic role of irradiation in utero remains unresolved, however, since there was no increased frequency seen in children exposed in utero during the Hiroshima and Nagasaki atomic bomb explosions, nor in a carefully controlled prospective study of prenatal irradiation.[124]

Individuals who have received irradiation to the spine for treatment of ankylosing spondylitis or radioactive phosphorus for polycythemia vera, have a higher incidence of leukemia than the general population. In addition, the increased incidence of leukemia in long-term survivors of childhood cancer and Hodgkin's disease may be partially attributable to radiation therapy.

Following the atomic bombing of Hiroshima and Nagasaki, a very high rate of leukemia, peaking 6 to 7 years later, was found among the survivors. The incidence was dose-related, correlating closely with the distance from the hypothetical center (hypocenter) of the blast. Among the adult population, myelogenous leukemia of both the acute and chronic types predominated, but children who were heavily exposed developed predominantly acute lymphocytic leukemia. Thus, the myeloid and lymphoid cell lines appear to have different susceptibilities to leukemogenesis at different ages, and irradiation appears to affect that line which is most susceptible at the age when one is exposed. No excess of leukemia has been found in children exposed to atomic bomb irradiation in utero or in children born of exposed survivors.[158]

Chemical Carcinogens

At present there is no evidence that chemicals are involved in a major way in the etiology of leukemia. Although a number of drugs have been implicated, the evidence is strongest for benzene,[97, 128] which is associated mainly with the development of acute myelogenous leukemia several years after pancytopenia accompanied by a hypoplastic bone marrow has been induced. The high rate of leukemia in shoemakers appears to represent an occupational hazard as a result of chronic benzene exposure.

Viral Agents

The case for a viral etiology of human acute leukemia rests upon two major lines of evidence: (1) the ability of viruses to produce leukemia in other mammalian species, and (2) the presence of biochemical markers of viral infection in human leukemia cells.

It now seems fairly certain that a variety of animal leukemias require the presence of a virus for their clinical expression.[217] In the mouse model, the virus is usually vertically transmitted from parent to offspring via infected ova, sperm,[49] or breast milk; external factors such as irradiation, chemicals, and immune system damage appear to hasten the onset of leukemia.[134] Thus, although the presence of the virus appears to be central in the etiology of these murine leukemias, it may require interaction with various genetic and environmental factors before expressing itself.[190]

Some animal leukemias are characterized by the presence of so-called C-type particles in the plasma and organs. These spherical particles are approximately 100 nm in diameter, contain an electron-dense, round, RNA-containing nucleoid separated by a clear circular zone from a thin external "unit membrane," and appear to represent one stage in the development of an RNA-type leukemia virus. Particles resembling these C-type particles have also been reported in human leukemia cells examined with the electron microscope,[77] (Fig. 8–3) but only in a small proportion of the specimens examined. Similar particles have also been found in spun plasma[187] or urine sediment[7] of leukemia patients, but have also been seen in an equivalent number of normal controls.[227] C-particles have also been found in monkey, rat, and human placentas leading to speculation that there may be vertical transmission of latent, oncogenic viruses from one generation to another.[125, 126]

In order for an RNA virus to produce a permanent genetic change in a given cell line, it must have the capacity to transcribe its "message" (provirus) into the DNA of the cell's genome. An enzyme capable of transcribing DNA from viral RNA has now been detected in a number of tumor viruses;[19, 310] this RNA-instructed DNA polymerase has also been called *"reverse transcriptase"* because it catalyzes a reaction (RNA → DNA) that is the reverse of the classic DNA → RNA transcription sequence (Fig. 8–4).

The detection of viral reverse transcriptase in the leukemic cells of virus-induced animal leukemias provides direct evidence of the presence of virus in these cells. Other indications of the viral presence are: RNA nucleotide sequences similar to those found in RNA tumor viruses, new surface membrane antigens, and high molecular weight (70S) RNA. The fact that these same viral "footprints" can also be found in human leukemia cells (but not in normal marrow cells) has been proposed as presumptive evidence of the presence of virus in these cells. Of course the fact that a virus is present in human leukemic cells does not necessarily prove that it is of etiologic significance; it is also possible that these viruses are merely "passengers."

If viruses are involved in the etiology of human leukemia, their role is much more subtle than it is in most virus-induced illnesses. There is no evidence that leukemia is a contagious disease for it does not appear to be spread by direct contact or by transfusion of leukemic cells,[34, 311] nor is there unequivocal evidence of time-space clustering of cases. Likewise, horizontal transmission of the disease from leukemic mothers to their offspring does not appear to occur as frequently as might be expected if a virus were involved, for only a handful of cases of leukemia have been reported in the children of leukemic mothers.[28, 70]

The "Oncogene" Hypothesis. A theory which reconciles the possibility of a viral etiology for human leukemia with its apparent nontransmissibility is the *"oncogene" hypothesis*.[319a] Stated simply, this theory proposes that RNA tumor provirus is present in all vertebrate cells, integrated into the genome, but it is maintained in an unexpressed form by repressors in normal cells. Various carcinogenic agents (chemicals, irradiation, other viruses)

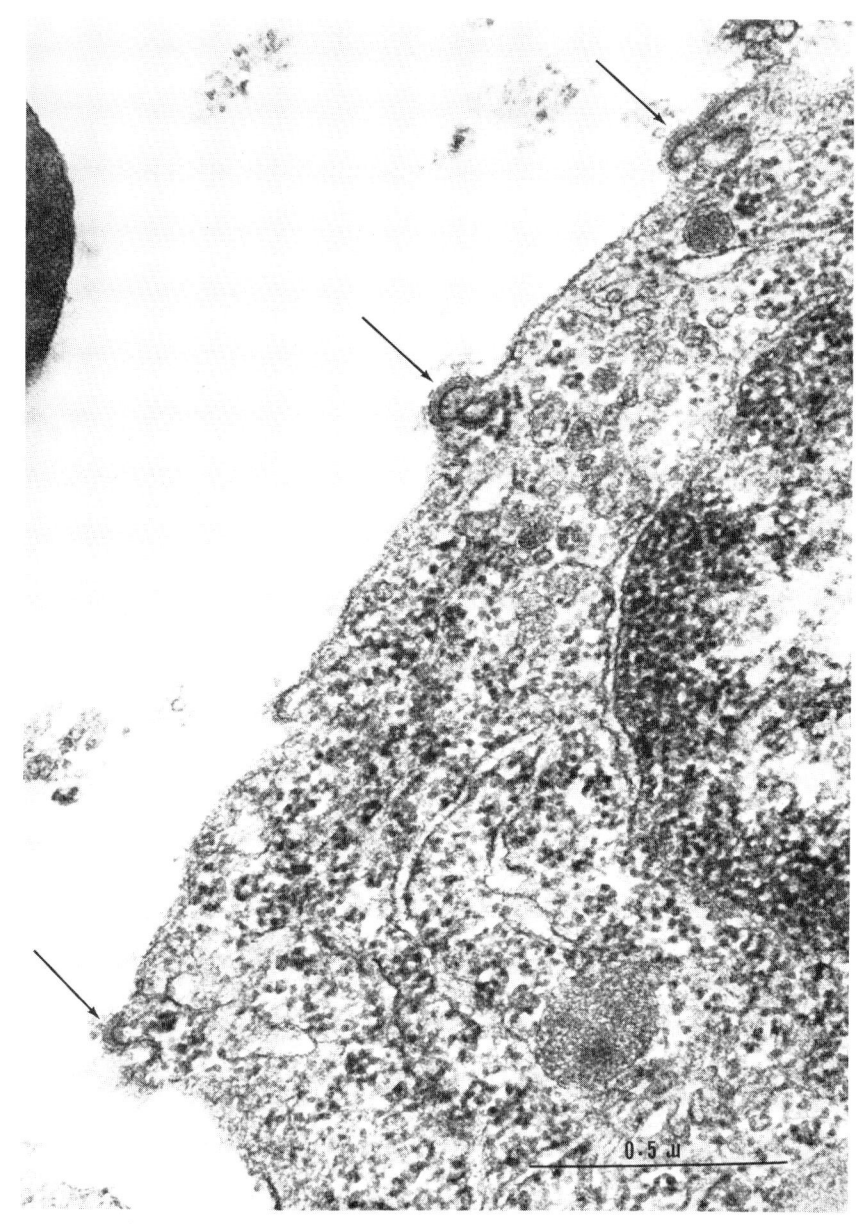

Figure 8-3 Budding of "virus-like" particles from the plasma membrane of a cell in the lymph node of a patient with acute lymphocytic leukemia (×90,000). (From Dmochowski, L., et al.: Cancer 20:760, 1967.)

may induce malignant transformation in cells by activating these endogenous virogenes; at this point the transformed cells produce detectable viral products, such as surface antigens, reverse transcriptase, and viral RNA.

Although the "oncogene" theory is an attractive one, it remains unproved. Moreover, the failure to detect DNA segments complementary to tumor virus RNA in nonleukemic humans casts doubts upon its validity. In particular, a study in which only the leukemic member of a pair of identical twins contained DNA segments com-

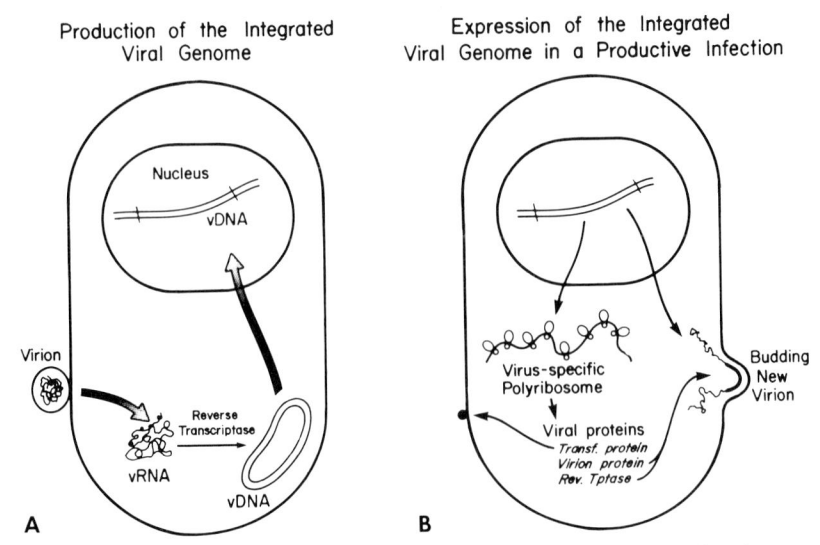

Figure 8-4 The life cycle of an RNA tumor virus. A, The virus infects the cell and inserts its RNA and reverse transcriptase into the cytoplasm. The reverse transcriptase then catalyzes the synthesis of a DNA copy of the viral RNA. B, The DNA transcript (provirus) may then integrate into the chromosomes of the host cell, where it may remain "silent" (unexpressed) or it may transcribe viral messenger RNA. The viral proteins specified by this viral messenger RNA have two known functions: (1) production of new viral particles which bud from the cell surface and infect other cells, or (2) transformation of the cell into a neoplastic cell. (From Baltimore, D.: Viruses, Polymerases, and cancer. © The Nobel Foundation, 1976.)

plementary to tumor virus RNA[23] suggests the provirus had not been vertically transmitted, but had been acquired after fertilization.

THE ACUTE LEUKEMIAS

PATHOGENESIS

Although the most diagnostic and dramatic findings of an acute leukemia relate to the presence of abnormal numbers of primitive or "blast" cells in the peripheral blood and bone marrow, the major problems faced by the patient are a manifestation of what is absent—i.e., mature, functional blood cells. Consequently, the clinical and pathologic findings of the acute leukemias are primarily a reflection of the consequences of the bone marrow failure resulting from a shift from the production of mature, functional cells to production of abnormal, undifferentiated cells.

Initially leukemia was considered to be a proliferative abnormality, with uncontrolled rapidly proliferating leukemic cells overgrowing the normal marrow precursor cells. This concept was challenged by Astaldi and Mauri[9] in 1954, when their studies demonstrated a low mitotic index for leukemic cells. This finding was considered more compatible with the concept that leukemia might result from accumulation of slowly dividing cells that fail to differentiate. More recent studies of cellular kinetics have confirmed their observations. At the time of diagnosis, the percentage of marrow blast cells in active cell cycle (as measured by the ^{3}H-thymidine labeling index) is in the range of 6.8 ± 3.5 per cent, while peripheral blast cells show an even lower percentage of label uptake.[94] These figures are well below those seen for normal marrow precursor cells (approximately 50 per cent in active cell cycle).

Another early misconception about leukemic cell kinetics was that proliferation of these cells was unresponsive to control mechanisms. Actually there is now evidence to suggest that the cells are indeed under the control of certain growth regulators. For example, the similarity of proliferative activity in various marrow sites sampled simultaneously or during different times of the day suggests regulation by systemic humoral substances.[199] Furthermore, in vitro proliferation of AML cells in agar is dependent upon the same humoral stimuli (colony stimulating activity) that regulate colony formation by normal granulocyte precursor cells.

Leukemia as an Accumulative Phenomenon

The primary problem in the leukemias appears to be an unregulated proliferation and continued accumulation of primitive cells that have lost the capacity to mature. Unlike most hematopoietic precursor cells that mature to end-stage functional cells (erythrocytes, neutrophils) with finite lifespan and limited proliferative potential, leukemic blast cells, by virtue of their inability to differentiate, may have unlimited proliferative potential and lifespan. Thus, the leukemic population may increase exponentially, and monopolize the available nutrients and "lebensraum" of the marrow. There are several mechanisms by which the expanding leukemic population might exert a selective growth advantage: (1) more successful competition for essential nutrients or vitamins, or both, (2) production of substances which inhibit enzyme synthesis or activity in normal hemic precursor cells, (3) contact inhibition, or (4) production of a growth inhibitor. Thus, in the untreated state and in relapse, not only may the hematopoietic precursor cells be physically crowded from the marrow, but also factors which biochemically interfere with their production may come into play.

Cytogenetics of the Acute Leukemias and the Clonal Hypothesis

When examined by standard techniques, approximately half the patients with acute leukemia show no abnormalities in chromosome number or appearance.[92] On the other hand, 30 to 50 per cent of patients with acute leukemia do show karyotypic aberrations. Those cases of acute leukemia who do have cytogenetic alterations show considerable diversity, ranging from translocations to abnormalities in chromosome number and morphology. In general, patients with ALL have hyperdiploid karyotypes with chromosome numbers of up to 90, while AML patients often manifest hypodiploid karyotypes and chromosome numbers rarely reach 50.[265] Among the myeloid leukemias certain nonrandom chromosomal patterns appear; these involve mainly the C group of chromosomes and include an additional #8 (trisomy 8), loss of #7 (monosomy 7), and a translocation between #8 and #21.[262a] The #8–#21 translocation has been termed the "prototypic karyotype" because it may turn out to be a basic chromosomal change in AML; a missing sex chromosome, particularly the Y, commonly accompanies this translocation.

At the time of diagnosis, all the dividing leukemic cells from a given patient's blood and marrow show virtually the same karyotypic alteration, suggesting evolution of the entire leukemic population from a clone of cells derived from a single abnormal stem cell.[229] In AML, erythroid cells in the bone marrow have been shown to possess the same abnormal karyotypes as cells of the granulocytic series, while lymphoid cells are cytogenetically normal.[160a] During periods of remission, the marrow karyotype reverts to normal (suggesting repopulation by normal hematopoietic elements), but with relapse of the disease, leukemic cells with the original aberrant karyotype reappear.[92, 229] This stability of the abnormal karyotype throughout the course of the illness suggests that relapse is due to persistence of the original leukemic clone of cells rather than re-induction by a persistent leukemogenic stimulus.

An alternative to the clonal hypothesis is that leukemia is multicentric in origin, arising from the transformation of many (possibly all) marrow cells by the leukomogenic event (virus, irradiation, etc.) According to this theory, the stability of karyotypic abnormalities results from the production of consistent chromosomal changes by the leukomogenic agent and, indeed, there is evidence that some murine leukemia viruses can induce identical chromosomal abnormalities within a given strain of mice.

Morphologic Classification of the Acute Leukemias

The hallmark of an acute leukemia is the "blast" cell, a relatively undifferentiated cell with diffusely distributed nuclear chromatin, one or more nucleoli, and basophilic cytoplasm. Blast cells are also part of the normal maturation sequence of hemic and lymphoid elements, but under normal conditions constitute less than 5 per cent of the nucleated cells of the bone marrow and are never seen in the peripheral blood. The presence of an increased number of these poorly differentiated cells is the sine qua non for diagnosis of an acute leukemia.

Since the blast cell is a primitive cell it is sometimes difficult to determine whether it is a lymphoid or a myeloid precursor cell. However, this distinction is critical for therapeutic and prognostic reasons, and consequently it is essential at the time of diagnosis to characterize the leukemic process morphologically as lymphocytic (lymphoblastic) or nonlymphocytic (myeloblastic). A number of cytologic criteria have been established to differentiate these two entities (Table 8-2).

Figure 8-5 demonstrates the morphologic features of the various forms of childhood leukemia; these will be discussed in detail below. When the blast cells contain primary (azurophilic) granules or rod-like aggregates of these granules (Auer rods), they are presumed to represent primitive granulocytic or monocytic precursor cells and are classified within the acute myelogenous leukemia (AML) spectrum. Special histochemical stains for granule enzymes (myeloperoxidase) or lipids (Sudan black) may serve to accentuate the granules or Auer rods when the routine staining techniques fail to demonstrate them. When neither granules nor Auer rods are demonstrable, the blast cells are presumed to represent acute lymphoblastic leukemia (ALL) or acute undifferentiated leukemia (AUL) cells.

There are also "softer" criteria which can be utilized to differentiate myeloblasts from lymphoblasts. Some of these are: the nature of the nuclear chromatin (clumped in lymphoblasts, spongy in myeloblasts), the nuclear/cytoplasmic ratio (higher in lymphoblasts than in myeloblasts), nature of nucleoli (more distinct and "punched out" in myeloblasts than in lymphoblasts), and nature of cytoplasm (blue and nongranular in lymphoblasts, blue-grey with granules or Auer rods in myeloblasts).

The relative frequency of the acute leukemia variants of childhood is as follows:[54, 96, 113]

	Per Cent
Acute lymphoblastic leukemia	60–70
Acute undifferentiated leukemia	0–10
Acute myelocytic leukemia*	20–30

*Including acute myelomonocytic leukemia (5 to 6 per cent) and acute monocytic leukemia (0.1 to 2.1 per cent).

Table 8-2 Morphologic Characteristics of ALL and AML*

	ALL	AML
Nuclear chromatin	Clumped	Spongy
Nuclear/cytoplasmic ratio	High	Low
Nucleoli	0–2	2–5
Auer rods	Absent	Present
Granules	Absent	Present
Cytoplasm	Blue	Blue-gray
Cytochemistry		
PAS	Positive	Negative
Myeloperoxidase	Negative	Positive
Sudan black	Negative	Positive
Esterases		
α-naphthyl acetate	Negative	Positive (AMML, AMoL)
Naphthol ASD chloroacetate	Negative	Positive (AML, AMML)

*The AML group includes acute myelocytic leukemia (AML), acute myelomonocytic leukemia (AMML), acute monocytic leukemia (AMoL), and erythroleukemia.

Acute Lymphoblastic Leukemia

Careful morphologic and immunologic evaluation has demonstrated that ALL of childhood is not a homogeneous entity, but actually comprises several subgroups. On morphologic grounds, ALL may be subdivided into three types (L1, L2, L3) according to the occurrence of individual cytologic features and the degree of heterogeneity in the distribution of these features among the leukemic blast cell population[25] (Table 8–3). The L1 type is the typical form of acute lymphoblastic leukemia of childhood (Fig. 8–5A). The L2 type (acute *undifferentiated* or *stem cell* leukemia) is characterized by blast cells that are large and manifest nuclear clefting, folding, and indentation; nucleoli are nearly always present and may be very large (Fig. 8–5B). The L3 type *(Burkitt type)* is characterized by a homogeneous population of primitive cells with deeply basophilic cytoplasm, prominent cytoplasmic vacuolation, and surface markers characteristic of B-lymphocytes (Fig. 8–5C).

Immunologic Classification of ALL. Studies of the blast cells of ALL patients using the immunologic markers discussed in Chapter Five have also distinguished three subclasses: T-cell leukemia, B-cell leukemia, and "null" cell leukemia (Table 8–4).

Several groups[44, 321] have now demonstrated that the T-cell subclass (Fig. 8–6) is frequently characterized by (1) occurrence in older children (usually boys), (2) high initial leukocyte count, and (3) mediastinal mass. These patients, in general, have a poorer response to therapy than the overall group of ALL patients.[321]

Blast cells with B-cell markers are unusual in ALL, representing only 2 per cent of cases. In several series such cells had the cytologic, cytochemical, and electron microscopic characteristics of Burkitt's tumor cells (L3) and ran a rapidly fatal course.[93, 344] In African patients this form of leukemia is frequently associated with a jaw tumor and in non-African patients, with an abdominal mass.

The majority of patients with ALL have blast cells which lack B- and T-cell surface markers and are considered to be "null" cells. This form of ALL is thought to represent a malignant proliferation of precursor lymphocytes. These patients have the best prognosis.

The Acute Myeloblastic Leukemias

The acute myeloblastic leukemia spectrum includes acute myeloblastic

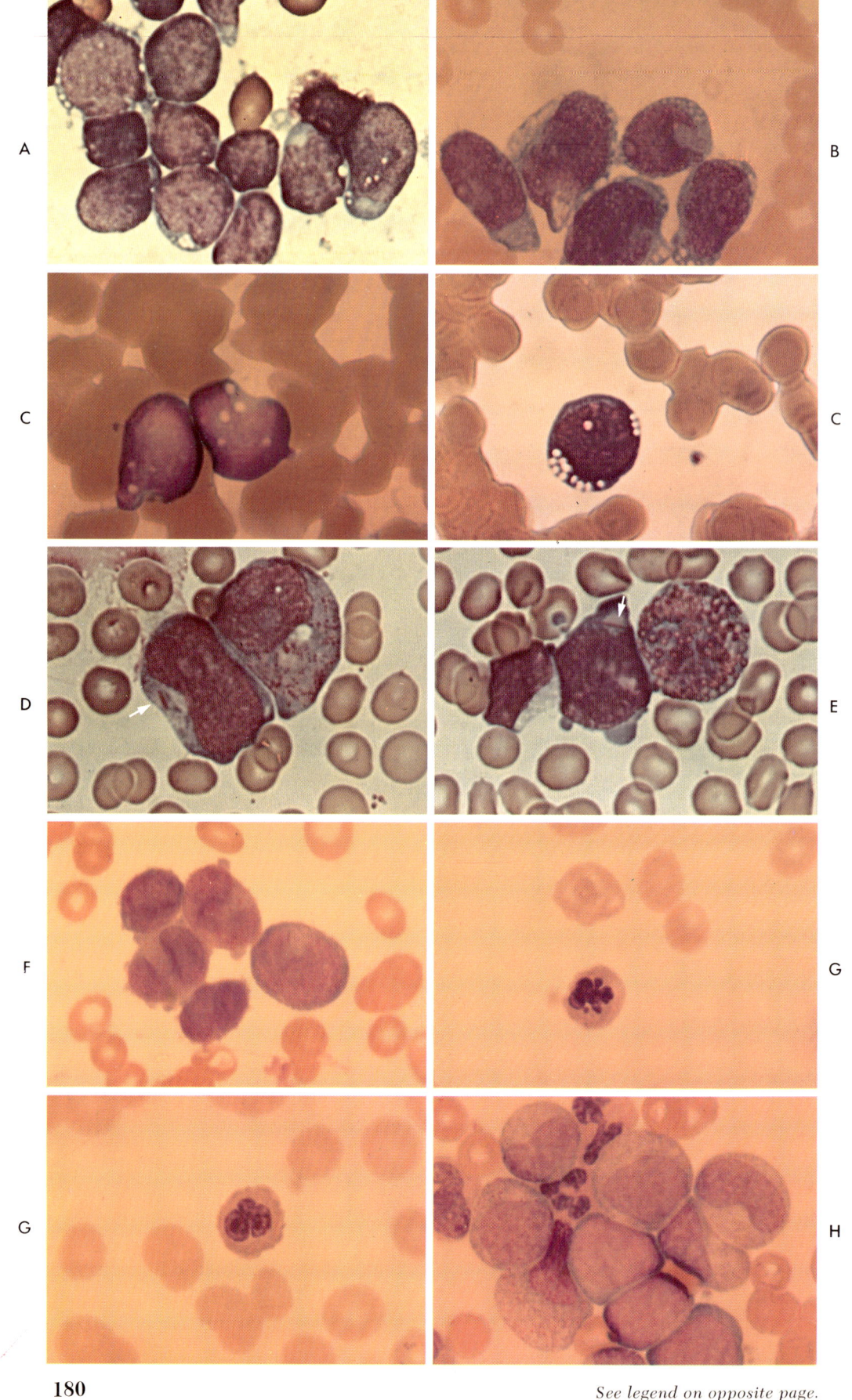

See legend on opposite page.

Table 8-3 Cytological Features of the "Lymphoblastic" Leukemias[25]

Cytological Features	L1	L2	L3
Cell size	Small cells predominate	Large, heterogeneous in size	Large and homogeneous
Nuclear chromatin	Homogeneous in any one case	Variable; heterogeneous in any one case	Finely stippled and homogeneous
Nuclear shape	Regular, occasional clefting or identation	Irregular; clefting and indentation common	Regular; oval to round
Nucleoli	Not visible, or small and inconspicuous	One or more present, often large	Prominent; one or more vesicular
Amount of cytoplasm	Scanty	Variable; often moderately abundant	Moderately abundant
Basophilia of cytoplasm	Slight or moderate, rarely intense	Variable; deep in some	Very deep
Cytoplasmic vacuolation	Variable	Variable	Often prominent

leukemia (AML), acute myelomonocytic leukemia (AMML), acute monocytic leukemia (AMoL), and erythroleukemia; eosinophilic leukemia and basophilic leukemia may also be included within this spectrum. The French-American-British Co-operative Group has subdivided the AML spectrum into six main types (M1 to M6).[25]

Acute Myeloblastic Leukemia (M1, M2)

M1 (MYELOBLASTIC LEUKEMIA WITHOUT MATURATION). These cells are difficult to identify as myeloblasts since they contain only a few azurophil granules. The *peroxidase* stain may help to accentuate these granules and differentiate this type from acute undifferentiated leukemia (L2).

M2 (MYELOBLASTIC LEUKEMIA WITH DIFFERENTIATION). Maturation at or beyond the promyelocyte state is present; Auer rods are visible (Fig. 8-5D, E).

Acute Promyelocytic Leukemia (M3)

M3 (HYPERGRANULAR PROMYELOCYTIC LEUKEMIA). The great majority of cells are abnormal promyelocytes, with more heavy granulation than is seen in M2 cells. Some cells may contain multiple Auer rods.

Clinically, M3 patients differ from those with other forms of acute leukemia by absence of hepatosplenomegaly and lymphadenopathy.[114] Their most distinguishing characteristic, however, is a marked propensity to develop hemorrhagic complications which do not respond to platelet transfusions. Accompanying thrombocytopenia in these patients are prolonged prothrombin time and thrombin time, hypofibrinogenemia, decreased levels of Factors V and VIII, shortened-euglobulin lysis time, and elevation of fibrin degradation products. These findings are consistent with disseminated intravascular coagulation (DIC), which appears to have been triggered by release into the circulation of tissue factor (tissue thromboplastin) from the cell membrane or granules of promyelocytes.[121]

Acute Myelomonocytic and Acute Monocytic Leukemia (M4, M5)

Leukemias with monocytic features manifest a continuous morphologic spectrum ranging from cases with a marked myeloblastic predominance

---

Figure 8-5 Morphology of leukemic cells. A, Acute lymphoblastic leukemia (L1); B, acute undifferentiated leukemia (L2); C, acute lymphoblastic leukemia—Burkitt type (L3); D, acute myeloblastic leukemia—a promyelocyte and a myeloblast (with an Auer rod); E, acute myeloblastic leukemia—an eosinophil with abnormally large granules and a myeloblast (with an Auer rod); F, acute myelomonocytic leukemia; G, erythroleukemia (diGuglielmo's syndrome)—these bizarre-appearing normoblasts with multilobulated nuclei were found in the peripheral smear; H, chronic granulocytic leukemia—granulocytic cells at all stages from myeloblast (extreme left corner) to mature polymorph are present.

Table 8–4 A Functional Classification of Acute Lymphocytic Leukemia

Surface Markers	Per Cent	Clinical Characteristics	Prognosis
T-cell	16–22	High white count Mediastinal mass	Poor
B-cell	2–3	Burkitt's tumor cells	Poor
Null cell	76–84		Good

and relatively few monocytoid cells (M4) (Fig. 8–5F) to those showing predominently monocytoid and histiocytic cells (M5). Clinically the leukemias with monocytic features are distinguishable by a high frequency of gum hypertrophy, lymphadenopathy, and ulceronecrotic lesions of the perirectal area. Also characteristic are elevated serum and urine muramidase levels. Monoblasts may be identified histochemically by the presence of fluoride-inhibitable nonspecific esterase activity in their cytoplasm.[347]

M4 (Myelomonocytic Leukemia). Both granulocytic and monocytic differentiation is present in varying proportions in the bone marrow and peripheral blood; the proportion of promonocytes and monocytes exceeds 20 per cent of the nucleated bone marrow cells. These monocytic cells stain heavily for nonspecific esterase histochemical activity (using naphthol AS- or ASD-acetate as substrate); also characteristic of these cells is almost complete inhibition of the esterase reaction by sodium fluoride.[270, 280] Auer rods may be seen.

M5 (Monocytic Leukemia). May contain poorly differentiated (monoblastic)

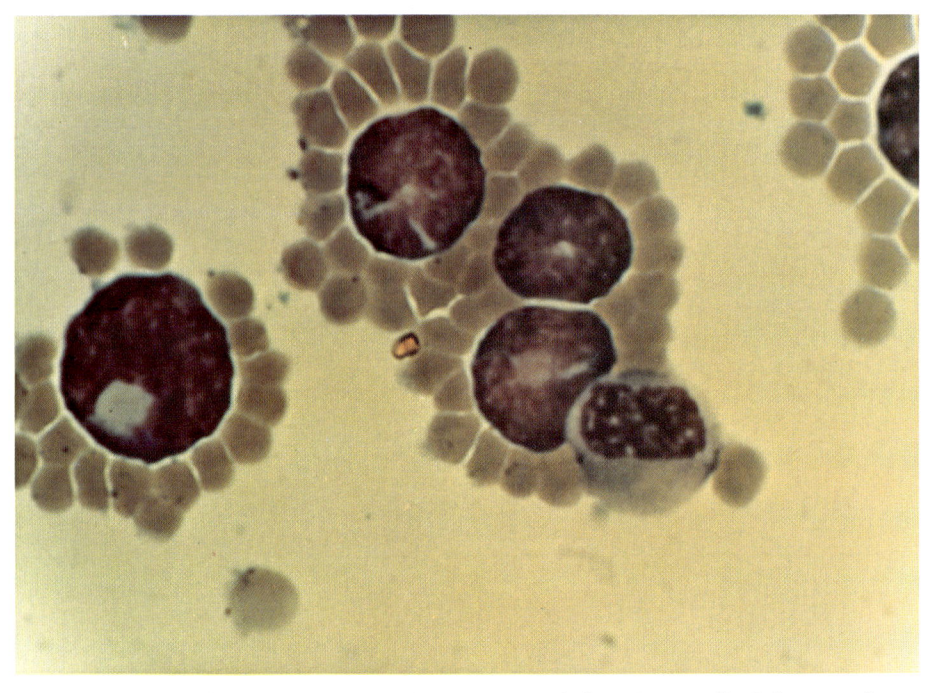

Figure 8–6 A T-cell leukemia. Blast cells are surrounded by "rosettes" of sheep erythrocytes. (Courtesy of Dr. John Quinn.)

consequences of leukemic infiltration. Acute myelocytic leukemia may present with a mass lesion (chloroma), particularly in the orbit[192] or spine, even when the peripheral blood appears normal. Gingival hypertrophy is seen predominantly in acute monocytic or acute myelomonocytic leukemia; ulceronecrotic lesions of the perirectal region are also characteristic of leukemias with monocytic features.

Differential Diagnosis of Acute Leukemia. Although acute leukemia in childhood is usually diagnosed without difficulty after examination of the peripheral blood and bone marrow, there are certain conditions which may mimic some of the physical and laboratory findings of acute leukemia. Among these are infectious mononucleosis, infectious lymphocytosis, pertussis, aplastic anemia, leukemoid reactions, neuroblastoma, idiopathic thrombocytopenic purpura, rheumatoid diseases, and various viral and bacterial infections.

INFECTIOUS MONONUCLEOSIS. Infectious mononucleosis is perhaps the illness which most commonly causes confusion in the differential diagnosis of acute leukemia. This condition may simulate leukemia in the presentation of generalized lymphadenopathy, splenomegaly, skin rash, purpuric lesions, and the presence of large immature cells in the peripheral blood.

The hallmark of infectious mononucleosis is the atypical lymphocyte. This cell is larger than the normal lymphocyte and may appear very immature. The cytoplasm is usually pale blue, with borders which stain more deeply basophilic than other areas; there is also usually striking vacuolation, which gives the cytoplasm a foamy appearance. The heterogeneity seen in the atypical lymphocytes of infectious mononucleosis contrasts with the homogeneous appearance presented by the blast cells of acute lymphoblastic leukemia. Anemia and significant thrombocytopenia, while occasionally occurring in mononucleosis, are much less frequent than in leukemia. The presence of heterophilic antibody, a positive mononucleosis spot test, or antibodies to Epstein-Barr (EB) virus also are more characteristic of infectious mononucleosis; however, these may not be present in the very young child with this illness. Examination of the bone marrow is rarely required to separate these two entities.

Although the classical form of infectious mononucleosis appears to be caused by the EB virus, it is now recognized that a number of other infectious agents, including cytomegalovirus, and toxoplasma have also been implicated etiologically.

INFECTIOUS LYMPHOCYTOSIS. Acute infectious lymphocytosis occurs sporadically as well as in epidemic form. This condition is associated with a very high leukocyte count. However, the lymphocytes seen are of the small, mature type rather than the large, immature type. Again, the mild clinical course and the absence of anemia and bleeding problems helps to distinguish this from acute leukemia.

PERTUSSIS. Children with pertussis may present with fever and a leukocyte count in excess of 50,000/mm^3 (all of which are mature lymphocytes). The condition can be differentiated from acute leukemia by the mature nature of the lymphocytes and by the absence of hepatosplenomegaly, anemia, and thrombocytopenia.

IDIOPATHIC THROMBOCYTOPENIC PURPURA (ITP). ITP is probably the most common cause of the acute onset of petechiae and purpura in childhood. This presentation may be distinguished from that of acute leukemia because the petechiae usually appear in a child who has been essentially well except for possibly a recent viral infection, whereas in acute leukemia the child has usually experienced increasing lethargy, pallor, and other signs of chronic illness. Unless there has been considerable bleeding, children with ITP have normal hemoglobin and hematocrit; the bone marrow shows normal hematopoiesis and adequate megakaryocytes.

APLASTIC ANEMIA. The fundamental pathophysiologic problem in both acute leukemia and aplastic anemia is a failure to produce normal mature blood cells. Consequently, these conditions may show a similar presentation, with pancytopenia, infection, and bleeding manifestations. Usually the patient with aplastic anemia does not have lymphadenopathy, hepatosplenomegaly, or blast cells in the peripheral blood. However, some patients with acute leukemia may not have circulating blast cells, hepatosplenomegaly, or lymphadenopathy either. Bone marrow examination should provide the definitive differentiation between these conditions since the hypocellular specimen seen in aplastic anemia contrasts markedly with the very cellular, homogeneous collection of blast cells seen in acute leukemia.

Occasionally the initial marrow aspirate in some leukemic patients may be hypoplastic and lack a significant increase in blast cells.[210] Although it may not be possible to diagnose leukemia with certainty in such patients, it should be strongly suspected when there is a rapid return of hematologic elements after a short course of corticosteroid therapy. The bone marrow should then be followed at frequent intervals to detect leukemic relapse; when clinically identifiable acute leukemia develops, it is usually of the lymphoblastic type.

RHEUMATIC DISEASES. In some patients with acute leukemia, musculoskeletal complaints, particularly arthritis, may so dominate the early course that a diagnosis of juvenile rheumatoid arthritis or rheumatic fever is made. The most helpful points distinguishing these patients from those with purely rheumatic disease appear to be severe excruciating joint pain, out of proportion to the degree of objective arthritis, and hematologic abnormalities (severe anemia, thrombocytopenia, abnormal leukocyte forms in the peripheral blood).[268]

LEUKEMOID REACTION (LEUKOERYTHROBLASTOSIS). Leukemoid reactions may produce a peripheral blood picture resembling acute leukemia by virtue of the presence of immature granulocytes, nucleated red cells, and an elevated leukocyte count. This constellation may occur in association with acute or subacute infections, massive hemolysis or hemorrhage, or involvement of the bone marrow by tumor metastases, myelofibrosis, vasculitis, or granuloma (tuberculosis, histoplasmosis, sarcoidosis). Bone marrow examination is useful in differentiating these conditions from acute leukemia.

NEUROBLASTOMA. Some patients with neuroblastoma may have extensive bone marrow involvement at the time of initial diagnosis. Such patients may present with pancytopenia and circulating neuroblastoma cells. These neuroblastoma cells may bear a strong resemblance to the blast cells of acute lymphoblastic leukemia. Bone marrow examination may be helpful in differentiating these two conditions if clumps of neuroblastoma cells (Fig. 8–8) or pseudo-rosettes are identifiable. Other clinical features, such as the presence of an abdominal mass, intraabdominal calcification observed on x-ray, or elevated catecholamine levels are also suggestive of neuroblastoma.

Laboratory Findings

PERIPHERAL BLOOD. In general, the degree of anemia, granulocytopenia, or thrombocytopenia does not correlate well with the apparent duration of symptoms or with the peripheral blast count.

Severe anemia (below 6 g/dl) is more likely to be present at the time of diagnosis in children under 4 years of age than it is in older children. The erythrocytes are usually normochromic/normocytic, and the reticulocyte count is inappropriately low for the degree of anemia, indicating fail-

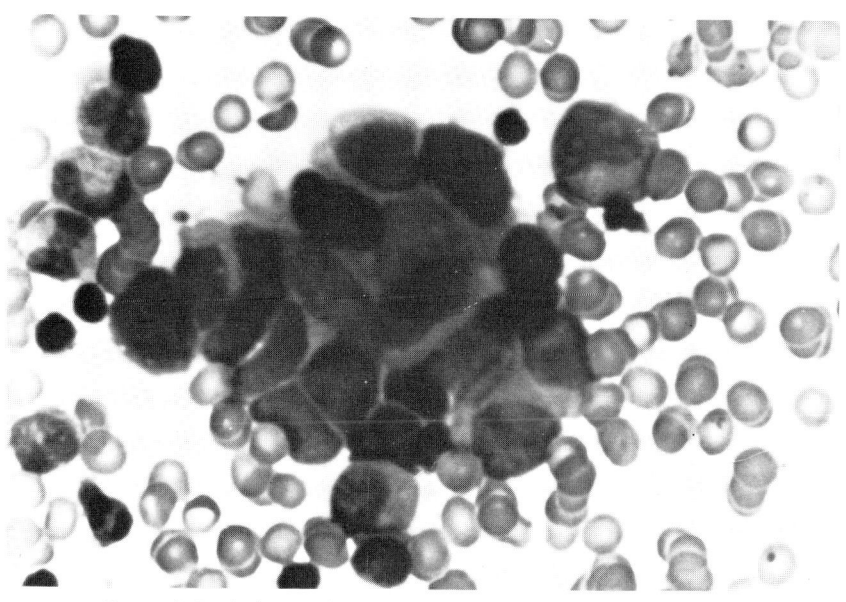

Figure 8-8 A clump of neuroblastoma cells in the bone marrow.

ure of the bone marrow to respond adequately.

The leukocyte count may vary from subnormal to markedly elevated levels; approximately 25 to 33 per cent of patients will have initial white cell counts of less than 5000/mm,³ whereas in 33 to 50 per cent the count will be in the range of 5000 to 20,000/mm,³ and in 20 to 33 per cent greater than 20,000/mm³.[200, 208] Approximately 5 to 20 per cent of patients will have an initial white count of 100,000/mm³ or greater.[200] Blast cells usually are easily detectable in the peripheral smear when the white count exceeds 5000/mm,³ but may not be seen when it is lower.

Both relative and absolute neutropenia is present, with the absolute neutrophil count below 1000/mm³ in the majority of patients. Thrombocytopenia is also almost invariably present at the time of diagnosis, but may not necessarily be sufficiently severe to cause hemorrhagic manifestations.

BONE MARROW. Bone marrow aspiration is the essential procedure for establishing a diagnosis of acute leukemia and also for identification of the cell line predominantly involved. The marrow specimen is usually markedly hypercellular and lacking the fat globules and bone particles characteristic of normal marrow.

Leukemia should be suspected whenever blast cells account for more than 5 per cent of the nucleated marrow cells, but a minimum of 25 per cent blast forms is usually considered necessary to establish the diagnosis. More frequently than not, the marrow contains from 60 to 100 per cent blast cells and presents a homogeneous picture when compared with the pleomorphic pattern seen in normal marrow specimens.

Occasionally bone marrow aspiration results in a "dry tap." This failure to obtain an adequate specimen is sometimes erroneously attributed to a "packed marrow;" however, other conditions leading to a "packed marrow" (e.g., chronic myelogenous leukemia, megaloblastic anemias) generally are not associated with difficulty in obtaining marrow samples by aspiration. A more likely explanation for this phenomenon in acute leukemia is the presence of reticulin fibrosis or bone infarction within the marrow cavity.[174] Marrow biopsy with a Jamshidi or Vim-Silverman needle will usually produce an adequate specimen; the sample obtained by this technique should be touched to glass slides before it is placed in fixative because such stained "touch-preparations" are very useful in assessing cellular morphology.

BLOOD CHEMISTRIES

Hyperuricemia. The serum uric acid level frequently is elevated at the time of diagnosis; even if it is normal initially, it may become elevated after therapy is initiated as the DNA of moribund leukemic cells is catabolized. When the hyperuricemia becomes extreme (20 to 55 mg per 100 ml) it may be accompanied by anorexia, nausea, persistent vomiting, extreme weakness, lethargy, convulsions, and coma.[291] Hyperuricemia may also result in obstruction of renal tubules by precipitated urate crystals and consequent acute renal failure. Management of this complication is discussed in Chapter Seven.

Hypocalcemia. Hypocalcemia may be present in as many as 10 per cent of children with acute leukemia;[160] this may be the result of acute renal failure or hypoalbuminemia in some cases, whereas in others the release of phosphate by lymphoblasts (which have high concentrations of this ion) may bind calcium and remove it from the serum.[349] Severe hypocalcemia may be accompanied by mental confusion, loss of appetite, nausea, vomiting, weakness, photophobia, carpopedal spasm, positive Chvostek sign, and convulsions.

Hypercalcemia. Hypercalcemia appears to be less common than hypocalcemia in children with acute leukemia.[231, 301] It is associated with nausea, vomiting, myalgia, polydipsia, polyuria, and hypertension and may result from the release by the leukemic cells of a substance with parathormone-like activity. Management of hypercalcemia is discussed in Chapter Seven.

Hypokalemia. Hypokalemia is especially frequent in acute myelocytic leukemia and all patients with this disease should be observed for this complication.[231] The proposed mechanisms for development of hypokalemia include: (1) renal tubular lesions induced by raised serum levels of muramidase, (2) malnutrition, (3) nephrotoxicity secondary to gentamicin/cephalothin combination therapy, (4) rapid cellular uptake of potassium, and (5) transcellular movement of potassium secondary to antibiotic therapy.

Hyperkalemia. Hyperkalemia is less frequently noted in acute leukemia than is hypokalemia. In general it is observed as a complication of cytotoxic therapy with subsequent massive lysis of neoplastic cells or acute renal failure secondary to hyperuricemia. If not recognized and treated appropriately, hyperkalemia may lead to cardiac arrest.

"Spurious" hyperkalemia has been reported in leukemic patients with very high white cell counts;[339] this may represent breakdown of leukocytes in vitro between the time of venipuncture and separation of serum or plasma for potassium determination. This phenomenon should be suspected in leukemic patients with hyperkalemia in the absence of appropriate clinical and EKG abnormalities (especially if there is a high peripheral white count).

Hyponatremia. Hyponatremia is infrequent in leukemic patients. It has on occasion been reported in association with the syndrome of inappropriate antidiuretic hormone secretion; this has been described as a complication of therapy with the cytotoxic agents vincristine and cyclophosphamide[75] and also in certain patients with AML.[215]

Hypernatremia. Hypernatremia is rare in leukemia patients; it has been reported in association with diabetes insipidus, an infrequent complication of central nervous system leukemia when there are infiltrates in the diencephalon and pituitary.

Hypoglycemia. Hypoglycemia is rarely seen in acute leukemia;[159] an entity known as *artifactual hypoglycemia* is seen in patients with very high blast counts when delay in running the test allows the cells to consume glucose in vitro.[89]

Muramidase. Muramidase or lysozyme is a hydrolytic enzyme that is present in the primary granules of primitive granulocyte and monocyte precursor cells. Elevated serum and urine levels of this enzyme are present in AML, but the highest levels are seen in AMML and AMoL. When renal muramidase excretion is particularly heavy, a nephropathy characterized by hypokalemia, hyperkaluria, and azotemia may develop.

Extramedullary Leukemia

Although leukemia is primarily a disease of bone marrow and peripheral blood, other tissues may also become infiltrated by the abnormal cells. This may be manifested overtly in some organs by clinically apparent enlargement or derangement of function; involvement of other organs may be clinically occult, but detectable by histologic sampling.

At the time of initial diagnosis, the organs most commonly showing clinical involvement are the liver, spleen, lymph nodes, and bones. However, microscopic foci are also present in other tissues and may persist after complete remission has been attained. Thus, approximately 40 per cent of living patients in complete marrow remission have had evidence of microscopic residual disease found in the liver, testes, CNS, and kidneys.[198a, 277] Autopsy studies of patients who have died while in complete remission have demonstrated an even higher incidence (over 50 per cent) of extramedullary leukemia with residual leukemic foci in the kidneys, liver, testes, spleen, brain, and meninges.[228, 288]

The significance of these occult extramedullary foci is twofold: (1) with prolonged duration of hematologic remission, they may become larger and eventually cause clinical morbidity, and (2) leukemic cells from these sites may metastasize to the bone marrow and produce a hematologic relapse.

CENTRAL NERVOUS SYSTEM. Few children with acute leukemia have overt central nervous system (CNS) involvement at the time of diagnosis. Since this complication becomes more frequent with prolonged duration of remission, it was rarely encountered in the era prior to chemotherapy, when survival times were very short. However, as chemotherapy began to produce long-term remissions, the incidence of this complication became more frequent particularly in children with ALL (50 to 70 per cent of cases). Prolonged survival alone is not the only determinant of CNS leukemia; a heavy burden of disease as measured by organomegaly and an initial white count greater than 50,000/mm^3 also increases the likelihood of its appearance.

Karyotypic studies suggest that CNS leukemia is a metastatic phenomenon resulting from seeding of the CNS by cells from the original leukemic clone at the time of initial diagnosis. Invasion of the CNS follows a specific anatomical route, which is determined by the structure of the leptomeninges[246, 247] (Fig. 8–9). Leukemic foci initially become apparent in the walls of the superficial arachnoid veins; they then extend sequentially into the arachnoid trabecular connective tissue, eventually destroying the mesothelial lining of the arachnoid channels and contaminating the cerebrospinal fluid.[247] With increasing leukemic cell mass, the deep arachnoid is infiltrated and the leukemic cells extend down around the cerebral vessels (Fig. 8–10). Leukemic cells invade the CNS parenchyma itself only after they have destroyed the pia-glial membrane.

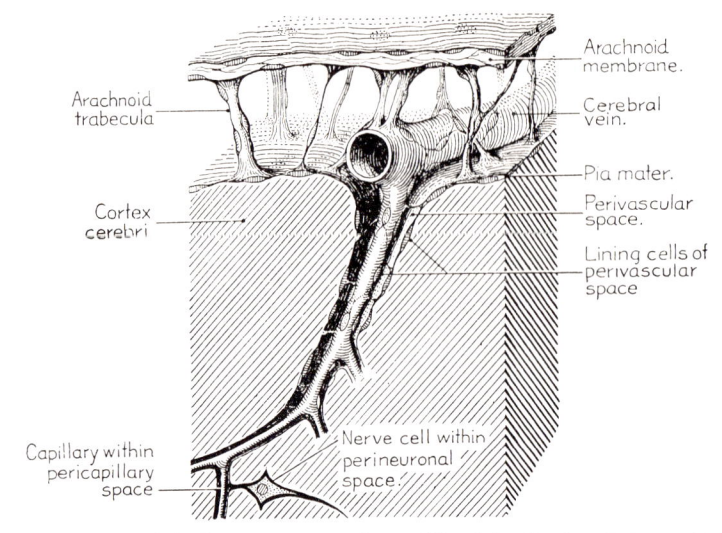

Figure 8-9 Anatomy of the leptomeninges. (From Weed, L. H.: Am. J. Anat. *31*:141, 1923.)

Leukemic cells may persist in the CNS throughout induction of hematologic remission because the "blood-brain barrier" provides a relative pharmacologic sanctuary which prevents the accumulation of systemic chemotherapy in sufficiently high concentrations to be cytotoxic. After months or years of dormancy these cells may resume proliferation and accumulate in sufficiently high numbers to cause clinical disease, the symptoms of which will reflect the anatomic pattern of CNS involvement—i.e., focal (parenchymal) or diffuse (meningeal).

Focal (Parenchymal) CNS Involvement. Infiltration of brain substance by leukemic cells may result in a mass lesion and the symptoms of increased intracranial pressure: headache, nausea, vomiting, lethargy, irritability, papilledema, and bilateral sixth nerve palsy. In addition, there may be localizing findings such as hemiparesis, isolated cranial nerve palsies, hemisensory loss, or convulsions. Hypothalamic involvement, with excessive weight gain, increased appetite, and diabetes insipidus, and cerebellar involvement, resulting in ataxia, dysmetria, hypotonia, and hyperreflexia, may occur as discrete entities.

Localized leukemic infiltrates involving the spinal cord are seen most frequently in acute myelogenous leukemia.[338] Because the presence of myeloperoxidase in these tumors frequently gives them a greenish hue, they are known as *chloromas*. The symptoms of cord compression include back and leg pain, numbness, weakness, Brown-Sequard syndrome, and bladder and bowel incontinence. Once these signs have appeared they progress very rapidly and may become irreversible unless treatment is initiated promptly. Unlike most other forms of CNS leukemia, spinal cord compression commonly occurs early in the course and may actually precede the systemic manifestations of leukemia by several months.

Along with the physical findings of cord compression, there may be increased CSF pressure and elevated CSF protein. Included in the differential diagnosis would be epidural hematoma (which has been observed following lumbar puncture in a severely thrombocytopenic patient[243]), vincristine neurotoxicity, and vertebral collapse.

Treatment. Intracerebral leukemic infiltrates are usually treated by ir-

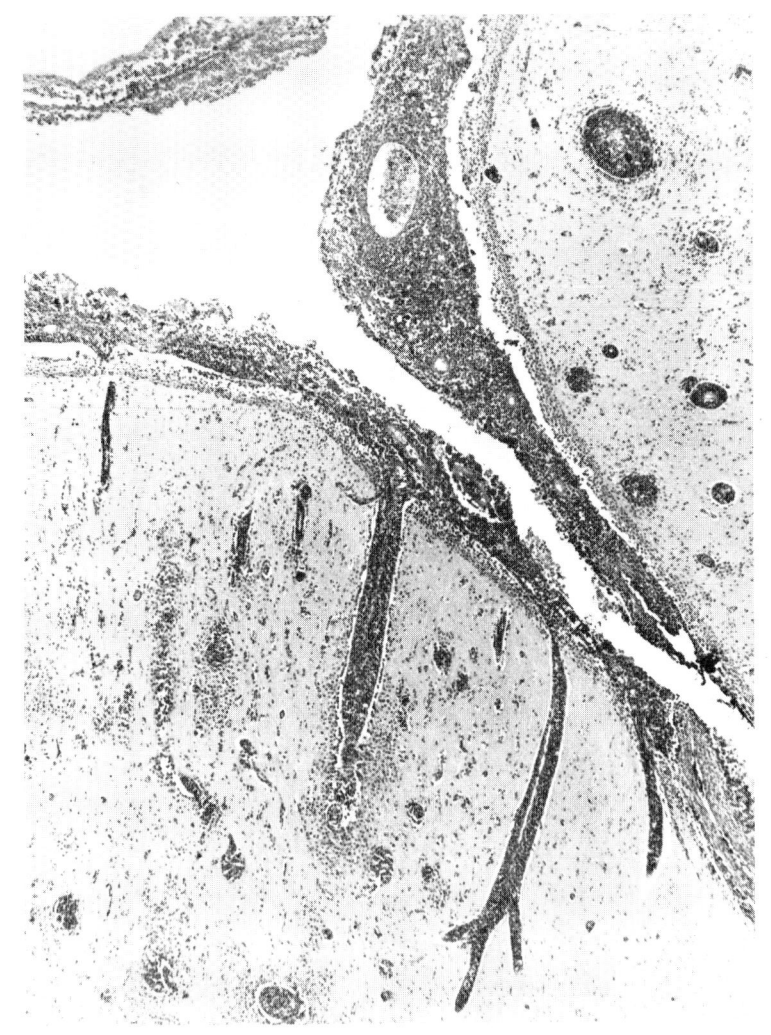

Figure 8-10 Leukemic meningitis. Leukemic infiltrate extends from subarachnoid space into CNS parenchyma along margins of the pia-glial membrane. (H & E, × 35.) (From Price, R.A., et al.: Cancer 31:520, 1973.)

radiation. Dexamethasone is useful in reducing cerebral edema secondary to the leukemic process and to the radiotherapy. Since intrathecal methotrexate does not enter the brain parenchyma in sufficiently high concentrations, it is not usually useful. Cord compression may be managed by decompression laminectomy or radiotherapy. Again dexamethasone may be useful to minimize edema.

Diffuse (Meningeal) Involvement. As in focal CNS involvement, the presenting signs and symptoms of meningeal leukemic infiltration are generally those of increased intracranial pressure. However, other nonspecific symptoms, such as diabetes insipidus, weight gain, and increased appetite should also cause this diagnosis to be suspected. In some patients the symptoms may be subtle and diagnosis is made either during routine follow-up lumbar puncture or on autopsy.

Diagnosis is usually based on CSF findings, which include elevated pressure, elevated protein, normal or decreased glucose level, and pleocytosis (from 10 to several thousand mononuclear cells/mm³). When the CSF is prepared for morphologic examination by cytocentrifugation, these mononuclear cells can be identified as blast cells (Fig. 8–11A). Such morphologic evaluation is useful in distinguishing the pleocytosis of leukemic meningitis from that induced as a reaction to intrathecal methotrexate (Fig. 8–11B) or CNS infection.

Treatment. The best treatment of leukemic meningitis is to eradicate it

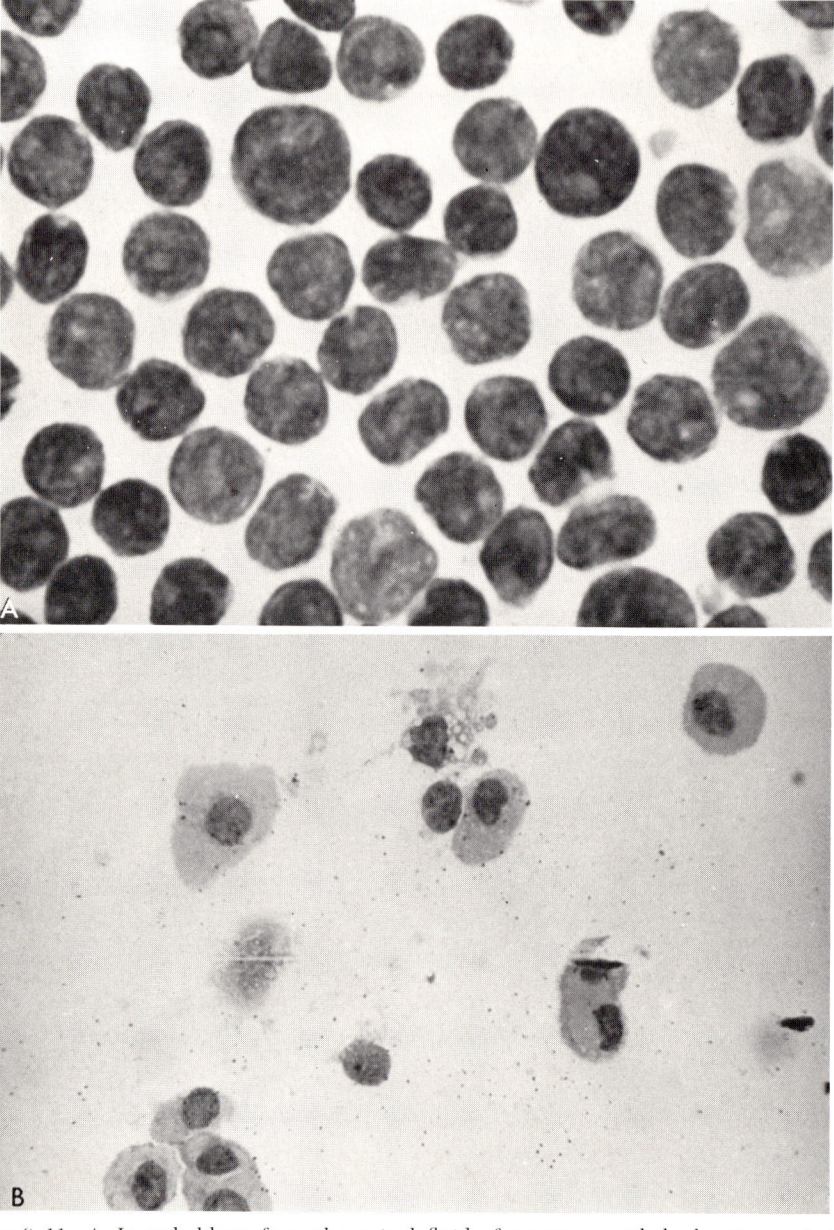

Figure 8-11 A, Lymphoblasts from the spinal fluid of a patient with leukemic meningitis. B, Histiocytes from the spinal fluid of a patient with a chemical arachnoiditis secondary to intrathecal methotrexate.

before it becomes clinically manifest. To this end, most ALL protocols incorporate CNS prophylactic therapy as an essential part of the regimen; this therapy usually combines intrathecal methotrexate administration with cranial irradiation (2000 to 2400 R) and will be discussed subsequently in this chapter.

When leukemic meningitis is clinically evident on physical or CSF examination, it is usually treated with intrathecal methotrexate injections (12 mg/m²/dose, up to maximum dose of 15 mg). Treatment is continued at 3-day intervals until the CSF returns to normal (usually within 1 to 2 weeks). Relatively high concentrations of methotrexate can be achieved in the CSF when it is given by the intrathecal route, and possibly, for this reason, methotrexate may be effective in controlling CNS leukemia even after blood and marrow leukemic cells have become resistant to it.

Intrathecal methotrexate can be given alone, in combination with cytosine arabinoside (30 mg/m²) or in combination with both cytosine arabinoside and hydrocortisone (15 mg/m²). Craniospinal irradiation and oral pyrimethamine[110] have also been used to treat leukemic meningitis.

Although CNS leukemia can be controlled temporarily by these methods, it can rarely be completely eradicated once it has become clinically manifest. Recurrences usually develop within a mean period of 3 to 6 months. The mean duration of CNS remission may be prolonged to 15.5 months by the use of triple (methotrexate, cytosine arabinoside, and hydrocortisone) intrathecal therapy for induction plus maintenance of remission.[243, 306] Recently Gribbin and co-workers have reported long-term control of CNS leukemia (median duration 2 years) by administering maintenance intrathecal methotrexate at 4-week intervals until the patient had been in continuous remission for 2 to 2½ years.[123a]

Since it is possible that failure of intrathecal chemotherapy to eradicate meningeal leukemia may be due in part to inadequate drug distribution in the CSF some authors now recommend intraventricular administration via an Ommaya reservoir.[243, 278] This has been shown to result in more reliable CSF drug levels than those achieved by lumbar puncture and has the additional advantage of allowing painless administration of the drug. However, this may be associated with a higher incidence of complications than seen following intrathecal administration.[123a]

TESTES. Like CNS leukemia, testicular involvement probably arises as a metastatic phenomenon in a "pharmacologic sanctuary" area. Although identified microscopically in 27 to 92 per cent[91, 116, 305] of male patients dying with widespread and extensive acute leukemia, clinical testicular leukemia is found in only about 1 to 16 per cent[91, 170, 175, 303, 305] of living male patients. Since this complication requires a median time of 13 months from diagnosis to develop, it has become more common as survival time has been lengthened by newer protocols.[116] In one recent study,[22a] testicular involvement accounted for 40 per cent of the leukemic relapses occurring in young males who had been in complete remission for 3 years or longer.

The clinical presentation is painless enlargement of the testicle; this may be either unilateral or bilateral (Fig. 8–12). In many cases this occurs while the bone marrow remains in complete remission and may be the first identifiable site of leukemic relapse, although bone marrow relapse usually follows within a median interval of 1 to 6.5 months.[175, 303]

While chemotherapy has been used to treat testicular leukemia, the drugs may not reach maximum concentration in this area because of a postulated "blood-gonad barrier." Radiation therapy (1200 R) appears to be successful in treating this complication;[303] both testes should be irradiated even when only one is clinically involved, since

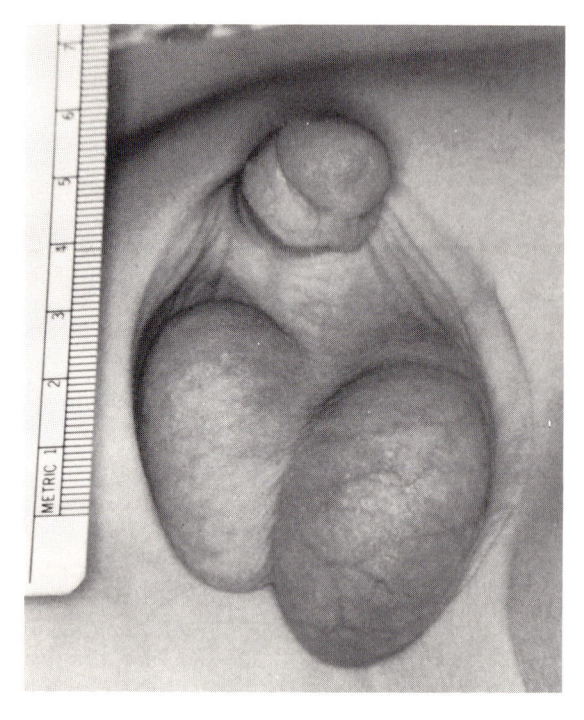

Figure 8–12 Testicular leukemia.

microscopic disease can usually be found in the "normal" gonad as well.[91, 305] An unfortunate side effect of testicular irradiation is permanent sterility. Fortunately, however, sexual maturation is not usually interfered with since the Leydig cells (which produce testosterone) are relatively radioresistant.[91, 305]

In view of the high proportion of the testicular relapses in young males who have been in complete remission for 3 years or more, the Children's Cancer Study Group investigated the ability of prophylactic radiotherapy to the testes to prevent subsequent testicular leukemia.[226a] Of 221 children who did not receive prophylactic therapy to their gonads, 13 subsequently had a testicular relapse, whereas of 76 who did receive gonadal radiotherapy (1200 rads), not one case of testicular relapse occurred.

OVARIES. Ovarian infiltrates appear with less frequency at autopsy than do testicular ones, the incidence being 11.5 per cent[305] to 36 per cent.[290] Although clinical involvement is difficult to detect, one patient with a pelvic mass resulting from leukemic infiltrates of the ovaries, tubes, uterus, broad ligaments, and pelvic nodes has been described.[305]

KIDNEYS. Asymptomatic leukemic infiltrates have been found in the kidneys of a few patients while in complete clinical remission,[227] and in 33 per cent of cases in an autopsy series. In this same autopsy series, another 33 per cent of cases had renal enlargement without demonstrable leukemic involvement.

Infiltration by leukemic cells, although producing renal enlargement, does not usually result in clinical symptomatology; however, hematuria, hypertension, or renal failure may occur. Local irradiation appears to be the treatment of choice for leukemic renal infiltrates.

Not all cases of renal enlargement in leukemic children are due to infiltration by tumor cells; some may be due to proximal tubular hypertrophy of unknown etiology. Noninfiltrative causes of renal failure in leukemic patients also include hyperuricemia, hemorrhage into the renal pelvis and ureters, pyelonephritis, sepsis, and severe dehydration.[183] Hypertension is more commonly associated with steroid therapy than due to leukemic renal involvement; it is also seen as a side effect of vincristine therapy. Hematuria also is more commonly associated with the complications of leukemia (e.g., thrombocytopenia) or its therapy (Cytoxan-induced hemorrhagic cystitis) than with direct leukemic infiltration of the kidneys.

GASTROINTESTINAL TRACT. Leukemic infiltrates in the gastrointestinal tract are common, but are usually clinically silent until the terminal stages of the disease. At this point necrotizing enteropathy may occur; this is characterized by necrosis of leukemic infiltrates, intramural hemorrhage, invasion of the gut wall by enteric microorganisms, perforation of the bowel wall, peritonitis, and sepsis.[8, 327] The most common site of necrotizing enteropathy is the cecum (sparing the appendix); this produces a catastrophic syndrome known as *"typhlitis"*[327] (Fig. 8–13) or *ileocecal syndrome*,[283] which has been found in 10 per cent of leukemic children at postmortem examination.[327] This condition may be suspected ante mortem by the progression of symptoms from vague right lower quadrant discomfort and fullness to development of a partially obstructive mass to signs of peritonitis and septic shock. Roentgenographically, a relative lack of gas in the right lower quadrant and minimal distention of the small bowel may be seen on plain films; barium enema may show severe mucosal irregularity, rigidity, loss of haustral markings, and occasional fistulation.[283]

Acute inflammatory states of the right lower abdominal quadrant accounted for half of the surgical indications in a recent series[282] of leukemic patients; of these the diagnoses were roughly evenly divided between appendicitis and typhlitis. The mortality of the acute surgical abdomen in this series was almost 100 per cent for patients in relapse. Consequently, surgery should be considered a last resort when an "acute surgical abdomen" develops in a child whose leukemia is in relapse.[282]

Other gastrointestinal lesions seen in children with acute leukemia may be related to neutropenia and/or chemotherapy. These include mouth ulcers (methotrexate toxicity), oral and esophageal moniliasis (prednisone, antibiotics), and perirectal abscesses (mainly in AMML and AMoL).

BONES AND JOINTS. Bone pain is one of the initial symptoms in 25 per cent of patients with acute leukemia;[316] migratory joint pain accompanied by swelling and tenderness occurs less frequently as a presenting symptom and may be misdiagnosed as rheumatic fever[294] or rheumatoid arthritis.[268] These symptoms may be the result of direct leukemic infiltration of the periosteum, periosteal elevation by underlying cortical disease, bone infarction, or expansion of the marrow cavity by the leukemic cells.

Radiologic changes are seen most easily in the long bones, especially around areas of rapid growth (knees, wrists, ankles).[340] Some patients may have characteristic radiologic changes in the absence of bone pain while others may have bone pain unaccompanied by radiologic changes.

The radiologic changes seen most frequently in acute leukemia are: (1) subperiosteal new bone formation, (2) transverse metaphyseal lucent bands, (3) osteolytic lesions involving the medullary cavity and cortex, (4) diffuse demineralization, and (5) transverse metaphyseal lines of increased density ("growth arrest" lines) (Fig. 8–14). The presence or absence of these findings at the time of initial diagnosis does not appear to influence the patient's prognosis for long-term survival.[17]

If the leukemia is responsive to chemotherapy, bone pain often regresses rapidly and bone lesions tend

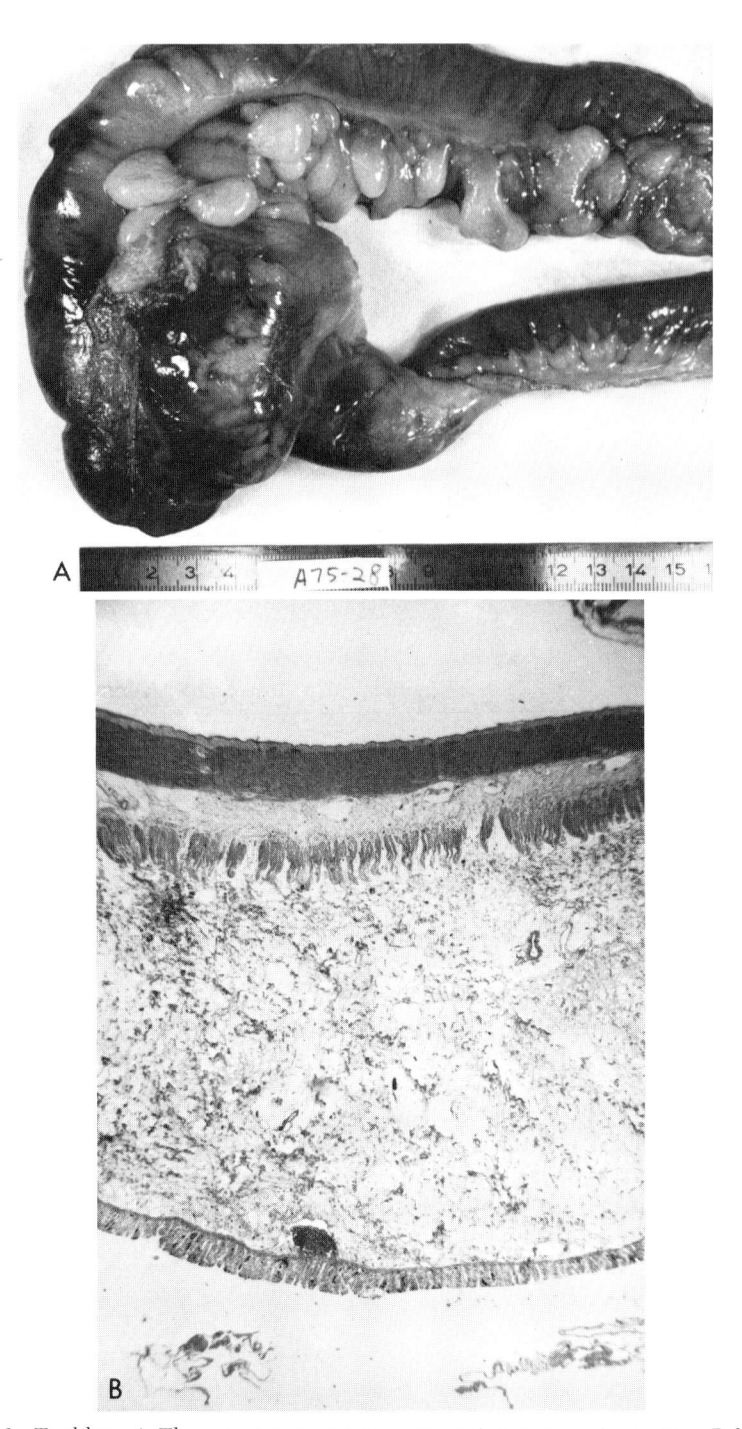

Figure 8-13 Typhlitis. *A,* The cecum is gangrenous-appearing on gross inspection. *B,* Microscopic section shows marked edema of bowel wall and absence of polymorphonuclear leukocytic infiltrate. (Courtesy of Dr. Ronald Maenza.)

THE LEUKEMIAS 199

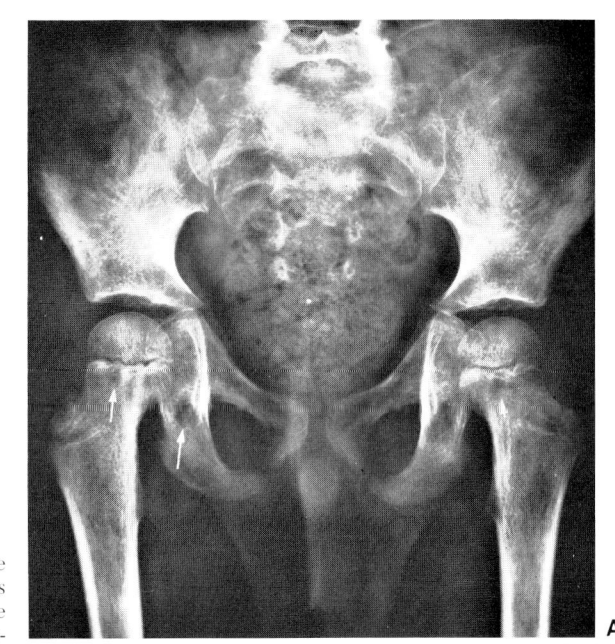

Figure 8–14 Bone changes in acute leukemia. *A*, Osteoporosis. The pelvis and femurs are demineralized and the trabeculae are coarsened. *B*, Submetaphyseal radiolucent bands in the bones of the knee. (From Teplick, J. G., and Haskin, M. E.: Roentgenologic Diagnosis. 3rd Ed. Philadelphia, W. B. Saunders Co., 1976.)

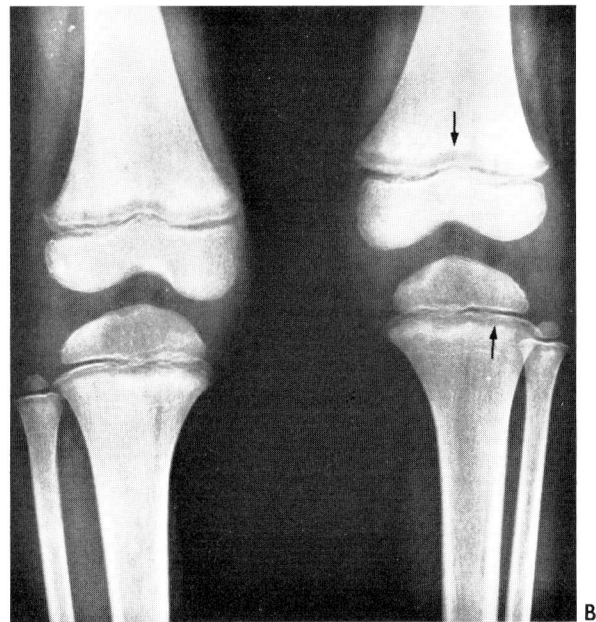

to heal when remission is attained.[316] When the leukemia is refractory to chemotherapy, bone pain may be treated symptomatically with analgesics, prednisone, or low-dose irradiation (200 to 600 R).

CHLOROMAS. Chloromas are localized solid tumor masses composed of poorly differentiated cells of the granulocytic series; although cellular morphology varies from nongranular mononuclear cells to myelocyte, the primary malignant cell is the myeloblast. The name chloroma derives from the greenish color of the surface of the freshly cut specimen, which results from the presence of myeloperoxidase in the primary granules of the cells.[4, 156]

These tumors are associated with AML and CML and may actually precede the peripheral blood and marrow manifestations by as much as 2 years.[194] The most common site of involvement is bone, particularly of the face, cranium, and orbit. Other flat bones (sternum, ribs, vertebrae, pelvis) may also be frequently involved, but long bone involvement is uncommon.

Parenchymal organs that have shown frequent chloroma involvement are kidney, lymph nodes, testes, and ovaries, but nearly any parenchymal organ can be affected. Often these tumors are clinically silent and are discovered unexpectedly at postmortem examination. One area in which they may cause serious symptoms is the spinal cord; lesions arising from vertebral bodies and meninges may cause cord compression, which should be treated by laminectomy and radiotherapy.[233] Scanning techniques using gallium may be of value in localizing myeloblastoma masses early in their course and might obviate the need for laminectomy if radiotherapy can be instituted before function is compromised.[181]

MANAGEMENT OF THE CHILD WITH ACUTE LEUKEMIA

The basic principles of management of the child with acute leukemia may be summarized as follows:

1. Prompt recognition and treatment of life-threatening complications at the time of initial diagnosis.
2. Induction of complete remission using combination chemotherapy.
3. "Consolidation" therapy—this may include prophylactic treatment of "sanctuary" areas or may involve the use of a short course of combination chemotherapy to further reduce the leukemic population.
4. Continuous maintenance therapy with combination chemotherapy for a fixed period of time.

The physicians caring for a child with acute leukemia must constantly bear in mind that *the predominant causes of morbidity and mortality from this disease (at any time in its course) are infection and hemorrhage*, and these should always be considered in the differential diagnosis of any of its manifestations.

Recognition and Treatment of Life-Threatening Complications at the Time of Initial Diagnosis

At the time of diagnosis many children with acute leukemia are acutely and dangerously ill. While many of their problems arise from their compromised hematologic status (*anemia, neutropenia, thrombocytopenia*), others may result from direct organ infiltration by leukemic cells (*hepatic dysfunction, leukemic meningitis*) or from the consequences of the breakdown of DNA from the large mass of leukemic cells (*hyperuricemia*). All of these complications should be assessed and controlled *before* consideration is given to specific antileukemic chemotherapy. The evaluation and management of these problems were discussed in Chapter Seven. Except in the rare instance when the leukocyte count is in excess of $100,000/mm^3$ (*"blast crisis"*), there is no urgent reason to commence chemotherapy immediately, and it may even be detrimental to the patient to do so.

"**Blast Crisis.**" When the white count is in excess of $100,000/mm^3$ there is a particularly high risk that the patient will develop an intracranial hemorrhage. This dire consequence is the result of rupture of intracerebral vessels that have been compromised by leukocyte sludging or by nodules of leukemic tissue. Hyperuricemia is also a likely complication of *blast cell crisis*, and the level of uric acid may reach extremely high levels following the initiation of cytoreductive chemotherapy. Consequently, urgent and effective medical therapy is indicated.

Vigorous intravenous hydration and alkalinization of the urine should be started immediately (see Chapter Seven); large doses of allopurinol should also be given. Once the leukemia has been classified according to morphologic type, specific chemotherapy should be initiated. If the diagnosis is ALL, treatment with vincristine (1.5 mg/m^2 I.V. weekly, not to exceed an individual total dose of 2 mg) and prednisone (40 mg/m^2 P.O. daily) has been recommended.[145] For AML or AMML treatment with daunorubicin (45 mg/m^2 I.V. push daily for 3 days) and cytosine arabinoside (100 mg/m^2 B.I.D., I.V. push for 5 days) can be used.[145] The level of circulating blast cells can also be rapidly reduced within 2 to 4 hours by leukapheresis.[145] An alternate mode of therapy for "blast crisis" of acute nonlymphocytic leukemia is radiotherapy (600 R) to the entire cranium and hydroxyurea (3.0 g/m^2 I.V.).[337]

Remission Induction

The goal of induction therapy is to reduce the leukemic cell burden and allow for repopulation of the marrow by normal stem cells. While single agents are capable of inducing remission in the acute leukemias, regimens which combine these agents are even more successful and today virtually all induction regimens involve the use of multiple agents simultaneously. Such regimens have been more successful for ALL than for AML primarily because of the ability of drugs such as vincristine, prednisone, and L-asparaginase to more or less selectively destroy ALL cells while causing little or no damage to normal hematopoietic stem cells. Although these drugs undoubtedly also kill some normal lymphocytes, the patient is better able to withstand this temporary insult than he can the severe depletion of granulocytes and platelets. The situation for AML is somewhat different. Since the leukemic population is biochemically, morphologically, and kinetically similar to normal hematopoietic precursors, there is relatively little sparing of normal erythroid, myeloid, and megakaryocyte stem cells, and consequently remission induction is accompanied by hazardous and sometimes fatal neutropenia and thrombocytopenia.

Remission may be defined as the absence of detectable stigmata of leukemia based on physical, hematologic, and bone marrow findings.

1. Physical examination: Absence of physical findings and symptoms directly attributable to leukemia.

2. Hematologic: Absence of blast cells on peripheral smear; neutrophil count greater than 500/mm^3; platelet count greater than 75,000/mm.^{3}

3. Bone marrow: 5 per cent or fewer blast cells and evidence of reappearance of erythroid, myeloid, and megakaryocytic elements around marrow particles.

Unfortunately, these criteria reflect the relatively insensitive methods we have for detecting leukemic cells rather than the fact that the leukemic population has been eradicated and the patient cured. Since approximately 10^{12} (1 trillion) leukemic cells are present at the time of diagnosis,[293] and destruction of 99.9 to 99.99 per cent of these cells is necessary to attain remission,[137] a large residual leukemic population (10^8 or 100 million cells) could still persist after the induction chemotherapy regimen. These cells, although clinically undetectable, could serve as a nidus for relapse of the disease at some later time.

The evidence that leukemic cells do indeed persist during remission may be summarized as follows:

1. Termination of Remission. If no further chemotherapy is given after remission induction with vincristine/prednisone, clinically apparent leukemia will recur within a median interval of 40 to 60 days. Since the doubling time of leukemic cells is approximately 4 days, this period of time would allow a residual population of 10^8 leukemic cells to expand to 10^{12} (1 trillion) cells, the number necessary for clinically evident disease. Unmaintained remission of longer than 60 days may result if a smaller residual leukemic cell population were present at the end of the induction course.

2. *Karyotypic Evidence.* At the time of relapse, the leukemic population frequently has the same chromosomal abnormalities as the original cells. This suggests that the "new" cells belong to the same clone as the original cells rather than to a new clone induced by a subsequent leukemogenic stimulus.

3. *Histologic Evidence.* Approximately 45 per cent of patients in clinical remission of acute leukemia have demonstrable foci of leukemic cells in visceral organs (liver, spleen, kidneys, gonads, bowel, lymph nodes, or central nervous system) when these organs are examined by needle biopsy or at postmortem[228, 288] (Fig. 8–15).

4. *Extramedullary Leukemia.* Relapse of leukemia does not always occur in the bone marrow or peripheral blood. Leukemic foci large enough to cause clinically apparent disease may develop in visceral organs or the central nervous system at a time when the peripheral blood and bone marrow appear to be perfectly normal. Such recurrences are thought to develop from small nests of leukemic foci persisting in these "sanctuary" areas after the induction course.

Why Do Leukemic Cells Persist During Remission? Leukemic cells can persist after induction chemotherapy only if they have been able to avoid the toxic effects of the drugs. The mechanisms for this may have a biochemical, kinetic, or anatomic basis.

BIOCHEMICAL BASIS. A small pro-

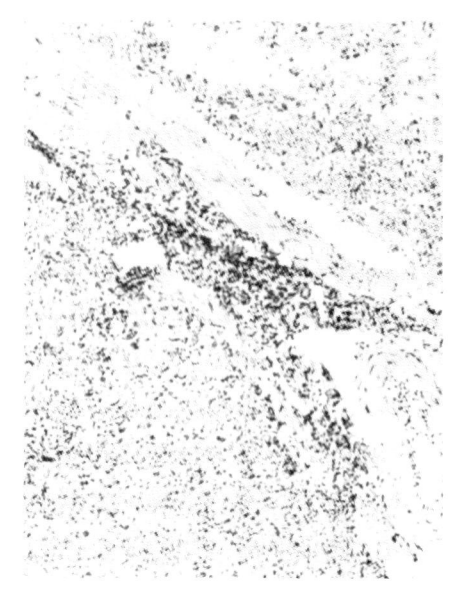

Figure 8–15 Occult leukemic focus in spleen of a patient who died of intercurrent infection while in "complete remission." Photomicrograph shows dense, dark collection of leukemic cells within perivascular lymphatics between splenic trabeculae. (From Simone, J. V., et al.: Blood 39:759, 1972.)

portion of the leukemic cell population may be inherently resistant to the drugs and consequently not eradicated with the rest of the leukemic cell population. These cells may then give rise to a new leukemic cell population that is resistant to chemotherapy.

KINETIC BASIS. Labeling experiments identify two functionally different leukemic blast cell populations with regard to proliferative activity. One population, composed of large blast cells with fine nuclear chromatin and deeply basophilic cytoplasm, is very heavily labeled by ^{3}H-thymidine and is apparently the actively proliferative compartment. The other population, consisting of smaller cells with more densely clumped chromatin and less basophilic cytoplasm, exhibits no proliferative activity. These "resting" or "sterile" cells eventually become labeled several hours after injection of ^{3}H-thymidine as they resume proliferative activity; they can therefore be conceptualized as a reserve or stem-cell pool for the larger cells. Since most antineoplastic drugs act during the cell cycle, cells that are in a resting or nondividing state (G_0) may not be susceptible to their actions. Such "sleeper" cells may resume active replication at a later time (when the drug is no longer present) and result in clinical relapse of leukemia.

ANATOMIC BASIS. Drugs are not distributed evenly throughout the entire body. In some areas, because of poor perfusion or physiologic barriers, the concentration of the drug may not be sufficiently high to kill leukemic cells. An example of such an anatomic "sanctuary" is the central nervous system, which excludes many drugs by virtue of the "blood-brain barrier." Sanctuaries presumably also exist in other visceral organs, such as the gonads, kidneys, liver, and spleen.

Central Nervous System Prophylaxis

Prophylactic treatment of the central nervous system is designed to eradicate residual leukemic foci in the meninges and brain parenchyma that may have persisted following remission induction. As mentioned earlier (section on CNS leukemia), failure to treat the central nervous system permits these occult foci of disease to produce clinical CNS leukemia and may eventually lead to hematologic relapse as well.

The complications of the CNS prophylactic regimen are cosmetic, hematologic, and neurologic. Total alopecia almost always follows cranial irradiation. Slow leakage of methotrexate from the CSF to the peripheral blood may suppress the bone marrow and lower the hemoglobin level, white cell count, and platelet count, leading some authors to recommend that folinic acid (citrovorum factor) be given systemically in a dose equal to the intrathecal methotrexate dose.

A wide spectrum of neurologic complications ranging from mild to lethal has been seen following CNS prophylactic treatment.[243a] Those commonly observed are headache, fever, nausea, and vomiting within several hours following lumbar puncture,[241] and a mild, temporary encephalopathy characterized by lethargy, somnolence, loss of appetite, and elevated CSF protein appearing several weeks after the CNS treatment.[203] Several follow-up studies show no evidence of permanent neurologic or psychologic dysfunction in most patients after periods varying from 18 months to 4 years.[11,297] However, some patients who had been given high-dose intravenous methotrexate as part of their maintenance regimens developed a high incidence of neurologic problems, including seizures, paraplegia, dementia, and multifocal leukoencephalopathy.[203,207,248] Occasional patients have developed chemical arachnoiditis,[36] encephalopathy,[203] and paraplegia[191] following intrathecal methotrexate. A distinctive group of neuropathologic lesions, chiefly affecting the cerebral white matter, may develop in children receiving therapy for leukemia; these alterations are at least partially attributable to vigorous chemotherapy and cranial irradiation.[75a,248]

Maintenance Therapy

Once remission has been achieved, it is important to maintain it without even the briefest of relapses. Most evidence indicates that relapse is associated with poorer long-term survival, even if remission can be successfully reinduced. Maintenance therapy appears to be necessary to prevent proliferation of persistent occult foci of leukemic cells. In most patients, failure to provide this maintenance therapy will result in relapse within 3 to 4 months.

Although several drugs have been found to be useful for maintenance therapy when administered as single agents, combination therapy with two or more drugs appears to be more effective. Methotrexate and 6-mercaptopurine form the cornerstones of most ALL maintenance regimens, since they are much more effective in maintaining than in inducing remission; other drugs, such as vincristine, prednisone, and L-asparaginase, although effective in inducing remission, are not satisfactory for maintaining remission. Developing effective maintenance therapy for AML has proved to be more difficult than for ALL; however, a number of drug regimens are being tested at the present time.

Management of Acute Lymphocytic Leukemia

Remission Induction. As shown in Table 8–5, many chemotherapeutic agents are capable of inducing remission in ALL when used singly. However, combinations of two (or more) of these agents have been even more successful (Table 8–6).

The combination used most frequently is vincristine/prednisone, both because of its relatively high success rate (80 to 95 per cent) and because of its bone marrow-sparing properties. The standard regimen is given as follows: vincristine, 1.5 mg/m² (maximum, 2.0 mg) I.V. on a weekly basis, and prednisone, 40 mg/m²/day orally.

Table 8–5 Effectiveness of Single Drugs for Remission Induction in Acute Lymphoblastic Leukemia

	PER CENT COMPLETE REMISSION RATE
Vincristine	55–85[82, 163a, 166, 200]
Prednisone	60–76[163a, 185, 200]
L-asparaginase	43–70[163a, 200, 307]
Daunorubicin	45–65[162, 163, 163a, 200]
Adriamycin	12.5–35[163a, 307, 308, 309]
Cytosine arabinoside	5–35[152, 163a, 200, 320]
Cyclophosphamide	25–35[163a, 200]
6-Mercaptopurine	25–35[100, 163a, 200]
Methotrexate	22–30[100, 163a, 200]

Table 8–6 Effectiveness of Drug Combinations for Remission Induction in Acute Lymphoblastic Leukemia

DRUG COMBINATION	PER CENT COMPLETE REMISSION RATE
Vincristine/Prednisone/ Daunorubicin	94–100[197, 333]
Vincristine/Prednisone	83–92[86, 163a, 275]
6-Mercaptopurine/ Prednisone	64–93[86, 87, 102, 171]
Methotrexate/Prednisone	75–85[163a, 171]
Daunorubicin/Prednisone	65–90[150, 163a]
Cyclophosphamide/ Prednisone	58–85[87, 163a]
6-Mercaptopurine/ Methotrexate	40–45[163a]

Although four weeks generally are required to achieve complete remission, in most cases there is a marked regression of symptoms and organomegaly within the first few days of treatment. Blast cells usually disappear from the peripheral blood within the first 1 to 2 weeks; however, the hemoglobin, hematocrit, neutrophil, and platelet counts may actually decrease below pretreatment levels during this period before beginning their return to normal levels in the second to third weeks.

While this regimen does not have the severe bone marrow toxicity seen in other ALL and AML regimens, other major side-effects can be troublesome. These include vincristine-induced peripheral neuropathy, jaw pain, abdominal pain, constipation, paralytic ileus, and hair loss. If vincristine is not properly injected intravenously, severe skin irritation and necrosis can result. Prednisone can cause gastrointestinal irritation, hypertension, excessive weight gain, and increased susceptibility to infections.

The addition of L-asparaginase as a third drug to the vincristine/prednisone regimen appears to result in a slight, but statistically significant, increase in the proportion of patients attaining complete remission.[234a] Moreover, the intensiveness of the initial therapy may influence the duration of the subsequent hematologic remission, possibly by decreasing the residual leukemic cell burden. Those patients who have had a three drug induction regimen (with daunorubicin or L-asparaginase as the third drug), or who have had an intensive phase of chemotherapy early in remission, appear to enjoy significantly longer remissions than those who had a two drug induction phase and no intensification phase.[287]

PATIENTS IN WHOM REMISSION IS NOT ATTAINED WITH THE INITIAL INDUCTION REGIMEN. If after the first four weeks of therapy, the bone marrow does not fulfill the criteria for complete remission, several alternatives are available. For those patients in whom the marrow findings represent a significant improvement over the initial sample, it is probably worth persisting with the vincristine-prednisone regimen for another 2 to 3 weeks in an effort to convert a partial remission to a complete one. On the other hand, if there is no improvement or a worsening of the hematologic findings occurs, other drug combinations should be utilized; these may include L-asparaginase, daunomycin, Adriamycin, 6-mercaptopurine, or methotrexate. Reconsideration of the original morphologic diagnosis is probably in order as well. Approximately 5 per cent of patients will die within the first weeks or months of treatment without ever attaining remission.[205]

Central Nervous System Prophylaxis. This phase of therapy is usually initiated as soon as bone marrow remission has been attained; the technique most frequently used is a combination of cranial irradiation (2400 rads) and intrathecal methotrexate.[13] This combination of therapy appears to be more effective than intrathecal methotrexate alone and less myelosuppressive and growth-retarding than craniospinal irradiation.[11]

CNS prophylaxis has proved to be a significant contribution to the management of children with ALL. Not only has the incidence of overt CNS leukemia been reduced from 50 per cent to below 10 per cent, but the durations of both hematologic remission and survival appear to be prolonged as well.[13, 161]

Maintenance Therapy. Today most maintenance regimens for ALL incorporate daily 6-mercaptopurine and intermittent methotrexate (with or without cyclophosphamide) in continuous administration until relapse occurs. Some regimens also include pulse doses of vincristine and prednisone given at monthly or trimonthly intervals.

The effects of maintenance therapy must be constantly monitored and drug dosages modified as the circumstances warrant. Among the indications for reduction or temporary discontinuation of maintenance drug dosages are: (1) *bone marrow suppression*—the dosages should be halved when the leukocyte count falls below 1000/mm^3 and the medications discontinued when the absolute neutrophil count falls below 500/mm^3, (2) *mouth ulcers*—methotrexate should be stopped until they are healed, (3) *diarrhea, persistent vomiting*—both 6MP and methotrexate should be stopped, (4) *active infection*—all maintenance medications should be discontinued until the infectious process has resolved, (5) *renal insufficiency*—methotrexate should be discontinued if BUN is > 20 mg/100 ml, (6) *liver dysfunction*—elevated transaminase or bilirubin levels are an indication for modifying the dosages of 6MP and methotrexate, (7) *neurotoxicity*—severe constipation, paresthesias, muscular weakness, foot drop, and severe abdominal cramps are indications for discontinuing vincristine, (8) *hematuria*—this may represent hemorrhagic cystitis when cyclophosphamide is used; the drug should be discontinued in this event.

DURATION OF MAINTENANCE THERAPY. The optimal conditions for discontinuing therapy of ALL are unknown. Simone, in a recent review of the subject, found that when therapy with single or multiple agents was stopped after 1½ to 14 months of remission, half the patients relapsed within 2 to 10 months.[286] A small study (involving only 15 patients), which maintained ALL patients on chemotherapy for 2½ to 3 years and then divided the patients randomly into further chemotherapy or cessation of therapy groups, found no difference in the relapse rate of the two groups over the next 5 years (approximately 50 per cent for both groups). A somewhat larger study, which stopped therapy after 2½ to 3½ years, found a subsequent 16 per cent relapse rate, with the risk of relapse being highest in the first year after cessation of therapy.[14] The proportion of patients remaining in complete remission then declined exponentially for the next 1 to 2 years and leveled off thereafter.[13, 286] More recently a group of 280 children with ALL who had been on various combinations of continuous chemotherapy were randomly allocated to either continued chemotherapy or discontinued chemotherapy after three years of complete remission.[22a] After a median follow-up period of 19 months, there were no significant differences in the relapse rates between those patients remaining on chemotherapy and those who had stopped chemotherapy. At this point, 14 per cent of the 280 patients had had some type of relapse; 52 per cent of these relapses occurred in the bone marrow, 13 per cent in the central nervous system, and 29 per cent in the testes (testicular relapses accounted for 40 per cent of the relapses in male patients).

These data appear to indicate that continued chemotherapy is useful in preventing leukemic cell proliferation or eradicating leukemic cells or both, up to a point (perhaps 2 to 3 years), but then ceases to be of significant value.[14] For this reason, as well as for the fact that maintenance therapy is accompanied by significant long-range toxicity (e.g., hepatic and pulmonary fibrosis, osteoporosis, bladder fibrosis, hemorrhagic cystitis, growth suppression, and immunologic suppression), it has been recommended that maintenance therapy be stopped at this point.

Reinduction After Bone Marrow Relapse. When a patient with ALL suffers a bone marrow relapse, the usual practice is to re-treat with vincristine, prednisone and possibly a third drug (Adriamycin, L-asparaginase); patients who have responded to this regimen previously, and have not been on maintenance therapy with these drugs, have a 70 to 80 per cent chance of achieving a second remission. With subsequent relapses, the chances of repeat remission induction with this regimen decrease to 60 to 70 per cent for a third remission, and 50 to 60 per cent for a fourth remission.[300]

When vincristine/prednisone fails to reinduce remission, L-asparaginase, either alone or in combination with other agents, would probably be the next choice;[324] this agent has produced remissions in 62 per cent of children with advanced ALL.[307] Other drugs that can be used at this point are Adriamycin, daunomycin, cytosine arabinoside, high-dose methotrexate, and cyclophosphamide.

Patients who experience relapse following cessation of prolonged maintenance therapy for ALL form a unique population. Reinduction of remission occurs with relatively high frequency; in one study, 15 of 17 such patients treated with vincristine, prednisone, and Adriamycin achieved hematologic remission without severe toxicity.[256] However, the tendency to develop another relapse is approximately 50 per cent, with the site of relapse occurring with equal frequency in the bone marrow and CNS.

Just as relapse in the central nervous system is likely to lead to bone marrow relapse, so too bone marrow relapse is likely to be followed by central nervous system relapse. In fact, central nervous system relapse appears to be as likely during a second marrow remission as it is in the first.[256a] Apparently, central nervous system therapy during one remission does not carry over to the next (probably because of reseeding of the meninges). Thus, patients who develop recurrent ALL in the bone marrow should be considered for a second course of prophylactic central nervous system therapy.[256, 256a]

Results of Therapy for ALL. In the era when no therapy was available, the median survival time for patients with ALL was approximately 3 months;[319] this was extended to 9 months by the use of supportive measures, such as blood transfusion and antibiotics.[34] With the use of chemotherapy capable of inducing and maintaining remission, the median survival was significantly prolonged, but only 7.8 per cent of patients survived for 5 or more years,[259] and only 3 per cent remained completely leukemia-free during this period.[171, 348] Interruption of remission by extramedullary leukemia, particularly of the CNS, was a significant impediment to long-term survival in these patients. The use of central nervous system prophylactic therapy in combination with aggressive multiagent chemotherapy has resulted in approximately 40 to 50 per cent of patients remaining alive and leukemia-free for 5 years.[289]

As of this writing, it is still not clear what the ultimate prognosis will be for leukemic patients who survive in complete remission for at least 5 years. Some cause for optimism, however, may be suggested by studies done before the era of "total therapy." By 1967, data on 158 cases of long-term remission had been collected, and studies of the subsequent relapse rate led to the prediction that at least half of those patients with acute leukemia surviving 5 years from diagnosis would survive indefinitely.[50] When these patients were reviewed again in 1971, 93 were still living and well, with no evidence of disease, from 9 to 21 years after diagnosis.[53]

PATIENTS WHO DIE WHILE IN COMPLETE REMISSION. Maintenance chemotherapy regimens for ALL patients may superimpose significant immunosuppression or neutropenia upon the immunologic dysfunction of the underlying disease. As a result, the patient's ability to resist infections of all types may become severely compromised. Since initiation of an aggressive "total therapy" regimen for ALL at St. Jude's Hospital (Memphis), 16 per cent of the deaths in ALL patients there have occurred as a result of complicating infections in patients who were in complete clinical remission.[288] The overwhelming majority of those infections were due to relatively nonpathogenic organisms, such as *Pneumocystis carinii*, cytomegalovirus, various fungi, and Herpes viruses.

POOR-RISK PATIENTS WITH ALL. ALL is not a homogeneous disease with respect to response to therapy. At the time of initial presentation, various clinical and laboratory findings have been useful in identifying subgroups of patients with a distinctly poorer prognosis than the overall group of ALL patients. Among the initial features which identify such poor-risk patients are:[58, 136, 289, 321, 328]

1. *Age.* Children under 2 years and over 10 years of age do not do as well as children between 2 and 10 years old.
2. *Race.* Black children have a relatively poorer response to therapy than do white children.
3. *Initial white count.* Over 50,000/mm³ indicates poorer prognosis.
4. *Spleen enlargement.* Spleen extending more than 5 cm below the costal margin has poorer outlook.
5. *Mediastinal mass on chest x-ray.*
6. *CNS involvement.*

As mentioned previously, many of

these high-risk factors have a high correlation with so-called T-marker leukemia and, as such, may represent a distinct subgroup of ALL.

Regimens involving more intensive and myelosuppressive chemotherapeutic combinations have been designed which appear to successfully induce remission in a large number of these high-risk patients.[16] However, it should also be emphasized not all patients exhibiting these findings at diagnosis do poorly. With the exception of patients with early CNS involvement, some individuals who have an excellent response to therapy may be found within each of the previously mentioned subgroups.[289] Thus, the risk of losing the small (but definite) chance for a good result in some of these patients must be considered when one is contemplating the use of grossly unconventional therapy in an effort to improve the prognosis of high-risk patients.[289]

Management of Acute Myelogenous Leukemia and its Variants

The initial management of leukemias within the AML spectrum, as with ALL, is directed toward the consequences of bone marrow failure (anemia, neutropenia, thrombocytopenia) and of hyperuricemia. Specific therapy, however, involves different drugs and the results are not as satisfactory as they are in ALL.

Acute Myelogenous Leukemia

REMISSION INDUCTION. Cytosine arabinoside (Ara-C) appears to be the most effective agent for remission induction. When used as a single agent it is capable of inducing remission in approximately 25 to 50 per cent of children with AML.[143, 178, 320] Other drugs which have been useful as single agents are daunorubicin,[43] 6-mercaptopurine,[100] Adriamycin, and methylglyoxal-bisguanylhydrazone (methyl GAG).[186]

The use of Ara-C in combination with other drugs has produced somewhat better rates of remission induction. The combinations of Ara-C, cyclophosphamide, and vincristine;[298] Ara-C and daunomycin;[71] Ara-C, vincristine, cyclophosphamide, and prednisone (COAP);[346] and Ara-C and 6-thioguanine[109] have induced remissions in 50 to 60 per cent of patients with AML. Even higher initial remission rates (66 to 78 per cent) have been attained when multidrug regimens (Ara-C, daunomycin, prednisone, mercaptopurine, thioguanine, and asparaginase) have been used.[83]

Since virtually all the drugs used in the treatment of AML are myelosuppressive, remission is rarely attained in the absence of a period of severe marrow hypoplasia. During this period, the patient remains highly susceptible to infections and hemorrhagic complications and must be supported with red cell and platelet transfusions, antibiotics, and occasionally granulocyte transfusions until marrow function returns.

Unlike the situation with ALL, there appears to be no good correlation between age of onset, height of the initial while cell count, or physical findings with the response to chemotherapy or survival of childhood AML patients.[98]

Because the duration of marrow remission has been relatively short (6 to 12 months) for AML, it has not been customary to give CNS prophylactic therapy following remission induction. However, now that the newer regimens are resulting in prolonged survival for AML patients, CNS leukemia is being seen with increasing frequency (23 per cent in one series)[242] and CNS prophylactic therapy may be indicated for these patients as well as for the ALL patients.[167]

RESULTS OF THERAPY FOR AML. Patients with AML treated during the years 1956 to 1968 rarely attained remission and had a median survival of only one month.[98] Now that effective induction regimens have been developed for AML, it is to be expected that over 50 per cent of patients will attain remission. Currently, the major obstacles to long-term survival in these patients are the lack of good maintenance regimens and the increasing appearance of CNS leukemia.

The median survival overall for AML is still considerably less than 1 year.[83, 109, 127] However, for those patients in whom complete remission is successfully induced, the median survival has varied from 1 to 3 years.[83, 127] The 3-year median survival was achieved in a small group of patients who received monthly 5-day continuous infusions of cytosine arabinoside.[127] It has been estimated that "cures" may be observed in 12 per cent of AML patients who achieve complete remission.[332]

Acute Monocytic Leukemia (AMoL). Patients with acute monocytic leukemia generally respond poorly to therapy and generally have a rapid demise;[80] however, some success has been achieved with regimens containing vinblastine[111] and combination chemotherapy with prednisone, vincristine, cytosine arabinoside, and anthracyclines.[279] More recently, daunorubicin and VP 16-213 have successfully induced remissions in patients with AMoL.[206] Since there is a high incidence of posttreatment disseminated intravascular coagulation, early institution of low-dose continuous heparin therapy along with large amounts of cryoprecipitate and fresh frozen plasma has been recommended to prevent significant bleeding.[206]

Acute Promyelocytic Leukemia (APL). Because of the high incidence of disseminated intravascular coagulation (DIC) associated with this condition, heparin therapy should probably be instituted, even prior to initiating chemotherapy (even when no evidence of DIC is present), since necrosis of the abnormal cells may result in release of tissue factor. Heparin should be continued until remission has been attained or the marrow promyelocyte percentage is less than 20 per cent.[121]

Daunomycin appears to be the most useful drug for treating APL; prior to its use, various drug combinations resulted in only a 13 per cent complete remission rate, but with daunomycin therapy the complete remission rate has risen to approximately 50 per cent.[31] This rate might be even higher were it not for the fact that approximately 50 per cent of patients die of sepsis or hemorrhage within the first two weeks after diagnosis. If remission is obtained it may have a remarkably long duration (median of 26 months[31]), and as many as 30 per cent of patients achieving complete remission may survive disease-free for more than 8 years.[332]

Eosinophilic Leukemia. Due to the rarity of this condition, the best therapy for it has not yet been established. However, a long term remission was achieved in one patient by induction with vincristine and maintenance with hydroxyurea.[61]

New Methods of Treatment of the Acute Leukemias

Immunotherapy. The basic principles of immunotherapy were discussed in Chapter 5. Its use in the acute leukemias is based on the premise that the leukemic cell population has acquired a new set of antigens which can be recognized as foreign or "not-self" by normal immunocytes. Evidence for the presence of such neoantigens on human leukemic blast cells has come from a number of laboratories.[48a, 60a, 79, 132, 325]

Active immunotherapy using BCG, irradiated leukemia cells, or both, has been successful in eradicating leukemia in experimental animals, provided that the leukemic cell burden has been reduced to a relatively low level (10^5 cells or less) by chemotherapy.[198] Since the leukemic cell population at the time of manifest clinical disease is at a much higher level (10^{12} cells) and can presumably overwhelm the immunologic defenses, immunotherapy would appear to be most beneficial when remission has been attained.

Following the principles enunciated above, Mathé and associates have utilized immunotherapy in an attempt to prolong remission of human ALL once the greatest possible reduction of leukemic cells was attained by combination chemotherapy, CNS irradiation, and intrathecal chemotherapy.[198] Immunotherapy consisted of repetitive BCG inoculations, pooled irradiated leukemic cells, or BCG and irradiated leukemic cells. Whereas all of the control patients had relapsed by day 130 of remission, 35 per cent of the immunotherapy group were still in remission after 3 years. Other groups,[144, 245] however, have been unable to confirm the beneficial effects of BCG. Indeed, it has been proposed that the apparent benefit of BCG in Mathé's patients may have been due to the exceptionally poor performance of a small group of control patients.[80a]

BCG has also been used in the treatment of acute myelogenous leukemia, again after the leukemic cell burden had been previously reduced with chemotherapy. In a study by Crowther and co-workers, immunotherapy with BCG and irradiated leukemic cells was found to be comparable to continuous chemotherapy for remission maintenance in AML patients (median duration, 5 months).[72] Powles and colleagues then attempted to increase duration of remission by giving both immunotherapy (BCG and irradiated allogeneic leukemic cells) and intermittent maintenance chemotherapy; the group of patients treated in this manner had a median remission duration of 10 months compared to 6 months for the control group treated with chemotherapy alone.[244] These results are considered promising in some circles[21] and have led to further studies, which are currently in progress.

Bone Marrow Transplantation. A major limitation on the amount of chemotherapy or radiotherapy that can be administered is the sensitivity of normal hematopoietic stem cells to these agents. In many instances, a leukemic cell population that has become resistant to conventional therapy can be eradicated by exceptionally high doses of the same agents. However, this is of little benefit to the patient, for unless a new source of normal marrow stem cells can be provided, he or she will die of the consequences of intractable bone marrow failure.

Bone marrow transplantation is a technique whereby hematopoietic stem cells are provided by intravenous infusion of a suspension of bone marrow cells from a normal donor (Fig. 8–16). Although it is technically feasible to obtain and infuse a sufficient quantity of donor cells to repopulate the patient's bone marrow, a major barrier to success has been immunologic incompatibility between donor and recipient.

HISTOCOMPATIBILITY. In humans two major histocompatibility loci, the "LA" (HLA-A) and the "4" (HLA-B) loci, have been identified by serologic means; these are controlled by a pair of autosomal genes located on chromosome 6.[164] Another major locus (HLA-D) in close relationship to these loci is identifiable by mixed lymphocyte studies. Due to the complex polymorphism of these loci, it is highly unlikely (chances of between 1:200 and 1:5000)[6] that unrelated individuals will be histocompatible.

Syngeneic transplants between identical twins involve donors and recipients carrying the same tissue antigens, and thus there is no immunologic barrier to transplantation. Similarly, autologous marrow taken from the patient when in remission and stored at −70° C involves no immunologic problems. However, an *allogeneic* graft involving a donor and recipient of different genetic origin (which is the type most

The Leukemias

How a Marrow Transplantation is Done

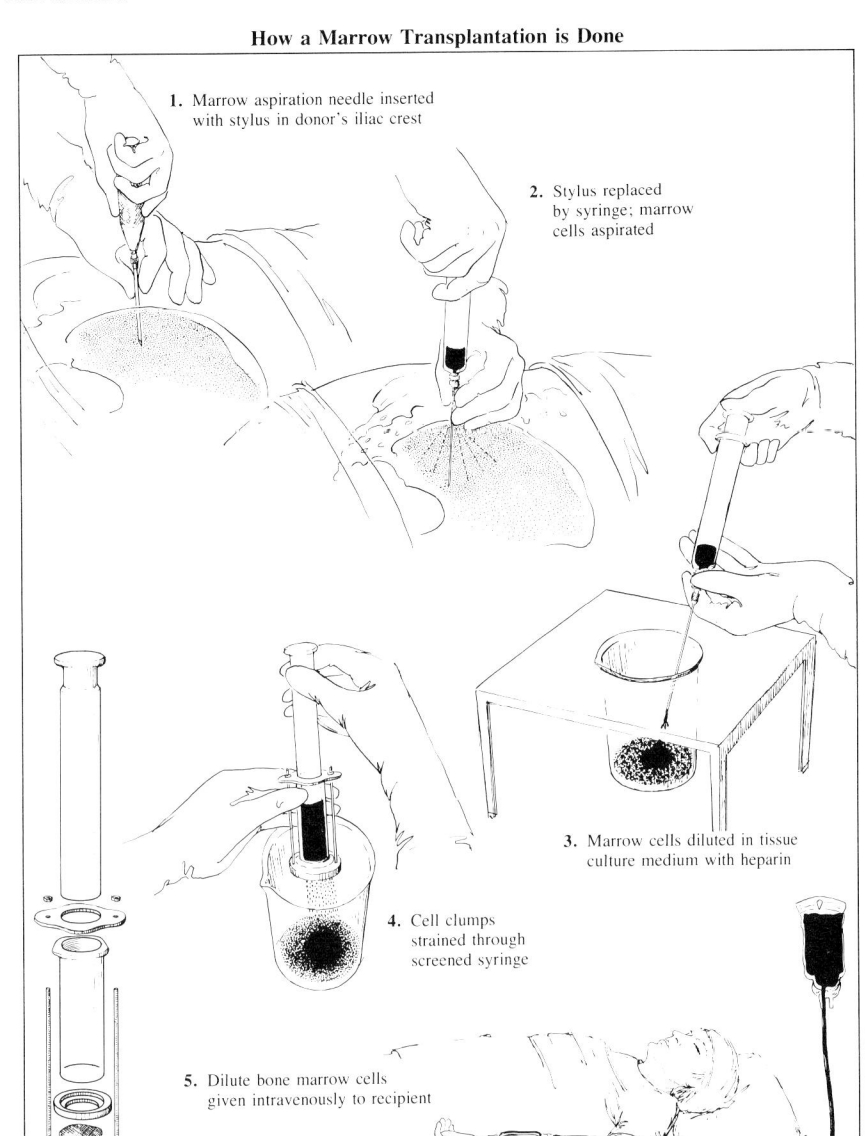

1. Marrow aspiration needle inserted with stylus in donor's iliac crest
2. Stylus replaced by syringe; marrow cells aspirated
3. Marrow cells diluted in tissue culture medium with heparin
4. Cell clumps strained through screened syringe
5. Dilute bone marrow cells given intravenously to recipient

Figure 8–16 Technique for bone marrow transplantation. (From Thomas E. D.: Resident and Staff Physician, June, 1976.)

commonly performed) will involve moderate to severe immunologic difficulties, depending upon the degree of histocompatibility between the donor and the recipient. Usually the best candidate for a satisfactory histocompatibility match will be a sibling of the patient; serologic testing (HLA typing) and mixed lymphocyte reactions permit detection of the sibling who is the best match for the patient. The chances of a given sibling being HLA compatible are roughly 1 in 4, but, because many patients have several siblings, there is approximately a 40 to 50 per cent chance that patients with at least one sibling will have an HLA matched sibling.

COMPLICATIONS OF BONE MARROW TRANSPLANTATION

Infectious Complications. Until the graft begins to function, the recipient of a bone marrow transplant is practically defenseless against all types of infections. Not only has immunosuppressive therapy rendered the patient immunologically incompetent against viral, fungal, and protozoal infections, but in addition severe granulocytopenia has rigorously compromised his or her ability to combat bacterial infections. The period of granulocytopenia persists for at least 10 to 20 days after grafting, while immunologic incompetence will last as long as immunosuppressive agents are administered.

Graft Rejection. Failure of the graft to survive in the recipient because of rejection by immunologic surveillance mechanisms is common to all forms of organ transplantation in allogeneic hosts. However, when patients are pretreated with immunosuppressive measures such as total body irradiation or cyclophosphamide, the incidence of marrow graft rejection is very low; in the series of Thomas and co-workers (100 cases of acute leukemia), only one patient rejected the graft.[315]

Graft Versus Host Disease (GVHD). Making use of immunosuppression in order to prevent rejection of a marrow graft is a two-edged sword, for donor marrow suspensions are invariably contaminated by immunologically competent peripheral blood lymphoid cells and marrow lymphoid precursor cells. These cells engraft the recipient along with the hematopoietic stem cells, and may produce a lethal immunologic reaction directed against him or her. In the recent series of Thomas and his colleagues, GVHD occurred in three fourths of the patients despite "perfect" matching of donor and recipient at the major human histocompatibility complex.[315]

The major target organs affected by this complication are the skin, the gut, and the liver. The earliest clinical manifestation of GVHD is a scaly erythematous skin reaction usually first noted on the forehead; this is followed by alopecia, intractable diarrhea, liver derangement, and death if the reaction is not brought under control with immunosuppressive agents. Interstitial pneumonia also occurs often in association with GVHD; approximately 50 per cent of these instances are associated with detectable infectious agents (cytomegalovirus, *Pneumocystis carinii*), while the remainder are idiopathic and may be related to intensive chemotherapy, radiotherapy, or the GVHD itself.[315a]

RESULTS OF BONE MARROW TRANSPLANTATION IN ACUTE LEUKEMIA

Syngeneic (monozygotic twin) Transplants. Thomas and associates, using "lethal" total body irradiation (sometimes preceded by administration of cytosine arabinoside) to eradicate the leukemic population, performed four transplants in identical twins with ALL; all relapsed within 7 to 12 weeks.[312] A subsequent regimen, adding high-dose cyclophosphamide before total body irradiation and marrow transplantation, produced eight relatively long-term (3 to 49 months) remissions in 20 patients with ALL and AML. More recently this regimen has been supplemented with intensive combination chemotherapy before giving cyclophosphamide and irradiation.

Allogeneic Transplants. Since most patients with leukemia are not fortunate enough to have an identical twin, the majority of marrow grafts have been performed between ABO-compatible, HLA-identical siblings. Despite the close histocompatibility matching in these cases, immunosuppressive therapy is still required to permit engraftment and to ameliorate graft-versus-host reactions.

Of the various regimens utilized, the best results have been attained with total body irradiation alone or in combination with cyclophosphamide.[314, 315]

Of 100 patients with acute leukemia, 13 have remained in remission on no maintenance antileukemic chemotherapy for 1 to 4½ years after transplantation.[315] A total of 31 patients had a relapse of leukemia, indicating that a significant residual leukemic cell burden was still present at the time of transplant.

Recurrence of leukemia in donor cells. In two patients, cytogenetic evidence has shown that the leukemic relapse following engraftment appeared to occur in donor cells.[88, 313] In both instances, the patients were females with ALL who had a marrow graft from an HLA-matched brother, and the recurrent leukemia was shown by cytogenetic analysis to be in male cells. This most intriguing development suggests that reinduction of a malignant cell population can occur in some patients with leukemia and that this phenomenon may be a factor in the relapse of leukemia after chemotherapy has brought about remission of the disease.

THE CHRONIC LEUKEMIAS

Of the chronic leukemias, only chronic granulocytic leukemia is seen with any frequency in childhood, accounting for approximately 2 to 5 per cent of cases of childhood leukemia.[69] Chronic lymphocytic leukemia has been reported in only a few children,[60, 148, 266] and chronic monocytic leukemia is very rare as well.

Since these disorders are, in their early phase, associated with the presence of increased numbers of mature cells in the peripheral blood, their mode of presentation, course, response to therapy, and complications are very different from those of the acute leukemias.

CHRONIC GRANULOCYTIC LEUKEMIA

Chronic granulocytic leukemia (CGL) is considered by most authors to constitute two distinct entities in childhood. One form, seen mainly in older children, is indistinguishable from classic adult-type CGL; the other form, so-called "juvenile" CGL, is seen mainly in infants and toddlers and is strikingly different with respect to clinical presentation, response to therapy, karyotypic findings, and prognosis. As will be discussed below, this "juvenile" form should more properly be considered a variant of myelomonocytic leukemia, rather than of CGL. A third or familial form of CGL has also been reported in two pairs of infant siblings.[149]

Adult-Type CGL

True CGL of childhood shares the following features with the adult form of the disease:

1. Leukocytosis with white blood cell counts of >50,000/mm.^{3}
2. A "shift to the left" of the differential, but an orderly sequenced maturation from myeloblasts to polymorphonuclear leukocytes; myeloblasts and promyelocytes usually account for less than 5 to 10 per cent of the peripheral white count.
3. Very low levels of leukocyte alkaline phosphatase (LAP).
4. A characteristic karyotypic abnormality, the Philadelphia (Ph^1) chromosome, in hematopoietic precursor cells.
5. Hypercellular bone marrow with predominance of myeloid cells in all stages of maturation; megakaryocytes often appear increased as well.
6. A mild normochromic, normocytic anemia.
7. Normal or elevated platelet count.
8. Response to busulfan.
9. A chronic course of several years, during which period the patient is asymptomatic and the disease is easily controlled with medication.

10. Eventual transformation into an acute leukemic phase (*blast cell transformation*).

THE PHILADELPHIA (PH¹) CHROMOSOME. CGL is the only human malignancy with a specific karyotypic marker. This consists of the loss of a portion of the long arm of chromosome G22. More recent studies have demonstrated that the missing piece may be translocated to chromosome C9[262] (Fig. 8–17).

The Ph¹ chromosome appears to be an acquired, rather than a congenital, abnormality. It is not present in non-affected twins of patients with CGL,[22, 118] nor is it present in all cells of CGL patients. Rather, its distribution appears to be limited to hematopoietic precursor cells;[334] thus, it is found in immature erythroid[253] and myeloid cells, as well as in megakaryocyte precursors,[151, 264] but not in peripheral lymphocytes or skin fibroblasts. These data suggest a clonal basis for CGL, with the disease arising in a common precursor cell for the erythroid, myeloid, and megakaryocytic lines.

At the time of diagnosis 90 to 100 per cent of dividing marrow cells contain the Ph¹ chromosome,[20] and it persists in nearly all marrow mitoses even after therapy has induced a clinical remission. Thus, although clinically well, the patient is living on an entirely leukemic bone marrow. In a few patients, in whom intensive chemotherapy has produced severe marrow hypoplasia, the karyotype may revert to normal for varying periods of time.

During blast cell transformation, the Ph¹ marker persists and is frequently accompanied by other karyotypic abnormalities, the most frequent of which is duplication of the Ph¹ chromosome.[151, 264, 335] These additional ab-

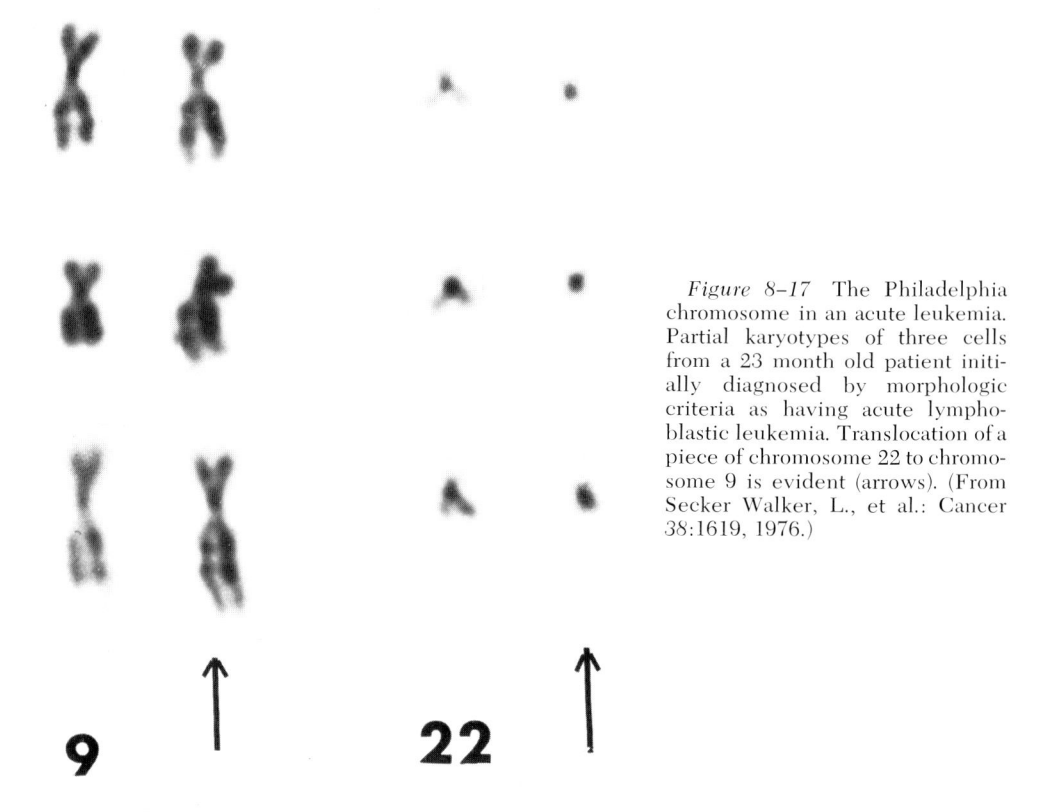

Figure 8–17 The Philadelphia chromosome in an acute leukemia. Partial karyotypes of three cells from a 23 month old patient initially diagnosed by morphologic criteria as having acute lymphoblastic leukemia. Translocation of a piece of chromosome 22 to chromosome 9 is evident (arrows). (From Secker Walker, L., et al.: Cancer 38:1619, 1976.)

normalities are lost if therapy successfully eradicates the excess blast cells, but return when blast cell crisis recurs.[304]

Pathogenesis. CGL appears to be a clonal disease arising in a pluripotent hematopoietic stem cell. This concept evolved from the above-mentioned studies of the Ph[1] chromosome. Studies performed on CGL patients who were heterozygous for glucose-6-phosphate dehydrogenase[20, 87a] or who had mosaicism of sex chromosomes[218] have also supported the notion that the disease probably originates from a single abnormal hematopoietic stem cell.

It has been postulated that the Ph[1] positive clone becomes predominant in the marrow because of either (1) a growth advantage over normal stem cells,[42] or (2) lack of response to normal growth-control mechanisms.[20] However, measurements of mitotic activity, DNA synthesis, and maturation time indicate that CGL precursor cells may actually be proliferating more slowly than normal marrow precursor cells.[234] Moreover, the presence of cyclic oscillation in CGL granulocyte production suggests the influence of the same regulatory mechanisms that regulate normal granulocytopoiesis.[326]

A possible clue to the selective growth advantage of Ph[1] positive cells is their resemblance to fetal hematopoietic cells. These similarities include size, density, cell-cycle characteristics, and ability to proliferate in extramedullary sites (liver, spleen).[220] The ability of Ph[1] positive cells to replicate in the liver and spleen as well as in the bone marrow may give them a better ability to expand their population than normal hematopoietic cells, whose replicative activity is limited to the bone marrow.

It is possible that extramedullary hematopoiesis may not merely reflect the expansion of the leukemic population but may also play an active role in the malignant evolution of CGL. The mechanism of granulopoiesis in the liver and spleen appears to be different and frequently more defective than that in the bone marrow.[18] Particularly intriguing in this regard is the fact that aneuploidy is found more commonly in spleen than in marrow cells.[18] As aneuploidy is a frequent accompaniment of blast cell transformation, it is possible that the new, more aggressive clone appears first in the spleen, and, indeed, there is evidence that morphologic signs of blast crisis are detected in spleen aspirates prior to being detectable in the bone marrow.[48]

Although initially granulocytopoiesis results in the production of predominantly mature granulocytes, eventually there is increasing failure of maturation, with continued overproduction of immature cells and underproduction of mature neutrophils, erythrocytes, and platelets. At this point the disease is considered to have entered its terminal or blast transformation phase and develops a picture closely resembling an acute leukemia.

Until recently, it had been commonly assumed that the acute leukemic phase of CGL represented transformation to acute myelogenous leukemia. However, certain differences in morphology and response to therapy are apparent. First, Auer rods are not usually seen in the blast cells of CGL, and second, the response to chemotherapy is generally poorer than that seen in AML. More recently, evidence has been presented which suggests that, in at least some cases, the blast cells may bear a closer resemblance to lymphoblasts than to myeloblasts. These results may be summarized as follows:

1. Morphologic Findings. Experienced hematologists have reviewed Wright-stained smears of three patients in the blastic phase of CGL and repeatedly called the blast cells lymphoblasts, even when the smears were mixed with smears from patients with AML and ALL.[42] In another study,[95] the blast cells of two children with Ph[1] positive CGL simultaneously expressed both lymphoid and myeloid properties.

2. *Biochemical Findings.* Approximately 20 per cent of patients in the blastic phase of CGL have terminal deoxynucleotidyl transferase activity in their blast cells.[202] This enzyme is considered to be a marker of thymus derived lymphocytes (T-cells) (Chapter Five).

3. *Immunochemical Findings.* A specific antigenic property of leukemic lymphoblasts is detectable in the blast cells of approximately one third of CGL patients in blast crisis.[201]

4. *Therapeutic Results.* Approximately 30 per cent of patients in the blastic phase of CGL have a good response to vincristine and prednisone, drugs which are considered to be effective for ALL, but not AML.[57]

How do these findings fit in with the hypothesis that CGL is a clonal disease arising in a pluripotent hematopoietic stem cell? How can the lymphoid line, which appears to lack the Ph[1] chromosome, become involved in the leukemia transformation? To answer these questions, Boggs has hypothesized that CGL may actually arise in a common hematopoietic-lymphoid precursor cell.[42] Since T-lymphocytes have an extraordinarily long intermitotic survival time (up to several years),[341] it might take several years before the Ph[1] chromosome appeared in a significant number of lymphocytes and, consequently, it would not be seen in the early phases of the disease, when most studies of lymphocyte karyotypes have been performed.

Clinical Features. The signs and symptoms of CGL usually develop insidiously over a period of several months. Early symptoms are related to the development of anemia, marrow hyperplasia, and splenomegaly. Anemia may lead to malaise, fatigue, decreased exercise tolerance, pallor, and irritability. Marrow hyperplasia may result in aching in the bones and sternal tenderness. The symptoms resulting from splenomegaly may be classified into two general categories: (1) mechanical problems, such as impingement on the stomach, a sensation of upper abdominal fullness, or a "dragging" sensation on the left side of the abdomen; or (2) sequestration of red cells and platelets (hypersplenism). There may also be "hypermetabolic" symptoms, such as fever, weight loss, and sweating. Rare presentations of CGL include priapism,[123] rheumatoid arthritis–like arthropathy, and prolonged or unusual infections.[263]

The characteristic physical signs at the time of initial presentation are pallor, warm, moist skin, low-grade fever, sternal tenderness, and hepatosplenomegaly. Mild to moderate lymphadenopathy may also be present.

Laboratory findings include a mild normochromic, normocytic anemia (approximately 9 g/100 ml), normal to slightly elevated reticulocyte count, marked leukocytosis (usually in excess of 100,000/mm^3), and a normal to elevated platelet count (unless hypersplenism has resulted in significant platelet sequestration). The differential count shows all forms of myeloid cells, from myeloblasts to polymorphonuclear leukocytes; the most mature elements are ordinarily present in the greatest number, and the less mature in diminishing frequency, with myeloblasts and promyelocytes not exceeding 10 per cent. A representative differential count at this point might show: 1 to 3 per cent myeloblasts, 2 to 4 per cent promyelocytes, 6 to 10 per cent myelocytes, 12 to 18 per cent metamyelocytes, 25 to 30 per cent bands, and 35 to 50 per cent mature polymorphs.[263] Mature and immature basophils and eosinophils may also appear in increased numbers.

Bone marrow aspiration yields a markedly hypercellular specimen which is composed predominantly of granulocytic cells in all stages of maturation. While the percentage of blast cells may be slightly higher than that seen in the peripheral blood, it is not much higher than that of normal bone marrow. Megakaryocytes are often found in normal or in increased numbers. However, the percentage of erythroid cells is markedly reduced in comparison to the granulocytic elements, and the myeloid/erythroid ratio may be as high as 10 to 50:1.

Decreased leukocyte alkaline phosphatase (LAP) activity is evident on histochemical and biochemical assays. Immunoassays, on the other hand, have shown normal quantities of LAP protein to be present in CGL leukocytes;[47] consequently, the molecular conformation of this enzyme may be altered in such a way as to result in low specific activity. Although the mechanism of the alteration is unknown, measurement of LAP activity provides a useful means of distinguishing the leukocytosis seen in CGL from that seen in various inflammatory and infectious processes, which are characteristically associated with significant elevations of LAP activity. A rise in LAP activity in a patient with CGL often suggests the presence of a concurrent disease, such as ulcerative colitis[258] or bronchopneumonia, or may herald the onset of blast cell transformation.[32] The LAP level may also increase during clinical remission of the disease.

CGL is associated with striking elevations of serum vitamin B_{12} levels (average increase is 15 times the normal mean concentration).[23a] This appears to be correlated with increased serum levels of transcobalamin I (TC I), the main carrier of endogenous vitamin B_{12}. This molecule is present in both normal and CGL granulocytes and is apparently released as the granulocytes break down.

Hyperuricemia and hyperuricuria occur frequently as a consequence of the rapid cellular turnover. This may lead to attacks of gout or urinary calculi.

BLAST CELL TRANSFORMATION AS AN INITIAL MANIFESTATION OF CGL. Occasionally patients with no previous history of CGL may present with a Ph^1 chromosome positive acute leukemia[46, 237] (Fig. 8–17). In some of these patients, the morphology of the blast cells may suggest AML, whereas others resemble those of ALL, AMML, eosinophilic leukemia, basophilic leukemia, or megakaryocytic leukemia.[151] These patients tend to have a higher median white count (135,000/mm³) and more basophils than do Ph^1 negative acute leukemia patients; they may also have minor changes in the peripheral blood including the Pelger-Huët anomaly, hypogranular neutrophils, and primitive monocytoid cells.[23b] The course is usually an acute one, with a poor response to chemotherapy (22 per cent complete remission rate).[237]

The relationship of these patients to CGL is unclear. Some authors consider them to represent variants of CGL;[335] others have suggested that they may be considered as Ph^1 chromosome positive acute leukemia.[237]

COURSE OF THE ILLNESS. Initially the disease can be kept under good control with therapy; busulfan is considered to be the drug of choice,[179] although hydroxyurea, melphalan,[274] and splenic irradiation are also useful. Usually, the white cell count is restored to normal within 4 to 6 weeks and the spleen has returned to normal size within 3 months. However, certain stigmata of the disease persist: the Ph^1 chromosome is still present in most of the bone marrow hematopoietic precursor cells, LAP level remains low in about 50 per cent of cases,[32] and the bone marrow remains hypercellular with myeloid predominance.

If the patient is not kept on maintenance doses of chemotherapy, clinical relapse usually reappears within 3 to

10 months. With maintenance therapy, clinical remission can be maintained for an average of 2 to 3 years, after which the patient may undergo blast cell transformation. This terminal phase may be heralded by reappearance of fatigue, fever, sweating, bone pain, thrombocytopenia, or the requirement of progressively higher drug dosages to maintain clinical remission. The diagnosis is usually confirmed by the presence of a relative increase in immature cells (the minimum level accepted for diagnosis of blast cell transformation is a combined blast cell and promyelocyte count in excess of 30 per cent in blood or marrow).

To a certain extent, the hemoglobin levels and platelet count appear to correlate with the morphology of the blast cells at the time of blast cell transformation. In one study,[259a] less than one third of patients with lymphoblastic morphology had a hemoglobin level below 10 g/100 ml, while two thirds of the myeloblastic patients were significantly more anemic. On the other hand, most of the lymphoblastic patients had significant thrombocytopenia, whereas the myeloblastic patients tended to have relatively adequate platelet counts.

Approximately 37 per cent of cases of blast cell transformation are complicated by extramedullary infiltrates;[259a] many of these involve the central nervous system. In this regard, blast cell transformation of CGL would seem to resemble the acute leukemias, with CNS leukemia as part of the natural history of the disease should the patient survive long enough for it to become clinically manifest.[10a]

Management

CHRONIC PHASE. Unlike the situation of the acute leukemias, anemia, infection, and hemorrhage are rarely problems in the initial management of CGL due to the differentiated nature of the neoplasm. However, hyperuricemia is usually present and should be brought under control before specific antileukemic therapy is initiated (Chapter Seven). Even when the initial uric acid level is within normal limits, prophylactic allopurinol therapy is advisable prior to initiation of chemotherapy since a great mass of granulocytic tissue will be lysed once treatment commences.

Chemotherapy. Busulfan is currently the drug used most widely for initial therapy of CGL.[32, 128, 179] The recommended initial dosage is 0.0625 mg/kg P.O. daily (adult dose, 4 mg daily). At this dosage there is a lag period of 10 to 14 days before the white count falls significantly and immature forms begin to disappear from the peripheral blood. The hemoglobin level begins to rise as the leukocyte count approaches normal levels, but splenic regression lags behind these changes, sometimes requiring 3 or more months before the spleen is no longer palpable.

When the white count has decreased to 30,000 to 40,000/mm,^{3} busulfan dosage should be decreased by 50 per cent, and the drug should be stopped entirely when the white count has fallen to 15,000 to 20,000/mm.^{3} A lag period is again seen after the drug is discontinued, and the blood count continues to fall for another 2 to 3 weeks. This delayed response makes it imperative that therapy be stopped *before* the white count becomes normal; otherwise, it may fall to subnormal levels as a consequence of severe, and possibly irreversible, bone marrow suppression. The platelet count should also be carefully monitored during the period of therapy.

The average patient requires 4 to 6 weeks of busulfan therapy initially in order to attain clinical remission. Once the white count has leveled off, most physicians initiate maintenance therapy with busulfan in continuous small doses designed to keep the white count between 7000 to 12,000/mm or in intermittent doses when the white count reaches 30,000/mm^3.[128]

TRANSFORMATION PHASE. At any

time after diagnosis, but most frequently between 1 to 4 years after, the patient may fail to respond to busulfan. This may be the first indication of metamorphosis from the chronic phase to a more accelerated or acute phase. This may be manifested in a number of ways:

1. Transformation to an acute leukemia.
2. Myelofibrosis.
3. Development of extramedullary solid tumors (chloromas).

Acute blastic transformation is responsible for at least 75 per cent of the deaths in CGL.[221] Therapy is less effective than in de novo AML or ALL. Since vincristine and prednisone may produce remission in approximately 30 per cent of these patients,[57] an initial 3 weeks' trial of this regimen has been recommended.[128] For patients who do not respond, there is probably no good alternative regimen, although a combination of hydroxyurea, 6-mercaptopurine, and prednisone may show promise.[32]

In patients with myelofibrosis only palliative measures can be taken.[120]

NEWER THERAPEUTIC ENDEAVORS. Although busulfan is an excellent agent for symptomatic management of CGL, it has improved survival in this disease minimally, if at all, since it has no effect on the time of appearance of blast cell transformation. Consequently, alternative measures have been sought which could postpone the terminal phase.

A group of patients with exceptionally long survival periods are those who show a significant number of Ph[1] negative cells in the bone marrow following recovery from busulfan induced marrow hypoplasia.[108] This is seen most often in patients who became hypoplastic after *small* doses of busulfan, suggesting that the Ph[1] positive population was unusually sensitive to the drug;[128] hypoplasia resulting from *excessive* doses of busulfan may actually eliminate the small Ph[1] negative population.

Some groups have attempted to eradicate the Ph[1] positive clone of cells by use of intensive multiagent chemotherapy and elective splenectomy at the time of initial diagnosis. Such an aggressive approach may result in enhancement of initial morbidity and mortality, but, it is hoped, will also improve long-term survival. Whether this will actually result will take time to determine.

An alternative approach to the problem is the harvesting and storage (in the frozen state) of peripheral blood or marrow stem cells while the patient is in the chronic stage, with the aim of using these cells for repopulating the marrow after total marrow aplasia has been induced by vigorous chemotherapy of blast transformation. Such treatment might be used on several occasions to keep the patient in the chronic phase of the disease. A palliative approach of this type might conceivably lengthen survival time.

Juvenile Type CGL

Although classic adult type Ph[1] chromosome positive CGL has been reported in the first year of life,[38] this is a very rare occurrence. A condition seen in infants and toddlers, characterized by leukocytosis, granulocyte hyperplasia, and low LAP has been called "juvenile CGL;" however, this condition manifests marked clinical, hematologic, and cytogenetic differences from classic CGL (Table 8–7). Among the major differences are: (1) absence of the Ph[1] chromosome;[255] (2) more prominent lymphadenopathy and skin lesions; (3) increased frequency of thrombocytopenia and hemorrhagic manifestations early in the course;[30, 69] (4) monocytosis in peripheral blood and marrow;[30] (5) increased fetal hemoglobin;[135] (6) a variety of red cell metabolic and immunologic characteristics associated with fetal red cells;[339] (7) poor response to busulfan;[135] (8) a much more acute course,

Table 8-7 Differences Between Adult and Juvenile Forms of Chronic Granulocytic Leukemia

	ADULT FORM	JUVENILE FORM
Chromosome studies	Ph^1 chromosome positive	Ph^1 chromosome negative
Age at onset	Usually above 2 years old	Usually less than 2 years old
Physical findings:		
Facial rash	Absent	Present
Lymphadenopathy	Occasional	Frequent with tendency to suppuration
Splenomegaly	Marked	Variable
Hemorrhagic manifestations	Absent	Frequent
Hematologic findings:		
WBC at onset	Usually > 100,000	Usually < 100,000
Monocytosis of peripheral blood and bone marrow	Absent	Usually present
Thrombocytopenia	Uncommon at onset	Frequent at onset
Red blood cell abnormalities:		
Ineffective erythropoiesis	Absent	Present
I antigen on red blood cell	Normal	Reduced
Fetal hemoglobin levels	Normal	15–50%
Normoblasts in peripheral blood	Unusual	Frequent
Other laboratory findings:		
Urinary and serum muramidase	Slightly elevated	Markedly elevated
Immunologic abnormalities	None	Strikingly high immunoglobulin levels, high incidence of anti-nuclear antibodies (52%) and anti-IgG antibodies (43%)
Nature of colonies produced in vitro from peripheral blood	Predominantly granulocytic	Almost exclusively monocytic
Response to busulfan	Uniformly good	Poor
Median survival	2½–3 years	<9 months

(From Altman, A. J., and Baehner, R. L.: J. Pediatr. 86:221, 1975.)

with significantly poorer median survival.[69, 135]

The striking involvement of the monocytic cell line in this disorder is exemplified by: (1) frequency of peripheral blood and bone marrow monocytosis, (2) elevated urine and serum muramidase levels, and (3) the production of large numbers of predominantly monocytic colonies in vitro from the peripheral blood of juvenile CGL patients.[5] Since this condition is neither a chronic nor a granulocytic leukemia, it should not be considered to represent a variant of CGL, but should instead be classified as a form of myelomonocytic leukemia.

Chemotherapy is of limited value either for remission induction or prolonging survival.[295] Some patients have apparently shown response to oral 6-mercaptopurine alone, but many have not. Most other agents (including busulfan) have been of no value. Recently three cases have been reported which showed a clinical and hematologic response to repeated cycles of sequential subcutaneous cytosine arabinoside and oral 6-mercaptopurine;[189] however, this response was mainly an improvement in well-being, rather than a prolongation of survival time. Supportive care may be as effective in management as vigorous chemotherapy.[295] Median survival time is less than 9 months.[135, 295]

REFERENCES

1. Acute Leukemia Group B: Acute lymphocytic leukemia in children: Maintenance

therapy with methotrexate administered intermittently. J.A.M.A. 207:923, 1969.
2. Adams, J. F., and Seaton, D. A.: Pathogenesis of megaloblastic anemia in diGuglielmo's disease. Scottish Med. J. 5:145, 1960.
3. Adamson, J. W., and Finch, C. A.: Erythropoietin and the regulation of erythropoiesis in diGuglielmo's syndrome. Blood 36:590, 1970.
4. Agner, K.: Verdoperoxidase. Adv. Enzymol. 3:137, 1943.
4a. Aksoy, M., Dinçol, K., Erdem, S., Dinçol, G.: Acute leukemia due to chronic exposure to benzene. Am. J. Med. 52:160, 1972.
5. Altman, A. J., Palmer, C. G., and Baehner, R. L.: Juvenile "chronic granulocytic" leukemia: a panmyelopathy with prominent monocytic involvement and circulating monocyte colony-forming cells. Blood 43:341, 1974.
6. Alvegard, T. A., Herzig, G. P., and Graw, R. G., Jr.: Allogeneic marrow transplantation for treatment of leukaemia. Scand. J. Haematol. 15:287, 1975.
7. Ames, R. P., et al.: Virus-like particles and cytopathic activity in urine of patients with leukemia. Blood 28:465, 1966.
8. Amromin, G. D., and Solomon R. D.: Necrotizing enteropathy. J.A.M.A. 182:23, 1962.
9. Astaldi, G., and Mauri, C.: Rechercher sur l'activite proliférative de l'hemocytoblaste de la leucémie aigue. Rev. Belge Path. Med. Exp. 23:69, 1954.
10. Athens, J. W., Bishop, C. R., and Cartwright, G. E.: The kinetics of neutrophilic granulocytes in chronic myelocytic leukemia—a review. In Zarafonetis, C. J. D. (ed.): International Conferences on Leukemia-Lymphoma. Philadelphia, Lea & Febiger, 1968.
10a. Atkinson, K., Kay, H. E. M., Lawler, S. D., et al.: Meningeal leukemia after blastic transformation of chronic myeloid leukemia. Cancer 35:529, 1975.
11. Aur, R. J. A., Hustu, H. O., Verzosa, M. S., Wood, A., and Simone, J. V.: Comparison of two methods of preventing central nervous system leukemia. Blood 42:349, 1973.
12. Aur, R. J. A., and Pinkel, D.: Total therapy of acute lymphocytic leukemia. Prog. Clin. Cancer 5:155, 1973.
13. Aur, R. J. A., Simone, J., Hustu, H. O., et al.: Central nervous system therapy and combination chemotherapy of childhood lymphocytic leukemia. Blood 37:272, 1971.
14. Aur, R. J. A., Simone, J. V., Hustu, H. O., et al.: Cessation of therapy during complete remission of childhood acute lymphocytic leukemia. N. Engl. J. Med. 291:1230, 1974.
15. Aur, R. J. A., Simone, J., Pinkel, D., and Hustu, H. O.: Results of stopping therapy during remission in 116 children with acute lymphocytic leukemia. Proc. Am. Assoc. Cancer Res. (Abstr.) 15:144, 1974.
16. Aur, R. J. A., Simone, J. V., and Pratt, C. B.: Successful remission induction in children with acute lymphocytic leukemia at high risk for treatment failure. Cancer 27:1332, 1971.
17. Aur, R. J. A., Westbrook, H. W., and Riggs, W., Jr.: Childhood acute lymphocytic leukemia. Initial radiological bone involvement and prognosis. Am. J. Dis. Child. 124:653, 1972.
18. Baccarani, M., Zaccaria, A., Santucci, A. M., et al.: A simultaneous study of bone marrow, spleen, and liver in chronic myeloid leukemia: evidence for differences in cell composition and karyotypes. Ser. Haematol. 8:81, 1975.
19. Baltimore, D.: Viral RNA-dependent DNA polymerase in virions of RNA tumor viruses. Nature 226:1209, 1970.
20. Barr, R. D., and Fialkow, P. J.: Clonal origin of chronic myelocytic leukemia. N. Engl. J. Med. 289:307, 1973.
21. Bast, R. C., Jr., Zbar, B., Borsos, T., and Rapp, H. J.: BCG and Cancer. N. Engl. J. Med. 290:1458, 1974.
22. Bauke, J.: Chronic myelocytic leukemia. Chromosome studies of a patient and his nonleukemic identical twin. Cancer 24:643, 1969.
22a. Baum, E., Land, V., Joo, P., et al.: Cessation of chemotherapy during complete remission of childhood acute lymphocytic leukemia. 13th Annual Meeting, American Society for Clinical Oncology, Abstract C-96, 1977.
23. Baxt, W., Yates, J. W., Wallace, H. J., Jr., et al.: Leukemia-specific DNA sequences in leukocytes of the leukemic member of identical twins. Proc. Natl. Acad. Sci. USA 70:2629, 1973.
23a. Beard, M. F., Pitney, W. R., and Sanneman, E. H.: Serum concentrations of vitamin B_{12} in patients suffering from leukemia. Blood 9:789, 1954.
23b. Beard, M. E. J., Durrant, J., Catovsky, D., et al.: Blast crisis of chronic myeloid leukaemia (CML). I. Presentation simulating acute lymphoid leukaemia. Brit. J. Haematol. 34:167, 1976.
24. Beck, W. S., and Valentine, W. N.: Biochemical studies on leukocytes. II. Phosphatase activity in chronic lymphatic leukemia, acute leukemia and miscellaneous hematologic conditions. J. Lab. Clin. Med. 38:245, 1951.
25. Bennett, J. M., Catovsky, D., Daniel, M.-T., et al.: Proposals for the classification of the acute leukaemias. French-American-British (FAB) Co-operative Group. Brit. J. Haematol. 33:451, 1976.
26. Bentley, H. P., Jr., Reardon, A. E.,

Knoedler, J. P., and Krivit, W.: Eosinophilic leukemia. Am. J. Med. 30:310, 1961.
27. Benvenisti, D. S., and Ultmann, J. E.: Eosinophilic leukemia. Ann. Intern. Med. 71:731, 1969.
28. Bernard, J., et al.: Leucémie aiguë d'une enfant de 5 mois née d'une mère atteinte de leucémie aiguë au moment de l'accouchement. Sem. Hôp. Paris 40:1233, 1964.
29. Bernard, J., Jacquillat, C., Chavalet, F., Boiron, M., Stoitchkov, Y., and Tanzer, J.: Leucémie aiguë d'une enfant de 5 mois née d'une mère atteinte de leucémie aiguë au moment de l'accouchement. Nouv. Rev. Fr. Hématol. 4:140, 1964.
30. Bernard, J., Seligmann, M., and Acar, J.: La leucémie myeloide chronique de l'enfant (étude de vingt observations). Arch. Fr. Pediatr. 19:881, 1962.
31. Bernard, J., Weil, M., Boiron, M., Jacquillat, C., Flandrin, G., and Gemon, M. F.: Acute promyelocytic leukemia: results of treatment by daunorubicin. Blood 41:489, 1973.
32. Bernard, J., and Tanzer, J.: Chronic myelocytic leukemia. In Holland, J. F., and Frei, E. J., III (eds.): Cancer Medicine. Philadelphia, Lea & Febiger, 1973.
33. Bernhard, W. G., Gore, I., and Kilby, R. A.: Congenital leukemia. Blood 6:990, 1951.
34. Bierman, H. R., Cohen, P., McClelland, J. N., and Shimkin, M. B.: The effect of transfusions and antibiotics upon the duration of life in children with lymphogenous leukemia. J. Pediatr. 37:455, 1950.
35. Bisel, H. F.: Criteria for evaluation of response to treatment in acute leukemia. Blood 11:676, 1956 (Letter).
36. Bleyer, W. A., Drake, J. C., and Chabner, B. A.: Neurotoxicity and elevated cerebrospinal fluid methotrexate concentration in meningeal leukemia. N. Engl. J. Med. 289:770, 1973.
37. Block, M., Jacobson, L. O., and Bethard, W. F.: Preleukemic acute human leukemia. J.A.M.A. 152:1018, 1953.
38. Bloom, G. E., Gerald, P. S., and Diamond, L. K.: Chronic myelogenous leukemia in an infant: serial cytogenetic and fetal hemoglobin studies. Pediatrics 38:295, 1966.
39. Bluming, A. Z.: Current status of clinical immunotherapy. Cancer Chemother. Rep. 59:901, 1975.
40. Bobrow, S. N., Smith, R. G., Reitz, M. S., et al.: Stimulated normal human lymphocytes contain ribonuclease-sensitive DNA polymerase distinct from viral RNA-dependent DNA polymerase. Proc. Natl. Acad. Sci. USA 69:3228, 1972.
41. Boggs, D. R., Wintrobe, M. M., and Cartwright, G. E.: The acute leukemias. Analysis of 322 cases and review of the literature. Medicine 41:163, 1962.
42. Boggs, D. R.: Editorial: Hematopoietic stem cell theory in relation to possible lymphoblastic conversion of chronic myeloid leukemia. Blood 44:449, 1974.
43. Boiron, M., Jacquillat, C. Weil, M., Tanzer, J., Levy, D., Sultan, C., and Bernard, J.: Daunorubicin in the treatment of acute myelocytic leukaemia. Lancet 1:330, 1969.
44. Borella, L., and Sen, L.: E receptors on blasts from untreated acute lymphocytic leukemia (ALL): Comparison of temperature dependence of E rosettes formed by normal and leukemic lymphoid cells. J. Immunol. 114:187, 1975.
45. Borella, L., Sen, L., and Green, A. A.: Cell surface markers and clinical features in acute lymphocytic leukemia. Proc. Am. Assoc. Cancer Res. 15:122, 1974.
46. Bornstein, R. S., Nesbit, M., and Kennedy, B. J.: Chronic myelogenous leukemia presenting in blastic crisis. Cancer 30:939, 1972.
47. Bottomly, R. H., Lovig, C. A., Holt, R., and Griffin, M. J.: Comparison of alkaline phosphatase from human normal and leukemic leukocytes. Cancer Res. 29:1866, 1969.
48. Brandt, L.: Comparative studies of bone marrow and extramedullary haemopoietic tissue in chronic myeloid leukemia. Ser. Haematol. 4:75, 1975.
48a. Brown, G., Capellaro, D., and Greaves, M.: Leukemia-associated antigens in man. J. Natl. Cancer Inst. 55:1281, 1975.
49. Buffett, R. F., et al.: Vertical transmission of murine leukemia virus. Cancer Res. 29:588, 1969.
50. Burchenal, J. H.: Formal discussion: long-term survival in Burkitt's tumor in acute leukemia. Cancer Res. 27:2616, 1967.
51. Burchenal, J. H.: Long-term survivors in acute leukemia and Burkitt's tumor. Cancer 21:595, 1968.
52. Burchenal, J. H.: Features suggesting curability in leukemia and lymphoma. In Leukemia-Lymphoma. Chicago, Yearbook Medical Publishers, 1970.
53. Burchenal, J. H.: Features suggesting curability in lymphoma and leukemia. CA 23:344, 1973.
54. Burgert, E. O., Jr., Nieri, R. L., Mills, S. D., et al.: Non-lymphocytic leukemia in childhood. Mayo Clin. Proc. 48:255, 1973.
55. Burgess, A. M.: Chloroma. J. Med. Res. 29:133, 1912–13.
56. Campbell, W. A. B., Macafee, A. L., and Wade, W. G.: Familial neonatal leukemia. Arch. Dis. Child. 37:93, 1962.
57. Canellos, G. P., De Vita, V. T., Whang-Peng, J., and Carbone, P. P.: Hematologic and cytogenetic remission of blastic transformation in chronic granulocytic leukemia. Blood 38:671, 1971.
58. Cangir, A., George, S., and Sullivan, M.:

Unfavorable prognosis of acute leukemia in infancy. Cancer 36:1973, 1975.
59. Carper, J. M., O'Donnell, W. M., and Monroe, J. H.: Neonatal leukemia. Detection of herpes virus in the mother and child. Am. J. Dis. Child. 115:61, 1968.
60. Casey, T. P.: Chronic lymphocytic leukemia in a child presenting at the age of two years and eight months. Aust. Ann. Med. 17:70, 1968.
60a. Chechik, B. E., and Gelfand, E. W.: Leukaemia-associated antigen in serum of patients with acute lymphoblastic leukaemia. Lancet 1:166, 1976.
61. Chusid, M. J., and Dale, D. C.: Eosinophilic leukemia. Remission with vincristine and hydroxyurea. Am. J. Med. 59:297, 1975.
62. Clarkson, B. D., in Boggs, D. R.: Hematopoietic stem cell theory in relation to possible lymphoblastic conversion of chronic myeloid leukemia. Blood 44:449, 1974.
63. Clarkson, B. D., and Boyse, E. A.: Possible explanation of the high concordance for acute leukemia in monozygotic twins. Lancet 1:699, 1971.
64. Clarkson, B. D., Dowling, M. D., Gee, T. S., et al.: Treatment of acute leukemia in adults. Cancer 36:775, 1975.
65. Clarkson, B. D., Okhita, T., Ota, K., and Fried, J.: Studies of cellular proliferation in human leukemia. I. Estimation of growth rates of leukemia and normal hematopoietic cells in two adults with acute leukemia given single injections of tritiated thymidine. J. Clin. Invest. 46:506, 1967.
66. Clough, P. W.: Monocytic leukemia. Bull. Johns Hopkins Hosp. 51:148, 1932.
67. Colebatch, J. H., Baikie, A. G., Clark, P., Jones, D. L., Lee, C. W. G., Lewis, I. C., and Newman, N. M.: Cyclic drug regimen for acute childhood leukaemia. Lancet 1:313, 1968.
68. Cooke, J. V.: Incidence of acute leukemia in children, J.A.M.A. 119:547, 1942.
69. Cooke, J. V.: Chronic myelogenous leukemia in children. J. Pediatr. 42:537, 1953.
70. Cramblett, H. G., Friedman, J. L., and Najjar, S.: Leukemia in an infant born of a mother with leukemia. N. Engl. J. Med. 259:727, 1958.
71. Crowther, D., Bateman, C. J. T., Vartan, C. P., et al.: Combination chemotherapy using L-asparaginase, daunorubicin, and cytosine arabinoside in adults with acute myelogenous leukemia. Brit. Med. J. 4:513, 1970.
72. Crowther, D., Powles, R. L., Bateman, C. J., et al.: Management of adult acute myelogenous leukaemia. Brit. Med. J. 1:131, 1973.
73. Cutting, H. O.: Inappropriate secretion of antidiuretic hormone secondary to vincristine therapy. Am. J. Med. 51:2691, 1971.
74. Darte, J. M. N., McClure, P. D., et al.: Congenital lymphoid hyperplasia with persistent hyperlymphocytosis. N. Engl. J. Med. 286:431, 1971.
75. DeFronzo, R. A., Colvin, O. M., Braine, H., et al.: Cyclophosphamide and the kidney. Cancer 33:483, 1974.
75a. De Vivo, D. C., Malas, D., Nelson, J. S., and Land, V. J.: Leukoencephalopathy in childhood leukemia. Neurology 27:609, 1977.
76. Djernes, B. W., Soukup, S. W., Bove, K. E., and Wong, K. Y.: Congenital leukemia associated with mosaic trisomy 9. J. Pediatr. 88:596, 1976.
77. Dmochowski, L., et al.: Electron microscopic studies of human leukaemia and lymphoma. Cancer 20:760, 1967.
77a. Draper, G. J., Heaf, M. M., and Kinnier Wilson, L. M.: Occurrence of childhood cancers among sibs and estimation of familial risks. J. Med. Genetics 14:81, 1977.
78. Doan, C. A., and Reinhart, H. L.: The basophil granulocyte, basophilcytosis, and myeloid leukemia, basophil and "mixed granule" types: an experimental, clinical and pathological study, with the report of a new syndrome. Am. J. Clin. Pathol. 11:1, 1941.
79. Dore, J. F., Motta, R., Markolev, W., et al.: New antigens in human leukaemic cells and antibody in the serum of leukaemic patients. Lancet 2:1396, 1967.
80. Dubowitz, V.: Acute monocytic leukemia with response to methotrexate. Arch. Dis. Child. 39:289, 1964.
80a. Editorial: Immunostimulation. Lancet 2:349, 1976.
81. Engfeldt, B., and Zetterstrom, R.: Disseminated eosinophilic collagen disease. Acta Med. Scand. 153:337, 1956.
82. Evans, A. E., Faber, S., Brunet, S., and Mariano, P. J.: Vincristine in the treatment of acute leukemia in children. Cancer 16:1302, 1963.
83. Evans, D. I. K., Morris Jones, P. H., and Morley, C. J.: Treatment of acute myeloid leukemia of childhood with cytosine arabinoside, daunorubicin, prednisolone, and mercaptopurine or thioguanine. Cancer 36:1547, 1975.
84. Evatt, B. L., Chase, G. A., Heath, C. W., Jr.: Time-space clustering among cases of acute leukemia in two Georgia counties. Blood 41:265, 1973.
85. Falletta, J. N., Starling, K. A., and Fernbach, D. J.: Leukemia in twins. Pediatrics 52:846, 1973.
86. Fernbach, D. J., George, S. L., Sutow, W. W., et al.: Long-term results of reinforcement therapy in children with acute luekemia. Cancer 36:1552, 1975.
87. Fernbach, D. J., Griffith, K. M., Haggard, M. E., et al.: Chemotherapy of acute leukemia in childhood: comparison of

cyclophosphamide and mercaptopurine. N. Engl. J. Med. 275:451, 1966.
87a. Fialkow, P. J., Jacobson, R. J., and Papayannopoulou, T.: Chronic myelocytic leukemia: clonal origin in a stem cell common to the granulocyte, erythrocyte, platelet, and monocyte/macrophage. Amer. J. Med. 63:125, 1977.
88. Fialkow, P. J., Thomas, E. D., Bryant, J. I., et al.: Leukaemic transformation of engrafted human marrow cells in vivo. Lancet 1:251, 1971.
89. Field, J. B., and Williams, H. E.: Artefactual hypoglycemia associated with leukemia. N. Engl. J. Med. 265:946, 1961.
90. Field, M., Block, J. B., et al.: Significance of blood lactate elevations among patients with acute leukemia and other neoplastic proliferative disorders. Am. J. Med. 40:528, 1966.
91. Finkelstein, J. Z., Dyment, P. G., and Hammond, G. D.: Leukemic infiltration of the testes during bone marrow remission. Pediatrics 43:1042, 1969.
92. Fitzgerald, P. H., Crossen, P. E., and Hamer, J. W.: Abnormal karyotypic clones in human acute leukemia: their nature and significance. Cancer 31:1069, 1973.
93. Flandrin, G., Brouet, J. C., Daniel, M. T., and Preud'homme, J. L.: Acute leukemia with Burkett's tumor cells: A study of six cases with special reference to lymphocyte surface markers. Blood 45:183, 1975.
94. Foadi, M. D., Cooper, E. H., and Hardisty, R. M.: Proliferative activity of leukemic cells at various stages of acute leukemia of childhood. Brit. J. Haematol. 15:269, 1968.
95. Forman, E. N., Padre-Mendoza, T., Smith, P. S., et al.: Ph[1]-positive childhood leukemias: spectrum of lymphoid-myeloid expressions. Blood 49:549, 1977.
96. Fraumeni, J. F., Jr., Manning, M. D., and Mitus, W. J.: Acute childhood leukemia: epidemiologic study by cell type of 1263 cases at the Children's Cancer Research Foundation in Boston, 1947–65. J. Natl. Cancer Inst. 46:461, 1971.
97. Fraumeni, J. F., Jr., and Miller, R. W.: Epidemiology of human leukemia. Recent observations. J. Natl. Cancer Inst. 38:593, 1967.
98. Freedman, M. H., Finkelstein, J. Z., Hammond, D. G., and Karon, M.: The effect of chemotherapy on acute myelogenous leukemia in children. J. Pediatr. 78:526, 1971.
99. Frei, E., III, and Freireich, E. J.: Progress and perspectives in the chemotherapy of acute leukemia. Adv. Chemother. 2:269, 1965.
100. Frei, E. III, Freireich, E. J., Gehan, E., et al.: Studies of sequential and combination antimetabolite therapy in acute leukemia: 6-mercaptopurine and methotrexate. From the Acute Leukemia Group B. Blood 18:431, 1961.
101. Freireich, E. J., Gehan, E., Frei, E., III, et al.: The effect of 6-mercaptopurine on the duration of steroid-induced remission in acute leukemia: a model for evaluation of other potentially useful therapy. Blood 21:699, 1963.
102. Frei, E. J., III, Karon, M., Levin, R. H., et al.: Effectiveness of combinations of antileukemic agents in inducing and maintaining remission in children with acute leukemia. Blood 26:642, 1965.
103. Fritz, R. D., Forkner, C. E., Jr., Freireich, E. J., et al.: The association of fatal intracranial hemorrhage and "blastic crisis" in patients with acute leukemia. N. Engl. J. Med. 261:59, 1959.
104. Furth, J., and Kahn, M. C.: Transmission of leukemia of mice with a single cell. Am. J. Cancer 4:276, 1937.
105. Gabuzda, T. G., Shute, H. E., et al.: Regulation of erythropoiesis in erythroleukemia. Arch. Intern. Med. 123:60, 1969.
106. Gallo, R. C., Miller, N. R., Saxinger, W. C., et al.: Primate RNA tumor virus-like DNA synthesized endogenously by RNA-dependent DNA polymerase in virus-like particles from fresh human acute leukemic blood cell. Proc. Natl. Acad. Sci. USA 70:3219, 1973.
107. Galton, D. A. G.: Chemotherapy of chronic myelocytic leukemia. Semin. Hematol. 6:323, 1969.
108. Galton, D. A. G., Spiers, A. S. D.: Progress in the leukemias. In Brown, E. B. and Moore, C. V. (eds.): Progress in Hematology. Vol. VII. New York, Grune & Stratton, 1971.
109. Gee, T. S., Yu, K. P., and Clarkson, B. D.: Treatment of adult acute leukemia with arabinosylcytosine and thioguanine. Cancer 23:1019, 1969.
110. Geils, G. F., Scott, C. W., Jr., Baugh, C. M., and Butterworth, C. E., Jr.: Treatment of meningeal leukemia with pyrimethamine. Blood 38:131, 1971.
111. Geiser, C. F., and Mitus, J. W.: Acute monocytic leukemia in children and its response to vinblastine (NSC-49842). Cancer Chemother. Rep. 59:385, 1975.
112. Gelfand, E. W., and Chechik, B. E.: Unmasking the heterogeneity of acute lymphoblastic leukemia. N. Engl. J. Med. 294:275, 1976.
113. George, S. L., Fernbach, P. J., Vietti, T. J., et al.: Factors influencing survival in pediatric acute leukemia. The SWCCSG experience, 1958–1970. Cancer 32:1542, 1973.
114. Ghitis, J.: Acute promyelocytic leukemia? Blood 21:237, 1963.
115. Gilliam, A. G., and Walter, W. A.: Trends of mortality from leukemia in the United

States 1921–55. Public Health Rep. 73: 773, 1958.
116. Givler, R. L.: Testicular involvement in leukemia and lymphoma. Cancer 23: 1290, 1969.
117. Glass, A. G., and Mantel, N.: Lack of time-space clustering of childhood leukemia, Los Angeles County 1960–64. Cancer Res. 29:1995, 1969.
118. Goh, K., Swisher, S. N., and Herman, E. C., Jr.: Chronic myelocytic leukemia and identical twins. Arch. Intern. Med. 120: 214, 1967.
119. Gordon, H. W.: Myeloid metaplasia masquerading as neonatal leukemia. Am. J. Dis. Child. 118:932, 1969.
120. Gralnick, H. R., Harbor, J., and Vogel, C.: Myelofibrosis in chronic granulocytic leukemia. Blood 37:152, 1971.
121. Gralnick, H., and Sultan, C.: Acute promyelocytic leukemia: haemorrhagic manifestation and morphologic criteria. Brit. J. Haematol. 29:373, 1975.
122. Graw, R. G., Jr., Lohrmann, H. P., Bull, M. I., et al.: Bone marrow transplantation following combination chemotherapy-immunosuppressive (B.A.C.T.) in patients with acute leukemia. Transplant. Proc. 2:349, 1974.
123. Graw, R. G., Jr., Skeel, R. T., and Carbone, P. P.: Priapism in a child with chronic granulocytic leukemia. J. Pediatr. 74:788, 1969.
123a. Gribbin, M. A., Hardisty, R. M., and Chessells, J. M.: Long-term control of central nervous system leukaemia. Arch. Dis. Child. 52:673, 1977.
124. Griem, M. L., Meier, P., and Dobben, G. D.: Analysis of the morbidity and mortality of children irradiated in fetal life. Radiology 88:347, 1967.
125. Gross, L.: The role of C-type and other oncogenic virus particles in cancer and leukemia. N. Engl. J. Med. 294:724, 1976.
126. Gross, L., Schidlovsky, G., Feldman, D., et al.: C-type virus particles in placenta of normal healthy Sprague-Dawley rats. Proc. Natl. Acad. Sci. USA 72:3240, 1975.
127. Grozea, P. N., Bottomly, R. H., Shaw, M. T., Tu, H., Chanes, R. E., and Condit, P. T.: The role of cytosine arabinoside maintenance in acute nonlymphoblastic leukemia. Cancer 36:855, 1975.
128. Gunz, F. W., and Baikie, A. G.: Leukemia. 3rd Ed. New York, Grune & Stratton, 1974.
128a. Gunz, F. W., Gunz, J. P., Veale, A.M.O., et al.: Familial leukaemia: a study of 909 families. Scand. J. Haematol. 15:117, 1975.
129. Gunz, F. W., and Spears, G. F. S.: Distribution of acute leukaemia in time and space. Studies in New Zealand. Brit. Med. J. 4:604, 1968.

130. Haahr, J., and Halveg, A. D.: Congenital leukemia. Acta Paediatr. Scand. 60:720, 1971.
131. Hall, J. G., Levin, J., Kuhn, J. P., Ottenheimer, E. J., van Berkum, K.A.P., and McKusick, V. A.: Thrombocytopenia with absent radius (TAR). Medicine 48:4, 1969.
132. Halterman, R. H., Leventhal, B. G., and Mann, D. L.: An acute-leukemia antigen: correlation with clinical status. N. Engl. J. Med. 287:1272, 1972.
133. Hanrahan, J. B., Sax, S. M., et al.: Factitious hypoglycemia in patients with leukemia. Am. J. Clin. Pathol. 40:43, 1963.
134. Haran-Ghera, N.: Influence of host factors on leukemogenesis by the radiation leukemia virus. Isr. J. Med. Sci. 7:17, 1971.
135. Hardisty, R. M., Speed, D. R., and Till, M. M.: Granulocytic leukaemia in childhood. Brit. J. Haematol. 10:551, 1964.
136. Hardisty, R. M., and Till, M. M.: Acute leukaemia 1959–64: factors affecting prognosis. Arch. Dis. Child. 43:107, 1968.
137. Hart, J. S., Shirakawa, S., et al.: The mechanism of induction of complete remission in acute myeloblastic leukemia in man. Cancer Res. 29:2300, 1969.
138. Hayes, D. M.: The seasonal incidence of acute leukemia. Cancer 14:1301, 1961.
139. Hayhoe, G. F. J., Quaglino, D., and Doll, R.: The cytology and cytochemistry of acute leukaemias. A study of 140 cases. M. R. C. Special Report Series, N. 304. London, Her Majesty's Stationery Office, 1964.
139a. Heath, C. W., Jr.: The epidemiology of leukemia. In Schottenfeld, D. (ed.): Cancer Epidemiology and Prevention. Springfield, Ill., Charles C Thomas, 1975.
140. Heath, C. W., Jr., Bennett, J. M., Whang-Peng, J., Berry, E. W., and Wiernick, P. H.: Cytogenetic findings in erythroleukemia. Blood 33:453, 1969.
141. Heath, C. W., Jr., and Hasterlik, R. J.: Leukemia among children in a suburban community. Am. J. Med. 34:796, 1963.
142. Hehlmann, R., Kufe, D., and Spiegelman, S.: RNA in human leukemic cells related to the RNA of a mouse leukemia virus. Proc. Natl. Acad. Sci. USA 69:435, 1972.
143. Henderson, E. S.: Treatment of acute leukemia. Semin. Hematol. 6:271, 1969.
144. Heyn, R., Borges, W., Joo, P., et al.: BCG in the treatment of acute lymphoblastic leukemia (ALL). Proc. Am. Assoc. Cancer Res. 14:45, 1973.
145. Hoagland, H. C., and Perry, M. C.: Blast cell crisis in acute or chronic leukemia. J.A.M.A. 235:1888, 1976.
146. Holland, J. F., and Glidewell, O.: Complementary chemotherapy in acute leukemia. In Mathé, G. (ed.): Recent results in

cancer research: advances in treatment of acute (blastic) leukemias. New York, Springer-Verlag, 1970.
147. Holland, J. F., and Glidewell, O.: Oncologists reply: survival expectancy in acute lymphocytic leukemia. N. Engl. J. Med. 287:769, 1972.
148. Holowach, J.: Chronic lymphoid leukemia in children. J. Pediatr. 32:84, 1948.
149. Holton, C. P., and Johnson, W. W.: Chronic myelocytic leukemia in infant siblings. J. Pediatr. 72:377, 1968.
150. Holton, C. P., Vietti, T. J., Nora, A. H., Donaldson, M. H., Stuckley, W. J., Jr., Watkins, W. L., and Lane, D. M.: Clinical study of daunomycin and prednisone for induction of remission in children with advanced leukemia. N. Engl. J. Med. 280:171, 1969,
151. Hossfeld, D. K., Tormey, D., and Ellison, R. R.: Ph[1]-positive megakaryoblastic leukemia. Cancer 36:576, 1975.
152. Howard, J. P., Albo, V., and Newton, W. A., Jr.: Cytosine arabinoside: results of a cooperative study in acute childhood leukemia. Cancer 21:341, 1968.
153. Hustu, H. O., and Pinkel, D.: Lymphosarcoma, Hodgkin's disease and leukemia in bone. Clin. Orthop. 52:83, 1967.
154. Hyman, C. B., Bogle, J. M., et al.: Central nervous system involvement by leukemia in children. Blood 25:1, 1965.
155. Hyman, C. B., Borda, E., Brubaker, C., Hammond, D., and Sturgeon, P.: Prednisone in childhood leukemia. Comparison of interrupted and continuous therapy. Pediatrics 24:1005, 1959.
156. Ioachim, H. L., Keller, S., Sabbath, M., Andersson, B., Dorsett, B., and Essner, E.: Myeloperoxidase and crystalline bodies in the granules of DMBA-induced rat chloroma cells. Am. J. Pathol 66:147, 1972.
157. Iverson, T.: Leukaemia in infancy and childhood. A material of 570 Danish cases. Acta Pediatr. Scand Suppl. 167:9, 1966.
158. Jablon, S., and Kato, H.: Childhood cancer in relation to prenatal exposure to atomic-bomb radiation. Lancet 2:1000, 1970.
159. Jaffe, N., and Kim, B. S.: Hypoglycemia and hypothermia in terminal leukemia. Pediatrics 48:836, 1971.
160. Jaffe, N., Kim, B. S., and Vawter, G. F.: Hypocalcemia—a complication of childhood leukemia. Cancer 29:392, 1972.
160a. Jensen, M. K., and Killmann, S.-A.: Chromosome studies in acute leukaemia. Evidence for chromosomal abnormalities common to erythroblasts and leukaemic white cells. Acta Med. Scand. 181:47, 1967.
161. Johnson, R. E.: An experimental therapeutic approach to L1210 leukemia in mice: combined chemotherapy and central nervous system irradiation. J. Natl. Cancer Inst. 32:1333, 1964.
162. Jones, B., Cuttner, J., Levy, R. N., Patterson, R. B., et al.: Daunorubicin (NSC-83142) versus daunorubicin plus prednisone (NSC-10023) versus daunorubicin plus vincristine (NSC-67574) plus prednisone in advanced childhood acute lymphocytic leukemia. Cancer Chemother. Rep. 56:729, 1972.
163. Jones, B., Holland, J. F., Morrison, A. R., et al.: Daunorubicin (NSC-82151) in the treatment of advanced childhood lymphoblastic leukemia. Cancer Res. 31:84, 1971.
163a. Jones, P. G., and Campbell, P. E.: Tumours of Infancy and Childhood. Oxford, Blackwell Scientific Publications, 1976.
164. Jongsma, A., Van Someren, H., Westervald, A., Hagemeier, A., and Pearson, P.: Localization of genes on human chromosomes using human chinese hamster cell hybrids. Humangenetik 20:195, 1973.
165. Kaplow, L. S.: A histochemical procedure for localizing and evaluating leukocyte alkaline phosphatase activity in smears of blood and marrow. Blood 10:1023, 1955.
166. Karon, M., Freireich, E. R., Frei, E., III, Taylor, R., et al.: The role of vincristine in the treatment of childhood acute leukemia. Clin. Pharmacol. Ther. 7:332, 1966.
167. Kay, H.E.M.: Development of CNS leukaemia in acute myeloid leukaemia in childhood. Arch. Dis. Child. 51:73, 1976.
168. Kersey, J. H., Sabad, A., Gajl-Peczalska, K., et al.: Acute lymphoblastic leukemic cells with T-(thymus-derived)lymphocyte markers. Science 182:1355, 1973.
169. Killmann, S. A.: Chronic myelogenous leukaemia: preleukaemia or leukaemia? Haematologica 57:641, 1972.
170. Koch, K., Reiquam, C. W., and Beatly, E. C.: Acute childhood leukemia—unusual complications. Rocky Mt. Med. J. 63:55, 1966.
171. Krivit, W., Brubaker, C., Hartmann, J., Murphy, M. L., Pierce, M., and Thatcher, S.: Induction of remission in acute leukemia of childhood by combination of prednisone and either 6-mercaptopurine or methotrexate. J. Pediatr. 68:965, 1966.
172. Krivit, W., Brubaker, C., Thatcher, G., Pierce, M., Perrin, E., and Hartmann, J.: Maintenance therapy in acute leukemia of childhood: comparison of cyclic vs. sequential methods. Cancer 21:352, 1968.
173. Krivit, W. Gilchrist, G., and Beatty, E. G.: The need for chemotherapy after prolonged complete remission in acute leu-

kemia of childhood. J. Pediatr. 76:138, 1970.
174. Kundel, D. W., Brecher, G., et al.: Reticulin fibrosis and bone infarction in acute leukemia. Implications for prognosis. Blood 23:526, 1964.
175. Kuo, T.-T., Tschang, T.-P., and Chu, J.-Y.: Testicular relapse in childhood acute lymphocytic leukemia during bone marrow remission. Cancer 38:2604, 1976.
176. Kyle, R. A., and Pease, G. L.: Basophilic leukemia. Arch. Intern. Med. 118:205, 1966.
177. Lampkin, B. C., McWilliams, N. B., et al.: The advantage of cell synchronization in therapy of myeloid leukemias in children. Blood 38:802, 1971.
178. Lampkin, B. C., McWilliams, N. B., and Mauer, A. M.: Treatment of acute leukemia. Pediatr. Clin. North Am. 19:1123, 1972.
179. Lane, D. M.: Chronic myelogenous leukemia and other myeloproliferative disorders. In Sutow, W. W., Vietti, T. J., and Fernbach, D. J. (eds.): Clinical Pediatric Oncology. St. Louis, C. V. Mosby Co., 1973.
180. Lanman, J. T., Bierman, H. R., and Byron, R. L., Jr.: Transfusion of leukemic leukocytes in man: hematologic and physiologic changes. Blood 5:1099, 1950.
181. Larson, S. M., Graff, K. S., Tretner, I., Zager, R. F., Henderson, E. A., and Johnston, G. S.: Positive Gallium 67 photoscan in myeloblastoma. J.A.M.A. 222:321, 1972.
182. Lascari, A.: Leukemia in Childhood. Springfield, Ill., Charles C Thomas, 1973.
183. Lascari, A. D., Givler, R. L., Soper, R. T., and Hill, L. F.: Portal hypertension in a case of acute leukemia treated with antimetabolites for ten years. N. Engl. J. Med. 279:303, 1968.
184. Lee, J. A. H.: Seasonal variation in leukaemia incidence. Brit. Med. J. 2:623, 1963.
185. Leikin, S., Brubaker, C., et al.: Varying prednisone dosage in remission induction of previously untreated childhood leukemia. Cancer 21:346, 1968.
186. Levin, R. H., Henderson, E., Karon, M., and Freireich, E. J.: Treatment of acute leukemia with methylglyoxal-bis-guanylhydrazone (methyl-GAG). Clin. Pharmacol. Ther. 6:31, 1965.
187. Levine, P. H., et al.: Relationship between clinical status of leukemic patients and virus-like particles in their plasma. Cancer 20:1563, 1967.
188. Levy, S. G.: Cat leukemia: a threat to man? N. Engl. J. Med. 290:513, 1974.
189. Lilleyman, J. S., Harrison, J. F., and Black, J. A.: Treatment of juvenile chronic myeloid leukemia with sequential subcutaneous cytarabine and oral mercaptopurine. Blood 49:559, 1977.
190. Lilly, F.: Guest editorial: Mouse leukemia—a model of multiple-gene disease. J. Natl. Cancer Inst. 49:927, 1972.
191. Luddy, R. E., and Gilman, P. A.: Paraplegia following intrathecal methotrexate. J. Pediatr. 83:988, 1973.
192. Lusher, J. M.: Chloroma as a presenting feature of acute leukemia. A report of two cases in children. Am. J. Dis. Child. 108:62, 1964.
193. Lynch, M. J.: Monocytic leukemia. Can. Med. Assoc. J. 70:670, 1954.
194. Mason, T. E., Demaree, R. S., Jr., and Margolis, C. I.: Granulocytic sarcoma (chloroma), two years preceding myelogenous leukemia. Cancer 31:423, 1973.
195. Mathé, G.: Immunotherapy in the treatment of acute lymphoid leukemia. Hosp. Pract. 6:43, 1971.
196. Mathé, G., Amiel, J. J., et al.: Active immunotherapy for acute lymphoblastic leukaemia. Lancet 2:697, 1969.
197. Mathé, G., Hayat, M., Schwarzenberg, L., et al.: Acute lymphoblastic leukemia treated with combination of prednisone, vincristine, and rubidomycin: value of pathogen-free rooms. Lancet 2:380, 1967.
198. Mathé, G., Pouillart, P., and Lapeyraque, F.: Active immunotherapy of L1210 leukemia applied after the graft of tumor cells. Brit. J. Cancer 23:814, 1969.
198a. Mathé, G., Schwarzenberg, L., Mery, A. M., et al.: Extensive histological and cytological survey of patients with acute leukaemia in "complete remission." Brit. Med. J. 1:640, 1966.
199. Mauer, A. M., and Fisher, V.: Characteristics of cell proliferation in four patients with untreated acute leukemia. Blood 28:428, 1966.
200. Mauer, A. M., Lampkin, B. C., and McWilliams, N. B.: The leukemias and reticuloendothelioses. In Nathan, D. G., and Oski, F. A. (eds.): Hematology of Infancy and Childhood. Philadelphia, W. B. Saunders Co., 1974.
201. McCaffrey, R., Greaves, M., Harrison, T. A., et al.: Biochemical and immunological evidence for lymphoblastic conversion in chronic myelogenous leukemia. Blood (Abstr.) 46:1043, 1975.
202. McCaffrey, R., Harrison, T. A., Parkman, R., et al.: Terminal deoxynucleotidyl transferase activity in human leukemic cells and in normal human thymocytes N. Engl. J. Med. 292:775, 1975.
203. McIntosh, S., and Aspnes, G. T.: Encephalopathy following CNS prophylaxis in childhood lymphoblastic leukemia. Pediatrics 52:612, 1973.

204. McIntosh, S., Klatskin, E. H., O'Brien, R. T., et al.: Chronic neurologic disturbance in childhood leukemia. Cancer 37:853, 1976.
205. McIntosh, S., and Pearson, H. A.: Treatment of childhood leukemia. J. Pediatr. 83:899, 1973.
206. McKenna, R. W., Bloomfield, C. D., Dick, F., Nesbit, M. E., and Brunning, R. D.: Acute monoblastic leukemia: diagnosis and treatment of ten cases. Blood 46:481, 1975.
207. Meadows, A. T., and Evans, A. E.: Effects of chemotherapy on the central nervous system. A study of parenteral methotrexate in long-term survivors of leukemia and lymphoma in childhood. Cancer 37:1079, 1976.
208. Meighan, S. S.: Leukemia in children. Incidence, clinical manifestations, and survival in an unselected series. Cancer 16:656, 1963.
209. Medical Research Council: Treatment of acute myeloid leukemia with daunorubicin, cytosine arabinoside, mercaptopurine, L-asparaginase, prednisone, and thioguanine: results of treatment with five multiple-drug schedules. Brit. J. Haematol. 27:373, 1974.
210. Melhorn, D. K., Gross, S., and Newman, A. J.: Acute childhood leukemia presenting as aplastic anemia: the response to corticosteroids. J. Pediatr. 77:647, 1970.
211. Miller, D. R., Newstead, G. J., and Young, L. W.: Perinatal leukemia with a possible variant of the Ellis-van Creveld syndrome. J. Pediat. 74:300, 1969.
212. Miller, J. F. A. P.: T-cell regulation of immune responsiveness. Ann. N.Y. Acad. Sci. 249:9, 1975.
213. Miller, R. W.: Persons with exceptionally high risk of leukemia. Cancer Res. 27:2420, 1967.
214. Miller, R. W.: Neoplasia and Down's syndrome. Ann. N.Y. Acad. Sci. 171:637, 1970.
215. Mir. M. A., and Delamore, I. W.: The syndrome of inappropriate sodium wasting and hyponatraemia in acute myeloid leukaemia. Brit. J. Haematol. 28:149, 1974.
216. Mitrakul, C., Othaganonda, B. O., et al.: Basophilic leukemia. Report of a case. Clin. Pediatr. 8:178, 1969.
217. Moloney, J. B.: The murine leukemias. Fed. Proc. 21:19, 1962.
218. Moore, M. A. S., Ekert, H., Fitzgerald, M. G., and Charmichael, A.: Evidence for the clonal origin of chronic myeloid leukemia from a sex chromosome mosaic: clinical cytogenetic, and marrow culture studies. Blood 43:15, 1974.
219. Moore, M. A. S., Spitzer, G., Williams, N., Metcalf, D., and Buckley, J.: Agar culture studies in 127 cases of untreated acute leukemia. The prognostic value of re- classification of leukemia according to in vitro growth characteristics. Blood 44:1, 1974.
220. Moore, M. A. S., Williams, N., and Metcalf, D.: In vitro colony formation by normal and leukemic human hematopoietic cells. Characterization of the colony-forming cell. J. Natl. Cancer Inst. 50:603, 1973.
221. Morrow, G. W., Jr., Pease, G. L., Stroebel, C. F., and Bennett, W. A.: Terminal phase of chronic myelogenous leukemia. Cancer 18:369, 1965.
222. Muggia, F. M., Heinemann, H. O., Farhangi, M., and Osserman, E. F.: Lysozymuria and renal tubular dysfunction in monocytic and myelomonocytic leukemia. Am. J. Med. 47:351, 1969.
223. Muss, H. B., and Moloney, W. C.: Chloroma and other myeloblastic tumors. Blood 42:721, 1973.
224. Nagao, T., Lampkin, B. C., and Mauer, A. M.: Maintenance therapy in acute childhood leukemia. J. Pediatr. 76:134, 1970.
225. Nau, R. C., and Hoagland, H. C.: A myeloproliferative disorder manifested by persistent basophilia, granulocytic leukemia, and erythroleukemic phases. Cancer 28:662, 1971.
226. Nelken, R. P., and Stockman, J. A., III: The hypereosinophilic syndrome in association with acute lymphoblastic leukemia. J. Pediatr. 89:771, 1976.
226a. Nesbit, M., Ortega, J., Donaldson, M., et al.: Prevention of testicular leukemia by prophylactic radiation in childhood acute lymphoblastic leukemia. 13th Annual Meeting, American Society for Clinical Oncology, Abstract C-201, 1977.
227. Newell, G. R., et al.: Evaluation of "virus-like" particles in the plasmas of 255 patients with leukemia and related diseases. N. Engl. J. Med. 278:1185, 1968.
228. Nies, B. A., Bodey, G. P., Thomas, L. B., Brecher, G., and Freireich, E. J.: The persistence of extramedullary leukemic infiltrates during bone marrow remission of acute leukemia. Blood 26:133, 1965.
229. Nowell, P. C.: Cytogenetics. In Becker, F. F. (ed.): Cancer: A Comprehensive Treatise. Vol. 1. New York, Plenum Press, 1975.
230. Nowell, P. C., and Hungerford, D. A.: Chromosome studies in human leukemia. II. Chronic granulocytic leukemia. J. Natl. Cancer Inst. 27:1013, 1961.
231. O'Regan, S., Carson, S., Chesney, R. W., and Drummond, K. N.: Electrolyte and acid-base disturbances in the management of leukemia. Blood 49:345, 1977.
232. Odeberg, B.: Eosinophilic leukemia and disseminated eosinophilic collagen disease — a disease entity? Acta Med. Scand. 177:129, 1965.
233. Oettgen, H. F., Stephenson, P. A.,

Schwartz, M. K., Leeper, R. D., et al.: Toxicity of *E. coli* L-asparaginase in man. Cancer 25:253, 1970.

234. Ogawa, M., Fried, J., Sakai, Y., Strife, A., and Clarkson, B. D.: Studies of cellular proliferation in human leukemia. The proliferative activity, generation time, and emergence time of neutrophilic granulocytes in chronic granulocytic leukemia. Cancer 25:1031, 1970.

234a. Ortega, J. A., Nesbit, M. E., Jr., Donaldson, M. H., et al.: L-asparaginase, vincristine, and prednisone for induction of first remission in acute lymphocytic leukemia. Cancer Res. 37:535, 1977.

235. Osgood, E. E.: Monocytic leukemia. Arch. Intern. Med. 59:931, 1937.

236. Osserman, E. F., and Lawlor, D. P.: Serum and urinary lysozyme (muramidase) in monocytic and monomyelocytic leukemia. J. Exp. Med. 124:921, 1966.

237. Peterson, L. C., Bloomfield, C. D., and Brunning, R. D.: Blast crisis as an initial or terminal manifestation of chronic myeloid leukemia. A study of 28 patients. Am. J. Med. 60:209, 1976.

238. Phair, J. P., Anderson, R. E., and Namiki, H.: The central nervous system in leukemia. Ann. Intern. Med. 61:863, 1964.

239. Pierce, M. I.: Leukemia in the newborn infant. J. Pediatr. 54:691, 1959.

239a. Pileri, A., Gabutti, V., et al.: Proliferative activity of the cells of acute leukemia in relapse and in steady state. Acta Haematol. 38:193, 1967.

240. Pinkel, D.: Five year follow-up of "total therapy" of childhood lymphocytic leukemia. J.A.M.A. 216:648, 1971.

241. Pizzo, P. A., Bleyer, W. A., Poplack, D. G., and Leventhal, B. G.: Reversible dementia temporally associated with intraventricular therapy with methotrexate in a child with acute myelogenous leukemia. J. Pediatr. 88:131, 1976.

242. Pizzo, P. A., Henderson, E. S., and Leventhal, B. G.: Acute myelogenous leukemia in children: a preliminary report of combination chemotherapy. J. Pediatr. 88:125, 1976.

243. Pochedly, C.: Treatment of meningeal leukemia. Hosp. Pract. 11:123, 1976.

243a. Pochedly, C.: Neurotoxicity due to CNS therapy for leukemia. Med. Ped. Oncol. 3:101, 1977.

244. Powles, R. L., Crowther, D., Bateman, C. J. T., et al.: Immunotherapy for acute myelogenous leukaemia. Brit. J. Cancer 28:365, 1973.

245. Preliminary Report to the Medical Research Council by the Leukaemia Committee and the Working Party on Leukaemia in Childhood: Treatment of acute lymphoblastic leukaemia, comparison of immunotherapy (BCG), intermittent methotrexate, and no therapy after a five-month intensive cytotoxic regimen (Concord Trial). Brit. Med. J. 4:189, 1971.

246. Price, R. A.: Histopathology of central nervous system leukemia. Med. Probl. Paediat. 16:80, 1975.

247. Price, R. A., and Johnson, W. W.: The central nervous system in childhood leukemia. I. The arachnoid. Cancer 31:520, 1973.

248. Price, R. A., and Jamieson, P. A.: The central nervous system in childhood leukemia. II. Subacute leukoencephalopathy. Cancer 35:306, 1975.

249. Pridie, C. H., and Dumitrescu-Pirvu, D.: Leucemie acuta si sindrom Bonnevie-Ullrich la un nou-nascut. Pediatria 10:345, 1961.

250. Prolla, J. C., and Kirsner, J. B.: Gastrointestinal lesions and complications of leukemias. Ann. Int. Med. 61:1084, 1964.

251. Quattrin, V. N., Dini, E., and Palumbo, E.: Basophile leukamien, Blut 5:166, 1959.

252. Rappaport, H.: Atlas of Tumor Pathology. Sect. 3, Fasc. 8. Washington, D.C., Armed Forces Institute of Pathology, 1966, pp. 239–285.

253. Rastrick, J. M.: A method for the positive identification of erythropoietic cells in chromosome preparations of bone marrow. Brit. J. Haematol. 16:185, 1969.

254. Reimann, D. L., Clemmens, R. L., and Pillsbury, W. A.: Congenital acute leukemia: skin nodules, a first sign. J. Pediatr. 46:415, 1955.

255. Reisman, L. E., and Trujillo, J. M.: Chronic granulocytic leukemia of childhood. Clinical and cytogenetic studies. J. Pediatr. 62:710, 1963.

255a. Rickles, F. R., and Miller D. R.: Eosinophilic leukemoid reaction. J. Pediatr. 80:418, 1972.

256. Rivera, G., Pratt, C. B., Aur, R. J., et al.: Recurrent childhood lymphocytic leukemia following cessation of therapy. Cancer 37:1679, 1976.

256a. Rivera, G., Aur, R. J., Pratt, C., et al.: Central nervous system relapse during second marrow remission of acute lymphocytic leukemia. 68th Meeting, American Association for Cancer Research, Abstract 364, 1977.

257. Roloff, J. N., Lukens, J. N.: Dissociation of erythroblastic and myeloblastic proliferation in erythroleukemia. Am. J. Dis. Child. 123:11, 1972.

258. Rosen, C. B., and Teplitz, R. L.: Chronic granulocytic leukemia complicated by ulcerative colitis: Elevated leukocyte alkaline phosphatase, and possible modifier gene deletion. Blood 26:148, 1965.

259. Rosen, R. B., and Nowack, J.: Survivals of 5 to 15 years in acute leukemia. Cancer 34:501, 1974.

259a. Rosenthal, S., Canneles, G. P., DeVita, V.

T., Jr., and Gralnick, H. R.: Characteristics of blast crisis in chronic granulocytic leukemia. Blood 49:705, 1977.
260. Rosner, F., and Lee, S. L.: Down's syndrome and acute leukemia: myeloblastic or lymphoblastic? Am. J. Med. 53:203, 1972.
261. Ross, J. D., Moloney, W. C., and Desforges, J. F.: Ineffective regulation of granulopoiesis masquerading as congenital leukemia in a mongoloid child. J. Pediatr. 63:1, 1963.
262. Rowley, J. D.: A new consistent chromosomal abnormality in chronic myelogenous leukemia identified by quinacrine fluorescence and Giemsa staining. Nature 243:290, 1973.
262a. Rowley, J. D., and Potter, D.: Chromosomal banding patterns in acute nonlymphocytic leukemia. Blood 47:705, 1976.
263. Rundles, R. W.: Chronic granulocytic leukemia. In Williams, W. J., Beutler, E., Erslev, A. J., Rundles, W. R. (eds.): Hematology. New York, McGraw-Hill Book Co., 1972.
264. Sandberg, A. A., Ishihara, T., Crosswhite, L. H., and Hauschka, T. S.: Comparison of chromosome constitution in chronic myelocytic leukemia and other myeloproliferative disorders. Blood 20:393, 1962.
265. Sandberg A. A., Ishihara, T., Kikuchi, Y., et al.: Chromosomal differences among acute leukemias. Ann. N.Y. Acad. Sci. 113:663, 1964.
266. Sardemann, H.: Chronic lymphocytic leukemia in an infant. Acta Pediatr. Scand. 61:213, 1972.
267. Schade, H., Schoeller, L., and Schultze, K. W.: D-trisomie (Paetau Syndrom) mit kongenitaler myeloischer Leukaemie. Med Welt 50:2690, 1962.
268. Schaller, J.: Arthritis as a presenting manifestation of malignancy in children. J. Pediatr. 81:793, 1972.
269. Schimpff, S. C., Wiernik, P. H., and Block, J. B.: Rectal abscesses in cancer patients. Lancet 2:844, 1972.
270. Schmalzl, F., and Braunsteiner, H.: On the origin of monocytes. Acta Haematol. 39:177, 1968.
271. Schultz, J., and Schwartz, S.: The chemistry of experimental chloroma. Cancer Res. 16:565, 1956.
272. Schwartz, A. D., Zelson, J. H., et al.: Acute myelogenous leukemia with compensatory but ineffective erythropoiesis: DiGuglielmo's syndrome. J. Pediatr. 77:653, 1970.
273. Scott, R. B., Ellison, R. R., and Ley, A. B.: A clinical study of 20 cases of erythroleukemia (DiGuglielmo's syndrome). Am. J. Med. 37:162, 1964.
274. Seeler, R. A., and Hahn, K. O.: Chronic granulocytic leukemia responding to melphelan. Cancer 27:284, 1971.
275. Selawry, O. S.: New treatment schedule with improved survival in childhood leukemia: Intermittent parenteral vs. daily oral administration of methotrexate for maintenance of induced remission. J.A.M.A. 194:75, 1965.
276. Selawry, O. S., Hananian, J., Wolman, I. J., et al.: Cooperative study: new treatment schedule with improved survival in childhood leukemia—intermittent parenteral vs. daily oral administration of methotrexate for maintenance of induced remission. J.A.M.A. 194:75, 1965.
277. Sharp, H. L., Nesbit, M. E., White, J. G., and Krivit, W.: Renal and hepatic pathology following initial remission of acute leukemia induced by prednisone. Cancer 20:1395, 1967.
278. Shapiro, W., Young, D., and Mehta, B.: Methotrexate distribution in cerebrospinal fluid after intravenous, ventricular, and lumbar injections. N. Engl. J. Med. 293:161, 1975.
279. Shaw, M. T.: "Pure" monocytic leukemia: a revised concept. Proc. Am. Assoc. Cancer Res. 15:162, 1974.
280. Shaw, M. T.: The cytochemistry of acute leukemia: A diagnostic and prognostic evaluation. Semin. Oncol. 3:219, 1976.
281. Sheets, R. F., Drevets, C. C., et al.: Erythroleukemia (DiGuglielmo's syndrome). A report of clinical observations and experimental studies in seven patients. Arch. Intern. Med. 111:295, 1963.
282. Sherman, N. J., Williams, K., and Wooley, M. M.: Surgical complications in the patient with leukemia. J. Pediatr. Surg. 8:235, 1973.
283. Sherman, N. J., and Wooley, M. W.: The ileocecal syndrome in acute childhood leukemia. Arch. Surg. 107:39, 1973.
284. Shohet, S. B., and Blum, S. F.: Coincident basophilic chronic myelogenous leukemia and pulmonary tuberculosis. Cancer 22:173, 1968.
285. Simmons, C. R., Harle, T. S., and Singleton, E. B.: The osseous manifestations of leukemia in children. Radiol. Clin. North Am. 6:115, 1968.
286. Simone, J. V.: Treatment of children with acute lymphocytic leukemia. Adv. Pediatr. 19:13, 1972.
287. Simone, J. V.: Factors that influence haematological remission duration in acute lymphocytic leukaemia. Brit. J. Haematol. 32:465, 1976.
288. Simone, J. V., Holland, E., and Johnson, W.: Fatalities during remission of childhood leukemia. Blood 39:759, 1972.
289. Simone, J. V., Verzosa, M. S., and Rudy, J.

A.: Initial features and prognosis in 363 children with acute lymphocytic leukemia. Cancer 36:2099, 1975.
290. Simonsen, L., and Fernbach, D. J.: Personal communication. In Sullivan, M. P. and Hrgovcic, M.: Extramedullary leukemia (Sutow, W. W., Vietti, T. J., Fernbach, D. J. (eds.): Clinical Pediatric Oncology.) St. Louis, C. V. Mosby Co., 1973.
291. Sinks, L. F., Newton, W. A., Jr., Nagi, N. A., and Stevenson, T. D.: A syndrome associated with extreme hyperuricemia in leukemia. J. Pediatr. 68:578, 1966.
292. Sinn, C. M., and Dick, F. W.: Monocytic leukemia. Am. J. Med. 20:588, 1956.
293. Skipper, H. E., and Perry, S.: Kinetics of normal and leukemic leukocyte populations — relevance to chemotherapy. Cancer Res. 30:183, 1970.
294. Smith, C. H.: Leukemia in childhood with onset simulating rheumatic disease. J. Pediatr. 7:390, 1935.
295. Smith, K. L., and Johnson, W.: Classification of chronic myelocytic leukemia in children. Cancer 34:670, 1974.
296. Smith, P. G., Pike, M. C., Till, M. M., and Hardisty, R. M.: Epidemiology of childhood leukaemia in greater London: a search for evidence of transmission assuming a possibly long latent period. Brit. J. Cancer 33:1, 1976.
297. Soni, S., Marten, G. W., Pitner, S. E., et al.: Effects of central nervous system irradiation on neuropsychologic functioning of children with acute lymphocytic leukemia. N. Engl. J. Med. 293:113, 1975.
298. Sonley, M. J., Nesbit, M. E., Samuels, L., Thatcher, L. G., Karon, M., and Hammond, G. D.: Cytosine arabinoside, cyclophosphamide, and vincristine in children with acute myelogenous leukemia. Thirteenth Annual Meeting of the American Society of Hematology, December, 1970, p. 104.
298a. Spitzer, G., and Garson, O. M.: Lymphoblastic leukemia with marked eosinophila: a report of two cases. Blood 42:377, 1973.
299. Stark, C. R., and Mantel, N.: Temporal-spatial distribution of birth dates for Michigan children with leukemia. Cancer Res. 27:1749, 1967.
300. Starling, K. L., Lane, D. M., Sutow, W. W., Monto, R. W., and Thurman, W. G.: Third and fourth remission induction with prednisone (NSC-10023) and vincristine (NSC-67574) in children with acute leukemia. Cancer Chemother. Rep. 54:293, 1970.
301. Stein, R. C.: Hypercalcemia in leukemia. J. Pediatr. 78:861, 1971.
302. Stewart, A., and Kneale, G. W.: Radiation dose effects in relation to obstetric x-rays and childhood cancers. Lancet 1:1185, 1970.
303. Stoffel, T. J., Nesbit, M. E., and Levitt, S. H.: Extramedullary involvement of the testes in childhood leukemia. Cancer 35:1203, 1975.
304. Strodes, C. H., Hyde, E. F., Pan, S. F., et al.: Cytogenetic studies during remission of blastic crisis in a patient with chronic myelocytic leukemia. Scand. J. Haemat. 10:130, 1973.
305. Sullivan, M. P., and Hrgovcic, M.: Extramedullay leukemia. In Sutow, W. W., Vietti, T. J., and Fernbach, D. J. (eds.): Clinical Pediatric Oncology. St. Louis, C.V. Mosby Co., 1973, pp. 227-251.
306. Sullivan, M. P., et al.: Combination interathecal therapy for meningeal leukemia: two vs. three drugs. American Association for Cancer Research, 66th Annual Meeting, San Diego, California, 1975 (Abstr. 340).
307. Tallal, L., et al.: E. coli L-asparaginase in the treatment of leukemia and solid tumors in 131 children. Cancer 25:306, 1970.
308. Tan, C., Etcubanas, E., Wollner, N., Rosen, G., Gilladoga, A., Showel, J., Murphy, M. L., and Krakoff, I. H.: Adriamycin — an antitumor antibiotic in the treatment of neoplastic diseases. Cancer 32:9, 1973.
309. Tanaka, K. R., Valentine, W. N., and Fredericks, R. E.: Diseases or clinical conditions associated with low leukocyte alkaline phosphatase. N. Engl. J. Med. 262:912, 1960.
310. Temin, H. M., and Mizutani, S.: RNA-dependent DNA polymerase in virions of Rous sarcoma virus. Nature 226:1211, 1970.
311. Thiersch, J. B.: Attempted transmission of human leukemia in man. J. Lab. Clin. Med. 30:866, 1945.
312. Thomas, E. D., Herman, E. C., Jr., Greenough, W. B., III, et al.: Irradiation and marrow infusion in leukemia. Arch. Intern. Med. 107:829, 1961.
313. Thomas, E. D., Bryant, J. I., Buckner, C. D., et al.: Leukaemic transformation of engrafted human marrow cells in vivo. II. Lancet 1:1310, 1972.
314. Thomas, E. D., Storb, R., Clift, R. A., et al.: Bone marrow transplantation. N. Engl. J. Med. 292:832, 895, 1975.
315. Thomas, E. D., Buckner, C. D., Banaji, M., et al.: One hundred patients with acute leukemia treated by chemotherapy, total body irradiation and allogenic marrow transplantation. Blood 49:511, 1977.
315a. Thomas, E. D., Fefer, A., Buckner, C. D., and Storb, R.: Current status of bone marrow transplantation for aplastic ane-

mia and acute leukemia. Blood 49:671, 1977.
316. Thomas, L. B., Forkner, C. E., Jr., Frei, E., III, Besse, B. E., Jr., and Stabenau, J. R.: The skeletal lesions of acute leukemia. Cancer 14:608, 1961.
317. Till, M. M., Hardisty, R. M., Pike, M. C., et al.: Childhood leukaemia in greater London: a search for evidence of clustering. Brit. Med. J. 3:755, 1967.
318. Till, M. M., Jones, J. H., Pentycross, C. R., Hardisty, R. M., Lawler, S. D., Harvey, B. A. M., and Soothill, J. F.: Leukaemia in children and their grandparents: studies of immune function in six families. Brit. J. Haematol. 29:575, 1975.
319. Tivey, H.: The natural history of untreated acute leukemia. Ann. N.Y. Acad. Sci. 60:322, 1954.
319a. Todaro, G. J., and Huebner, R. J.: The viral oncogene hypothesis: new evidence. Proc. Natl. Acad. Sci. USA 69:1009, 1972.
320. Traggis, D. G., Dohlwitz, A., Das, L., Jaffe, N., Moloney, W. C., and Hall, T. C.: Cytosine arabinoside in acute leukemia in childhood. Cancer 28:815, 1971.
321. Tsukimoto, I., Wong, K. Y., and Lampkin, B. C.: Surface markers and prognostic factors in acute lymphoblastic leukemia. N. Engl. J. Med. 294:245, 1976.
322. Van Eys, J., and Flexner, J. M.: Transient spontaneous remission in a case of untreated congenital leukemia. Amer. J. Dis. Child. 118:507, 1969.
323. Verzosa, M., and Fite, A.: Efficacy and morbidity of daunomycin (NSC-82151) added to vincristine (NSC-67574) and prednisone (NSC-10023) for remission induction of childhood acute lymphocytic leukemia. Cancer Chemother. Rep. 55:79, 1971.
324. Vietti, T. J., Ragab, A. H., and Land, V. J.: Management of acute leukemia. In Sutow, W. W., Viette, T. J., and Fernbach, D. J. (eds.): Clinical Pediatric Oncology. St. Louis, C. V. Mosby Co., 1973, pp. 194–226.
325. Viza, D. C., Bernard-Degani, O., Bernard, C., and Harris, R.: Leukemia antigens. Lancet 2:493, 1969.
326. Vodopick, H., Rupp, E. M., Edwards, C. L., Goswitz, F. A., and Beauchamp, J. J.: Spontaneous cyclic leukocytosis and thrombocytosis in chronic granulocytic leukemia. N. Engl. J. Med. 286:284, 1972.
327. Wagner, M. L., Rosenberg, H. S., Fernbach, D. J., and Singleton, E. B.: Typhlitis: a complication of leukemia in childhood. Am. J. Roentgenol. Radium Ther. Nucl. Med. 109:341, 1970.
328. Walters, T. R., Bushmore, M., and Simone, J.: Poor prognosis in Negro children with acute lymphocytic leukemia. Cancer 29:210, 1972.
329. Wang, J. J., Cortes, E., Sinks, L. F., and Holland, J. F.: Therapeutic effect and toxicity of Adriamycin in patients with neoplastic disease. Cancer 28:837, 1971.
330. Weatherall, D. J., Edwards, J. A., and Donohoe, W. T. A.: Haemoglobin and red cell enzyme changes in juvenile myeloid leukaemia. Brit. Med. J. 1:679, 1968.
331. Weil, M., Jacquillat, C., Boiron, M., et al.: Combination of arabinosyl cytosine, methyl-glyoxalbis-guanylhydrozone, 6-mercaptopurine, and prednisone in the treatment of acute myelocytic leukemia. Eur. J. Cancer 5:271, 1969.
332. Weil, M., Jacquillat, C. I., and Gemon-Auclerc, M. F.: Acute granulocytic leukemia. Treatment of the disease. Arch. Intern. Med. 136:1389, 1976.
333. Weinberger, M. M., and Oleinick, A.: Congenital marrow dysfunction in Down's syndrome. J. Pediatr. 77:273, 1970.
334. Whang, J., Frei, E., III, Tjio, J. H., Carbone, P. P., and Brecher, G.: The distribution of the Philadelphia chromosome in patients with chronic myelocytic leukemia. Blood 22:664, 1963.
335. Whang-Peng, J., Canellos, G. P., Carbone, P. P., and Tjio, J. H.: Clinical implications of cytogenetic variants in chronic myelocytic leukemia (CML). Blood 32:755, 1968.
336. Whitehouse, J. M. A., Crowther, D., Bateman, C. J. T., Beard, M. E. J., and Malpas, J. S.: Adriamycin in the treatment of acute leukaemia. Brit. Med. J. 1:482, 1972.
337. Wiernik, P. H.: Management of the acute leukemia patient. Conn. Med. 39:681, 1975.
338. Wilhyde, D. E., Jane, J. A., and Mullan, S.: Spinal epidural leukemia. Am. J. Med. 34:281, 1963.
339. Wills, M. R., and Fraser, I. D.: Spurious hyperkalemia. J. Clin. Pathol. 17:649, 1964.
340. Willson, J. K. V.: The bone lesions of childhood leukemia. A survey of 140 cases. Radiology 72:672, 1959.
341. Wilson, J. D., and Nossal, G. J. V.: Identification of human T and B lymphocytes in normal peripheral blood and in chronic lymphocytic leukemia. Lancet 2:788, 1971.
342. Windeyer, B. W., and Stewart, J. W.: The leukaemias. In Cade, S.: Malignant Disease and Its Treatment by Radium. Baltimore, Williams & Wilkins Co., 1952.
343. Wolcott, G. J., Grunnet, M. L., and Lahey,

M. E.: Spinal subdural hematoma in a leukemia child. J. Pediatr. 77:1060, 1970.
344. Wolff, L. J., Richardson, S. T., Neiburger, J. B., et al.: Poor prognosis of children with acute lymphocytic leukemia and increased cell markers. J. Pediatr. 89:956, 1976.
345. Wolk, J. A., Stuart, M. J., Davey, F. R., and Nelson, D. A.: Congenital and neonatal leukemia—lymphocytic or myelocytic? Amer. J. Dis. Child. 128:864, 1974.
346. Whitecar, J. P., Jr., Bodey, G. P., Freireich, E. J., III: Combination chemotherapy (COAP) of adult acute leukemia. Proc. Am. Assoc. Cancer Res. 11:83, 1970.
347. Yam, L. T., Li, C. Y., and Crosby, W. H.: Cytochemical identification of monocytes and granulocytes. Am. J. Clin. Pathol. 55:283, 1971.
347a. Young, J. L., Jr., and Miller, R. W.: Incidence of malignant tumors in U.S. Children. J. Pediatr. 86:254, 1975.
348. Zuelzer, W. W.: Implications of long-term survival in acute stem cell leukemia in childhood treated with composite cyclic therapy. Blood 24:477, 1964.
349. Zusman, J., Brown, D. M., et al.: Hyperphosphatemia, hyperphosphaturia, and hypocalcemia in acute lymphoblastic leukemia. N. Engl. J. Med. 289:1335, 1973.

Chapter Nine

HODGKIN'S DISEASE

Hodgkin's disease is a disorder of unknown etiology affecting lymphoid tissue. For a lymphoma to be characterized as Hodgkin's disease, abnormal giant binucleate cells (Reed-Sternberg cells, to be described below) must be present in association with significant distortion of lymphoid architecture. The diversity of the morphologic findings, however, in both the number and the appearance of Reed-Sternberg cells and in the accompanying inflammatory cellular proliferation and degree of fibrosis are such that one may question whether Hodgkin's disease may be regarded as a single entity.

Hodgkin's disease is considered to be of neoplastic nature because: (1) if untreated, it will spread throughout the lymphatic system and eventually involve nonlymphoid tissues, (2) it responds to treatment with agents usually utilized for the treatment of malignancies, (3) fresh biopsy material and short term cultures of such biopsies show aneuploidy and marker chromosomes in Hodgkin's cells, and (4) inoculation of cultured Hodgkin's cells into congenitally athymic ("nude") mice results in the development of neoplastic infiltrates.[72, 139]

EPIDEMIOLOGY

Hodgkin's disease has a unique bimodal distribution curve with peaks in young adults (15 to 34 years) and in older adults (over 50 years).[85] The annual incidence in United States children under 15 years is 0.4 per 100,000, with approximately equal rates in black and white children.[135]

Unlike most childhood neoplasms, there is no peak in incidence of Hodgkin's disease in children under 5 years of age—indeed, it is unusual for the disease to occur in a child of less than 5 years of age and rare under 2 years of age. The incidence increases with advancing age through childhood and the pattern of this increase appears to correlate with the economic development of the community. Three different patterns have been described:[26a]

Pattern I Seen in developing countries or in communities with a low economic level; characterized by an early incidence peak before the age of 15 years with only a moderate increase through adolescence and young adulthood.

Pattern II Seen in rural areas of developed countries and in Central Europe; characterized by moderate rates in both childhood and adolescence.

Pattern III Seen in urban areas of developed countries; characterized by a low incidence in childhood followed by a sharp increase during adolescence and reaching a peak by age 30.

The incidence of Hodgkin's disease increases more rapidly among boys than girls until 10 to 12 years of age, when the frequencies tend to converge[42] (Fig. 9–1); this results in approximately a 3:1 preponderance of males in the under-14-years age group with Hodgkin's disease (85 per cent of patients 10 years of age or younger are male), while in older age groups both sexes appear to be equally represented.[85]

Some epidemiologic features (particularly of pediatric Hodgkin's disease) suggest an infectious etiology. These include (1) an overall positive association between Hodgkin's disease and prior tonsillectomy (risk factor between 1.2- and 3.6-fold)[130] and possible relationship between tonsillar involution and the sharp increase seen in Hodgkin's disease mortality rates after 11 years of age,[87] (2) the occurrence of Hodgkin's disease clusters — the best known of these is the grouping of 31 cases of Hodgkin's disease and three cases of other lymphomas in a group of students at one Albany, New York, high school between the period 1948 and 1971,[128] (3) higher mortality from Hodgkin's disease in teachers[86] and physicians (in upstate New York,[129] but not Great Britain[113]) who would presumably have above-average contact with Hodgkin's disease patients, and (4) evidence from family studies of a three- to sevenfold increase in risk of developing the disease for children, parents, and siblings of Hodgkin's disease patients.[55, 103] The fact that the time intervals between diagnoses are shorter than the age differences between the family members (particularly for family members living in the same household) has been interpreted as indicative of an environmental (?infectious) rather than genetic influence to explain the familial incidence of the disease;[130] evidence that siblings of the

Figure 9–1 Age at diagnosis of Hodgkin's disease of 314 children in a multi-hospital series. (From Fraumeni, J. F., Jr., and Li, F. P.: J. Nat. Cancer Inst. 42:681, 1969.)

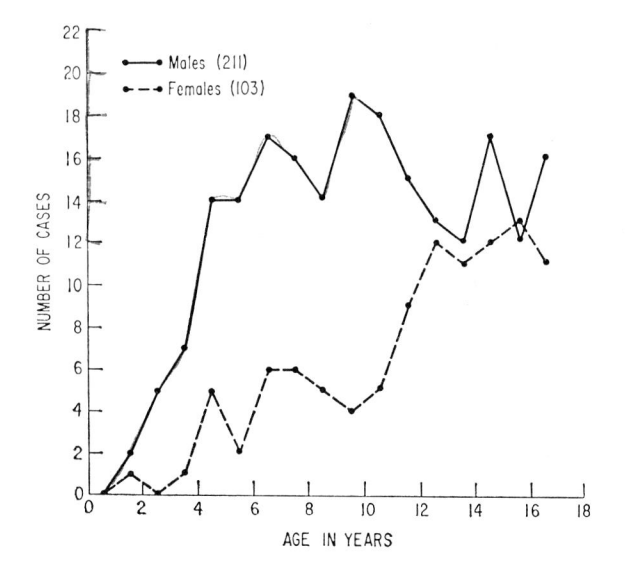

same sex as the patient have twice the risk of developing the disease as siblings of the opposite sex also may be interpreted as favoring an infectious rather than a genetic mechanism, since siblings of the same sex may have more acquaintances and experiences in common than do those of the opposite sex.[55]

Many of the above studies have been questioned from a statistical standpoint on the basis of a possible underascertainment of cases and inappropriate use of proportionate mortality analysis,[114] and none of them provides unequivocal evidence for an infectious or environmental basis for Hodgkin's disease or for transmission by person-to-person contact. Even if an infectious agent is eventually implicated in Hodgkin's disease, the chance of acquiring the disease by contact seems to be extremely slight, as is demonstrated by the absence of high frequency among marital partners exposed to the condition.

Gutensohn and Cole[55a] have recently proposed an infectious disease model for Hodgkin's disease based on the epidemiologic similarities between it and paralytic poliomyelitis. For both diseases there is an increased incidence associated with higher social class and small family size, and the age-incidence pattern varies according to the economic development of the community. In the case of poliomyelitis, paralysis rarely accompanies infection before the age of 5 years, but the probability that this complication will develop increases if the infection is acquired during adolescence or early adulthood. Likewise, Hodgkin's disease may be a rare manifestation of a common infection with the probability of developing the disease increasing as age at time of infection is delayed.

Other factors that may be associated with increased risk of developing Hodgkin's disease are: genetic susceptibility,[83] presence of certain HL-A antigens of the 4C group,[38] Italian and Jewish ancestry,[85] and certain congenital immunodeficiency states (ataxia-telangiectasia, Swiss-type agammaglobulinemia).[130]

ETIOLOGY AND PATHOGENESIS

Many of the clinical features of Hodgkin's disease suggest an infectious etiology. Patients frequently suffer from fevers, night sweats, and weight loss; there may also be an accompanying leukocytosis as well as the presence of inflammatory cells in the involved tissues. Although many infectious agents, including bacteria (mycobacteria, diphtheroids, spirochetes, brucella), parasites, fungi, and viruses have been proposed as the etiologic agent of Hodgkin's disease, none has been conclusively implicated. Recently, significant elevations in the mean antibody titer to Epstein-Barr (EB) virus have been found in a group of patients with Hodgkin's disease;[75] this relationship is intriguing, since EB virus has also been associated with Burkitt's lymphoma and infectious mononucleosis—diseases in which Reed-Sternberg cells have also been found. However, an etiologic relationship cannot be determined at the present time and it is possible that the virus may infect the cells secondarily after the malignant transformation has taken place.

Order and Hellman have proposed a hypothesis to relate viral infection to the pathogenesis of Hodgkin's disease by means of a chronic immune reaction.[98] According to this hypothesis, viral infection of T-lymphocytes (thymus-derived) leads to antigenic alteration of their surfaces, causing them to appear "foreign" to the rest of the lymphoid system. Normal immunocompetent T-cells then react against these antigenically altered cells and produce a chronic immune reaction, with wasting, anemia, lymphocyte depletion, immunologic defects, and susceptibility to infections similar to graft-versus-host disease.[65] Chronic graft-versus-host disease in experimental animals is known to induce malignant lymphoma and the appearance of abnormal "reticulum" cells,[110] and a similar mechanism is proposed for the appearance of neoplastic "reticulum" cells (including their end-stage multinucleated form, the Reed-Sternberg cell) in Hodgkin's disease. The progressive involvement of T-cells by viral transformation and in the chronic immune reaction could also result in the T-cell depletion and impairment of T-cell function seen in Hodgkin's disease.

Tindle and associates have also suggested that Hodgkin's disease is the culmination of a chronic immune reaction. However, they regard the neoplastic Hodgkin's cells as a persistent clone of abnormal transformed B-lymphocytes ("immunoblasts"), whose proliferative reaction has gone out of control.[124] DeVita, on the other hand, has suggested that the B-cell population in patients with Hodgkin's disease is basically normal, but is reacting to a T-lymphocyte that has been antigenically altered and transformed (into a malignant cell) by a virus.[30] Indeed, the fact that spleen fragments from patients with Hodgkin's disease produce immunoglobulins which have a high affinity for homologous peripheral blood lymphocytes[78] suggests that a tumor-associated antigen may be binding to T-lymphocytes.[30]

HISTOPATHOLOGY

Lymph nodes involved by Hodgkin's disease may exhibit a variety of cell types. It is possible to categorize these into two major groups: (1) reactive, inflammatory, or stromal cellular elements, and (2) malignant cellular elements (Hodgkin's cells) — one variant of which is the Reed-Sternberg cell.

REACTIVE, INFLAMMATORY, OR STROMAL CELLULAR ELEMENTS

Unlike the case for most other malignancies, the malignant mononuclear elements of Hodgkin's disease rarely occur in solidly packed sheets. Instead they occur singly or in small clusters, surrounded by a much larger mass of inflammatory and stromal elements. Thus, the obliteration of normal lymph node architecture is due predominantly to the accumulation of "nonmalignant" cells, among which are lymphocytes of various sizes, transformed lymphocytes ("immunoblasts"), histiocytes, eosinophils, plasma cells, and fibroblasts.

The role of these reactive cells is obscure. It has been speculated that the lymphoid elements (a high proportion of which are actively synthesizing DNA) represent an immune response to a powerful antigenic stimulus, a situation somewhat analogous to the benign, self-limiting proliferation seen in infectious mononucleosis;[69, 99] the histiocytes, on the other hand, do not appear to be engaged in a proliferative response. The fibroblasts are responsible for the bands of connective tissue deposited in the nodular sclerosis variant and are also seen in increased numbers in the lymphocyte depletion variant. Connective tissue is observed in two distinctive forms: (a) orderly distributed interconnecting collagen bands (nodular sclerosis type) and (b) irregularly distributed finely fibrillar connective tissue or compact proteinaceous material that resembles precollagen (lymphocyte depletion type).[80]

In addition to the cellular infiltrates, necrosis is a not infrequent feature of some forms of Hodgkin's disease, varying in extent from minute foci of fibrinoid necrosis to large areas of granular tissue destruction. These foci of necrosis are frequently surrounded by Hodgkin's cells.

MALIGNANT CELLULAR ELEMENTS (HODGKIN'S CELLS)

The mitotically active Hodgkin's cell is a large mononuclear cell with abundant, vacuolated pale blue cytoplasm, large basophilic nucleoli, and a strong affinity for methyl green–pyronine (*pyroninophilia*). Since morphologically similar mononuclear cells occasionally are found in reactive and inflammatory lymphadenopathies (particularly those of viral etiology), these cells cannot be considered diagnostic per se of Hodgkin's disease. The diagnostic cell is the *Reed-Sternberg cell* (Fig. 9–2), a large cell with abundant acidophilic to amphophilic cytoplasm and a bilobed (or multilobed) nucleus containing large, prominent nucleoli; both the nucleoli and the cytoplasm are vividly pyroninophilic. This cell appears to be a nonproliferating, end-stage derivative of the Hodgkin's cell.[99] The Reed-Sternberg cell, however, is not unique to Hodgkin's disease, for cells of similar appearance have been reported in infectious mononucleosis, "pseudolymphomatous" adenopathy associated with chronic phenytoin (Dilantin) administration, rubeola, thymoma, and non-Hodgkin's lymphomas;[119] its presence therefore is necessary, but not sufficient, for the diagnosis of Hodgkin's disease. An appropriate stromal reaction must be present as well.

The majority of the large abnormal cells found in Hodgkin's disease are not typical Reed-Sternberg cells but are variants of it, and these variants appear to correlate with the histologic patterns of the disease (to be discussed in a subsequent section). In general, the number of typical Reed-Sternberg cells varies inversely with the intensity of lymphocyte proliferation. Thus, when lymphocyte proliferation is prominent, characteristic Reed-Sternberg cells are rare, whereas when lymphocyte numbers are depleted, typical Reed-Sternberg cells become more apparent.

Lineage of the Hodgkin's Cell

The lineage of the Hodgkin's cell remains controversial. The three candidates for its precursor are the histio-

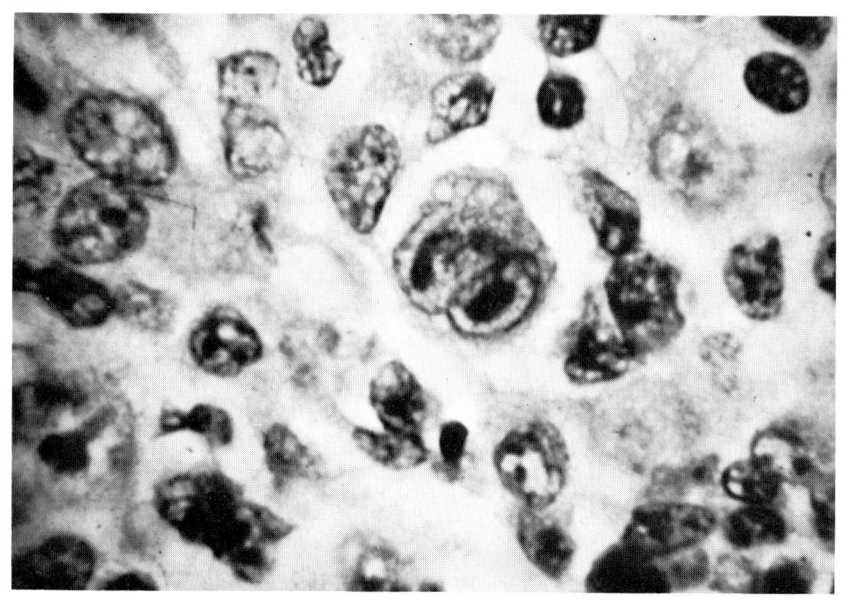

Figure 9–2 A Reed-Sternberg cell.

cyte (monocyte/macrophage), the B-lymphocyte, and the T-lymphocyte.

In the past the Hodgkin's cell was considered to be a "histiocytic" or "reticulum" cell on the basis of its morphologic appearance.[41] Studies by Kaplan and co-workers have tended to support this hypothesis because their cultures of cell suspensions and tissue mince fragments from spleens involved by Hodgkin's disease have produced a population of cells in vitro which have the morphologic appearance of macrophages as well as many of their functional attributes (phagocytic activity, surface markers, adherence properties).[72, 72a] On the other hand, histochemical studies of the mononuclear Hodgkin's cell and of the Reed-Sternberg cell fail to demonstrate significant activity of the enzymes considered characteristic of the histiocyte line (acid phosphatase, nonspecific esterases, and other lysozomal enzymes);[32, 134] instead these cells exhibit the strong reaction with methyl green–pyronine (pyroninophilia) that is characteristic of lymphoid cells.[134]

Tindle and associates, in observing the evolution of Reed-Sternberg-like cells in infectious mononucleosis, suggested that this cell could be traced from an innocuous-appearing small transformed B-lymphocyte precursor ("immunoblast").[124] The demonstration of intracellular immunoglobulin components within some Reed-Sternberg cells,[122] as well as the demonstration of surface immunoglobulins on Hodgkin's cells grown in vitro from pleural effusions,[12] provides further evidence for a relationship to the B-lymphocyte line.

Evidence for a T-cell origin for the Hodgkin's cell has come from ultrastructural studies that show marked similarities between Reed-Sternberg cells and the "transformed" lymphocytes found in normal lymph node follicular centers and in T-cell lymphomas.[49]

LYMPH NODE ARCHITECTURE

Lymph nodes involved by Hodgkin's disease show either partial or total obliteration of normal follicular and sinusoidal architecture by a diffuse and frequently mixed infiltration of lymphocytes, histiocytes, plasma cells, eosinophils, neutrophils, and Hodgkin's cells. The histologic subclassification of the disease is based primarily on the variations in the cellular composition of this infiltrate and particularly on the degree of lymphocytic or histiocytic involvement (Table 9–1).

The four subclassifications of Hodgkin's disease are: (1) *lymphocyte pre-*

Table 9–1 Histologic Subtypes of Hodgkin's Disease[81]

	LYMPHOCYTE PREDOMINANCE	NODULAR SCLEROSIS	MIXED CELLULARITY	LYMPHOCYTE DEPLETION
Lymph node architecture	Obliterated	Focal, partial, or total obliteration	Diffusely obliterated	Partially to totally obliterated
Cellularity	Lymphocytes and histiocytes in varying proportions	Lymphocytic, mixed with fibrosis and lacunar type R-S cells	Varies widely; lymphocytes, histiocytes, eosinophils, plasma cells, and neutrophils may be seen	Generally decreased
Fibrosis	Absent	Varies from a single collagen band to total sclerosis; birefringent	Disorderly	Disorderly, non-birefringent
Necrosis	None	Some	Usually focal	Considerable
Diagnostic R-S cells	Rare	Often rare	Numerous	Rare
R-S cell variant	Polypoid type	Lacunar type	—	Pleomorphic type
Prognosis	Excellent	Good	Fair	Poor

Table 9–2 Distribution of Histologic Subtypes in Pediatric Hodgkin's Disease[52]

Histology Diagnosis	Frequency (Per Cent)
Lymphocyte predominance	19
Nodular sclerosis	50*
Mixed cellularity	26
Lymphocyte depletion	5

*In the very young child the preponderance of this histologic type is even more marked; in one study, 63 per cent of children in the first decade of life had nodular sclerosis histology.[120]

dominance, (2) *nodular sclerosis*, (3) *mixed cellularity*, (4) *lymphocyte depletion*. Their relative frequency in childhood is shown in Table 9–2.

Lymphocyte Predominance (Fig. 9–3)

This form of Hodgkin's disease is characterized by an abundant proliferation of mature lymphocytes and reactive histiocytes and a relative paucity of Reed-Sternberg cells. Commonly seen, however, are abnormal large cells with polypoid, twisted nuclei, delicate nuclear chromatin, and small nucleoli. These are considered variants of the Reed-Sternberg cell.[80] A nodular or diffuse pattern may be present. Necrosis is not evident. The disease is usually localized at discovery and frequently presents as cervical adenopathy in young males; the prognosis is the most favorable of the Hodgkin's subtypes.

Nodular Sclerosis (Fig. 9–4)

The lymph nodes contain nodules of lymphoid tissue partially or completely separated by orderly bands of collagen of variable width; typical Reed-Sternberg cells are difficult to find, but a variant form of large size with a delicate nucelar chromatin pattern, small eosinophilic nucleoli, a tendency to hyperlobation, and abundant pale cytoplasm with sharply demarcated borders is more frequently found. In formalin-fixed sections these cells give the appearance of being situated in a large, clear space (lacuna); this lacunar effect is produced by apparent collapse of the cytoplasm, creating an artifactual space between the retracted cytoplasm and the plasma membrane. Recently it has been suggested that the presence of lipids in the cytoplasm of these lacunar cells is responsible for their marked cytoplasmic pallor and retraction with formalin fixation.[5a]

Nodular sclerosis is generally a disease of young females. It is usually localized at discovery, being most frequently found in the neck and me-

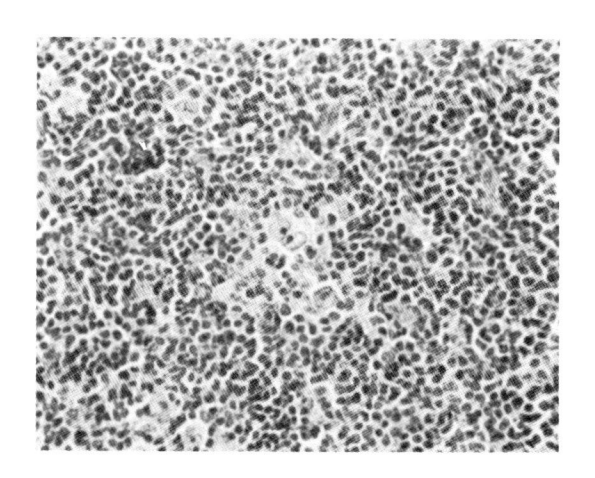

Figure 9–3 Hodgkin's disease. Lymphocyte predominance type (×360), showing abundance of mature lymphocytes, occasional atypical histiocytes, and a rare typical Reed-Sternberg cell. (From Rosenberg, S. A., and Kaplan, H. S.: Calif. Med. *113*:23, 1970. Courtesy of the Western Journal of Medicine.)

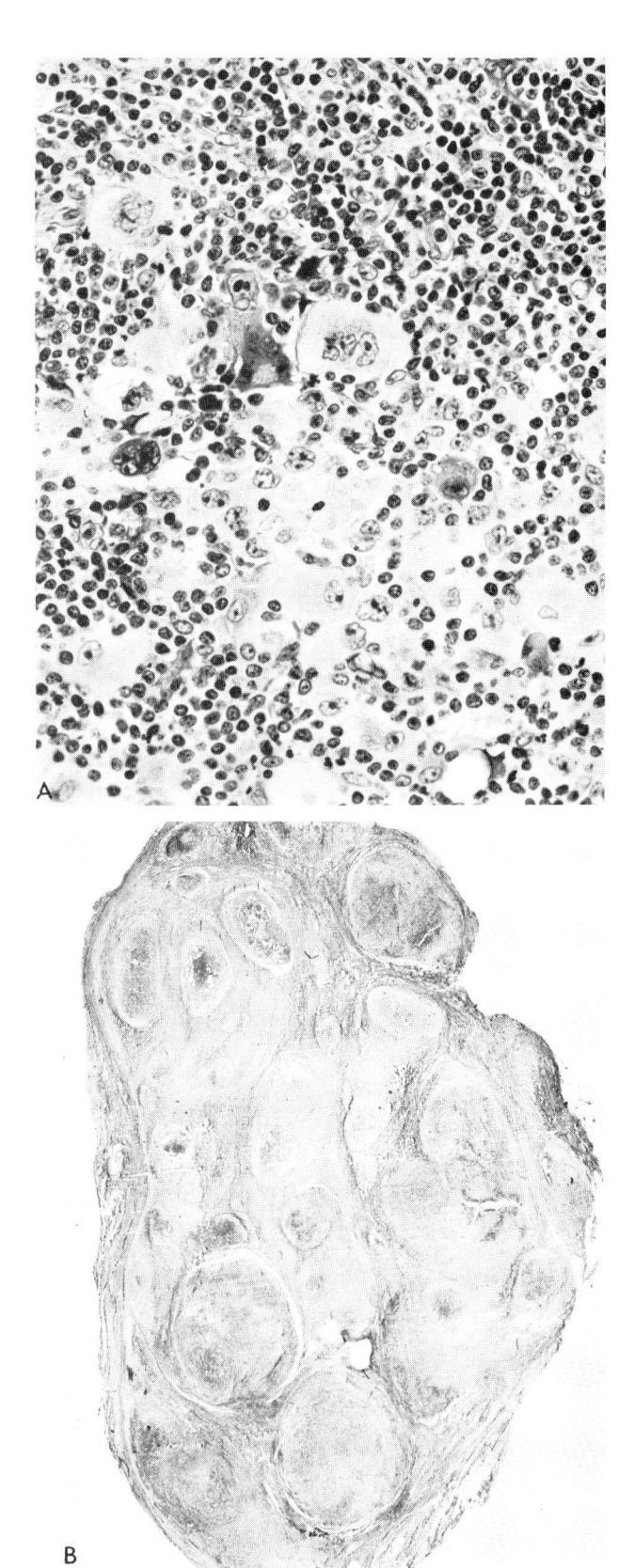

Figure 9–4 Hodgkin's disease. Nodular sclerosis type. *A*, Low power view showing broad collagen bands which divide the lymph node into smaller nodes (H & E, ×8). *B*, High power view showing "lacunar" cells with sharply defined borders and pale cytoplasm (H & E, ×350). (From Lukes, R. J., et al.: Cancer *19*:317, 1966.)

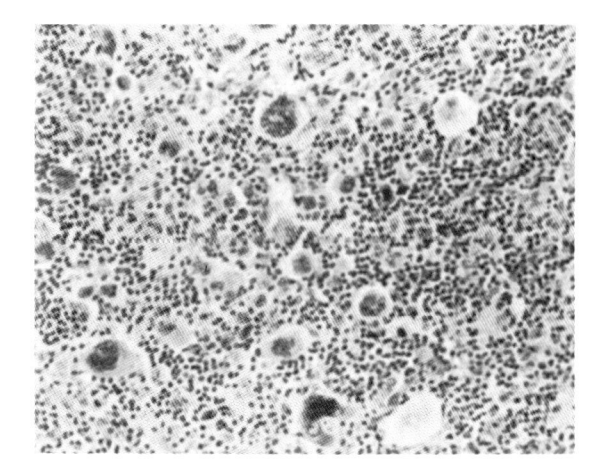

Figure 9–5 Hodgkin's disease. Mixed cellularity type (×360) with pleomorphic cellular infiltrate and frequent Reed-Sternberg cells. (From Rosenberg, S. A., and Kaplan, H. S.: Calif. Med. *113*:23, 1970. Courtesy of The Western Journal of Medicine.)

diastinum (particularly the anterior-superior mediastinum). The prognosis is relatively favorable.

Mixed Cellularity (Fig. 9–5)

This form of Hodgkin's disease is the most pleomorphic variant; its infiltrate consists of numerous neutrophils, eosinophils, lymphocytes, histiocytes, plasma cells, and typical Reed-Sternberg cells. Foci of necrosis are also commonly seen; these may be surrounded by reactive histiocytes and Langhans's giant cells. The prognosis for these patients is less favorable than for the lymphocyte predominance or nodular sclerosis variants.

Lymphocyte Depletion (Fig. 9–6).

This form of Hodgkin's disease manifests diffuse fibrosis and necrosis and a paucity of lymphocytes; Reed-Sternberg cells and large "histiocytic" mononuclear cells are usually numerous. The fibrosis, unlike that seen in nodular sclerosis, is disorderly in character and without collagen band formation. Lymphocyte depletion Hodgkin's disease is associated with a pleomorphic variant of the Reed-Sternberg cell; this variant exhibits a wide range of bizarre morphologic expressions, including extreme variations in nuclear number and configuration and giant nucleoli. Lymphocyte

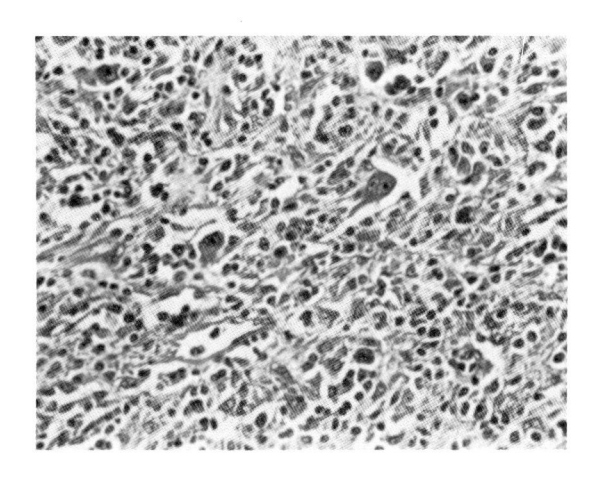

Figure 9–6 Hodgkin's disease. Lymphocyte depletion type (×360) with numerous malignant "histiocytes" and Reed-Sternberg cells but paucity of lymphocytes. (From Rosenberg, S. A., and Kaplan, H. S.: Calif. Med. *113*:23, 1970. Courtesy of The Western Journal of Medicine.)

depletion Hodgkin's disease has the poorest prognosis and may run a very rapid, fulminant course.

EVOLUTION OF HISTOLOGIC PATTERNS

Hodgkin's disease is a complex, evolving process with an apparent overlapping spectrum of the histologic types.[81] Thus, the lymphocyte predominance type of Hodgkin's disease may be transformed into the mixed cellularity type by the addition of other cellular elements (eosinophils, plasma cells, neutrophils), the development of disorderly fibrosis, and a prominent increase in the number of diagnostic Reed-Sternberg cells; this may herald the onset of a change in the disease pattern that is associated with more aggressive behavior and widespread lesions. Mixed cellularity Hodgkin's disease may evolve into lymphocyte depletion type by loss of cellular components other than Reed-Sternberg cells; this usually signals systemic progressive disease of brief duration. This histologic evolution may thus be an expression of the natural history of the disease.

The nodular sclerosis type of Hodgkin's disease appears to be a distinctive variant and does not appear to enter into the orderly progression seen with lymphocyte predominance→ mixed cellularity → lymphocyte depletion. However, nodular sclerosis Hodgkin's disease does have its own progression from a cellular phase with "lacunar" cells through progressive fibrosis to a stage of total sclerosis. In the early phase (cellular phase) of nodular sclerosis, the nodules are composed mainly of lymphocytes and "lacunar" Reed-Sternberg cells, and there is minimal formation of collagen bands. The next phase is associated with the appearance of numerous eosinophils or mature granulocytes and more prominent collagen bands. Eventually the nodule undergoes total sclerosis.

CLINICAL PRESENTATION

In childhood, Hodgkin's disease usually presents as a painless, enlarged, firm (but not hard) superficial lymph node; in 90 per cent of cases the cervical area is primarily involved, but other nodal groups (mediastinal, inguinal, axillary) can occasionally be the initial presenting site.[52] When the right cervical nodes are affected, the mediastinal or hilar nodes appear to be also involved in about 25 per cent of cases, whereas when the left cervical nodes are affected, the abdominal nodes are more likely to be affected and the mediastinum spared. These enlarged nodes may fluctuate in size and frequently the patient will have received one or more courses of antibiotic therapy for presumed infectious lymphadenitis. Unlike the other lymphomas, Hodgkins's disease rarely appears in Waldeyer's ring, Peyer's patches, or epitrochlear nodes.

Not infrequently (10 to 15 per cent) the diagnosis of Hodgkin's disease is made only after a second node is removed weeks or months after an initial node biopsy showed "nondiagnostic" changes.[57] This may reflect poor selection of the initial node or inability of the pathologist to discern the early changes of Hodgkin's disease. In this regard, nodes from cervical and axillary regions (preferably the largest node that has recently enlarged) are more likely to be diagnostic than are those from inguinal, femoral, or submaxillary regions, where chronic infections or inflammatory processes may distort the histologic picture.[57] Likewise, pathologic changes in very small satellite nodes are likely to be secondary to a reactive lymphoid hyperplasia rather than to the tumor itself.

Systemic symptoms such as *malaise, fever, night sweats*, and *weight loss* may also be present in approximately 30 per cent of children;[57] these are much more likely to be seen in advanced stages of the disease. The *fever* of Hodgkin's disease may be intermittent, erratic, recurrent, or sustained; the classic *Pel-Ebstein* cyclic fever with intermittent evening temperature elevations alternating with afebrile periods lasting days or weeks is only rarely seen. Not all fevers in patients with Hodgkin's disease are due to the disease per se—the frequently associated immunologic deficiencies may predispose the patient to infectious complications (Herpes zoster and other viral, protozoal, and opportunistic bacterial infections). *Pruritus* is seen in approximately 15 per cent of adults (particularly in young women with mediastinal nodular sclerosis), but occurs relatively infrequently in children.

Complaints relating to extranodal disease such as cough (pulmonary infiltration), jaundice (hepatic involvement), or abdominal pain (bowel involvement) are unusual as initial presenting complaints. Occasionally a patient will present with obstructive respiratory symptoms secondary to a mediastinal mass (superior vena caval syndrome) or with the serendipitous discovery of a mediastinal mass on chest x-ray.

LABORATORY FEATURES

HEMATOLOGIC FINDINGS

Anemia is a frequent finding and, in most patients, appears to result from a combination of shortened red cell survival time and abnormalities in the utilization of iron for erythropoiesis.[26] The red cells may be either normochromic/normocytic or hypochromic/microcytic in character. Ferrokinetic studies show a picture similar to that seen in patients with chronic inflammatory diseases—i.e, low serum iron, normal iron-binding capacity, and increased stainable iron stores in bone marrow, liver, and spleen, which are poorly mobilized for red cell production.[26, 46] The mechanism for the shortened erythrocyte survival time is not always evident; in some patients it appears to be related to increased red cell destruction by reticuloendothelial cells, particularly those in the spleen. Rarely a Coombs' positive autoimmune hemolytic anemia develops.

Leukocyte abnormalities are also evident in Hodgkin's disease. Neutrophilia occurs in about 50 per cent of patients,[125] and eosinophilia in about 15 to 20 per cent.[63] In some cases the elevations in the granulocyte count may be so extreme as to suggest chronic granulocytic leukemia; however, the fact that leukocyte alkaline phosphatase (LAP) is usually elevated during active phases of Hodgkin's disease is helpful in distinguishing the two conditions. Lymphocytes may be normal in number early in the course, but lymphopenia is a sign of advanced disease. An absolute lymphocytosis is rarely, if ever, seen in Hodgkin's disease and should always prompt reevaluation of the diagnosis.

Many types of large atypical mononuclear cells may be found in the peripheral blood of patients with Hodgkin's disease. Some of these, such as the dark basophilic lymphoid "immunoblasts," are not specific for Hodgkin's disease, for they can be found in normal subjects as well as in patients with infectious mononucleosis, cytomegalovirus disease, and non-Hodgkin's lymphomas.[56] Other large, atypical, moderately basophilic cells with large nucleoli (some of which resemble Reed-Sternberg cells) appear to be more specific for Hodgkin's disease and to be indicative of disseminated disease.[56, 108] The presence of these cells indicates a poor prognosis and may represent final host failure to neutralize circulating tumor cells.[108]

When the bone marrow is diffusely infiltrated by Hodgkin's disease, the picture of a myelophthisic anemia with leukoerythroblastosis may be found. In general, however, the marrow involvement is focal (Fig. 9–7) and often associated with fibrosis due to in-

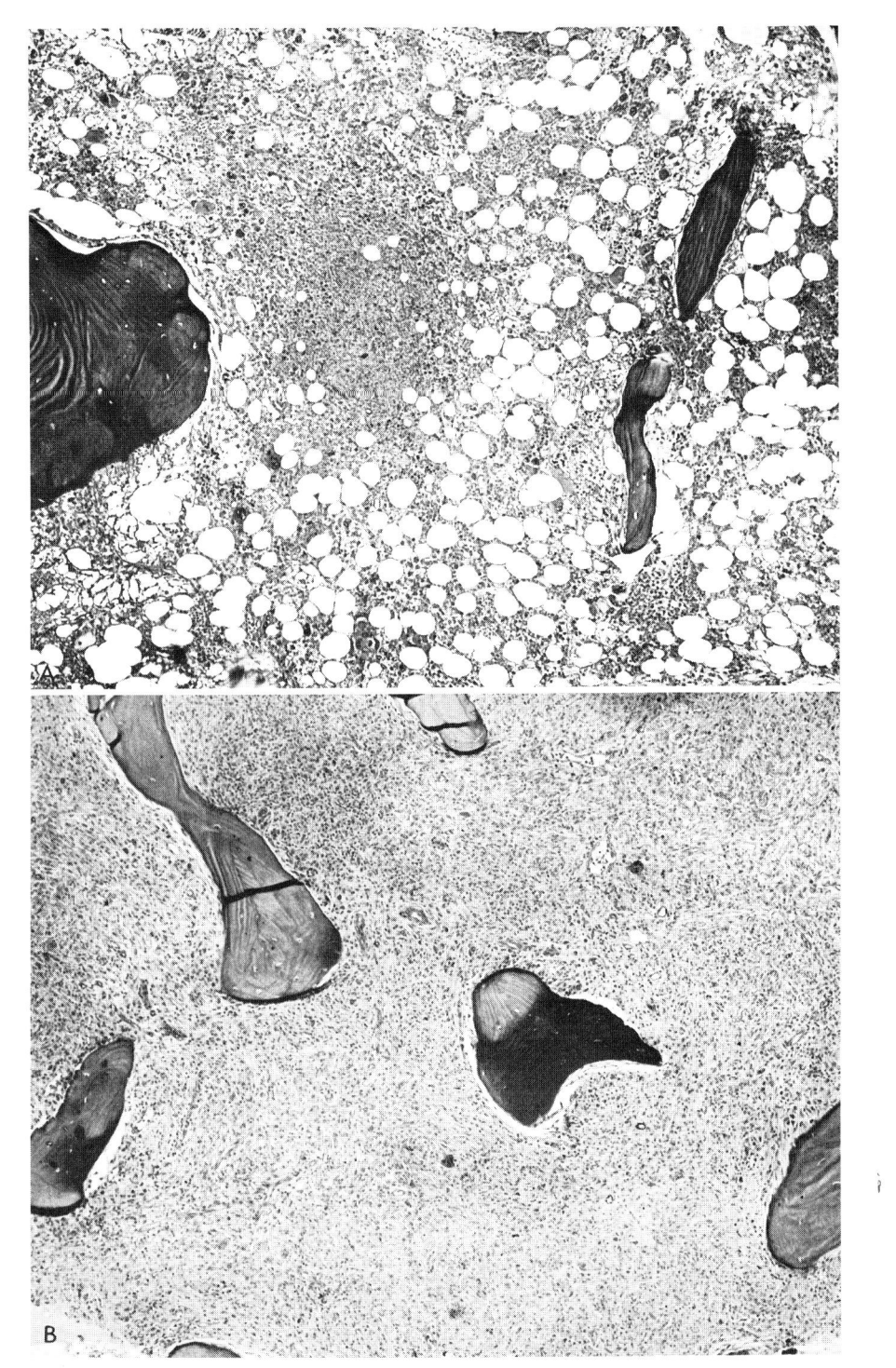

Figure 9-7 *A*, Focal involvement of the bone marrow by Hodgkin's disease (H & E, ×40). *B*, Diffuse involvement of the bone marrow by Hodgkin's disease (H & E, ×40). (From O'Carroll, D. I., et al.: Cancer 38:1717, 1976.)

creased collagen or reticulin. Surprisingly, the diffuse myelofibrosis associated with Hodgkin's involvement is frequently reversible with intensive chemotherapy.[93, 131]

Needle aspiration is usually not satisfactory for diagnosing bone marrow involvement by Hodgkin's foci owing to the patchy nature of the disease and the fact that making smears of the aspirate distorts the granuloma-like architecture of the lesions; furthermore, the fibrous nature of the lesions may make it difficult to aspirate marrow particles. The marrow is, therefore, best studied by multiple needle biopsies or open surgical biopsy. Marrow involvement is found most commonly when the disease is widespread and frequently is accompanied by systemic symptoms, elevated serum alkaline phosphatase, radiologic evidence of bone lesions, or otherwise unexplained pancytopenia.

SEROLOGIC FINDINGS

Among the wide spectrum of serologic studies utilized, the *serum copper level* and the *erythrocyte sedimentation rate* (ESR) are of particular value in evaluating and following patients with Hodgkin's disease.

The *serum copper level* prior to treatment correlates with the stage of the disease and consequently probably reflects the volume (or activity) of involved tissue. It is also of value in the recognition of residual or recurrent disease. Since, with almost no exceptions, the serum copper value returns to normal in complete remission, it has been recommended that this parameter be included in the criteria for complete remission.[123] The serum copper level is also correlated to some extent with the histology of the tumor, the lymphocyte depletion type having the highest values, while the lymphocyte predominance type may not affect the serum copper level at all.[60, 123]

When following the serum copper level in adolescent girls and young women, one must be aware of the fact that estrogens increase the level (often considerably), and consequently contraceptive pills and pregnancy must be considered when there is a sudden increase in serum copper values.[123]

The *ESR* is commonly elevated in patients with active Hodgkin's disease and may fall to normal levels during remission. However it is important to remember that patients with Hodgkin's disease who have been treated with radiotherapy may have higher ESR values (even when they are in remission) than normal, nonirradiated individuals. Thus, while normal children may have an ESR of 4.7 mm/hr, irradiated Hodgkin's disease patients may have values up to 30 mm/hr.[73a] In one study in which this latter value was used as the upper limit of normal, 90 per cent of Hodgkin's disease patients who demonstrated an ESR in excess of this figure (after remission induction) developed clinical evidence of relapse within 4.5 months.[73a] Sometimes an elevated ESR may be the only sign of persistent or recurrent disease; the ESR is persistently elevated when bone is involved with Hodgkin's disease. However, it is a nonspecific finding and may not always be elevated in the face of active disease.

Serum *alkaline phosphatase levels* also correlate to some extent with stage and activity of the disease. With advancing disease the proportion of patients with elevated enzyme levels increases from 14 per cent in Stages I and II to 81 per cent in Stage IV.[3] In the afebrile patient, an elevated serum alkaline phosphatase level may indicate bone or liver involvement; the hepatic isoenzyme is by far the most important cause of the elevation of alkaline phosphatase seen at the onset of Hodgkin's disease.[3] An elevated level of this enzyme must be interpreted with caution, however, as fever may be associated with a nonspecific elevation of the hepatic isoenzyme; this frequently subsides with defervescence. Elevation of the bone isoenzyme in teenagers usually represents a physiologic concomitant of the rapid bone growth of adolescence rather than osseous pathology.[3]

Hypoalbuminemia at the time of diagnosis implies an advanced stage and a resultant debilitated state. The serum protein pattern returns to normal, however, with remission of the disease.[13]

IMMUNOLOGIC FEATURES

Many patients with Hodgkin's disease display a defect in T-lymphocyte cell-mediated immunity which may be manifested by defective delayed hypersensitivity reactions, failure of homograft rejection, and poor response of lymphocytes in vitro to mitogens such as phytohemagglutinin (PHA). B-lymphocyte function, on the other hand, is relatively unimpaired and humoral immunity (as measured by serum immunoglobulin levels and specific antibody synthesis) is preserved until the disease is far advanced.

The impairment of T-cell function in Hodgkin's disease patients appears to be relative rather than absolute. With adjustment of antigen doses one can find a defect in skin-test reactivity and PHA response early in the course of the disease, but total anergy and extensive defects in PHA responsiveness are infrequently found until the disease is far advanced.[77,137] Patients with mixed cellularity and lymphocyte depletion types are more likely to show anergy than are those with the lymphocyte predominance or nodular sclerosis types.[5]

Since absolute T-lymphocyte counts (as measured by cytotoxicity with an anti–T-cell serum) are generally not diminished in patients with untreated Hodgkin's disease until the disease is far advanced, it would thus appear that the defective cellular immunity seen in early Hodgkin's disease is more a consequence of altered T-cell function than of actual absence of these cells. The alteration in function may be related to the masking of the surface of a sizable fraction of peripheral blood T-lymphocytes by a serum low-density lipoprotein factor.[45] Several other potential inhibitors are also increased in the sera of patients with Hodgkin's disease; these include antilymphocyte antibodies,[78] ferritin,[36] and chemotactic-factor inhibitor.[132]

The T-cell defect becomes more severe as the disease advances. Lymphopenia also occurs almost invariably with symptomatic and advanced disease; this lymphopenia, however, does not reflect selective T-cell depletion, but rather a combined T- and B-cell reduction.[10] Thus, humoral immunity becomes impaired as the disease becomes more advanced and the consequent defective antibody synthesis leads to a further compromise of immune function, rendering the patient highly susceptible to a wide variety of infections.

There are three clinical situations in which immunologic testing (Table 9–3) might prove to be of value in Hodgkin's disease patients: (1) as a guide to prognosis and treatment at the onset of the disorder; (2) in following the patient's status while the disease is in apparent remission; and (3) in differentiating Hodgkin's disease from other causes of unexplained fever, lymphadenopathy, or hepatosplenomegaly.

Table 9–3 Immunologic Testing in Hodgkin's Disease

Lymphocyte count
Skin tests
  1. Tuberculin
  2. Streptokinase-streptodornase
  3. Mumps
  4. *Candida albicans*
  5. Histoplasmin
  6. Dinitrochlorobenzene (active sensitization)
In vitro response to phytohemagglutinin and antigens
Immunoglobulin levels

Roentgenographic Features

Since much of the visceral involvement of Hodgkin's disease is beyond the limits of physical examination, a complete radiologic survey is essential for staging the extent of involvement and for following the patient's response to therapy.

Chest. Enlarged mediastinal nodes are the most common intrathoracic manifestations of Hodgkin's disease (Fig. 9–8). The anterior and middle mediastinal compartments are affected most frequently; posterior mediastinal involvement usually indicates disease below the diaphragm.[54] Among the various histologic subtypes, the nodular sclerosis type has a striking predilection for mediastinal involvement while the lymphocyte predominance type rarely involves the mediastinum.

Routine full-lung tomograms have an extremely low yield of pertinent additional information if the stereo posteroanterior and lateral chest films are unequivocally normal;[23] However, whole lung tomography may be of value if bulky mediastinal adenopathy obscures hilar regions and lung parenchyma or if tortuous superior mediastinal vessels, thoracic cage deformities, or other equivocal changes cause difficulties in interpreting the plain films.

Skeletal System. Skeletal disease is unusual as a presenting feature of Hodgkin's disease but may appear in the later stages of the illness. The two most frequently involved areas in both adults and children are the lower dorsal and lumbar spine and the pelvis. Lesions are usually lytic in appearance and are usually suggested by clinical signs or symptoms. It has been speculated that bone involvement may occur as a result of direct invasion of those portions of the skeleton in closest proximity to affected groups of lymph nodes.[89]

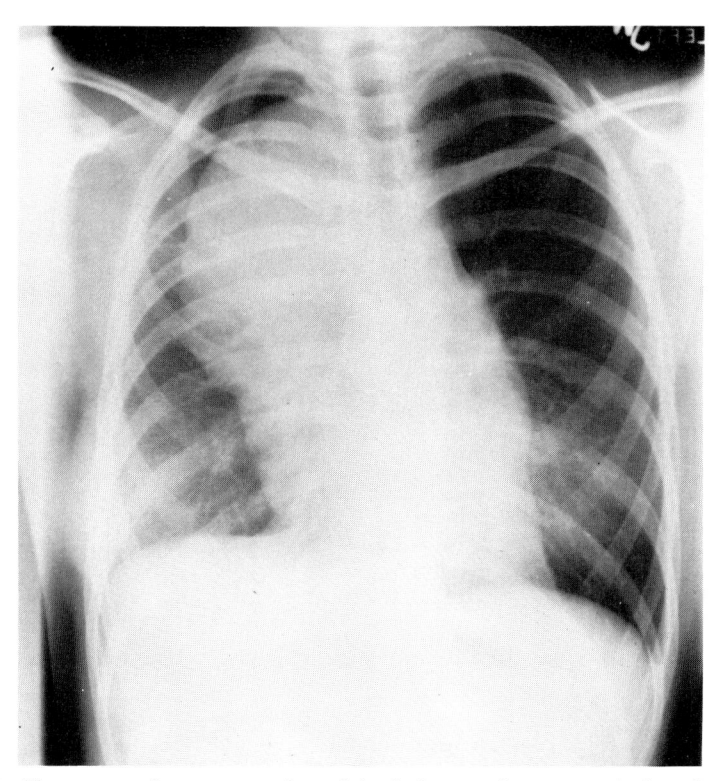

Figure 9–8 Chest x-ray of a patient with Hodgkin's disease showing marked mediastinal lymphadenopathy.

Intravenous Pyelography and Inferior Venacavography. These procedures are of some value in detecting retroperitoneal Hodgkin's disease, but are probably not as reliable as lymphangiography. The most common abnormality found on IVP is extrinsic compression by adjacent enlarged lymph node groups; major obstructive manifestations are not common.[54] Pyelography also allows for accurate localization of the kidneys prior to radiotherapy.

The inferior venacavogram is felt to be of value in assessing the upper portion of the retroperitoneal space (above the celiac node group) and may be useful in identifying subdiaphragmatic disease; in this regard the technique is a useful supplement to lymphangiography, which is unable to detect disease in these areas.

Gastrointestinal Examination. Intrinsic involvement of the gastrointestinal tract by childhood Hodgkin's disease is uncommon; likewise, abnormalities seen in contrast studies of the intestinal tract are uncommon and are usually related to compression by adjacent soft tissue masses.

STAGING

Staging is the process of determining the location and extent of disease; it is of critical importance for determining the patient's prognosis and for planning a therapeutic protocol. Table 9-4 lists the procedures which are considered useful for staging of patients with Hodgkin's disease.

A note of caution must be raised before discussing the major invasive staging procedures, *lymphangiography* and *exploratory laparotomy*. The patient who has significant mediastinal or hilar lymphadenopathy is not a good candidate for either of these procedures until the lymphoid masses have been reduced in size by administration of part of the planned course of mantle radiotherapy (1500 to 2000 rads in 2 to 2½ weeks).[70] Otherwise the enlarged nodes may compromise ventilation during anesthesia or postoperatively or may produce superior vena caval compression.

Table 9-4 Staging Procedures in Hodgkin's Disease

History (ask especially about fever, night sweats, weight loss)
Physical Examination
Hematologic Studies
  Complete blood count
  Platelet count
  Erythrocyte sedimentation rate
Biochemical studies
  Liver function tests (including fibrinogen and protein electrophoresis)
  Renal function tests
  Serum copper
  Alkaline phosphatase
Immunologic evaluation
Radiologic studies
  Chest x-ray
  Skeletal survey
  Lymphangiogram
  Consider: Mediastinal tomography
          Inferior venacavogram with intravenous pyelography
Nuclear medicine studies
  Liver-spleen scan
  Bone scan
  Total body gallium scan
Exploratory laparotomy
  Multiple lymph node biopsies
  Splenectomy
  Liver biopsy
  Bone marrow biopsy
  Relocation of ovaries

LYMPHANGIOGRAPHY

This technique is the most important radiologic method for detecting Hodgkin's disease below the diaphragm. The procedure is performed as follows: a blue dye is injected subcutaneously into several of the intercarpal spaces of the foot, thereby rendering the lymphatic vessels of the foot visible through the skin. One of the lymph vessels is then cannulated and an oily contrast medium is injected slowly. Shortly after its injection the contrast material reveals the lymph vessels and nodes of the legs,

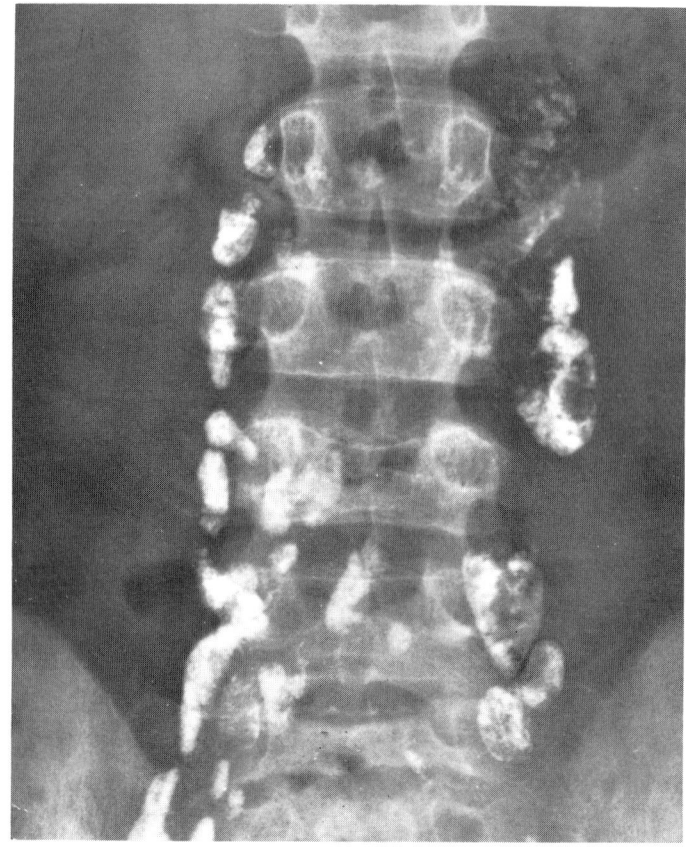

Figure 9-9 Hodgkin's disease of retroperitoneal lymph nodes. Lymphangiogram shows enlargement and a granular or foamy appearance of lymph node groups adjacent to L-2 region and well-defined filling defects in a laterally displaced periaortic lymph node to the left of L-3. (From Grossman, H., et al.: Am. J. Roentgenol. *108*:354, 1970.)

pelvis, and retroperitoneal areas (Fig. 9-9). The value of lymphangiography is limited, however, by failure to demonstrate disease in the superior periaortic, periportal, or splenic hilar nodes as well as in the spleen or liver.

In some centers there is a reluctance to perform lymphangiography in small children because of technical difficulties with sedation of the patient and cannulating small lymphatic vessels as well as difficulties in interpreting the results. The prolonged immobilization required makes the use of heavy sedation or a general anesthetic necessary in such patients. In one series at a large cancer center, however, 80 per cent of the lymphangiograms in children were successful, and nearly 50 per cent revealed abnormalities.[54]

The criteria for interpreting a positive lymphangiogram are based on: (1) *increase in lymph node size;* (2) *foamy or granular appearance of lymph nodes;* and (3) *filling defects in the lymph nodes;* the latter is the principal cause of interpretative difficulties with pediatric lymphangiograms, since inadequate doses of contrast material and incomplete filling, as well as occasional normal variants, can produce spurious conclusions.[54]

The surgeon contemplating a staging procedure should be aware of and attempt to verify the state of any node groups in which lymphangiography has demonstrated possible tumor involvement; this may require taking x-rays in the operating room to make sure that the abnormal-appearing nodes have been removed.

Not only is lymphangiography useful for staging and pinpointing likely pathologic nodes for the surgeon, but in addition serial abdominal films frequently permit evaluation of the patient's response to therapy. This is not as true for children as for adults, however, since the oily contrast material is mobilized from their lymph nodes in a shorter period of time and often is no longer visible after 1 to 3 months. For this reason some groups are resorting to repeat lymphangiograms if there is clinical suspicion of relapse or if insufficient residual contrast material remains to permit adequate routine surveillance.[22] These repeat studies were positive for tumor in seven of 11 children with clinical suspicion of relapse and in three of 11 asymptomatic children.

Lymphangiography is contraindicated if parenchymal pulmonary pathology (infection, previous irradiation, pulmonary hypertension, or Hodgkin's involvement) is present, if there is a significant right-to-left shunt, or if there is a history of allergy to iodine-containing dyes. It is also relatively contraindicated in patients with obstruction of the superior vena cava or jugular veins.[6] It is not necessary to perform lymphangiography if Stage III or IV disease has already been documented.

Complications of this procedure include: (1) *symptomatic pulmonary oil embolism* secondary to injection of an excessive amount of the oil, too rapid injection of the oil, lymphaticovenous anastomoses (usually when there is extensive retroperitoneal node involvement), or inadvertent injection of oil into a small venule instead of a lymphatic vessel; (2) *oil embolism to other organs* (kidney, brain, liver); (3) *cellulitis* at cutdown site; (4) *allergic reaction* to the iodine-containing dye mixed with the oil or to the blue dye used to expose the lymphatic vessels; (5) occasional *fever* lasting from 12 to 36 hours after injection of the oil (this may be a result of excessive pulmonary oil embolism); (6) transient *pain*, usually at the site of involved abdominal or pelvic nodes; and (7) *scars* on the dorsal surfaces of both feet.

EXPLORATORY LAPAROTOMY

Exploratory laparotomy has become an important part of the evaluation process because of our inability to determine the presence or absence of abdominal disease with more limited procedures.

Ultmann[126] has compiled the results of several studies and has demonstrated the limitations of nonsurgical approaches to staging of Hodgkin's disease: (1) 12 per cent of patients with negative lymphangiograms had abdominal disease revealed at laparotomy; (2) 32 per cent of patients with positive lymphangiograms were found to be free of abdominal disease at laparotomy; (3) 27 per cent of patients with "clinically negative" spleens were subsequently found to have Hodgkin's disease in the spleen; (4) 38 per cent of patients with enlarged spleens had no evidence of splenic involvement after careful histologic sectioning; (5) 3 per cent of patients with "clinically negative" livers had Hodgkin's disease demonstrable in open wedge biopsy of the liver; (6) of patients with "clinically positive" livers (hepatomegaly, abnormal liver function tests, abnormal liver scan), 90 per cent had no evidence of histologic Hodgkin's involvement after careful examination of wedge biopsy of the liver. As a result, laparotomy improves staging and alters therapy for approximately 14 to 40 per cent of patients.[39, 57, 58]

At laparotomy, all nodes which appear abnormal on lymphangiogram are biopsied; random para-aortic, porta hepatic, and splenic hilar nodes are also biopsied. Splenectomy, open wedge biopsy of the liver, and bone marrow biopsy are also performed. In girls the ovaries may be relocated to shield them from subsequent radiotherapy; with this technique, ovarian function is retained in two thirds of young female patients receiving total nodal radiotherapy for Hodgkin's disease, and successful pregnancies have also been made possible.[74]

Splenectomy, at the time of staging laparotomy, has both diagnostic and therapeutic advantages. Because of its apparent key role in predicting liver and bone marrow involvement, careful sectioning of the spleen (3 to 5 mm sections) provides important information on which to base therapy and prognosis. Furthermore, removal of the spleen eliminates the need to irradiate the splenic bed and thereby spares the left kidney and left lower lung field from the effects of radiation.

On the other hand, splenectomy increases the susceptibility of children with Hodgkin's disease (who may already have immunologic impairment) to infectious complications. Primary among these are overwhelming bacterial infections—in one recent report there were 20 episodes of meningitis or septicemia (50 per cent of which were fatal) in 18 of 200 children with Hodgkin's disease after splenectomy. These infections generally were caused by penicillin-sensitive organisms (pneumococcus, streptococcus);[25] but infections with *Hemophilus influenzae, Listeria, Pseudomonas,* and meningococcus have also been reported. Approximately 80 per cent of the infections occur within the first two years after splenectomy, and there is a tendency to recurrent episodes.[59] Since the illness is usually abrupt in onset, with a fulminant course, *any febrile episode in a child splenectomized for staging of Hodgkin's disease should be considered as a possible life-threatening bacterial infection and treated with high-dose antibiotic therapy.* Penicillin prophylaxis may also be considered for such patients.

In addition to the infectious complications arising as a result of splenectomy, there is also a 5 per cent incidence of postoperative bowel obstruction and a 1 to 2 per cent incidence of wound infection in children undergoing staging laparotomy.[106] Less common complications are: small left pleural effusion, transient mild pancreatitis, retroperitoneal hematoma, subphrenic abscess, and thrombotic episodes.

STAGING CLASSIFICATION

The current staging classification for Hodgkin's disease was defined at the Ann Arbor Symposium[18] and is summarized in Table 9-5. This classification is based on the conception of Hodgkin's disease as a unifocal illness with contiguous lymphoid spread. When the disease is confined to a single lymph node area or to closely contiguous lymph node groups (Stages I and II), the prognosis is relatively good, whereas widespread lymphoid involvement or spread to extranodal organs connotes advanced disease and has a relatively poor prognosis. The one exception to this rule is the situation where extranodal disease occurs by direct extension from a contiguous lymphoid focus, e.g., a single focus of pulmonary disease as a direct extension of hilar adenopathy. Such patients have essentially the same prognosis as those with hilar adenopathy alone.[92] Consequently, extranodal involvement by extension is recognized by staging the disease as if the patient had only nodal involvement, but adding the designation (E).

Table 9-6 demonstrates the results of staging in 289 pediatric Hodgkin's disease patients accumulated by Gottlieb[52] from a variety of references; it may be seen that 65 per cent of chil-

Table 9-5 Clinical Staging of Hodgkin's Disease

Stage I: Involvement of a single lymph node region (I) or of a single extralymphatic organ or site (I$_E$) by direct extension.

Stage II: Involvement of two or more lymph node regions (number to be stated) on the same side of the diaphragm (II), or localized involvement (by direct extension) of extralymphatic organ or site and of one or more lymph node regions on the same side of the diaphragm (II$_E$).

Stage III: Involvement of lymph node regions on both sides of the diaphragm (III), which may also be accompanied by localized involvement (by direct extension) of extralymphatic organ or site (III$_E$), by involvement of the spleen (III$_S$), or both (III$_{SE}$).

Stage IV: Diffuse or disseminated involvement of one or more extralymphatic organs or tissues with or without associated lymph node enlargement. The site of involvement is identified as follows:
N — Lymph nodes   S — Spleen
H — Liver   L — Lung
M — Marrow   O — Bone
P — Pleura   D — Skin
                                    CNS — Central nervous system

Systemic Symptoms
Each stage is subdivided into A and B categories, B for those with defined general symptoms and A for those without. The B classification will be given to those patients with unexplained weight loss of more than 10% of the body weight in the 6 months before admission, or unexplained fever with temperatures above 38°C, or night sweats, or any combination of these.

Note: Pruritus alone does not qualify for B classification; also, a short febrile illness associated with a known infection will not qualify for B classification.

Table 9-6 Distribution of Pediatric Hodgkin's Disease Patients by Clinical Stage[52]

STAGE	FREQUENCY (PER CENT)
I	28
II	37
III	23
IV	12

dren present with relatively limited disease (Stages I and II).

NATURAL HISTORY

Hodgkin's disease appears to arise in a unifocal manner and extension occurs mainly via the lymphatic system involving contiguous lymph node groups in a predictable fashion.[105] Thus, about 90 per cent of initial distributions (as well as later extension) of disease involve lymph node chains that may be considered contiguous by the criterion of direct lymphatic communication.[68] This is exemplified by the high incidence of mediastinal disease in patients presenting with cervical adenopathy (particularly on the right side), a reflection of the important lymphatic trunks connecting the two areas.

Less immediately obvious as a manifestation of contiguous lymphatic spread of Hodgkin's disease is the "mediastinal skip" pattern in which the disease involves the left lower cervical or supraclavicular (Virchow's) nodes as well as the para-aortic lymph node chain without intervening mediastinal or intrathoracic involvement;[68] this relationship, however, is thought to result from dissemination of Hodgkin's cells through the thoracic duct, which is a direct channel between the upper para-aortic area and the left neck. Indeed, in several studies, Reed-Sternberg cells (and their mononuclear precursors) have been demonstrated in thoracic duct lymph of patients with involvement of the para-aortic nodes.[34, 35] Thus, extension from the lymph nodes at the base of the neck by way of the thoracic duct to the upper lumbar para-aortic lymph nodes is a major "escape route" for the disease and is probably the single most important cause of failure of localized or regional radiotherapy.[68] Since the thoracic duct empties into the left subclavian vein, dividing Hodgkin's tumor cells may also reach the bloodstream via this route.

Splenic involvement is usually accompanied (or preceded) by the evidence of involvement of the upper lumbar para-aortic lymph nodes, and it has been suggested that disease tends to spread from the upper lumbar para-aortic lymph nodes (presumably via lymphatic channels) to the spleen.[68] However, the filter action of the spleen makes a hematogenous mechanism for spread possible as well.

Splenic involvement appears to occupy a unique position as an indicator of extranodal (particularly hepatic) dissemination of Hodgkin's disease; indeed, the larger the spleen and the greater its involvement, the more likely is there to be demonstrable involvement of the liver, whereas liver involvement rarely occurs in the absence of splenic involvement. Spread to the liver probably occurs via the splenic vein and the portal system.

The probability of spread to the bone marrow also appears to be strongly correlated with prior or concomitant involvement of the para-aortic lymph nodes and the spleen. Hodgkin's disease may gain access to the vertebral marrow by direct extension from the para-aortic nodes, but it is probable that in most instances it reaches the bone marrow in many areas simultaneously by hematogenous dissemination.[68]

When extranodal sites have become involved, extension may occur via hematogenous routes; such random spread is more characteristic of the less favorable histologic subtypes (mixed cellularity, lymphocyte depletion). Support for the notion that Hodgkin's disease may spread via the bloodstream comes from the correlation between extranodal disease, unfavorable outcome, and histologic evidence of vascular invasion in lymph nodes or spleens of patients with Hodgkin's disease,[102] as well as the observation of circulating Reed-Sternberg cells in some patients with Hodgkin's disease.[15]

PARENCHYMAL ORGAN INVOLVEMENT

Mediastinal and Pulmonary Disease

The mediastinal and hilar nodes are the pathway to the lungs for Hodgkin's disease; essentially there is no pulmonary Hodgkin's disease without mediastinal or hilar disease. There is a striking predilection of the nodular sclerosis type for mediastinal involvement—over 90 per cent of patients presenting with only mediastinal involvement have this histopathologic picture.[80] It might be expected that a high percentage of pulmonary involvement would also involve this variant, and indeed, 90 per cent of the cases are of the nodular sclerosis type; lymphocyte predominant Hodgkin's disease, on the other hand, rarely involves the lungs.

Anatomically there are four forms of pulmonary involvement: (1) contiguous, (2) lymphatic peribronchovascular, (3) lymphatic subpleural, and (4) intraparenchymal.[54, 118, 125, 127]

Contiguous lesions or solitary pulmonary lesions may occur as a result of the direct invasion of the lung from mediastinal or hilar nodes. These are now considered to represent Stage II$_E$ disease and do not have the same ominous connotation as true hematogenous Stage IV lesions.

Peribronchovascular disease occurs due to spread of tumor along the lymphatics radiating from the hilar nodes. The discrete infiltrations of the interstitial septa have a characteristic fanlike pattern of radiating streaks.

Subpleural spread most commonly occurs with involvement of the anterior mediastinum;[40] plaque-like pleural thickening or effusion may be evident on x-ray.

Intraparenchymal involvement may be either nodular or alveolar (pneumonic) in nature; when multiple lesions are present, this represents true Stage IV disease of presumably hematogenous spread. Nodular lesions may appear as single or multiple densities (usually bilateral), with indistinct margins. The alveolar form, on the other hand, strongly resembles a pneumonitis and is sometimes difficult to distinguish from an infectious process.

Pleural effusion is common in patients with Hodgkin's disease. When, as often occurs, it is due to lymphatic obstruction in the mediastinum or hilus, mediastinal irradiation may provide rapid relief. Small left pleural effusions are sometimes seen after staging laparotomy. Actual pleural invasion by Hodgkin's disease also does occur, but relatively rarely in comparison to the incidence of this complication in non-Hodgkin's lymphoma.

A dramatic consequence of the mediastinal adenopathy that sometimes occurs in Hodgkin's disease patients is the *superior vena cava syndrome*. The clinical manifestations and treatment of this condition are discussed in Chapter 7.

Neurologic Complications

Neurologic dysfunction is usually a late manifestation of Hodgkin's disease and may be considered under two major headings: (1) complications arising as a result of actual metastatic invasion of the nervous system by the tumor, and (2) complications related to the presence of the tumor elsewhere in the body.

Neurologic Complications Resulting from Metastatic Spread to the Nervous System. Hodgkin's disease may reach the nervous system by a variety of routes. One such route involves spread from paravertebral lymph nodes along nerve roots, blood vessels, or perineural lymphatics into the spinal canal by way of the intervertebral foramina. Tumor involving the nasopharynx or cervical lymph nodes may enter the cranial vault by direct extension along cranial nerves and meningeal vessels to produce epidural and subdural deposits along the base of the brain. Alternatively, osseous involvement of the vertebral bodies or the skull may directly extend into the epidural space and produce deposits which compress the spinal cord or brain. Another mode of spread may involve hematogenous dissemination.

In general, Hodgkin's involvement of the central neuraxis is epidural in location and produces compressive symptoms, which vary according to the area of the nervous system involved. The clinical manifestations and treatment of spinal cord compression are discussed in Chapter 7. Of interest is a recent study which shows that despite (or perhaps because of) the high incidence of Hodgkin's disease in the cervical lymph nodes, spinal cord compression in Hodgkin's disease rarely involves the cervical region.[44] This may reflect the fact that a very high fraction of Hodgkin's disease patients often have irradiation to the neck as the initial treatment, and thus elective or therapeutic courses of radiation to lymph node–bearing areas may prevent or reduce the incidence of spinal cord compression.[44]

Intracranial disease may present with signs and symptoms of increased intracranial pressure or with hemiparesis, hemisensory defects, focal seizures, or, occasionally, papilledema.[61] When the base of the brain is involved, there may be palsies of the cranial nerves (most commonly cranial nerves III, VI, and VII). Intracranial Hodgkin's disease may be treated by radiation therapy; this should be preceded by dexamethasone (Decadron) to relieve cerebral edema.

Leptomeningeal metastasis (diffuse seeding of the meninges) is rare in Hodgkin's disease. The diagnosis may be suggested by: (1) simultaneous occurrence of signs and symptoms involving more than one anatomic level of the neuraxis (i.e., focal seizures, cranial nerve palsies, spinal root signs, and lower motor neuron weakness), (2) neurologic signs, which are more common and widespread on examination than suspected from the patient's complaints, and (3) signs of meningeal irritation. The diagnosis can usually be made by cerebrospinal fluid examination, which reveals increased pressure, a pleocytosis, elevated protein, and low glucose level. Occasionally malignant cells may be demonstrated in the CSF and will be helpful in differentiating this condition from infectious meningitis caused by opportunistic organisms.[97]

Neurologic Complications Related to the Presence of the Tumor Elsewhere in the Body. Nonmetastatic neurologic complications may occur as the result of metabolic and nutritional disorders, infections, chemotherapy, radiotherapy, or the remote effects of Hodgkin's disease on the nervous system. These are briefly reviewed below. A full discussion of these is beyond the scope of this book, but an excellent account may be found in the review by Somasundaram and Posner.[117]

METABOLIC DISORDERS. Among the specific metabolic causes of neurologic dysfunction in Hodgkin's patients are *hypercalcemia, hypoglycemia, hyponatremia, hepatic and renal failure,* and *pulmonary insufficiency.* Hypercalcemia occurs in about 20 per cent of patients with Hodgkin's disease, but to a clinically significant extent in only 1 to 2 per cent.[127] It usually occurs with advanced disease and in the presence of widespread bone destruction. The clinical manifestations and treatment of this problem are discussed in Chapter 7.

INFECTIONS. Infections of the nervous sytem in Hodgkin's disease patients may involve the usual bacterial and viral pathogens; in addition, however, the immunologic incompetence (both innate and iatrogenic) of these patients predisposes them to infection by a wide variety of opportunistic agents.

Herpes zoster is a well-known complication of Hodgkin's disease, whose incidence appears to be increasing as staging and therapeutic maneuvers become more aggressive. In 1965 a review of 600 patients with Hodgkin's disease showed an 8 per cent overall incidence of Herpes zoster;[115] since then the incidence has risen in some series to 15 to 25 per cent[28] (versus 0.2 per cent in the general population and 7 to 8 per cent in patients with other lymphomas).[109] The incidence in pediatric Hodgkin's patients may be even higher than for the overall Hodgkin's patient population; a recent series reported an incidence of 52 per cent in Stages I to III pediatric Hodgkin's disease patients who had undergone a staging laparotomy (with splenectomy) followed by aggressive radiation therapy and chemotherapy.[51]

Zoster may occur before the disease is diagnosed or at any time during its course (including quiescent periods). In some instances radicular pain caused by Herpes zoster may be the initial symptom of intraspinal involvement, and cord compression may subsequently develop at the same spinal segment.[50] In typical zoster infections ("shingles") sensory findings (hyperalgesia and hypoalgesia) are always present along the involved nerve root and are followed by the development of a crop of vesicles limited to the dermatome supplied by the affected nerve (Fig. 9–10). Occasionally the process spreads to the anterior horn cells of the same

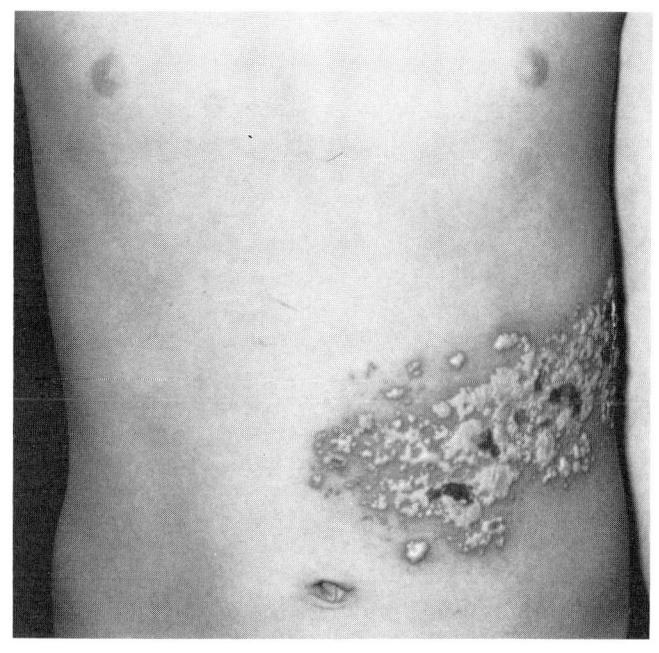

Figure 9-10 Herpes zoster ("shingles") eruption.

segment and produces a segmental motor paresis (usually temporary). The zoster lesions may also generalize from the unilateral primary area and produce a "chickenpox" syndrome, which usually subsides if the patient is in good condition; however, if the patient is debilitated or has active, uncontrolled Hodgkin's disease, the illness may progress and be fatal.

Meningitis of bacterial, viral, fungal, or protozoal origin must be considered in every patient with headache, stiff neck, or unexplained fever. The most common organisms are *Cryptococcus neoformans, Listeria monocytogenes, Diplococcus pneumoniae, Toxoplasma gondii,* and *Herpes zoster.* Because many of these organisms tend to be relatively indolent, the onset of symptoms may be subacute and the classic signs of meningeal irritation (e.g., nuchal rigidity) may be lacking.

Brain abscess is uncommon in Hodgkin's disease, but may be associated with (1) *Cryptococcus,* (2) gram-negative bacteria, (3) fungi *(Aspergillus, Candida),* or (4) *Toxoplasma gondii.* The latter is particularly treacherous since it frequently occurs in patients whose Hodgkin's disease is quiescent and who are not on steroids or other chemotherapeutic agents;[117] diagnosis may be made by the presence of elevated *Toxoplasma* antibodies in the blood and CSF or a positive Sabin-Feldman dye test (although these are sometimes absent or negative). If a mass lesion is demonstrable on contrast study, but the antibody tests are negative, diagnostic biopsy should be performed to distinguish between brain abscess and intraparenchymal Hodgkin's disease.

CHEMOTHERAPY. Many of the agents used to treat Hodgkin's disease can produce neurologic side effects. The most common of these occurs with vincristine therapy, but steroids, procarbazine, methotrexate, and vinblastine may also produce neurologic dysfunction. These agents are discussed in Chapter Three.

RADIOTHERAPY. In general, the nervous system is relatively resistant to damage by ionizing radiation, but some parts of it are more sensitive than others. The spinal cord is perhaps the most susceptible area and radiation myelopathy occurs not infrequently because the spinal cord is often included in the radiation field. In about 10 to 15 per cent of patients receiving treatment to the cervical, supraclavicular, and mediastinal regions, a *transient myelopathy* develops; this is characterized by brief tingling and electric shock–like sensations extending down the back into the extremities upon flexion or extension of the neck *(Lhermitte's sign)*. This condition is not associated with motor dysfunction, and permanent myelopathy does not develop.

A more serious complication of spinal radiation, *radiation necrosis* of the cord, occurs following dosages in excess of 4000 rads over 4 weeks.[117] It can appear any time between 6 months and 5 years following radiation treatment, and the early signs are paresthesias, sensory changes, pain, and motor weakness. There may then be progression over the next several months to an incomplete or complete sensorimotor transverse cord lesion with paraplegia or tetraplegia. Since this condition cannot be distinguished clinically from epidural cord compression with certainty, myelography may be indicated.

Bones

Bones are frequently involved by Hodgkin's disease; this may occur by hematogenous spread or by contiguous spread from regional lymph nodes. The thoracic and lumbar vertebrae are the bones most frequently involved, probably as a result of contiguous spread from neighboring lymph nodes (in 29 per cent of these patients paravertebral masses can be observed);[53] the major complication of vertebral involvement is spinal cord compression resulting from collapse of a vertebral body (Fig. 9–11) or from extension of the tumor into the epidural area.

Bone lesions may be osteoblastic or osteolytic; osteoblastic lesions are invariably accompanied by an elevated serum alkaline phosphatase. Skeletal Hodgkin's disease has an ominous prognosis; 50 to 60 per cent of patients die within 2 years of discovery of bone lesions.[53, 127]

Liver

Since the spleen appears to be the portal of entry for Hodgkin's disease into the liver, there is rarely (if ever) Hodgkin's disease of the liver without concomitant splenic disease.[48] If the spleen is not palpable, there is a 50 per cent chance of splenic involvement and a 5 per cent chance of liver involvement. If the spleen is palpable, the likelihood of splenic involvement is greater than 75 per cent and that of liver involvement is more than 50 per cent.[127]

It is unusual for marked and obvious liver involvement to occur early in the course of the disease. Mild hepatomegaly, nonspecific abnormalities on liver scan, and abnormal liver function tests (BSP retention and elevated transaminase or alkaline phosphatase levels) are not uncommon; however, these show little correlation with actual histologic involvement of the liver by Hodgkin's disease. Furthermore, liver function tests and scans frequently revert to normal following irradiation of active Hodgkin's foci in other anatomic locations.[62]

Apparently the presence of Hodgkin's foci in other anatomic locations can produce a reactive process in the liver associated with nonspecific functional and histologic changes. Among the nonspecific histologic findings are (1) lymphocytic infiltration in the portal tracts, (2) occasional eosinophils and plasma cells (but not Reed-Sternberg cells) admixed with the lymphocytic infiltrates, (3) abnor-

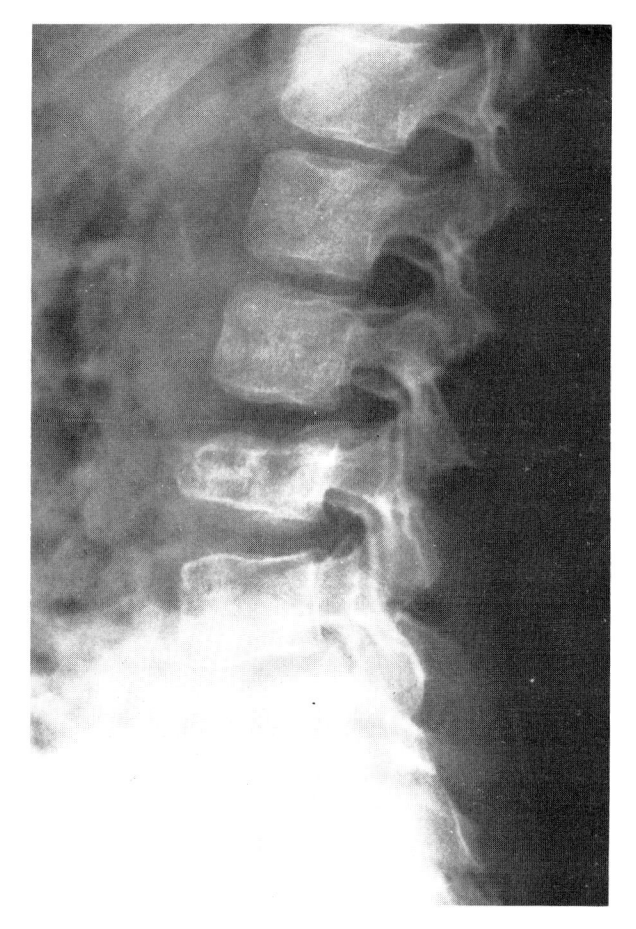

Figure 9–11 Hodgkin's disease of bone. X-ray shows collapse of fourth lumbar vertebral body by a mixed lytic and blastic process. (From Grossman, H., et al.: Am. J. Roentgenol. *108*:354, 1970.)

malities of the hepatic cells, including fatty metamorphosis, (4) cholestasis, and (5) isolated noncaseating epithelioid granulomas of unknown significance. In one series of 57 patients with Hodgkin's disease who underwent liver biopsy, all manifested some form of nonspecific mesenchymal reaction; these changes showed no correlation with stage, symptoms, age, sex, liver function tests, or life expectancy.[96]

In order to establish actual Hodgkin's involvement of the liver, two criteria must be met:[81] (1) evidence of a discrete lesion with features of one of the histologic Hodgkin's subtypes, (2) conclusive evidence of a Reed-Sternberg cell or one of its variants. The anatomic pattern of involvement may be diffuse or nodular—the nodular pattern may be demonstrable by liver scan.

Jaundice. The presence of jaundice in patients with Hodgkin's disease is an ominous prognostic sign and may be a terminal or preterminal event in as many as 90 per cent of patients.[111] However, jaundice may not necessarily be directly related to tumor involvement of the liver; other causes include: (1) hemolytic anemia, (2) viral hepatitis, (3) toxic hepatitis, (4) toxoplasmosis, (5) cytomegalic inclusion virus, and (6) cholestasis of unknown etiology and other nonspecific associated hepatic changes.

When jaundice is due to hepatic involvement by Hodgkin's disease it is important to differentiate between parenchymal Hodgkin's disease and obstruction of the porta hepatis by lymph nodes, since, in extrahepatic obstructive jaundice, hepatic portal radiotherapy may be beneficial. From a review of published cases it appears, however, that in most instances the jaundice is secondary to intrahepatic obstruction by portal peribiliary infiltration.[76, 125, 127]

THERAPY

The recommended therapy for a patient with Hodgkin's disease must be individualized on the basis of age, extent of disease, and histopathology of the lesions. In general, however, the improving results of aggressive therapy suggest that, in the future, many patients will be treated by a combination of chemotherapy and radiotherapy.

RADIATION THERAPY

Radiation therapy is an effective method of treating Hodgkin's disease provided that (1) "tumoricidal" dosage is utilized, and (2) adequate radiation doses are delivered to all sites of involvement with tumor.

Radiation Dosage

Following radiation therapy, the risk of "true"* recurrence of Hodgkin's disease within the field of treatment is inversely proportional to radiation dosage:[66, 69]

Dosage†	Risk Per Cent of "True" Recurrence
<1000 rads	78
1000–2000 rads	48
2000–3000 rads	26
3000–3500 rads	12
3500–4000 rads	4
4400 rads	1.3

---

*A "true" recurrence is defined as "the reappearance of lymphadenopathy or other evidence of activity in a treated field as the first new manifestation of Hodgkin's disease."[66]

†Delivered at approximately 1000 rads per week.

The optimal tumoricidal dose level of radiotherapy necessary to totally eradicate a focus of Hodgin's disease is considered to be 3500 to 4000 rads, given at a rate of 1000 to 1100 rads per week[4, 69] (exceptionally large or slowly regressing lymph node masses may be treated with a local "boost" to 5000 rads over 5 to 6 weeks[70, 71]). Such dosages of megavoltage x-rays, delivered to large fields encompassing multiple lymph node chains, are well tolerated by normal skin, connective tissue, and mucous membranes; they may even be delivered safely to small volumes of vital organs such as the liver, lungs, and kidney.[69]

Radiation Fields

Radiotherapy is delivered both to areas of clinically evident disease ("involved" fields) and to all contiguous lymphatic structures to which microscopic spread of disease is likely to have occurred ("extended" fields). In some instances, extended field treatment may entail irradiation of virtually all lymph node chains ("total nodal"), as well as other lymphatic structures — e.g., Waldeyer's ring ("total lymphoid"). The necessity for "extended field" irradiation became evident when it was noted that the sites of first recurrence of disease after local radiotherapy were in lymph nodes initially uninvolved clinically, but adjacent to those with disease.

It is highly desirable to treat multiple lymph node chains in continuity with as few fields as possible. The reason for this is the difficulty in calculating radiation dosimetry at the junction of adjacent fields — errors in such calculations can lead to (1) undertreatment of diseased lymph nodes when inadequate dosage is applied at the junction or (2) serious damage to normal structures when adjacent fields overlap and produce

Hodgkin's Disease

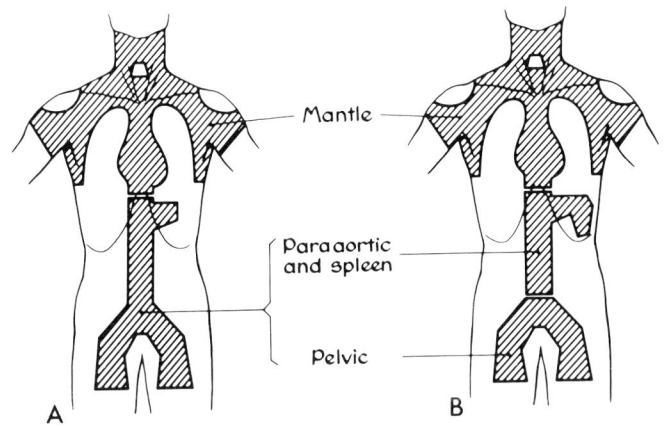

Figure 9–12 The "mantle" and "inverted Y" fields used in radiotherapy of Hodgkin's disease patients. In splenectomized patients (A) the splenic pedicle is marked by metallic clips at the time of surgery and included in the inverted Y field. (From Kaplan, H. S.: Cancer Res. 36:3863, 1976.)

"hot spots." Since it is possible, with megavoltage beams, to encompass all of the major lymph node chains above the diaphragm (cervical, supraclavicular, infraclavicular, axillary, hilar, and mediastinal) in a single *"mantle"* field and all of the major lymph node chains below the diaphragm (para-aortic, splenic pedicle, and pelvic) in a single *"inverted Y"* field* (Fig. 9–12), only a single junction is required—this occurs at approximately the level of the eleventh or twelfth thoracic vertebrae, where there are relatively few lymph nodes.[69]

The "mantle" field irradiates about 15 per cent of the total bone marrow distribution while the "inverted Y" field encompasses another 50 per cent; thus "total nodal" irradiation encompasses about 65 per cent of the total marrow (in the adult).[7,33] Children may tolerate total nodal irradiation better than adults because they still have a significant proportion of their active marrow in the femur and tibia.

Complications of mantle irradiation include symptomatic pulmonary radiation reaction (20 per cent), pericarditis (13 per cent), Lhermitte's syndrome (15 per cent), and thyroid dysfunction (13 per cent).[19]

Chemotherapy

Although many chemotherapeutic agents show individual therapeutic efficacy in Hodgkin's disease (Table 9–7), it is only when these agents are

Table 9–7 Chemotherapeutic Agents Which Show Activity Against Hodgkin's Disease

Alkylating Agents
Nitrogen Mustard (HN$_2$)
Chlorambucil
Cyclophosphamide
Nitrosoureas (CCNU)
Vinca Alkaloids
Vincristine (VCR)
Vinblastine (VBL)
Antibiotics
Adriamycin (ADM)
Bleomycin (BLM)
Miscellaneous
Procarbazine (PCB)
Imidazole carboxamide (DTIC)
Corticosteroids (PRD)

---

*The inverted Y field does not effectively encompass the mesenteric lymph nodes; however, these are seldom involved in Hodgkin's disease.

used as part of a combination chemotherapy protocol that a significant increase in complete remissions and improvement in survival is attainable. With drugs used singly or sequentially, the rate of complete remission is between 10 and 30 per cent,[17, 79] with a median duration of 10 weeks,[33] whereas combination chemotherapy has produced complete remission rates in the range of 70 to 80 per cent, with a median duration of 29 to 42 months.[29]

Of these combinations, the standard of comparison remains the MOPP protocol of DeVita (Table 9-8); however a number of other four- and five-drug programs are currently under investigation (Table 9-8). These new combinations may prove useful not only for initial management but also for treatment of the patient who relapses after MOPP treatment.

Currently a major question regarding chemotherapy of Hodgkin's disease is its duration. The standard MOPP protocol involves six monthly cycles followed by no maintenance therapy. In several series, the duration of complete remission has been prolonged by maintaining patients with chemotherapy for longer periods,[43] but other studies suggest that there is no further benefit from maintenance therapy provided that the patients really have attained complete remission.[136] It would thus appear that, rather than administering a predetermined, set number of courses of therapy, strict attention should be paid to the time at which complete remission occurs, and chemotherapy should be continued for a short finite period following that time.

COMBINED MODALITY THERAPY

Both radiotherapy and chemotherapy have their limitations with regard to eradicating Hodgkin's disease. Radiotherapy (in "tumoricidal dosage") is capable of destroying all Hodgkin's foci *in the treated fields*; however, it obviously has no effect on disease which is outside the radiation field. Consequently, relapse, when it occurs in patients treated by irradiation alone, usually results from occult microscopic foci outside of the treatment field. Chemotherapy, on the other hand, is not limited by anatomic considerations and is able to eradicate foci of disease throughout the body. Nonetheless, approximately

Table 9-8 Combination Chemotherapy Regimens[71]

MOPP[29]
HN$_2$	6 mg/m^2, I.V., days 1 and 8
VCR	1.0–1.4 mg/m^2, I.V., days 1 and 8
PCB	100 mg/m^2/day, P.O., days 1 to 14
PRD	40 mg/m^2/day, P.O., days 1 to 14

14 day cycles separated by 14 day rest periods; usually six or more cycles; PRD in cycles 1 and 4 only.

MVPP[94]
HN$_2$	6 mg/m^2, I.V., days 1 and 8
VBL	6 mg/m^2, I.V., days 1 and 8
PCB	100 mg/m^2, P.O., days 1 to 14
PRD	40 mg/day, P.O., days 1 to 14

14 day cycles separated by 28 day rest periods; usually six or more cycles; PRD given in all cycles.

ABVD[14]
ADM	25 mg/m^2, I.V., days 1 and 14
BLM	10 mg/m^2, I.V., days 1 and 14
VBL	6 mg/m^2, I.V., days 1 and 14
DTIC	150 mg/m^2, I.V., days 1 to 5

14 day cycles and 14 day rest periods. Advantage: no cross-resistance against MOPP; high rate of response in MOPP failures (≈75–80 per cent).

CAVe[104]
CCNU	100 mg/m^2, P.O., day 1
ADM	60 mg/m^2, I.V., day 1
VBL	5 mg/m^2, I.V., day 1

Cycles repeated every 6 weeks (if blood counts permit) to total of nine cycles; about 50 per cent response rate in MOPP failures.

MOP

Same as MOPP, except for the omission of prednisone in all cycles in patients previously treated with mantle field radiotherapy.

60 per cent of patients with advanced Hodgkin's disease (Stages IIIB and IV) who achieve complete remission with MOPP eventually relapse. Since 88 per cent of these relapses occur in sites of previously active Hodgkin's involvement, it would appear that chemotherapy is limited with regard to its ability to totally eradicate bulk disease (especially for the nodular sclerosis and mixed cellularity types).[138]

Since radiotherapy is effective in eliminating defined areas of bulk disease and chemotherapy has its major effect against small microscopic foci of clinically occult disease, it would appear logical that a combination of these modalities would be very effective for total treatment of Hodgkin's disease. Hence, the recent trend in the treatment of Hodgkin's disease has been to develop combined radiotherapy/chemotherapy protocols.

While it is technically possible to deliver total lymphoid radiotherapy followed by a complete course of six cycles of chemotherapy,[69] there may be significant problems with bone marrow suppression and vincristine neuropathy. The incidence of Herpes zoster and secondary malignancies may also be increased in patients treated with combination chemotherapy/radiotherapy.

In an effort to minimize the potential problems associated with combined chemotherapy/radiotherapy one group has attempted to lower the dose of radiotherapy in patients who are also being treated with chemotherapy and has achieved "encouraging results."[101] There is now some evidence to indicate that supplementary chemotherapy may allow the physician to limit the dose of irradiation in selected pediatric patients as well.[31] This would be desirable, since radiotherapy has much more damaging effects on growing structures than it does on fully formed ones, and altered bone growth (kyphoscoliosis, aseptic necrosis, arrested growth) is a significant complication in terms of quality of survival in pediatric Hodgkin's patients.[100]

RESULTS OF THERAPY

With the development of radiotherapy and combination chemotherapy and the realization that they must be utilized in an aggressive manner, Hodgkin's disease is no longer considered an inexorably fatal condition. Indeed, prolonged remissions may be achieved in many patients, and it is even possible now to consider that a considerable portion may be "cured." As shown in Table 9–9, 5-year survival (in a predominantly adult group of patients) is now high not only in Stages I and II but in Stage III disease as well. These patients were treated with high-dose total lymphoid radiotherapy in Stages I, II, and III$_S$ A; total lymphoid radiotherapy supplemented with either hepatic radiotherapy or MOPP chemotherapy in Stages III$_S$B and IV$_{H+}$ A or B; and MOPP chemotherapy ± supplementary radiotherapy in Stages IV$_M$A or B and IV$_L$A or B. Since the curve for relapse-free survival flattens out at 10 years at about 50 per cent, this represents a minimum estimate of the permanent cure rate which can now be achieved in Hodgkin's disease.[70] For pediatric patients, treated by varying combinations of radiotherapy

Table 9–9 Prognosis in Patients with Hodgkin's Disease* (Stanford Data)[70]

STAGE	PER CENT 5-YEAR SURVIVAL	PER CENT 5-YEAR RELAPSE-FREE
I	86	72.5
II	93.6	69.0
III	81.3	61.1
IV	39.0	26.9
All Cases	81.3	61.5

*See text for details of treatment.

and chemotherapy, median survival is also in excess of 10 years.[31]

The therapeutic approach to pediatric Hodgkin's disease remains controversial. On the one hand, it is considered desirable to be as aggressive as possible with the initial therapy in order to completely eradicate all foci of disease and prevent recurrence. On the other hand, the deleterious effects of radiotherapy and chemotherapy on developing bone, muscle, and parenchymal organs are well recognized, as are the possible oncogenic sequelae of these therapeutic modalities.

A recent progress report after 8 years of trials at Stanford demonstrates that, overall, patients treated with combined modality therapy do indeed have improved survival compared with patients who were treated with radiotherapy alone.[105a] This difference in survival curves is not apparent until patients have been followed for at least three years and is most significant for symptomatic (B) patients and for patients with Stage IIIB disease; the survival curves for patients with Stage IA, IIA, and IIB disease have not yet been found to be affected by combined modality therapy (although relapse-free survival time is longer for these patients).

Some authors contend that children with Stage I and IIA Hodgkin's disease may be adequately controlled by involved field[24] or extended field (mantle plus para-aortic)[12a] irradiation, whereas others feel that the combination of low-dose radiation plus MOPP chemotherapy will result in excellent survival with minimal morbidity.[31] A major point of dispute is whether all patients with relatively localized disease should be subjected to intensive combined modality therapy in order to prevent the relatively small number of relapses that might occur if all such patients were treated with more limited therapy. It has been argued that there exists a very real second chance of cure by radiotherapy when nodal disease becomes evident in previously unirradiated areas or by chemotherapy when relapse occurs in parenchymal organs or previously irradiated nodal areas. Other authors believe that the best hope for cure of Hodgkin's disease depends on aggressive initial treatment and that reliance on a second treatment course to salvage the patients who relapse may significantly reduce the likelihood of therapeutic success.[105a, 133]

FOLLOW-UP EXAMINATION

In most patients who are not cured, the initial relapse tends to occur predominantly during the first 2 years after completion of the first course of treatment (Fig. 9–13), and patients who survive 5 years without relapse have at least 95 per cent chance of being permanently cured.[72] Accordingly, follow-up examinations should be scheduled more frequently in the initial period after therapy—one recommended schedule is to see the patient every 2 months for the first year following chemotherapy, every 3 months during the second year, every 4 months during the third year, every 6 months during years four and five, and annually thereafter.[31]

Follow-up examination should consist of:
Physical examination (with particular attention to lymphadenopathy or hepatomegaly)
Hematologic studies
    Complete blood count
    Erythrocyte sedimentation rate
Biochemical studies
    Liver function tests
    Serum copper
    Alkaline phosphatase
Radiologic studies
    Chest x-ray
    Abdominal film

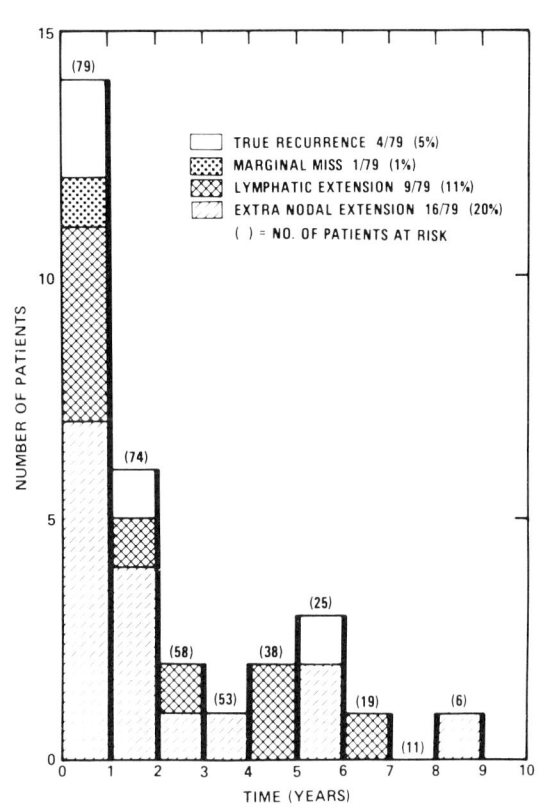

Figure 9-13 Histogram showing the types of relapse of Hodgkin's disease as a function of time. (From Donaldson, S. S., et al.: Cancer 37:2436, 1976.)

Relapses

Relapse may be heralded by constitutional symptoms, elevations of serum copper level or erythrocyte sedimentation rate, palpable lymphadenopathy, widening of the mediastinal shadow, change in the residual lymphangiogram dye in abdominal nodes, or dysfunction of parenchymal organs. However, one must not automatically assume that any new symptom or sign is due to relapse of Hodgkin's disease; biopsy confirmation is highly desirable in all instances. This should be followed by a complete diagnostic re-evaluation (including repeat lymphangiogram and laparotomy, if necessary).

Treatment of relapse in lymphoid structures or localized osseous sites calls for high-dose radiotherapy to the site(s) of relapse and previously untreated lymphoid areas, supplemented, in most instances, by six cycles of MOP chemotherapy. Relapse in parenchymal organs may be treated with MOP chemotherapy, supplemented in some instances with low/moderate doses of radiotherapy to sites of relapse.[70] When relapse occurs in a patient who has received MOPP chemotherapy for initial therapy, the choice of chemotherapeutic regimen for relapse treatment is dependent on the timing of the relapse—patients who develop "late" relapses (more than 12 months after completion of the last MOPP cycle) usually do well on another course of MOPP, while those relapsing earlier should be regarded as MOPP failures and treated with one of the new combinations.[71]

Second Malignancies

In a series of more than 1000 patients with Hodgkin's disease, 35 associated cancers have been reported by Berg.[9] This incidence rate was considered to be above that expected for an age- and sex-matched population. A similar incidence (3.4 to 3.5 per cent) of second malignancies has also been reported for a series of 116 pediatric Hodgkin's patients[95] and for a group of 452 patients treated at the National Cancer Institute (NCI).[16] The NCI patients were analyzed according to mode of treatment and the group who had received intensive treatment with both radiation and combination chemotherapy (either concurrently or sequentially) appeared to be the most susceptible to second malignancies; this group had a 14.5-fold greater risk of developing a second malignancy than would be expected for a similar age- and sex-matched control population.

Although a variety of second malignancies have been seen (including breast carcinoma, thyroid carcinoma, fibrosarcoma, squamous cell carcinoma), there appears to be an especially high incidence of leukemia in Hodgkin's disease patients; Crosby has described an incidence of 17 per 100,000 per year for subsequent acute granulocytic leukemia in Hodgkin's disease, which he estimated to be a tenfold excess over that of the general population.[27] Rosner and Grünwald, in an extensive review of the literature, found 74 cases of acute myelocytic leukemia or one of its variants, 11 cases of acute lymphocytic leukemia, 12 cases of chronic myelocytic leukemia, and 37 cases of chronic lymphocytic leukemia associated with Hodgkin's disease.[107] They, as well as a number of other authors, have concluded that the development of acute leukemia during the course of Hodgkin's disease is most likely related to radiation therapy and it has been estimated that the risk of radiation-induced leukemia in this condition is in the range of 1:1000.[37]

The development of acute leukemia is also related to the intensity of therapy administered; the observed-to-expected ratio of acute myelogenous leukemia varies from 262.2 with intensive chemotherapy to 1333.3 with combined intensive chemotherapy and intensive radiotherapy.[124a] Thus, it would appear that chemotherapy may potentiate the effect of radiotherapy. It is also possible that acute leukemia is part of the natural history of Hodgkin's disease and is now being seen with greater frequency because of the prolonged survival associated with more aggressive therapy.

REFERENCES

1. Abt, A. B., Kirschner, R. H., Belliveau, R. E., et al.: Hepatic pathology associated with Hodgkin's disease. Cancer 33:1564, 1974.
2. Aisenberg, A. C.: Lymphocytopenia in Hodgkin's disease. Blood 25:1037, 1965.
3. Aisenberg, A. C., Kaplan, M. M., Rieder, S. V., and Goldman, J. M.: Serum alkaline phosphatase at the onset of Hodgkin's disease. Cancer 26:318, 1970.
4. Aisenberg, A. C.: Primary management of Hodgkin's disease. N. Engl. J. Med. 278:93, 1968.
5. Aisenberg, A. C.: Malignant lymphoma. N. Engl. J. Med. 288:883, 935, 1973.
5a. Anagnostou, D., Parker, J. W., Taylor, C. R., et al.: Lacunar cells of nodular sclerosing Hodgkin's disease. An ultrastructural and immunohistologic study. Cancer 39:1032, 1977.
6. Andersen, O. F., Fogelberg, M. G., Rosencrantz, N. M., et al.: Postlymphographic cerebral lipid embolization in the vena cava superior syndrome. Cancer 39:79, 1977.
7. Atkinson, H. R.: Bone marrow distribution as a factor in estimating radiation to the blood-forming organs: A survey of present knowledge. J. Coll. Radiol. Aust. 6:149, 1962.
8. Azzam, S. A.: High incidence of Hodgkin's disease in children in Lebanon. Cancer Res. 26:1202, 1966.
9. Berg, J. W.: The incidence of multiple primary cancers: I. Development of further cancers in patients with lymphomas, leukemias, and myeloma. J. Natl. Cancer Inst. 38:741, 1967.
10. Bobrove, A. M., Fuks, Z., Strober, S., and Kaplan, H. S.: Quantitation of T and B lymphocytes and cellular immune func-

tion in Hodgkin's disease. Cancer 36: 169, 1975.
11. Bodie, J. F., and Linton, D. S.: Hepatic oil embolization as a complication of lymphangiography. Radiology 99:317, 1971.
12. Boecker, W. R., Hossfeld, D. K., Gallmeier, W. M., and Schmidt, C. G.: Clonal growth of Hodgkin's cells. Nature 258:235, 1975.
12a. Botnick, L. E., Goodman, R., Jaffe, N., et al.: Stages I–III Hodgkin's disease in children. Cancer 39:599, 1977.
13. Boggs, D. R., and Fahey, J. L.: Serum protein changes in malignant disease. II. The chronic leukemias, Hodgkin's disease and malignant melanoma. Natl. Cancer Inst. Monogr. 25:1381, 1960.
14. Bonadonna, G., Monfardini, S., DeLena, M., et al.: Adriamycin, bleomycin, vinblastine, and imidazole carboxamide (ABVD) — a new combination effective in advanced Hodgkin's disease. In Proceedings of the XI International Cancer Congress, Florence, Italy, Vol. 1, pp. 271–272, 1974.
15. Bouroncle, B. A.: Sternberg-Reed cells in the peripheral blood of patients with Hodgkin's disease. Blood 27:544, 1966.
16. Canellos, G. P., DeVita, V. T., Arsenau, J. C., et al.: Second malignancies complicating Hodgkin's disease in remission. Lancet 1:947, 1975.
17. Carbone, P. P., Spurr, C., Schneiderman, N., et al.: Management of patients with malignant lymphoma: A comparative study with cyclophosphamide and vinca alkaloids. Cancer Res. 28:811, 1968.
18. Carbone, P. P., Kaplan, H. S., et al.: Report of the Committee on Hodgkin's disease staging classification. Cancer Res. 31:1860, 1971.
19. Carmel, R. J., and Kaplan, H. S.: Mantle irradiation in Hodgkin's disease. An analysis of technique, tumor eradication, and complications. Cancer 37:2813, 1976.
20. Cassady, J. R.: Discussion in Case Records of the Massachusetts General Hospital, Case 27–1975. N. Engl. J. Med. 293:86, 1975.
21. Castellino, R. A., Glatstein, E., Turbow, M. M., et al.: Latent radiation injury of lungs or heart activated by steroid withdrawal. Ann. Intern. Med. 80;593, 1974.
22. Castellino, R. A., Bergiron, C., and Markovits, P.: Repeat lymphography in children with Hodgkin's disease. Cancer 38:90, 1976.
23. Castellino, R. A., Filly, R., and Blank, N.: Routine full-lung tomography in the initial staging and treatment planning of patients with Hodgkin's disease and non-Hodgkin's lymphoma. Cancer 38: 1130, 1976.
24. Cham, W. C., Tan, C. T. C., Martinez A., et al.: Involved field radiation therapy for early stage Hodgkin's disease in children. Preliminary results. Cancer 37:1625, 1976.
25. Chilcote, R. R., Baehner, R. L., Hammond, D., et al.: Septicemia and meningitis in children splenectomized for Hodgkin's disease. N. Engl. J. Med. 295:798, 1976.
26. Cline, M. J., and Berlin, N. I.: Anemia in Hodgkin's disease. Cancer 16:526, 1963.
26a. Correa, P., and O'Conor, G. T.: Epidemiologic patterns of Hodgkin's disease. Int. J. Cancer 8:192, 1971.
27. Crosby, W. H.: Acute granulocytic leukemia, a complication of therapy in Hodgkin's disease? Clin. Res. 17:463, 1969.
28. Currie, S., and Henson, R. A.: Neurological syndromes in the reticuloses. Brain 94:307, 1971.
29. DeVita, V. T., Jr., Serpick, A. A., and Carbone, P. P.: Combination chemotherapy in the treatment of advanced Hodgkin's disease. Ann. Intern. Med. 73:881, 1970.
30. DeVita, V. T., Jr.: Lymphocyte reactivity in Hodgkin's disease: A lymphocyte civil war. N. Engl. J. Med. 289:801, 1973.
31. Donaldson, S. S., Glatstein, E., Rosenberg, S. A., and Kaplan, H. S.: Pediatric Hodgkin's disease. II. Results of therapy. Cancer 37:2436, 1976.
32. Dorfman, R. F.: Enzyme histochemistry of normal, hyperplastic, and neoplastic lymphoreticular tissue. Lymph Tumors in Africa (Symposium), Paris, 1963. Basel, S. Karger, 1964.
33. Einhorn, L.: Evaluation and treatment of Hodgkin's disease in the 70's. Connecticut Med. 39:694, 1975.
34. Engeset, A., Höeg, K., Höst. H., et al.: Thoracic duct lymph cytology in Hodgkin's disease. Int. J. Cancer 4:735, 1969.
35. Engeset, A., Cooper, E. H., Brennhovd, I., Höeg, K.: The thoracic duct lymph in Hodgkin's disease. II. Quantitative analysis of the cellular composition of the lymph. Int. J. Cancer 8:113, 1971.
36. Eshhar, Z., Order, S. E., and Katz, D. H.: Ferritin, a Hodgkin's disease associated antigen. Proc. Natl. Acad. Sci. USA 71: 3956, 1974.
37. Ezdinli, E. Z., Sokal, J. E., Aungst, C. W., et al.: Myeloid leukemia in Hodgkin's disease: Chromosomal abnormalities. Ann. Intern. Med. 7:1097, 1969.
38. Falk, J., and Osoba, D.: HL-A antigens and survival in Hodgkin's disease. Lancet 2:1118, 1971.
39. Filler, R. M., Jaffe, N., Cassady, J. R., et al.: Experience with clinical and operative staging of Hodgkin's disease in children. J. Pediatr. Surg. 10:321, 1975.

40. Fleischner, F. G., Bernstein, C., and Levine, B. E.: Retrosternal infiltration in malignant lymphoma. Radiology 51:350, 1948.
41. Frajola, W. J., Greider, M. H., and Bouroncle, B. A.: Cytology of the Sternberg-Reed cell as revealed by the electron microscope. Ann. N.Y. Acad. Sci. 73:221, 1958.
42. Fraumeni, J. F., Jr., and Li, F. P.: Hodgkin's disease in childhood: An epidemiologic study. J. Natl. Cancer Inst. 42:681, 1969.
43. Frei, E., III, Luce, J. K., Gamble, J. F., et al.: Combination chemotherapy in advanced Hodgkin's disease. Ann. Intern. Med. 79:376, 1973.
44. Friedman, M., Kim, T. H., and Panahon, A. M.: Spinal cord compression in malignant lymphoma. Treatment and results. Cancer 37:1485, 1976.
45. Fuks, Z., Strober, S., and Kaplan, H. S.: Interaction between serum factors and T lymphocytes in Hodgkin's disease. Use as a diagnostic test. N. Engl. J. Med. 295:1273, 1976.
46. Giannopoulos, P. P., and Bergsagel, D. E.: The mechanism of anemia associated with Hodgkin's disease. Blood 14:856, 1959.
47. Givler, R. L., Brunk, S. F., Hass, C. A., and Gulfessarian, H. D.: Problems of interpretation of liver biopsy in Hodgkin's disease. Cancer 28:1335, 1971.
48. Glatstein, E., Guernsey, J. M., Rosenberg, S. A., and Kaplan, H. S.: The value of laparotomy and splenectomy in the staging of Hodgkin's disease. Cancer 24:709, 1969.
49. Glick, A. D., Leech, J. H., Flexner, J. M., and Collins, R. D.: Ultrastructural study of Reed-Sternberg cells. Comparison with transformed lymphocytes and histiocytes. Am. J. Pathol. 85:195, 1976.
50. Goldman, L. B.: Hodgkin's disease: An analysis of 212 cases. J.A.M.A. 114:1611, 1940.
51. Goodman, R., Jaffe, N., Filler, R., and Cassady, J. R.: Herpes zoster in children with Stages I–III Hodgkin's disease. Radiology 118:429, 1976.
52. Gottlieb, J. A.: Malignant lymphoma. In Nathan, D. G., and Oski, F. A.: Hematology of Infancy and Childhood. Philadelphia, W. B. Saunders Co., 1974.
53. Granger, W., and Whitaker, R.: Hodgkin's disease in bone, with special reference to periosteal reaction. Brit. J. Radiol. 40:939, 1967.
54. Grossman, H., Winchester, P. H., Bragg, D. G., et al.: Roentgenographic changes in childhood Hodgkin's disease. Am. J. Roentgenol. 108:354, 1970.
55. Grufferman, S., Cole, P., Smith, P., and Lukes, R. J.: Hodgkin's disease in siblings. N. Engl. J. Med. 296:248, 1977.
55a. Gutensohn, N., and Cole, P.: Epidemiology of Hodgkin's disease in the young. Int. J. Cancer 19:595, 1977.
56. Halie, M. R., Huiges, W., and Niewig, H. O.: Abnormal cells in the peripheral blood of patients with Hodgkin's disease. I. Observations with light microscopy. Brit. J. Haematol. 28:317, 1974.
57. Hays, D. M.: The staging of Hodgkin's disease in children reviewed. Cancer 35:973, 1975.
58. Hellman, S.: Current studies in Hodgkin's disease. What laparotomy has wrought. N. Engl. J. Med. 290:894, 1974.
59. Horan, M., and Colebatch, J. H.: Relation between splenectomy and subsequent infection. A clinical study. Arch. Dis. Child. 37:398, 1962.
60. Hrgovcic, M., Tessmer, C. F., Thomas, F. B., et al.: Significance of serum copper levels in adult patients with Hodgkin's disease. Cancer 31:1337, 1973.
61. John, H. T., and Nabarro, J. D. N.: Intracranial manifestations of malignant lymphoma. Brit. J. Cancer 9:386, 1955.
62. Johnson, R. E., Thomas, L. B., Johnson, S. K., and Johnston, G. S.: Correlation between abnormal baseline liver tests and long term clinical course in Hodgkin's disease. Cancer 33:1123, 1974.
63. Jones, P. G., and Campbell, P. E.: Tumours of Infancy and Childhood. Oxford, Blackwell Scientific Publications, 1976, pp. 182–202.
64. Kadin, M. E., Glatstein, E., and Dorfman, R. R.: Clincopathologic studies of 117 untreated patients subjected to laparotomy for the staging of Hodgkin's disease. Cancer 27:1277, 1971.
65. Kaplan, H. S., and Smithers, D. W.: Autoimmunity in man and homologous disease in mice in relation to the malignant lymphomas. Lancet 2:1, 1959.
66. Kaplan, H. S.: Evidence of a tumoricidal dose level in the radiotherapy of Hodgkin's disease. Cancer Res. 26:1221, 1966.
67. Kaplan, H. S.: On the natural history, treatment, and prognosis of Hodgkin's disease. Harvey Lect. 1968–1969.
68. Kaplan, H. S.: Contiguity and progression in Hodgkin's disease. Cancer Res. 31:1811, 1971.
69. Kaplan, H. S., Hodgkin's Disease. Cambridge, Mass., Harvard University Press, 1972.
70. Kaplan, H. S., and Rosenberg, S. A.: The management of Hodgkin's disease. Cancer 36:796, 1975.
71. Kaplan, H. S., and Rosenberg, S. A.: Hodgkin's disease: Current recommendations for management. CA 25:306, 1975.
72. Kaplan, H. S.: Hodgkin's disease and other human malignant lymphomas: Advances and prospects. G.H.A. Clowes

Memorial Lecture. Cancer Res. 36: 3863, 1976.
72a. Kaplan, H. S., and Gartner, S.: "Sternberg-Reed" giant cells of Hodgkin's disease: Cultivation in vitro, heterotransplantation, and characterization as neoplastic macrophages. Int. J. Cancer 19:511, 1977.
73. Kaufman, S. D.: Case Records of the Massachusetts General Hospital, Case 16–1971. N. Engl. J. Med. 284:899, 1971.
73a. Le Bourgeois, J. P., and Tubiana, M.: The erythrocyte sedimentation rate as a monitor for relapse in patients with previously treated Hodgkin's disease. Int. J. Radiation Oncology Biol. Phys. 2:241, 1977.
74. LeFloch, O., Donaldson, S. S., and Kaplan, H. S.: Pregnancy following oophoropexy and total nodal irradiation in women with Hodgkin's disease. Cancer 38:2263, 1976.
75. Levine, P. H., Ablashi, D. V., Berard, C. W., et al.: Elevated antibody titers to Epstein-Barr virus in Hodgkin's disease. Cancer 27:416, 1971.
76. Levitan, R., Diamond, H. D., and Craver, L. F.: The liver in Hodgkin's disease. Gut 2:60, 1961.
77. Levy, R., and Kaplan, H. S.: Impaired lymphocyte function in untreated Hodgkin's disease. N. Engl. J. Med. 290:181, 1974.
78. Longmire, R. L., McMillan, R., Yelenosky, R., et al.: In vitro splenic IgG synthesis in Hodgkin's disease. N. Engl. J. Med. 289:763, 1973.
79. Luce, J. K., Frei, E., III, Gehan, E. A., et al.: Chemotherapy of Hodgkin's disease. Maintenance therapy vs. no maintenance after remission induction with combination chemotherapy. Arch. Intern. Med. 131:391, 1973.
80. Lukes, R. J., Butler, J. J., and Hicks, E. B.: Natural history of Hodgkin's disease as related to its pathological picture. Cancer 19:317, 1966.
81. Lukes, R. J.: Criteria for involvement of lymph node, bone marrow, spleen, and liver in Hodgkin's disease. Cancer Res. 31:1755, 1971.
82. Lukes, R. J.: Updated Hodgkin's disease: Prognosis and relationship of histologic features to clinical stage. J.A.M.A. 222:1294, 1972.
83. Lynch, H. T., Saldivar, V. A., Guirgis, H. A., et al.: Familial Hodgkin's disease and associated cancer. A clinical-pathologic study. Cancer 38:2033, 1976.
84. MacLeod, M., and Stalker, A. L.: Diagnosis of Hodgkin's disease by liver biopsy. Brit. Med. J. 1:1449, 1962.
85. MacMahon, B.: Epidemiology of Hodgkin's disease. Cancer Res. 26:1189, 1966.
86. Milham, S.: Hodgkin's disease as an occupational disease in teachers. N. Engl. J. Med. 290:1329, 1974.
87. Miller, R. W.: Mortality in childhood Hodgkin's disease: An etiologic clue. J.A.M.A. 198:1216, 1966.
88. Moore, M. R., Bull, J. M., Jones, S. E., et al.: Sequential radiotherapy and chemotherapy in the treatment of Hodgkin's disease. A progress report. Ann. Intern. Med. 77:1, 1972.
89. Mosely, J. E.: Bone Changes in Hematologic Disorders. New York, Grune & Stratton, 1963, p. 203.
90. Muggia, F. M., and Heinemann, H. O.: Hypercalcemia associated with neoplastic disease. Ann. Intern. Med. 73:281, 1970.
91. Mullins, G. M., Flynn, J. P. G., El-Mahdi, A. M., et al.: Malignant lymphoma of the spinal epidural space. Ann. Intern. Med. 74:416, 1971.
92. Musshoff, K.: Prognostic and therapeutic implications of staging in extranodal Hodgkin's disease. Cancer Res. 31:1814, 1971.
93. Myers, C. E., Chabner, B. A., DeVita, V. T., and Gralnick, H. R.: Bone marrow involvement in Hodgkin's disease: Pathology and response to MOPP chemotherapy. Blood 44:197, 1974.
94. Nicholson, W. M., Beard, M. E. J., Crowther, D., et al.: Combination chemotherapy in generalized Hodgkin's disease. Brit. Med. J. 3:7, 1970.
95. Norris, D. G., Burgert, E. O., Jr., Cooper, H. A., and Harrison, E. G., Jr.: Hodgkin's disease in childhood. Cancer 36:2109, 1975.
96. Oehlert, W., Musskoff, K., Wunsch, B., et al.: Unspezifische Mesenchymreaktionen und Parenchymschaden der Leber bei Patienten mit Morbus Hodgkin. Klin. Wochenschr. 48:126, 1970.
97. Olson, M. E., Chernik, N. L., and Posner, J. B.: Infiltration of the leptomeninges by systemic cancer. A clinical and pathologic study. Arch. Neurol. 30:122, 1974.
98. Order, S. E., and Hellman, S.: Pathogenesis of Hodgkin's disease. Lancet 1:571, 1972.
99. Peckham, M. J., and Cooper, E. H.: Proliferation characteristics of the various classes of cells in Hodgkin's disease. Cancer 24:135, 1969.
100. Probert, J. C., and Parker, B. R.: The effects of radiation therapy on bone growth. Radiology 114:155, 1975.
101. Prosnitz, L. R., Farber, L. R., Fischer, J. J., et al.: Long term remissions with combined modality therapy for advanced Hodgkin's disease. Cancer 37:2826, 1976.
102. Rappaport, H., Strum, S. B., Hutchison,

G., et al.: Clinical and biological significance of vascular invasion in Hodgkin's disease. Cancer Res. 31:1794, 1971.
103. Razis, D. V., Diamond, H. D., and Craver, L. F.: Familial Hodgkin's disease: Its significance and implications. Ann. Intern. Med. 51:933, 1959.
104. Rosenberg, S. A.: CCNU, Adriamycin, and vinblastine (CAVe) combination chemotherapy for advanced Hodgkin's disease (in preparation).
105. Rosenberg, S. A., Kaplan, H. S.: Evidence for an orderly progression in the spread of Hodgkin's disease. Cancer Res. 26:1225, 1966.
105a. Rosenberg, S. A., Kaplan, H. S., and Glatstein, E.: The role of adjuvant MOPP in the radiation therapy of Hodgkin's disease: a progress report at eight years of the Stanford trials. Amer. Soc. Clin. Oncology, 13th Annual Meeting, 1977 (Abstr. C–304).
106. Rosenstock, J. G., D'Angio, G., and Kiesewetter, W. B.: The incidence of complications following staging laparotomy for Hodgkin's disease in children. Am. J. Roentgenol. Radium Ther. Nucl. Med. 120:531, 1974.
107. Rosner, F., Grünwald, H.: Hodgkin's disease and acute leukemia. Report of eight cases and review of the literature. Am. J. Med. 58:339, 1975.
108. Schiffer, C. A., Levi, J. A., and Wiernik, P. H.: The significance of abnormal circulating cells in patients with Hodgkin's disease. Brit. J. Haematol. 31:177, 1975.
109. Schimpff, S., Serpick, A., Stoler, B., et al.: Varicella-zoster infection in patients with cancer. Ann. Intern. Med. 76:241, 1972.
110. Schwartz, R. S., and Andre-Schwartz, J.: Malignant lymphoproliferative diseases: Interactions between immunological abnormalities and oncogenic viruses. Ann. Rev. Med. 19:269, 1968.
111. Sherlock, P., Winawer, S. J., Lacher, M. J., and Ehrlich, A. N.: Gastrointestinal manifestations of Hodgkin's disease. In Lacher, M. J. (ed.): Hodgkin's Disease. New York, John Wiley & Sons, 1976.
112. Shipley, W. U., Piro, A. J., and Hellman, S.: Radiation therapy of Hodgkin's disease: Significance of splenic involvement. Cancer 34:223, 1974.
113. Smith, P. G., Kinlen, L. J., and Doll, R.: Hodgkin's disease mortality among physicians. Lancet 2:525, 1974.
114. Smith, P. G., and Pike, M. C.: Current epidemiological evidence for transmission of Hodgkin's disease. Cancer Res. 36:660, 1976.
115. Sokal, J. E., and Firat, D.: Varicella-zoster infection in Hodgkin's disease. Am. J. Med. 39:452, 1965.
116. Solidoro, A., Guzman, C., et al.: Relative increased incidence of childhood Hodgkin's disease in Peru. Cancer Res. 26:1204, 1966.
117. Somasundaram, M., and Posner, J. B.: Neurological complications of Hodgkin's disease. In Lacher, M. J. (ed.): Hodgkin's Disease. New York, John Wiley & Sons, 1976.
118. Stolberg, H. O., Patt, N. L., MacEwen, K. F., et al.: Hodgkin's disease of lung: Roentgenologic-pathologic correlation. Am. J. Roentgenol. 92:96, 1964.
119. Strum, S. B., Park, J. K., et al.: Observation of cells resembling Sternberg-Reed cells in conditions other than Hodgkin's disease. Cancer 26:176, 1970.
120. Strum, S. M., and Rappaport, H.: Hodgkin's disease in the first decade of life. Pediatrics 46:748, 1970.
121. Strum, S., and Rappaport, H.: Interrelations of the histologic types of Hodgkin's disease. Arch. Pathol. 91:127, 1971.
122. Taylor, C. R.: The nature of Reed-Sternberg cells and other malignant "reticulum" cells. Lancet 2:802, 1974.
123. Thorling, E. B., and Thorling, K.: The clinical usefulness of serum copper determinations in Hodgkin's disease. A retrospective study of 241 patients from 1963–1973. Cancer 38:225, 1976.
124. Tindle, B. H., Parker, J. W., and Lukes, R. J.: "Reed-Sternberg cells" in infectious mononucleosis? Am. J. Clin. Pathol. 58:607, 1972.
124a. Toland, D. M., and Coltman, C. A., Jr.: Second malignancies complicating Hodgkin's disease: the Southwest Oncology Group experience. Amer. Soc. Clin. Oncology. 13th Annual Meeting, 1977 (Abstr. C–340).
125. Ultmann, J. E., Cunningham, J. K., and Gellhorn, A.: The clinical picture of Hodgkin's disease. Cancer Res. 26:1047, 1966.
126. Ultmann, J. E.: Current status: The management of lymphoma. Semin. Hematol. 7:441, 1970.
127. Ultmann, J. E.: Clinical course and complications in Hodgkin's disease. Arch. Intern. Med. 131:332, 1973.
128. Vianna, N. J., Greenwald, P., Brady, J., et al.: Hodgkin's disease: Cases with features of a community outbreak. Ann. Intern. Med. 77:169, 1972.
129. Vianna, N. J., Polan, A. K., Keogh, M. D., and Greenwald, P.: Hodgkin's disease mortality among physicians. Lancet 2:131, 1974.
130. Vianna, N. J.: Evidence for infectious component of Hodgkin's disease and related considerations. Cancer Res. 36:663, 1976.
131. Viola, M. D., Kovi, J., and Mykhopadhyay, M.: Reversal of myelofibrosis in

Hodgkin's disease. J.A.M.A. 223:1145, 1973.
132. Ward, P. A., and Berenberg, J. L.: Defective regulation of inflammatory mediators in Hodgkin's disease. N. Engl. J. Med. 290:76, 1974.
133. Weller, S. A., Glatstein, E., Kaplan, H. S., and Rosenberg, S. A.: Initial relapses in previously treated Hodgkin's disease. I. Results of second treatment. Cancer 37:2846, 1976.
134. Yam, L. T., and Li, C.-Y.: Histogenesis of splenic lesions in Hodgkin's disease. Am. J. Clin. Pathol. 66:976, 1976.
135. Young, J. L., Jr., and Miller, R. W.: Incidence of malignant tumors in U.S. children. J. Pediatr. 86:254, 1975.
136. Young, R. C., Canellos, G. P., Chabner, B. A., et al.: Maintenance chemotherapy for advanced Hodgkin's disease in remission. Lancet 1:1339, 1973.
137. Young, R. C., Corder, M. P., Berard, C. W., and DeVita, V. T.: Immune alterations in Hodgkin's disease. Arch. Intern. Med. 131:446, 1973.
138. Young, R. C., Canellos, G. P., Chabner, B. A., and DeVita, V. T.: Patterns of relapse after complete remission in Hodgkin's disease treated with MOPP chemotherapy. Proceedings of the Eleventh Annual Meeting of the American Society of Clinical Oncology, May, 1975 (Abstr. 1114).
139. Zamecnik, P. C., and Long, J. C.: Growth of cultured cells from patients with Hodgkin's disease and transplantation into nude mice. Proc. Natl. Acad. Sci. U.S.A. 74:754, 1977.

Chapter Ten

NON-HODGKIN'S LYMPHOMAS

The non-Hodgkin's lymphomas occur about 1.3 times more frequently and cause twice the number of deaths than Hodgkin's disease in children under 15 years of age.[60, 61, 94] They are a difficult group of tumors to categorize clearly, and a discouraging group to treat. The differences in the incidence and manner of presentation of these neoplasms reported from a number of large treatment centers probably reflects, at least in part, variations among oncologists in classifying a disease as leukemia or lymphoma. Some consider a disease to be leukemia if there is any evidence of bone marrow involvement, whereas others may term the same malignancy Stage IV non-Hodgkin's lymphoma or lymphoma with leukemic conversion, especially if there is marked extramedullary tumor involvement. The differences in incidence of mediastinal involvement among a number of larger series most likely reflects the tendency for mediastinal disease to infiltrate bone marrow and to be subject to classification as either leukemia or lymphoma. The criteria used to separate leukemia from lymphoma in many centers is the presence of 25 per cent or more blast cells in the bone marrow. Thus, the diagnosis can change with a second differential cell count or can vary with the technician who does the count.

In comparison to adult non-Hodgkin's lymphomas, the childhood forms have long been known to involve the anterior mediastinum or the intestinal tract more frequently, to disseminate to the meninges, bone marrow, and peripheral blood, and to follow a rapidly progressive and fatal course. Despite these obvious clinical differences between adult and childhood lymphomas, there has been a tendency to apply to children the knowledge obtained from treating adults with non-Hodgkin's lymphoma. It is now apparent that a number of histologic types of lymphomas with a good prognosis are common in adults, but rarely occur in children, while certain histologic types occur primarily in childhood. The non-Hodgkin's lymphomas of childhood are now emerging as a heterologous group of disorders with different clinical patterns and prognoses, and a distribution of histologic types that are different from that found in adults.

ETIOLOGY

Lymphoreticular malignancies have been shown to be of viral origin in a number of animals, including the mouse, rat, chicken, and cat. In addition to the presence of the oncogenic virus, induction of lymphoma in the animal model also usually requires the presence of susceptible lymphoid tissue and an animal with a genetic predisposition to the development of the disorder. It is believed that thymectomy in the AKR mouse[47] and bursectomy in the chicken[28] prevent the development of virally induced lymphoid malignancy by removing the target organ upon which the virus acts. It has also been found that a single gene locus is of importance in determining the susceptibility of certain mouse strains to a number of oncogenic viruses.[71] Other factors which appear to precipitate the development of virally induced lymphoreticular malignancies in certain animal models include radiation exposure,[47] chronic graft-versus-host reactions,[4] immunosuppressive agents,[35] and a variety of immunologic factors.[51]

A number of observations indicate that a virus may also play an etiologic role in the development of lymphoreticular malignancies in man. African children with Burkitt's lymphoma invariably have antibodies against Epstein-Barr virus (EBV). This lymphotrophic Herpes virus, which has as its main target the B-lymphocyte,[44] is also associated with nasopharyngeal carcinoma and infectious mononucleosis. In the geographic areas of Africa where this tumor occurs, EBV infections are acquired at an early age, and 80 to 90 per cent of healthy subjects have antibodies. The antibody titers, however, are much lower in control subjects than in patients with Burkitt's lymphoma, and the sera of about 70 per cent of patients have a unique antibody directed against the so-called EBV early antigen.[34] This antibody is found in all patients who experience a short and lethal course, but in only 43 per cent of those who survive for more than 2 years.[33] The high incidence of African Burkitt's lymphoma in geographic areas where malaria is endemic has led to theories that malaria or some other insect-borne infection may in some way predispose the patient to the development of lymphoma from an EBV infection or act with EBV as a co-carcinogen.[23, 91] It is of interest that concurrent infection with a murine plasmodium increases the incidence of malignant lymphomas following injection of Moloney virus in adult mice.[86]

Despite the accumulating serologic evidence that EBV plays an etiologic role in the development of African Burkitt's lymphoma, about 15 to 50 per cent of children in the United States with a histologically similar tumor do not have antibodies to EBV,[36, 54] and, when present, the levels of antibodies are in the range found in normal persons.[36] Hirshaut and associates[36] interpret these findings to mean either that African and American Burkitt's lymphoma have different etiologies or that EBV is not the etiologic agent of Burkitt's lymphoma in Africa or America. The most incriminating evidence that EBV may be an oncogenic virus are the reports of the development of malignant lymphoma in marmosets that received EBV of infectious mononucleosis origin.[79, 87]

There is a marked increase in the incidence of lymphoreticular malignancies in children with inherited immunodeficiency disorders including those with the Bruton type of sex-linked agammaglobulinemia, combined immunodeficiency, the Wiskott-Aldrich syndrome, and ataxia-telangiectasia.[25, 70] It has been estimated that the incidence of malignancies in patients with primary immunodeficiency disorders is about 10,000 times that of the general age-matched population.[25] Iatrogenic immunosuppression also appears to predispose to the development of malignant neoplasms of the lymphoreticular system. These tumors have occurred in patients treated with immunosuppressive agents who were the recipients of renal transplants, or who have been treated for a number of other nonmalignant conditions, including psoriasis, collagen-vascular diseases, and chronic renal disease.[70] It has been proposed that alterations in the immune system caused by malaria[67] or its therapy[76] may make a subject more susceptible to Burkitt's lymphoma.

Therapy with the hydantoin drugs, including phenytoin (Dilantin) and mephenytoin (Mesantoin), has been known to produce a reaction characterized by lymphadenopathy, eosinophilia, fever, skin rash, and hepatosplenomegaly. The histology of the enlarged lymph nodes in this so-called pseudolymphoma syndrome often simulates that seen in Hodgkin's disease and malignant lymphomas.[21, 78] This hydantoin-induced syndrome usually clears rapidly after withdrawal of the medication and recurs if the drug is given again.[68] However, several reports have now described the occurrence of true malignant lymphoma in patients who have received hydantoin for long periods of time, some of whom initially had the pseudolymphoma syndrome which regressed following drug withdrawal.[24, 39, 55] There is also evidence that patients with convulsive disorders treated with hydantoin drugs have a small but statistically significant increased incidence of malignant lymphoma.[3] The mechanism by which hydantoin-associated lymphomas are produced is unknown, but it may be related to impaired humoral and cell-mediated immune responses which have been demonstrated in patients following long-term therapy.[81] It is of interest that the hydantoins have also been reported to produce a mononucleosis-like syndrome,[1] a disorder usually caused by EBV.

There is also evidence that radiation exposure results in an increased incidence of lymphoma in addition to leukemia and other malignant diseases. Children who received radiation to the thymus, persons irradiated for ankylosing spondylitis, and atomic bomb survivors from Hiroshima have about twice the expected incidence of lymphoma.[2, 66]

PATHOLOGY

Pathologic terms that have been used for decades, such as "lymphosarcoma," "reticulum-cell sarcoma," and "giant follicular lymphoma" are seldom used at most treatment centers today because of their lack of prognostic significance and poor correlation with response to therapy. Rappaport's classification[73, 74] of the non-Hodgkin's lymphomas or modifications of it (Table 10-1) has now gained considerable acceptance, and, at least in adults, appears to have clinical usefulness in determining prognosis[45, 69] and defining treatment.[46] It replaces the older terminology with histologic subgroups called undifferentiated, histiocytic, well differentiated and poorly differentiated lymphocytic, and mixed histiocytic-lymphocytic lymphomas. Each subgroup is further separated into a nodular or a diffuse type. However, histologic evaluations of childhood lymphomas seldom show nodular varieties. A review of 178 children reported from four large series revealed only 5 to have a nodular pattern.[64] The histologic distribution of these tumors according to a modification of Rappaport's classification is shown in Table 10-2. In addition to the paucity of nodular lymphomas, other differences in distribution of lymphomas in adults and children are the occurrence of Burkitt's tumor mainly in children and of a diffuse, poorly differentiated lymphocytic lymphoma of the convoluted cell type[7] almost exclusively in children. Furthermore, well differentiated lymphocytic lymphomas do not seem to occur during childhood. The preponderance of histologic types in children that have been known to have a poor prognosis in adults explains the past observation that children with non-Hodgkin's lymphomas usually do poorly compared to adults. Because of these findings, other classifications for non-Hodgkin's lymphomas in children have been proposed (Table 10-1).

Burkitt's lymphoma is composed of

Table 10–1 Histologic Classifications of Non-Hodgkin's Lymphomas

COMMONLY USED CLASSIFICATIONS		PROPOSED CHILDHOOD CLASSIFICATIONS	
Rappaport[73,74]	*Lukes and Collins*[56]	*Sullivan**[82,83]	*Murphy et al.*[64]
I. Undifferentiated	I. Undefined cell	I. Burkitt's tumor	I. Undifferentiated Burkitt's tumor

II. Lymphocytic— poorly differentiated	II. T-cell types
	  1. Convoluted lymphocyte
	  2. Immunoblastic sarcoma (T-cell)
		II. Non-Burkitt's tumor lacking leukemia propensity	II. Undifferentiated non-Burkitt's tumor

III. Lymphocytic— well differentiated	III. B-cell types
	  1. Small lymphocyte (CLL)
	  2. Plasmacytoid lymphocytic
	  3. Follicular center cell (follicular, diffuse, follicular and diffuse, and sclerotic)
	    a. Small cleaved
	    b. Large cleaved
	    c. Small non-cleaved
	    d. Large non-cleaved
	  4. Immunoblastic sarcoma (B-cell)
		III. Non-Burkitt's tumor with leukemic propensity	III. Convoluted lymphocyte

IV. Mixed		IV. Histiocytic	IV. Lymphocytic–poorly differentiated
V. Histiocytic			V. Lymphocytic–well differentiated
(Each type has nodular and diffuse subgroups)			VI. Large basophilic cell (immunoblast)
	IV. Histiocytic		VII. Mixed
	V. Unclassifiable		VIII. Histiocytic

*Histologic types culled from the M. D. Anderson Hospital classification which were found in children.

Table 10-2 Histologic Distribution of 178 Childhood Non-Hodgkin's Lymphomas*

Histology	Per Cent
Diffuse	
Undifferentiated	
Non-Burkitt's	46.2
Burkitt's	9.5
Lymphocytic, poorly differentiated	9
Mixed	1.7
Histiocytic	28
Nodular	
Lymphocytic, poorly differentiated	1.1
Histiocytic	1.7
Unclassifiable	2.8

*Based on the data compiled by Murphy and associates from four series.[26, 64, 72, 83]

cells of a relatively uniform size which are no larger than the nucleus of the reactive histiocyte. The cytoplasm is well-defined and contains small vacuoles. The nucleus has coarse chromatin and multiple nucleoli.[9] It is included in the general category of diffuse undifferentiated lymphomas in the Rappaport classification, but does not have a nodular form.

Sullivan[82, 83] has separated the non-Burkitt's undifferentiated lymphomas into two types. One has staining characteristics similar to Burkitt's lymphoma, but the cells show more variation in size and shape of their nucleus and amount of cytoplasm than does the Burkitt type. The second type has cells with little or no cytoplasm, marked variation in nuclear size, and frequent folding or clefts in the nuclei. This second type usually arises in the mediastinum or cervical lymph nodes, has a high incidence of involvement of the central nervous system, and often progresses to acute lymphoblastic leukemia. This tumor appears to be similar in histology to the convoluted lymphocytic form in the classification proposed by Murphy and coworkers[64] or the convoluted T-cell malignant lymphoma described by Lukes and Collins.[57]

Nathwani and associates[65] have proposed the term malignant lymphoma, lymphoblastic type, for a group of tumors composed of immature lymphoid cells that are indistinguishable from the cells of acute lymphoblastic leukemia. They can be further divided into those with and those without convoluted nuclei, but both groups frequently occur in children and adolescents, often present with mediastinal masses, have a high incidence of bone marrow and blood involvement during the course of the disease, and have a rapid and usually fatal course. The convoluted cell types of non-Hodgkin's lymphomas proposed by other classifications[57, 64, 83] appear to be included in this more comprehensive grouping.

One tumor type composed of large basophilic cells similar in appearance to those that occur in immunologically stimulated lymph nodes made up over 35 per cent of the cases of one series in which this histologic classification was used.[64] This type is usually included in the histiocytic category of Rappaport. This so called "immunoblastic" type usually arose in tonsils, adenoids, or Peyer's patches, and, although it involved about one-third of the patients, was the histologic type in 60 per cent of the survivors. The poor prognosis associated with localized mediastinal disease contrasted with the good prognosis noted in localized disease originating in Waldeyer's ring or the intestinal tract in this same series.[64] Children with disseminated disease had a poor prognosis irrespective of the tumor histology.

In summary, it is clear that the Rappaport classification has its limitations when applied to children. Nodular lymphomas are rare during this period of life, and over 90 per cent of tumors in most series fall into the categories of diffuse undifferentiated, diffuse poorly differentiated, or diffuse histiocytic lymphomas. The modifications of the Rappaport classification and newer subgroupings at a number of institutions have made comparisons with older reports and between a number of centers most difficult, despite their usefulness at the local institution. Universal acceptance of a histologic classification system appropriate for non-Hodgkin's lymphomas of childhood is clearly needed.

CLINICAL PRESENTATIONS

The non-Hodgkin's lymphomas may present in a variety of ways. The symptoms usually depend upon the location of the tumor, and location is often associated with a particular histologic type. In most series, males are affected two to three times more commonly than females.[60]

LYMPHADENOPATHY

About 20 to 30 per cent of children with non-Hodgkin's lymphomas present with enlarged lymph nodes, usually of the cervical region,[6, 29] (Fig. 10-1), but axillary, inguinal, epitrochlear, or preauricular lymph node enlargement may also be the first sign of disease. Involved nodes are often very firm and nontender, and in about 75 per cent of cases the nodes are unilateral.[40] The children are usually asymptomatic, are brought to their physician because of the lymphadenopathy, and are sent to an oncologist or to a surgeon for node biopsy because of the large size of the node or its lack of response to antibiotic therapy.

MEDIASTINAL MASS

Involvement of the mediastinum, with dyspnea and cough, is a common presentation for lymphoma (Fig. 10-2). There may be evidence of a superior vena caval syndrome, with obstruction to venous return resulting in distended neck veins, and edema of

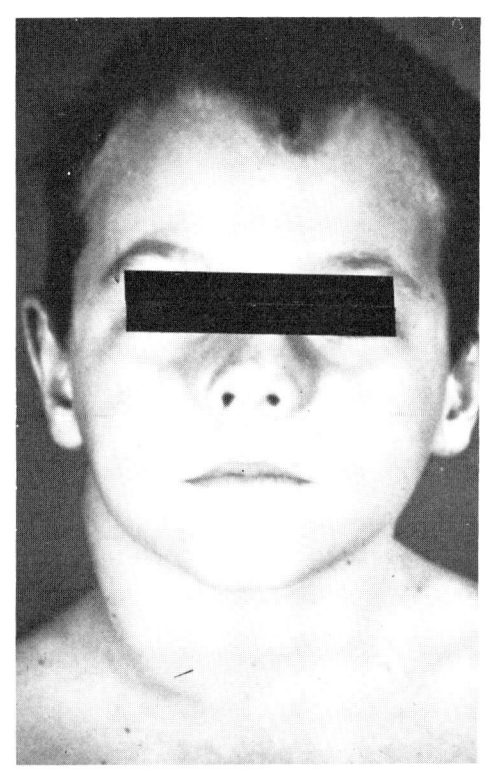

Figure 10-1 Marked cervical lymphadenopathy as the presenting finding in a child with non-Hodgkin's lymphoma.

the neck and face.[17] Pleural effusions are often present, and cytologic examination of pleural fluid may sometimes confirm the diagnosis. Lymphoma in the mediastinum may present as an emergency situation when there is significant airway obstruction. These lymphomas often are histologically of the diffuse lymphoblastic type[65] and the cells often have cleft nuclei. Despite the different terminology used in many centers, all agree that the mediastinal tumor has a marked tendency to involve the bone marrow and progress to an acute lymphocytic leukemia. Many of these tumors have been found to be composed of T-lymphocytes (thymus-derived). It is of major interest that children with acute lymphocytic leukemia and marked mediastinal involvement often have malignant T-lymphocytes in their peripheral blood, suggesting that we are

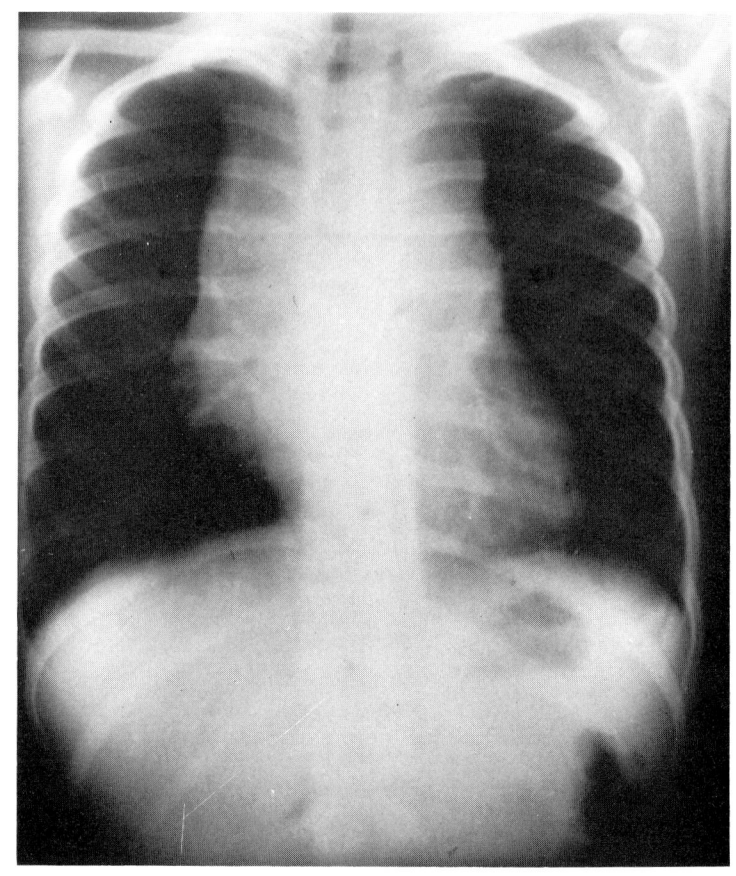

Figure 10–2 Mediastinal lymphoma. This patient developed acute lymphocytic leukemia 6 months following the initial diagnosis.

looking at a spectrum of the same disease.[78a, 84a] This group of children with leukemia has a prognosis that is much worse than that for the child with ALL who lacks these findings.

PRIMARY GASTROINTESTINAL LYMPHOMA

The gastrointestinal tract is not an uncommon primary site of non-Hodgkin's lymphoma in children. In one series of 196 children, Jenkin and associates[43] found 75 to have Hodgkin's disease and 121 to have non-Hodgkin's lymphoma. In this latter group, 39 (32 per cent) had the primary site of origin in the gut. In 35 of these 39 children, the primary site was in the lower ileum, cecum, appendix, ascending colon, or some combination of these sites. The lower portions of the intestinal tract were seldom involved. This observation has been made by many investigators and is believed to be due to more abundant lymphoid tissue in those areas of the gastrointestinal tract that are most commonly involved. Jenkin's observations are similar to the incidence of primary gastrointestinal involvement reported in other childhood series; Baily and associates[6] reported a 19 per cent incidence, Zea and co-workers[95] a 20 per cent incidence, and Murphy and associates[64] a 32 per cent incidence. These patients usually present with abdominal pain, vomiting, and diarrhea. Occasionally there is abdominal distention, and a palpable mass. Other presentations include intussusception and acute gastrointestinal bleeding.[95] Lymphoma is the most frequent anatomic lesion causing intussusception in children over 6 years of age.[85] Occasional instances of malignant lymphoma of the small intestine have been reported in more than one child in the same family.[58] Primary gastrointestinal lymphomas occur less commonly in adults than children.

BURKITT'S TUMOR

This neoplasm makes up over half of all childhood malignancies in the areas of Africa where it is endemic.[88] The African variety has a marked predilection for one or more quadrants of the jaw. It commonly involves the maxilla or orbit, and often reaches massive size before the patient seeks medical aid (Fig. 10–3). Another frequent presentation is abdominal swelling due to tumor in the retroperitoneum, bowel, mesentery, or ovary. Paraplegia is the presenting complaint in nearly 20 per cent of children.[15] The paraplegia is usually of sudden onset and does not respond to chemotherapy. It is thought to be caused by infarction of the spinal cord due to compression of the radicular arteries by retroperitoneal tumor masses.[92] There is usually little local invasiveness, and, although there may be marked local tissue destruction, few symptoms result except from those caused by tumor bulk. Leukemic transformation is uncommon, and there is little involvement of superficial lymph nodes. However, central nervous system involvement with malignant cells in the spinal fluid is a frequent occurrence.[41, 96]

The American equivalent of Burkitt's tumor less often involves the jaw, and usually presents with abdominal disease involving both ovaries or the gastrointestinal tract.[16] The bone marrow appears to be more frequently involved than in the African variety, but there is a lower incidence of central nervous system disease. Despite these clinical differences and the previously mentioned serologic differences, the American and African varieties appear to be histologically identical.

OTHER PRIMARY SITES

A small number of lymphomas arise from the lymphatic tissue in the pharynx made up of the adenoid, lateral band, faucial tonsil, and lingual tonsil (Waldeyer's ring). This was the primary site in five of 48 children in one series[6] and four of 31 in another.[64] Less common sites of primary involvement include bone, brain, retroperitoneal or mesenteric lymph nodes, salivary glands, skin, and gonads.

DIFFERENTIAL DIAGNOSIS

The child has a number of normal findings which reflect an active and prominent lymphoreticular system. Lymphocytes outnumber polymorphonuclear leukocytes during the early childhood years; the normal thymus is often interpreted as being enlarged when viewed on roentgeno-

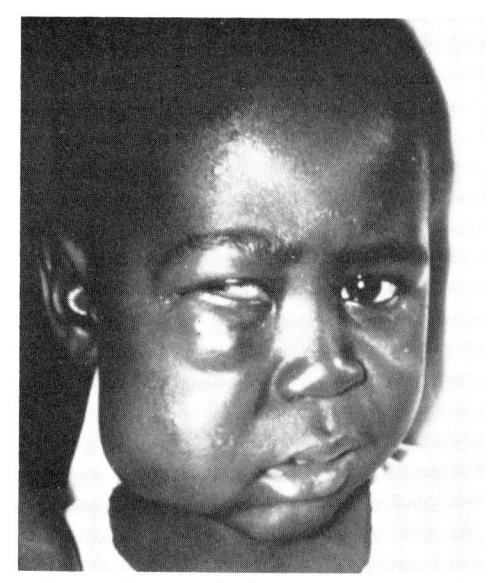

Figure 10–3 Burkitt's tumor arising in the right maxilla of an African child.

grams early in life; "enlarged tonsils" in a child are a common finding and, unfortunately, are too often surgically removed because of their size; and the "two-finger breadth" spleen may no longer be palpable one to two days following recovery from a nonspecific infection. In addition to these normal variations and responses, a number of common and some rare disorders may simulate a malignant lymphoma and present a diagnostic challenge, even to the experienced physician.

CERVICAL LYMPHADENITIS

Cervical lymphadenopathy is a common pediatric problem and, in most instances, is infectious in etiology. Often there is an associated pharyngitis, purulent tonsillitis, fever, dental problem, leukocytosis, or other evidence of infection. In 1963, Dajani and co-workers[18] studied 34 consecutive cases of children with enlarged cervical lymph nodes and found 25 to be attributable to Group A streptococcus, five to *Staphylococcus aureus*, and two to mycobacteria. A similar study of 74 children by Barton and Feigin[8] in 1974 found only 19 to be due to Group A beta-hemolytic streptococcus, but 27 to be due to *Staphylococcus aureus*. The remainder had other or mixed bacterial infections, and in about 25 per cent no organism was identified. Other infectious diseases which cause cervical adenopathy include toxoplasmosis, infectious mononucleosis, cytomegalovirus infection, tuberculosis, atypical mycobacteria infection, histoplasmosis, cat-scratch fever, and infections from anaerobic bacteria.

Seldom is a child referred to an oncologist with an obvious infectious cervical lymphadenitis, or without having previously been treated with antibiotics. If there has been a history suggestive of an infectious etiology, and the patient has been treated with penicillin, a short 10 day to 2 week course of an antibiotic which treats the penicillin-resistant staphylococcus often produces a favorable response, and biopsy can be avoided. Biopsy is indicated, however, when suspicion is high or there is lack of response to antibacterial therapy. Appropriate cultures for bacteria, mycobacteria, and fungal agents at the time of biopsy may determine the cause of lymphadenopathy interpreted histologically as compatible with a nonspecific inflammatory process. If the clinical suspicion for malignant disease remains high, it is not unusual for a second biopsy specimen to confirm the diagnosis of lymphoma despite the initial nonspecific or nondiagnostic pathologic report.

DRUG-INDUCED ADENOPATHY

Lymphadenopathy, hepatosplenomegaly, eosinophilia, skin rash, and fever may occur following therapy with one of the hydantoin drugs (page 274). A similar condition has been reported that may be due to sulfisoxazole.[13]

MUCOCUTANEOUS LYMPH NODE SYNDROME

An apparently new disease, first described by Kawasaki in Japan in 1967,[48] has been termed the mucocutaneous lymph node syndrome. Patients range in age from 2 months to 9 years, but the majority have been under 2 years of age. The major clinical features include nonsuppurative cervical lymphadenopathy, prolonged fever, conjunctivitis, a polymorphous rash with intense erythema, edema of the hands and feet, hyperemia of the lips, pharynx, and tongue, and desquamation of the skin of the palms and soles. About 1 to 2 per cent of the patients die suddenly from acute heart failure. Death is usually due to myocardial infarction secondary to coronary thromboarteritis.[49] Over 6000 cases have been reported in Japan and a small number of cases have now been reported in Hawaii[59] and the continental United States.[10] At the present time the etiology of this disorder is unknown. Recently, rickettsia-like bodies were found by electron microscopy in biopsy specimens from the skin or lymph nodes of a number of patients.[32] Despite the marked lymphadenopathy, the full-blown syndrome should seldom be confused with a malignant process.

SINUS HISTIOCYTOSIS WITH MASSIVE LYMPHADENOPATHY[22, 52]

Over 50 cases have now been reported of a pseudolymphomatous syndrome which is characterized by bilateral, painless, and often massive cervical lymphadenopathy. Occasionally axillary or inguinal nodes are involved. The majority of patients are under 10 years of age. Fever, anemia, neutrophilia, and hypergammaglobulinemia are usually present, but most patients appear to be in good health. The condition is progressive or stable over a period of years, and then usually subsides. The characteristic histology of the lymph nodes reveals many monocytes and large histiocytes, which are often foamy and clumped together. The histiocytes usually contain phagocytized lymphocytes or other blood cells, but should be distinguishable from the histiocytic type of malignant lymphoma. The etiology of the disorder remains unknown.

INTESTINAL DISORDERS WITH LYMPHOID HYPERPLASIA[30]

Diffuse lymphoid polyposis of the colon is a rare, benign disorder that involves the entire colon or rectum. Recurrent abdominal pain or rectal bleeding may be the presenting symptoms. The disorder may easily be misdiagnosed as familial polyposis because several members of the same family may be affected.

Benign lymphoid hyperplasia of the terminal ileum is found most commonly in adolescents, and consists of discrete polypoid lesions composed of hyperplastic lymphoid tissue, which may be pedunculated. The lesions may be asymptomatic, but sometimes cause recurrent abdominal pain. The etiology of these disorders is unknown.

OTHER LYMPHOMA-LIKE DISORDERS

In 1967 Canale and Smith[11] reported a number of children with generalized lymphadenopathy and hepatosplenomegaly. A number of these patients also had a Coombs' positive hemolytic anemia and thrombocytopenia. The histology of the lymph nodes was variable, but sometimes resembled a malignant process. We are aware of two families in which a similar disorder existed. In one, a daughter, mother, and grandmother were affected from early childhood. In the second family, one child had chronic lymphadenopathy, splenomegaly, thrombocytopenia, and a Coombs' positive hemolytic anemia, while his father and brother had only a mild, compensated Coombs' positive hemolytic anemia.

A rare disorder characterized by lymphadenopathy, splenomegaly, and marked lymphocytosis has been reported in two young children, which resembles chronic lymphocytic leukemia but is apparently benign.[14, 19] The white cell count may be as high as 160,000/mm.^{3} In one child the disorder was diagnosed at birth.

EVALUATION OF THE PATIENT

Once the diagnosis of lymphoma is suspected, a tissue diagnosis must be made. Occasionally a complete blood count will determine that the patient has leukemia, and node biopsy is then unnecessary. If there is a generalized lymphadenopathy or any evidence that the bone marrow may be involved, such as bone pain, the presence of anemia, granulocytopenia, or thrombocytopenia, bone marrow aspiration should first be performed despite the absence of abnormal cells in the peripheral blood. Node biopsy adds little additional information if the bone marrow is infiltrated with malignant lymphocytes. Once a decision is made to obtain a tissue specimen, a biopsy of the mass lesion, or excisional biopsy of the lymph node, should be carried out. A needle biopsy should not be performed, nor should a diagnosis be made on the interpretation of a frozen tissue section. When the patient presents with abdominal or mediastinal symptoms that require immediate therapeutic intervention, there may be little time to pick the most appropriate node or tissue to biopsy, and a histologic diagnosis is often made first from tumor tissue obtained at the time of laparotomy or cells obtained from a pleural effusion.

The staging systems used for Hodgkin's disease are based on the premise that the disorder is unicentric in origin and follows a predictable pattern of spread along the lymphatic system. The extent of disease determined by a staging system has prognostic significance and often dictates therapy, which in many instances consists of radiation therapy alone. Extrapolation of the information learned from the clinical staging, including celiotomy and splenectomy, in patients with Hodgkin's disease and adult non-Hodgkin's lymphoma may not lead to valid conclusions regarding appropriate therapy in children with non-Hodgkin's lymphoma. This appears to be due to the preponderance in childhood of the undifferentiated, poorly differentiated, and histiocytic cell types of lymphoma (Rappaport system), which belong to the diffuse subgroup—tumors which have a poor prognosis even in the adult—and which have a tendency for early systemic spread. It is therefore not surprising that radiation therapy alone, with fields determined by an anatomic staging system, has not produced the excellent results in children that have been reported in many series of adult patients. The statement that "the general indications for chemotherapy for patients with the non-Hodgkin's lymphomas are much the same as for those with Hodgkin's disease,"[75] does not generally hold true in children, and probably is questionable in adults with tumors of a histologic type known to have a poor prognosis and a tendency to disseminate widely, despite their apparent localization. We have therefore not used staging laparotomy routinely in children with non-Hodgkin's lymphoma, nor limited therapy to radiation alone.

Once the diagnosis of non-Hodgkin's lymphoma is made, a number of diagnostic studies are indicated to determine both degree of tumor dissemination and the status of organ function which may be affected by disease or by subsequent therapy. Recommendations vary among institutions, but complete blood count, bone marrow aspiration or biopsy, chest x-rays, and studies of renal and hepatic function are essential prior to initiation of therapy. Bone marrow biopsy has been reported to be markedly superior to aspiration for the detection of focal lymphoma.[27] A high incidence of central nervous system involvement occurs in children, especially in those with diffuse, poorly differentiated lymphocytic lymphoma. This may occur prior to the development of leukemic transformation of the bone marrow.[38] It therefore seems prudent to evaluate the status of the central nervous system with a lumbar puncture and cytologic examination of the spinal fluid as part of the initial workup. The determination of a serum uric acid level is extremely important, because it may be elevated prior to the initiation of therapy, and, once rapid lysis of malignant lymphocytes occurs, uric acid nephropathy may result.[50] Hyperuricemia and renal failure may sometimes be the presenting manifestations of occult lymphoma.[93] The extent of the evaluation to be performed

Table 10-3 Suggested Evaluation of the Child With Non-Hodgkin's Lymphoma

---

Routine Evaluation:
   Tissue diagnosis
   Complete blood count, platelet count, erythrocyte sedimentation rate
   Bone marrow examination
   Spinal fluid examination
   Serum uric acid
   Evaluation of hepatic function, including alkaline phosphatase, SGOT, SGPT, BSP
   Evaluation of renal function, including urinalysis, BUN, creatinine
   Chest roentgenograms
   PPD or Tine Test
If indicated in the individual case:
   Intravenous pyelogram
   Lymphangiogram
   Contrast studies of gastrointestinal tract
   Skeletal survey or scan
   Soft tissue views of the nasopharynx
   Liver-spleen scan
   Cytologic evaluation of ascitic or pleural fluid

---

for each patient often depends on the individual situation, but a suggested guideline is outlined in Table 10-3.

Some studies have indicated a high correlation between serum copper levels and disease activity, and it has been reported that elevated levels in active disease have decreased as the disease has responded to therapy.[37]

THERAPY AND PROGNOSIS

The best methods of treating children with non-Hodgkin's lymphoma are still under intensive investigation, and, unlike the treatment of Hodgkin's disease, the state of the art has not progressed to the point where definite guidelines can be recommended. The majority of children tend to have rapidly progressive disease which cannot usually be controlled by radiation therapy alone despite the fact that the neoplasm often appears localized at the time of diagnosis.[77] One review of 221 previously reported cases noted only a 9 per cent 5-year survival rate.[5] Aur and co-workers have reported that 33 per cent of children with lymphoma subsequently develop acute lymphocytic leukemia, and the frequency is even higher when the primary tumor is in the anterior mediastinum.[5] Although children with lymphoma, including those who have had leukemic transformation, often have a dramatic initial response to radiation therapy and antileukemic chemotherapy, the improvement is usually transient. The long-term remissions and possible cures now being reported in many children with acute lymphoblastic leukemia seldom are achieved in those with lymphomas that have undergone leukemic transformation, and the latter group appears to be less responsive to the usual antileukemic chemotherapy.[5]

Few would disagree that the child with apparently localized mediastinal disease, localized disease of a poor prognostic histologic type, or advanced, widespread disease should be treated with chemotherapy. There is some disagreement regarding the treatment of localized disease of the gastrointestinal tract. Jenkin and associates[43] have stated that primary malignant lymphoma in childhood, when limited to the gut and mesenteric nodes, is associated with a good prognosis when treated by surgical excision and postoperative radiation to the whole abdomen. They reported five of six cases alive at 5 years, compared with only one of 12 treated with surgery alone. Of those with more advanced gastrointestinal disease, however, only one in 18 survived. Zea and colleagues,[95] however, believe the most important treatment modality to be combination chemotherapy, and treated only one of six patients with completely resected bowel disease with radiation and all of them with chemotherapy. All six survived. Of those with unresectable disease, however, only one in 15 survived despite the use of aggressive chemotherapy and irradiation. It therefore appears that the child with resectable intestinal disease has a good prognosis if treated with either radiation or chemotherapy to destroy residual, microscopic disease, but those with extensive tumor left behind have a poor prognosis despite the addition of further therapy. Unfortunately, the majority of patients with gastrointestinal lesions in most series have nonresectable disease and a poor prognosis.

A number of drugs are effective in treating non-Hodgkin's lymphoma, and combination chemotherapy has generally proved to be superior to single drug regimens.[12] Various chemotherapeutic combinations used in a number of studies in adults, such as COP[80] (cyclophosphamide, vincristine, prednisone) or COPP[62] (cyclophosphamide, vincristine, prednisone, procarbazine) have been most successful in those with nodular and well differentiated lymphomas, histologic types that are rare in children.

Some recent reports of the therapeutic results in the treatment of childhood lymphomas have been more encouraging. Jenkin[42] recently reported a 19 per cent 3-year survival, Murphy and associates[64] noted a 32 per cent survival, and Lemerle and co-workers[53] a 27 per cent survival. Traggis and associates[84] reported a survival rate of 51.7 per cent of pediatric patients with disease localized to the head and neck. The factors which influenced survival in this latter report were the stage of lymphoma (Ann Arbor staging system), the histology, and the anatomic location of the tumor. Twelve of 17 Stage I patients survived and all of seven patients with tumors showing nodular histology survived. This is one of the few series having a number of children with tumors showing a nodular histology, including one 11 month old boy, and indicates that a nodular pattern is associated with a good prognosis in the child as well as the adult. In addition, those patients with non-Hodgkin's lymphomas limited to the tonsils and adenoids had a better survival rate than expected, although the numbers in this series were small. All 4 children with Stage I disease in this anatomic area survived, including two with the diffuse, undifferentiated lymphomas.

Aur and associates[5] reported that six of eight children with localized disease in various anatomic sites who were treated with radiation therapy and intensive combination chemotherapy were free of disease 16 to 27 months following diagnosis. Djerassi and Kim,[20] using high doses of intravenous methotrexate given in pulse infusions, achieved 16 complete and five partial remissions in 21 patients they were able to evaluate. Fifty per cent of patients (six of 12) who had no previous chemotherapy were entered into a maintenance program of combination chemotherapy, including monthly high-dose methotrexate, and were alive and disease-free 2½ to 4½ years after discontinuing therapy and 4½ to 8½ years after the diagnosis was first made. Five of these six patients had advanced disease at the time of diagnosis. It is of interest that the more conventional use of methotrexate has been of limited value in the treatment of non-Hodgkin's lymphoma.

Because of the high conversion rate of those with diffuse lymphoma to leukemia, especially in patients with mediastinal lymphoma, and because a significant number of such patients develop central nervous system involvement, it has been proposed that prophylactic central nervous system treatment be given in a manner similar to that now used for children with lymphocytic leukemia.[38] A number of centers have now been using central nervous system prophylaxis.[63, 83]

Wollner and colleagues have used massive doses of cyclophosphamide followed by a regimen previously used in the treatment of acute lymphoblastic leukemia, including intrathecal methotrexate (Memorial Sloan-Kettering L-2 protocol).[89] These investigators reported a complete remission in 28 of 29 children with 23 remaining in complete remission for periods up to 18 months. A more recent report of the results of this treatment protocol revealed 80 per cent of 35 patients to be alive, with a median observation time of over 14 months.[90] These results were much better than those achieved by previous treatment regimens used by these investigators.

In summary, at present we do not know the best methods of treating non-Hodgkin's lymphoma. In those with the diffuse histologic varieties, which constitute the majority of patients, we have been using radiation therapy delivered to massive lesions, combination chemotherapy similar to that used in treating acute lymphocytic leukemia, and central nervous system prophylactic treatment. Although the rationale for aggressive therapeutic regimens appears sound and the preliminary reports following their use are encouraging, the impact of such treatment programs on the ultimate course of the disease remains to be determined.

REFERENCES

1. Abbott, J. A., and Schwab, R. S.: Mesantoin in the treatment of epilepsy: A study of its effect on the leukocyte count in seventy-nine cases. N. Engl. J. Med. 250:197, 1954.
2. Anderson, R. E., Nishiyama, H., Ii, Y., et al.: Pathogenesis of radiation-related leukemia and lymphoma: Speculations based primarily on the experience of Hiroshima and Nagasaki. Lancet 1:1060, 1972.
3. Anthony, J. J.: Malignant lymphoma associated with hydantoin drugs. Arch. Neurol. 22:450, 1970.
4. Armstrong, M. Y. K., Gleichman, E., Gleichman, H., et al.: Chronic allogenic disease. II. Development of lymphomas. J. Exp. Med. 132:417, 1970.
5. Aur, R. J. A., Hustu, H. O., Simone, J. V., et al.: Therapy of localized and regional lymphosarcoma of childhood. Cancer 27:1328, 1971.
6. Bailey, R. J., Jr., Burgert, E. O., Jr., and Dahlin, D. C.: Malignant lymphoma in children. Pediatrics 28:985, 1961.
7. Barcos, M. P., and Lukes, R. J.: Malignant lymphoma of convoluted lymphocytes—a new entity of possible T-cell type. In Sinks, L. F., and Goddens, J. O. (eds.): Conflicts in Childhood Cancer. An Evaluation of Current Management. Vol. 4. New York, Alan R. Liss, Inc., 1975, p. 147.
8. Barton, L. L., and Feigin, R. D.: Childhood cervical lymphadenitis: a reappraisal. J. Pediatr. 84:846, 1974.
9. Berard, C., O'Conor, G. T., Thomas, L. B., et al.: Histopathological definition of Burkitt's tumor. Bull. WHO 40:601, 1969.
10. Brown, J. S., Billmeier, G. J., Jr., Cox, F., et al.: Mucocutaneous lymph node syndrome in the continental United States. J. Pediatr. 88:81, 1976.
11. Canale, V. C., and Smith, C. H.: Chronic lymphadenopathy simulating malignant lymphoma. J. Pediatr. 70:891, 1967.
12. Carbone, P. P.: Management of patients with non-Hodgkin's lymphomas. Arch. Intern. Med. 131:455, 1973.
13. Case Records of the Massachusetts General Hospital. Case 33–1972. N. Engl. J. Med. 287:349, 1972.
14. Casey, T. P.: Chronic lymphocytic leukemia in a child presenting at the age of two years and eight months. Aust. Ann. Med. 17:70, 1968.
15. Cockshott, W. P., and Evans, K. T.: Childhood paraplegia in lymphosarcoma (Burkitt's tumour). Brit. J. Radiol. 36:914, 1963.
16. Cohen, M. H., Bennett, J. M., Berard, C. W., et al.: Burkitt's tumor in the United States. Cancer 23:1259, 1969.
17. D'Angio, G. J., Mitus, A., and Evans, A. E.: The superior mediastinal syndrome in children with cancer. Am. J. Roentgenol. 93:536, 1965.
18. Dajani, A. S., Garcia, R. E., and Wolinsky, E.: Etiology of cervical lymphadenitis in children. N. Engl. J. Med. 268:1329, 1963.
19. Darte, J. M. M., McClure, P. D., Saunders, E. F., et al.: Congenital lymphoid hyperplasia with persistent hyperlymphocytosis. N. Engl. J. Med. 284:431, 1971.
20. Djerassi, I., and Kim, J. S.: Methotrexate and citrovorum factor rescue in the management of childhood lymphosarcoma and reticulum cell sarcoma (non-Hodgkin's lymphomas): prolonged unmaintained remissions. Cancer 38:1043, 1976.
21. Doyle, A. P., and Henderson, H. R.: Mesantoin lymphadenopathy morphologically simulating Hodgkin's disease. Ann. Intern. Med. 59:363, 1963.
22. Editorial: A new lymphoma syndrome. Lancet 1:139, 1973.
23. Editorial: Burkitt lymphoma and malaria. Lancet 2:300, 1970.
24. Gans, R. A., Neal, J. A., and Conrad, F. G.: Hydantoin-induced pseudo-pseudolymphoma. Ann. Intern. Med. 69:557, 1968.

25. Gatti, R. A., and Good, R. A.: Occurrence of malignancy in immunodeficiency diseases: a literature review. Cancer 28:89, 1971.
26. Glatstein, E., Kim, H., Donaldson, S. S., et al.: Non-Hodgkin's lymphomas. VI. Review of treatment in childhood. Cancer 34:204, 1974.
27. Goffinet, D. R., Castellino, R. A., Kim, H., et al.: Staging laparotomies in unselected previously untreated patients with non-Hodgkin's lymphomas. Cancer 32:672, 1973.
28. Good, R. A., and Finstad, J.: Essential relationship between the lymphoid system, immunity, and malignancy. Natl. Cancer Inst. Monogr. 31:41, 1969.
29. Grundy, G. W., Creagan, E. T., and Fraumeni, J. F.: Non-Hodgkin's lymphoma in childhood: Epidemiological features. J. Natl. Cancer Inst. 51:767, 1973.
30. Gryboski, J.: Miscellaneous diseases affecting the small bowel and colon. In Gastrointestinal Problems in the Infant. Philadelphia, W. B. Saunders Co., 1975, p. 685.
31. Haghbin, M., Tan, C. C., Clarkson, B. D., et al.: Intensive chemotherapy in children with acute lymphocytic leukemia (L-2 protocol). Cancer 33:1491, 1974.
32. Hamashima, Y., Kishi, K., and Tasaka, K.: Rickettsia-like bodies in infantile acute febrile mucocutaneous lymph node syndrome. Lancet 2:42, 1973.
33. Henle, W., Henle, G., Gunvén, P., et al.: Patterns of antibodies to Epstein-Barr virus induced early antigens in Burkitt's lymphoma. Comparison of dying patients with long-term survivors. J. Natl. Cancer Inst. 50:1163, 1973.
34. Henle, W., Henle, G., Zajac, B. A., et al.: Differential reactivity of human serums with early antigens induced by Epstein-Barr virus. Science 169:188, 1970.
35. Hirsch, M. S., Black, P. H., and Proffitt, M. R.: Immunosuppression and oncogenic virus infections. Fed. Proc. 30:1852, 1971.
36. Hirshaut, Y., Cohen, M. H., and Stevens, D. A.: Epstein-Barr virus antibodies in American and African Burkitt's lymphoma. Lancet 2:114, 1973.
37. Hrgovcic, M., Tessmer, C. F., Thomas, F. B., et al.: Serum copper observations in patients with malignant lymphoma. Cancer 32:1512, 1973.
38. Hutter, J. J., Jr., Favara, B. E., Nelson, M., et al.: Non-Hodgkin's lymphoma in children: correlation of CNS disease with initial presentation. Cancer 36:2132, 1975.
39. Hyman, G. A., and Sommers, S. C.: The development of Hodgkin's disease and lymphoma during anticonvulsant therapy. Blood 28:416, 1966.
40. Jaffe, B. F., and Jaffe, N.: Head and neck tumors in children. Pediatrics 51:731, 1973.
41. Janota, I.: Involvement of the nervous system in malignant lymphoma in Nigeria. Brit. J. Cancer 20:47, 1966.
42. Jenkin, R. D. T.: The management of malignant lymphoma in childhood. In Deeley, T. J. (ed.): Modern Radiotherapy—Malignant Disease in Children. London, Butterworths, 1974.
43. Jenkin, R. D. T., Sonley, M. J., Stephens, C. A., et al.: Primary gastrointestinal tract lymphoma in childhood. Radiology 92:763, 1969.
44. Jondal, M., and Klein, G.: Surface markers of human B and T lymphocytes. II. Presence of Epstein-Barr virus receptors on B lymphocytes. J. Exp. Med. 138:1365, 1973.
45. Jones, S. E., Fuks, Z., Bull, M., et al.: Non-Hodgkin's lymphomas. IV. Clinicopathologic correlations in 405 cases. Cancer 31:806, 1973.
46. Jones, S. E., Fuks, Z. Kaplan, H. S., et al.: Non-Hodgkin's lymphomas. V. Results of radiotherapy. Cancer 32:682, 1973.
47. Kaplan, H. S.: On the natural history of murine leukemias: presidential address. Cancer Res. 27:1325, 1967.
48. Kawasaki, T.: Acute febrile mucocutaneous syndrome with lymph node involvement with specific desquamation of the fingers and toes in children. Jap. J. Allergy 16:178, 1967.
49. Kawasaki, T., Kosaki, F., Okawa, S., et al.: A new infantile acute febrile mucocutaneous lymph node syndrome (MLNS) prevailing in Japan. Pediatrics 54:271, 1974.
50. Kiely, J. M., Wagoner, R. D., and Holley, K. E.: Renal complications of lymphoma. Ann. Intern. Med. 71:1159, 1969.
51. Klein, G.: Experimental studies in tumor immunology. Fed. Proc. 28:1739, 1969.
52. Lampert, F., and Lennert, K.: Sinus histiocytosis with massive lymphadenopathy: fifteen new cases. Cancer 37:783, 1976.
53. Lemerle, M., Gerard-Marchant, R., Sarrazin, D., et al.: Lymphosarcoma and reticulum cell sarcoma in children. A retrospective study of 172 cases. Cancer 32:1499, 1973.
54. Levine, P. H., O'Conor, G. T., and Berard, C. W.: Antibodies to Epstein-Barr virus (EBV) in American patients with Burkitt's lymphoma. Cancer 30:610, 1972.
55. Li, F. P., Willard, D. R., Goodman, R., et al.: Malignant lymphoma after diphenylhydantoin (Dilantin) therapy. Cancer 36:1359, 1975.
56. Lukes, R. J., and Collins, R. D.: New approaches to the classification of the lymphoma. Brit. J. Cancer 31 (Suppl. 2): 1, 1975.
57. Lukes, R. J., and Collins, R. D.: Immunologic characterization of human malignant lymphomas. Cancer 34:1488, 1974.
58. Maurer, H. S., Gotoff, S. P., Allen, L., et al.:

Malignant lymphoma of the small intestine in multiple family members. Cancer 37:2224, 1976.
59. Melish, M. E., Hicks, R. H., and Larsen, E.: Mucocutaneous lymph node syndrome (MCLS) in the U.S. (Abstr.). Pediatr. Res. 8:427, 1974.
60. Meyers, M. H., Heise, H. W., Li, F. P., et al.: Trends in cancer survival among U.S. white children, 1955–1971. J. Pediatr. 87:815, 1975.
61. Miller, R. W., and Dalager, N. A.: U.S. childhood cancer deaths by cell type, 1960–68. J. Pediatr. 85:664, 1974.
62. Morgenfeld, M. C., Pavlovsky, A., Suarez, A., et al.: Combined cyclophosphamide, vincristine, procarbazine, and prednisone (COPP) therapy of malignant lymphoma. Cancer 36:1241, 1975.
63. Murphy, S. B., and Davis, L. W.: Hodgkin's disease and the non-Hodgkin's lymphomas in childhood. Semin. Oncol. 1:17, 1974.
64. Murphy, S. B., Frizzera, G., and Evans, A. E.: A study of childhood non-Hodgkin's lymphoma. Cancer 36:2121, 1975.
65. Nathwani, B. N., Kim, H., and Rappaport, H.: Malignant lymphoma, lymphoblastic. Cancer 38:964, 1976.
66. Nishiyama, H., Anderson, R. E., Ishimaru, T., et al.: The incidence of malignant lymphoma and multiple myeloma in Hiroshima and Nagasaki atomic bomb survivors: 1945–1965. Cancer 32:1301, 1973.
67. O'Conor, G. T.: Persistent immunologic stimulation as a factor in oncogenesis, with special reference to Burkitt's tumor. Am. J. Med. 48:279, 1970.
68. Oates, R. K., and Tonge, R. E.: Phenytoin and the pseudolymphoma syndrome. Med. J. Aust. 2:371, 1971.
69. Patchefsky, A. S., Brodovsky, H. S., Menduke, H., et al.: Non-Hodgkin's lymphomas: A clinicopathologic study of 293 cases. Cancer 34:1173, 1974.
70. Penn, I.: Occurrence of cancer in immune deficiencies. Cancer 34:858, 1974.
71. Pincus, T., Hartley, J. W., and Rowe, W. P.: A major genetic locus affecting resistance to infection with murine leukemia viruses. I. Tissue culture studies of naturally occurring viruses. J. Exp. Med. 133:1219, 1971.
72. Pinkel, D., Johnson, W., and Aur, R. J. A.: Non-Hodgkin's lymphoma in children. Brit. J. Cancer (Suppl. 2) 31:298, 1975.
73. Rappaport, H.: Tumors of the hematopoietic system. Atlas of Tumor Pathology, Sect. 3, Fasc. 8. Washington, D.C., Armed Forces Institute of Pathology, 1968.
74. Rappaport, H., Winter, W. J., and Hicks, E. B.: Follicular lymphoma: A re-evaluation of its position in the scheme of malignant lymphoma based on a survey of 253 cases. Cancer 9:792, 1956.
75. Rosenberg, S., and Kaplan, H. S.: Hodgkin's disease and other malignant lymphomas. California Med. 113:23, 1970.
76. Sadoff, L.: Aetiology of Burkitt's lymphoma. Lancet 2:1414, 1972.
77. Sageman, R. H., Wolff, J. A., Sitarz, A., et al.: Radiation therapy for lymphoma in children. Radiology 86:1096, 1966.
78. Saltzstein, S. L., and Acherman, L. V.: Lymphadenopathy induced by anticonvulsant drugs and mimicking clinically and pathologically malignant lymphomas. Cancer 12:164, 1959.
78a. Sen, L., and Borella, L.: Clinical importance of lymphoblasts with T markers in childhood leukemia. N. Engl. J. Med. 292:828, 1975.
79. Shope, T., Dechairo, D., and Miller, G.: Malignant lymphoma in cotton-top marmosets after inoculation with Epstein-Barr virus. Proc. Natl. Acad. Sci. USA 70:2487, 1973.
80. Skarin, A. T., Pinkus, G. S., Myerowitz, R. L., et al.: Combination chemotherapy of advanced lymphocytic lymphoma: Importance of histologic classification in evaluating response. Cancer 34:1023, 1974.
81. Sorrell, T. C., Forbes, I. J., Burness, F. R., et al.: Depression of immunological function in patients treated with phenytoin sodium (sodium diphenylhydantoin). Lancet 2:1233, 1971.
82. Sullivan, M. P.: Non-Hodgkin's lymphoma of childhood. In Sutow, W. W., Vietti, T. J., and Fernback, D. J. (eds.): Clinical Pediatric Oncology. St. Louis, C. V. Mosby Co., 1973, p. 313.
83. Sullivan, M. P.: Treatment of lymphoma. Cancer 35:991, 1975.
84. Traggis, D., Jaffe, N., Vawter, G., et al.: Non-Hodgkin's lymphoma of the head and neck in childhood. J. Pediatr. 87:933, 1975.
84a. Tsukimoto, I., Wong, K. Y., and Lampkin, B. C.: Surface markers and prognostic factors in acute lymphoblastic leukemia. N. Engl. J. Med. 294:245, 1976.
85. Wayne, E. R., Campbell, J. B., Kosloske, A. M., et al.: Intussusception in the older child—suspect lymphosarcoma. J. Pediatr. Surg. 11:789, 1976.
86. Wedderburn, N.: Effect of concurrent malarial infection on development of virus-induced lymphoma in Balb/c mice. Lancet 2:1115, 1970.
87. Werner, J., Wolf, H., Apodaca, J., et al.: Lymphoproliferative disease in cotton-top marmoset after inoculation with infectious mononucleosis-derived Epstein-Barr virus. Int. J. Cancer 15:1000, 1975.
88. Williams, A. O.: Tumors of childhood in Ibadan, Nigeria. Cancer 36:370, 1975.

89. Wollner, N., D'Angio, G., Burchenal, J. H., et al.: Treatment of non-Hodgkin's lymphoma in children with multiple drug leukemia regimen and radiation therapy. Proc. Am. Ass. Cancer Res. 14:97, 1973.
90. Wollner, N., Lieberman, P., Exelby, P., et al.: Non-Hodgkin's lymphoma in children: Results of treatment with LSA_2-L_2 protocol. Brit. J. Cancer 31 (Suppl. 2): 337, 1975.
91. Wright, D. H.: Burkitt's lymphoma and malaria. Lancet 2:881, 1970.
92. Wright, D. H.: Burkitt's tumour: A post-mortem study of 50 cases. Brit. J. Surg. 51:245, 1964.
93. Yolken, R. H., and Miller, D. R.: Hyperuricemia and renal failure — presenting manifestations of occult hematologic malignancies. J. Pediatr. 89:775, 1976.
94. Young, J. L., and Miller, R. W.: Incidence of malignant tumors in U.S. children. J. Pediatr. 86:254, 1975.
95. Zea, J. M., Exelby, P. R., and Wollner, N.: Abdominal non-Hodgkin's lymphoma in children. J. Pediatr. Surg. 11:363, 1976.
96. Ziegler, J. L., and Bluming, A. Z.: Intrathecal chemotherapy in Burkitt's lymphoma. Brit. Med. J. 3:508, 1971.

Chapter Eleven

THE HISTIOCYTOSES

The histiocytoses (*reticuloendothelioses*) are a group of diseases whose basic pathology is the localized or disseminated infiltration of normal tissues by morphologically recognizable histiocytes.[61] Included within this grouping are: *histiocytic medullary reticulosis* (malignant histiocytosis), *familial erythrophagocytic lymphohistiocytosis, sex-linked reticulohistiocytosis with hypergammaglobulinemia* and *histiocytosis X*.

The histiocytic cell series (reticuloendothelial system) may be viewed as a continuum of highly phagocytic mononuclear cells of mesenchymal origin. The progenitor cells arise in the bone marrow as monoblasts and promonocytes, intermediate forms circulate in the peripheral blood as monocytes, and the mature forms are the fixed tissue histiocytes (macrophages) of the liver, spleen, lungs, lymph nodes, adrenal cortex, and bone marrow, and the free histiocytes of connective tissue[9] (Fig. 11-1). Closely related to these cells in both mesenchymal origin and in histochemistry is the Langerhans cell of the epidermis, which forms a reticulo*epithelial* network of scavengers for molecular matter.[59]

Cline and Golde[9] have formulated a classification of the histiocytic disorders (Table 11-1) based on the following principles: (1) histiocytic diseases with the least cellular differentiation will have the highest degree of cellular proliferative activity and will be clinically most acute, (2) histiocytic diseases in which mature macrophages of low proliferative capacity predominate will be clinically more chronic, (3) although one cell type will predominate in a given patient, there may be a spectrum of cells at different levels of maturation, thereby giving rise to a certain overlap in the clinical and pathologic features among the disease syndromes.

Although diseases characterized by proliferation of the less mature elements of the reticuloendothelial system, such as *acute monocytic leukemia* and *poorly differentiated histiocytic lymphoma* (reticulum cell sarcoma), may be considered to be part of the continuum of histiocytic diseases, they will be considered in separate chapters.

Histiocytic Medullary Reticulosis (Malignant Histiocytosis)

This is a nonhereditary, rapidly fatal illness characterized clinically by (1)

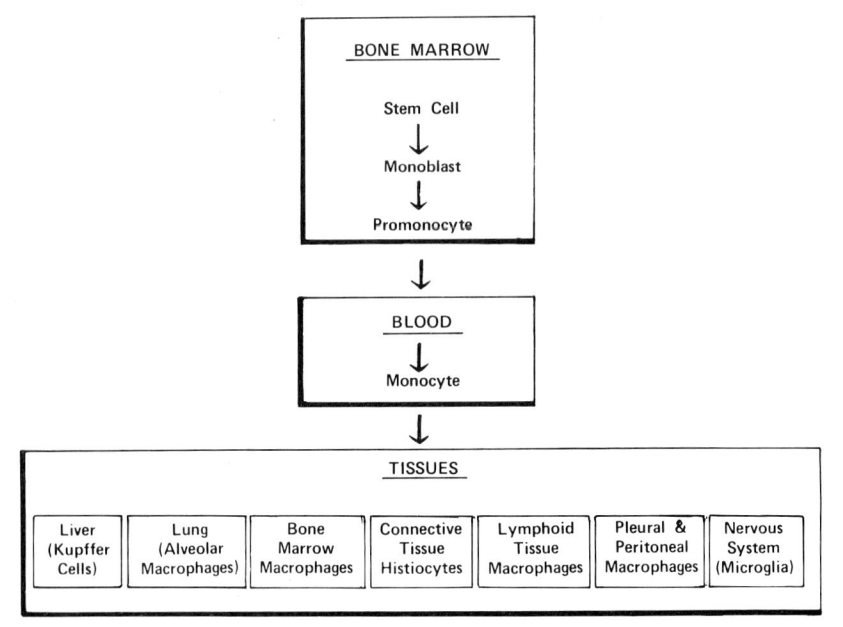

Figure 11-1 Maturation of the histiocytic cell series.

fever, (2) hepatosplenomegaly, (3) lymphadenopathy, (4) pancytopenia, and (5) Coombs' negative hemolytic anemia.[9, 54, 61] The disease derives its name from the characteristic focal proliferation of moderately well differentiated histiocytes within the subcapsular or medullary portion of lymph nodes.[57] The bone marrow and other tissues also contain histiocytic infiltrates; these characteristically manifest varying degrees of erythrophagocytosis, and occasionally phagocytosis of erythroblasts, platelets, lymphoid cells, and nuclear debris may be seen as well (Fig. 11-2).[52] The histiocytic nature of the cells is also expressed by the presence of characteristic membrane receptor sites[24] and elevated urinary muramidase levels.[12] More recent reviews have considered this condition to be a malignant histiocytosis[6, 9, 65] or a lymphoreticular lymphoma with a histiocytic function.[52]

This disease is seen most frequently in young adults and the aged.[69] In general it responds poorly to therapy, although transient responses to steroids and cytotoxic agents have been reported;[9] one patient has sur-

Table 11-1 Classification of the Histiocytic Disorders[9]

Predominant Cell	Clinical Disorder
Monoblast, promonocyte	Acute monocytic leukemia
Promonocyte, immature macrophage	Histiocytic lymphoma (poorly differentiated)
Monocyte, immature macrophage	Letterer-Siwe disease
Immature macrophage	Histiocytic medullary reticulosis
Immature and mature macrophages	Multifocal eosinophilic granuloma*
	Unifocal eosinophilic granuloma
	Localized histiocytoma

*Also known as Hand-Schüller-Christian disease.

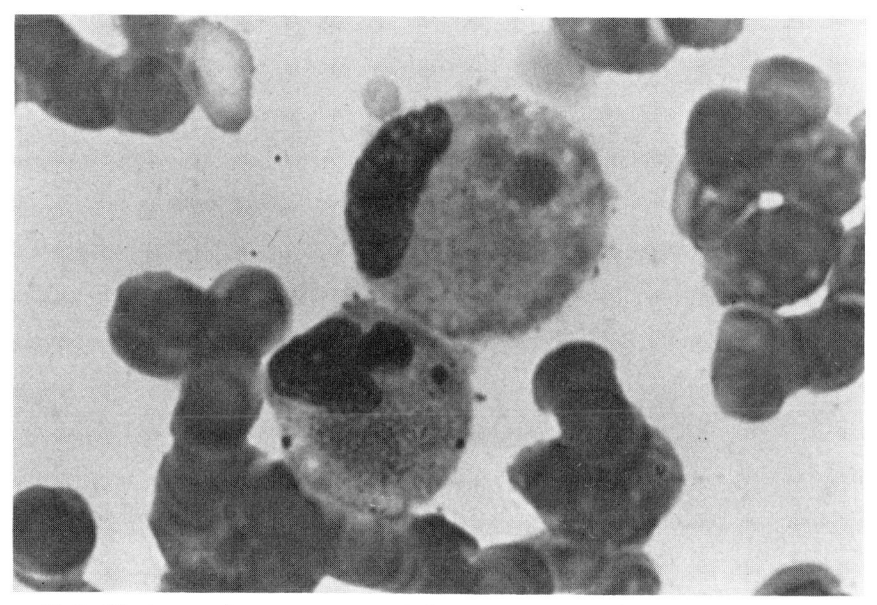

Figure 11–2 Histiocytes from a patient with histiocytic medullary reticulosis showing ingested erythrocytes and nuclear debris.

vived for more than 4 years after treatment with cyclophosphamide, vincristine, procarbazine, and prednisone (COPP).[62] Median survival is usually less than 6 months.

Familial Erythrophagocytic Lymphohistiocytosis (FEL) (Familial Hemophagocytic Reticulosis)

This unusual syndrome is characterized initially by the acute onset of relatively nonspecific symptoms: irritability, anorexia, vomiting, diarrhea, fever and pallor.[51, 61] Lymphadenopathy and hepatosplenomegaly are usually apparent on initial evaluation or develop soon thereafter. The course then consists of intermittent fevers, progressive pancytopenia, and liver dysfunction (including jaundice).

Perry and co-workers have recently reviewed a total of 38 children in 21 families afflicted with FEL and have concluded that the inheritance follows an autosomal recessive pattern;[51] as many as five siblings in a single family have died of this disease.[43] In patients with a compatible family history and clinical presentation, the diagnosis can be supported by liver, lymph node, or bone marrow examination; the characteristic pathologic finding is a diffuse mixed lymphocytic-histiocytic infiltration with prominent erythrophagocytosis.

While this disorder shares many of the clinical features of infantile histiocytosis X (Letterer-Siwe type), the majority of the cases differ in several important features:[66] (1) the typical skin lesions of Letterer-Siwe disease are absent, (2) erythrophagocytosis is a prominent feature of FEL, but not of Letterer-Siwe disease, (3) involvement of the central nervous system is common in FEL and uncommon in Letterer-Siwe disease, (4) in FEL the histiocytes are mixed with lymphocytes, whereas Letterer-Siwe disease is characterized by a mixed histiocytic-eosinophilic reaction.

The distinction between FEL and histiocytic medullary reticulosis is less clear-cut. The major points of difference are the familial nature of FEL and its propensity for occurring in infancy and early childhood (almost two thirds of reported cases have occurred within the first 3 months of life).[51] It has been suggested that these two entities may represent infantile and adult forms of the same disorder.[29]

FEL is a progressively fatal disorder in most cases, the average length of life being 6 weeks from the onset of the illness.[51] Frequently the terminal event is hemorrhagic in nature.[29, 42, 48, 66] In one series of six patients, hemorrhage was due to hypofibrinogenemia and thrombocytopenia, but this could not be related to liver disease, dysfibrinogenemia, or disseminated intravascular coagulation (DIC);[42] in another patient, however, documented DIC was present and was attributed to blockage of the reticuloendothelial clearance system of the liver, which thus failed to adequately remove activated clotting factors from the circulation.[48] Other patients have succumbed to sepsis or to a peculiar lymphocytic meningitis accompanied by seizures.[51]

Some patients have improved slowly with ACTH, steroids with antibiotics, or antibiotics alone; more recently, Fullerton and associates have achieved rapid responses to therapy with intravenous vinblastine and oral prednisolone.[17]

Sex-linked Reticulohistiocytosis With Hypergammaglobulinemia

This disorder is characterized by: (1) fever, (2) hepatosplenomegaly, (3) lymphadenopathy, (4) purpura, (5) jaundice, (6) hypergammaglobulinemia, and (7) X-linked recessive pattern of inheritance.[14] The characteristic histologic finding is the widespread infiltration of bizarre mononuclear cells accompanied by mature plasma cells; erythrophagocytosis is not evident. The course is progressive and rapidly fatal, with infection being the major terminal event.

HISTIOCYTOSIS X

In 1953 Lichtenstein identified the interrelationship between the clinically overlapping syndromes known as Letterer-Siwe disease, Hand-Schüller-Christian disease, and eosinophilic granuloma and classified them as variants of a single entity, which he called histiocytosis X.[35]

The characteristic histologic feature of histiocytosis X is a dense infiltrate of moderately differentiated, pale-staining histiocytes which are relatively benign and uniform in appearance.[53] Phagocytosis by the proliferating histiocytes is not a prominent feature in the early stages of the disease.

"Benign" Versus "Malignant" Histiocytosis—Pathologic Classification

Recently, Newton and Hamoudi[46] have proposed a pathologic classification for histiocytosis X which correlates clinical prognosis with histologic criteria. Their criteria are based on the study of tissues other than skin, since it was thought that skin biopsies did not provide reliable results. In this system, patients with a so-called "malignant" lesion had a relatively poor prognosis, while those with "benign" lesions had a relatively good prognosis.

"Malignant" lesions were characterized by diffuse infiltration of large individual histiocytes throughout the reticuloendothelial system, with relative preservation of normal architecture. Multinucleated giant cells, eosinophils, necrosis, and fibrosis were rarely seen. "Benign" lesions, on the other hand, contained a mixture of eosinophils and histiocytes. The histiocytes were usually predominant and appeared in sheets, giving a syncytial appearance. Fibrosis, focal necrosis, and multinucleated giant cells were also often observed.[32, 46]

Ultrastructure of Histiocytosis X Cells

The characteristic electron microscopic feature of the histiocytes in this group of disorders is the Langerhans granule, a five-layered membrane with central periodicity which has continuity with the cytoplasmic membrane (Fig. 11–3). These structures have been found in the skin lesions of Letterer-Siwe disease,[7] the pulmonary lesions of multifocal eosinophilic granuloma,[63] and unifocal eosinophilic granuloma of bone.[3] However, not all cases of histiocytosis manifest these granules.[64]

Apparently identical structures have also been found in the Langerhans cell of the human epidermis.[45] Recent reports indicate that the Langerhans cell is a specialized mesenchymal scavenger which engulfs and processes chemicals entering the epidermal intercellular spaces and forms a reticulo-*epithelial* system which shares many of the histochemical and biochemical features of the reticulo*endothelial* system.[59] Although this remarkable resemblance between histiocytosis X cells and Langerhans cells is intriguing, its exact significance is still unclear. It is unlikely that histiocytosis X cells are directly derived from Langerhans cells, since the normal Langerhans cell is confined to the epidermis, while the skin lesions of histiocytosis are primarily in the dermal layer.[1, 7] Moreover, it is difficult to see how bone and pulmonary lesions could occur in the absence of initial cutaneous involvement, as they do in some cases of histiocytosis X, if the cell of origin were the Langerhans cell. It would, therefore, appear to be more likely that the ultrastructural and histochemical similarities between these cell types reflect their origin from a common progenitor.

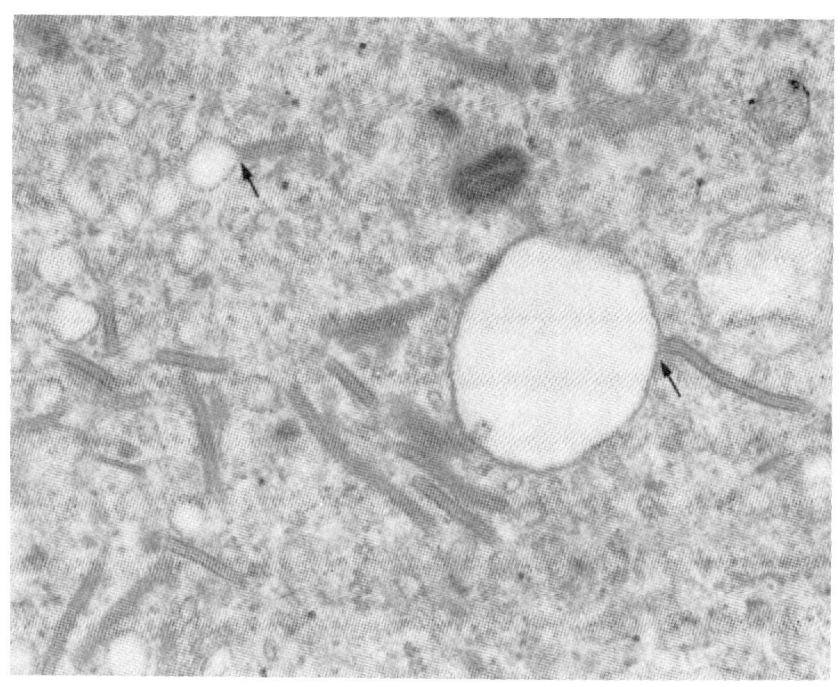

Figure 11–3 Langerhans granules in histiocytes from a patient with Letterer-Siwe disease; saccular dilatations are present at one end of some granules (arrows) (×40,000). (From Cancilla, P. A., et al.: Cancer 20:1986, 1967.)

LETTERER-SIWE DISEASE

Letterer-Siwe disease is the acute disseminated form of the histiocytosis X spectrum and is characterized by: (1) onset in infancy, (2) hepatosplenomegaly, (3) lymphadenopathy, (4) thrombocytopenic purpura, (5) generalized proliferation of nonlipid-storing histiocytes in multiple organs, including skin, bone, liver, spleen, and bone marrow, and (7) a rapidly fatal course if untreated.

Characteristically, the earliest presenting sign is a scaly, greasy, seborrhea-like skin eruption which begins on the scalp, behind the ears, and in the axillary, inguinal, or perineal areas[22] (Fig. 11-4); reddish-brown or purpuric papules, which are the basic lesions of histiocytosis, may be visible on close inspection. Other findings early in the course may include prominent cervical adenopathy, chronically draining otitis media, and gingival ulcerations. Nonspecific complaints, such as persistent fever, progressive weight loss, irritability, lethargy, or diarrhea, may also be early manifestations.

The complications of this disorder are related to the organ dysfunction resulting from histiocytic infiltration. In general, the response to therapy decreases and the mortality rate increases in proportion to the number of organs involved.[32] Of particular importance in this regard are the liver, lung, and bone marrow.

Liver dysfunction is manifested by hypoproteinemia, edema, ascites, and hyperbilirubinemia. Pulmonary dysfunction results in tachypnea, dyspnea, cyanosis, cough, pneumothorax, or pleural effusion; radiographic densities or infiltrates (diffuse cystic change, punctate nodular infiltrations, or extensive fibrosis)[27] can also occur. Bone marrow involvement can lead to anemia, leukopenia, or thrombocytopenia; however, the presence of excessive numbers of histiocytes in the marrow per se does not necessarily result in marrow dysfunction.[32] Pancytopenia may result from hypersplenism as well as from bone marrow failure.

Bony involvement of the mandible and maxilla and soft tissue involvement of the gingivae may result in loss

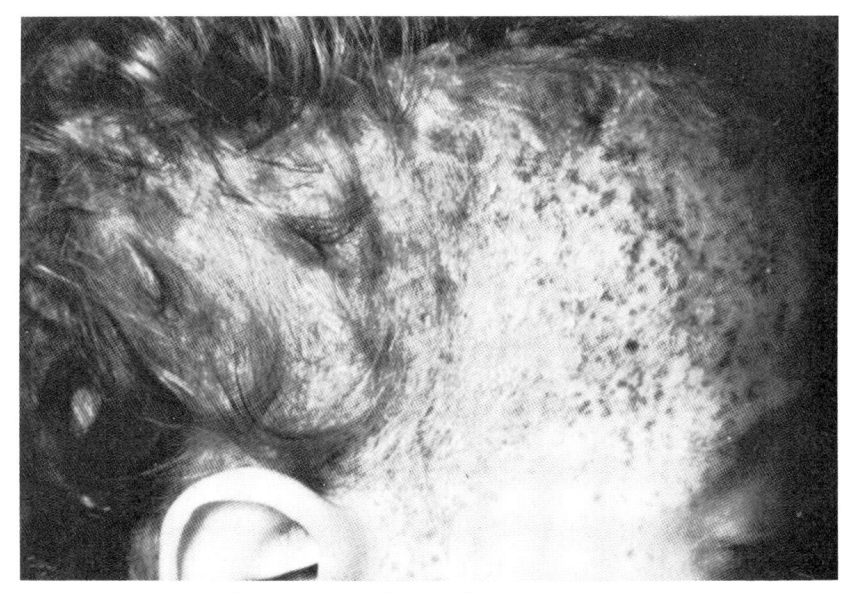

Figure 11-4 Patient with Letterer-Siwe disease showing characteristic papular, crusting seborrheic, and hemorrhagic skin eruption. (From Leikin, S.: Pediatr. Ann. 4:85, 1975.)

of or damage to the teeth. Lesions in the long bones may produce a limp, pain, or pathologic fracture. Mastoid involvement may extend to the middle ear, with resultant chronic otitis media. Orbital lesions are associated with exophthalmos. Vertebral collapse can cause scoliosis or neurologic damage.[67] Sphenoid involvement or pituitary infiltration can lead to diabetes insipidus, delayed puberty,[56] and growth retardation.[33] Other CNS manifestations include seizures,[55] papilledema,[16] and cerebellar ataxia.[40]

Pathology

The skin lesion of Letterer-Siwe disease has a distinctive histologic appearance, with relatively large focal aggregates of mononuclear histiocytes characteristically limited to the upper dermis (subepidermal zone)[53] (Fig. 11-5). By contrast, histiocytic lymphomas which involve the skin localize to the deep layers of the dermis, around skin appendages, and in the subcutis.

Letterer-Siwe disease of the lymph nodes is characterized by histiocytic proliferation originating in the sinuses; in the spleen the proliferation originates from histiocytic elements in the red pulp and only gradually encroaches upon the Malpighian corpuscles.[53] The bone marrow may also be extensively replaced by proliferating histiocytes.

HAND-SCHÜLLER-CHRISTIAN DISEASE (MULTIFOCAL EOSINOPHILIC GRANULOMA)

Hand-Schüller-Christian disease (multifocal eosinophilic granuloma) has a later onset (usually between 1 and 3 years of age) and a less severe clinical course than Letterer-Siwe disease. The major clinical manifestations relate to skeletal involvement (particularly the skull) (Figs. 11–6 and 11–7); however, soft tissue lesions (skin, lungs, ear) may also occur, resulting in chronic mastoiditis, loss of teeth, hypothyroidism, and adrenal insufficiency.[40, 70]

The triad of exophthalmos, diabetes insipidus, and skeletal lesions, once considered characteristic of this variant, is actually rarely seen.[38, 40, 47] Although the skeletal lesions are invariably present, only 50 per cent of patients have diabetes insipidus, and exophthalmos is even less common (10 per cent).[22] When skin lesions occur (in 30 to 50 per cent of patients), they usually consist of coalescing scaling or crusted brown to flesh-colored papules; purpura is less common than in Letterer-Siwe disease.

Pathology

Unlike Letterer-Siwe disease, which involves primarily the major reticuloendothelial organs (liver, spleen, lymph nodes, bone marrow), Hand-Schüller-Christian disease spares these organs and involves the perivascular connective tissue of the osseous and visceral organs, where peripheral lymphatics are abundant.[68] Common locations for early lesions are periosteum of bone, pleurae of the lungs, the capsules of the liver, spleen, and kidney, and the epicardium of the right atrium.

In this form of the disease, the cytoplasm of the histiocytes is more abundant and contains large amounts of lipid material (cholesterol and its esters). This accumulation of intracellular fat is thought to be derived from the phagocytosis of lipids that are normally present in the blood and tissue rather than being indicative of a primary disorder of lipid metabolism. Many of the histiocytes are multinucleated giant cells. Mature eosinophils may also be present in the lesions.

The appearance of the lesions varies according to the duration of the disease process.[10] Early bone lesions show foci of osseous destruction infiltrated by aggregates of cells, most of

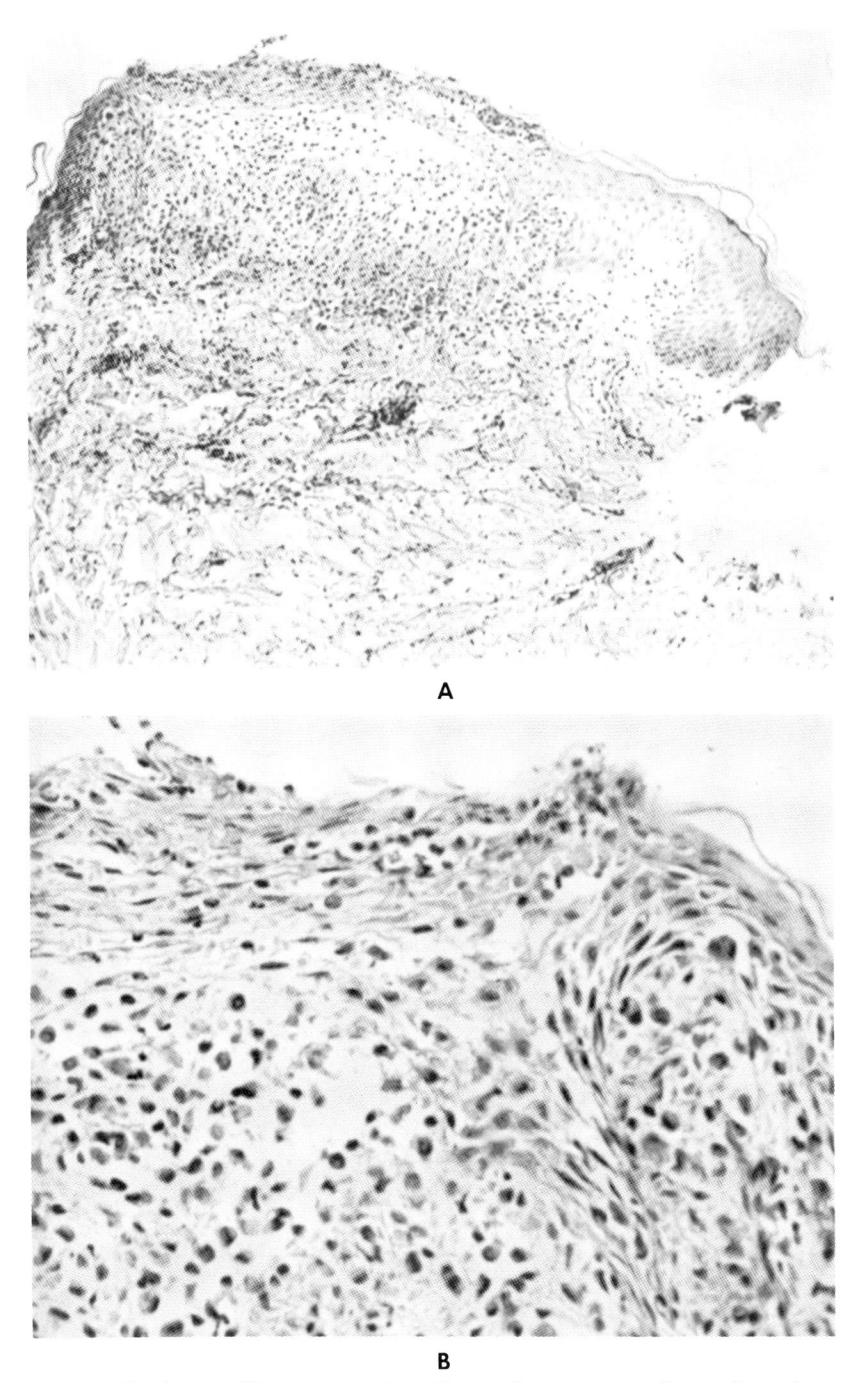

Figure 11-5 Skin lesion of histiocytosis X. *A*, The epidermis shows a focus of atrophy overlying a heavy infiltration of mononuclear cells in the dermis (H & E, ×130). *B*, Higher magnification shows mononuclear cells to have abundant cytoplasm and ovoid, kidney-shaped, and deeply indented nuclei (H & E, ×500). (From Doede, K. G., and Rappaport, H.: Cancer *20*:1782, 1967.)

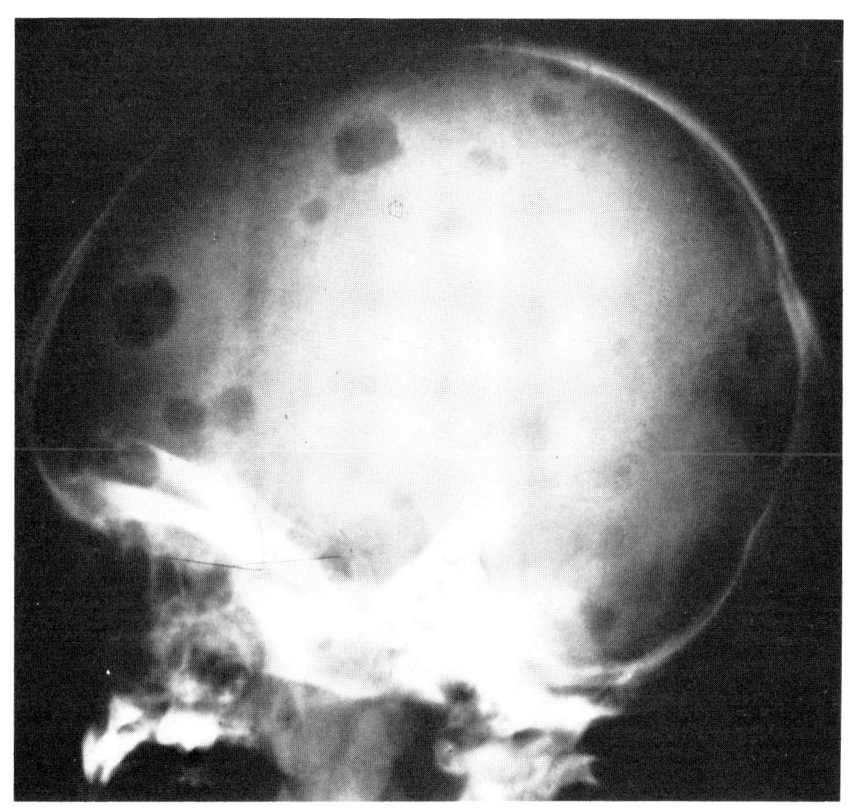

Figure 11–6 Skull film from patient with multifocal eosinophilic granuloma (Hand-Schüller-Christian disease). (From Leikin, S.: Pediatr. Ann. 4:85, 1975.)

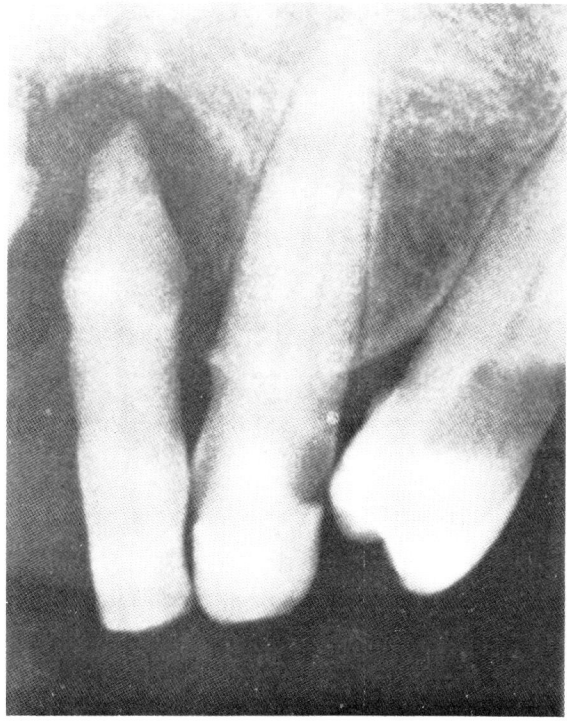

Figure 11–7 Dental film from a patient with multifocal eosinophilic granuloma, demonstrating classic "floating-in-air" appearance of teeth. (From Kaufman, A., et al.: Am. J. Med. 60:541, 1976.)

which are eosinophils and histiocytes; varying numbers of plasma cells, lymphocytes, monocytes, and occasional giant cells may also be present (Fig. 11–8).

In lesions of a few months' duration, eosinophils are few or absent, whereas giant cells and fibrosis become evident. The histiocytes are vesicular, with prominent nucleoli and foamy cytoplasm; when large destructive lesions are present, abundant amounts of lipid are found in the cytoplasm of the histiocytes (Fig. 11–9).

In still later stages of the disease, the entire granulomatous process becomes replaced with connective tissue.

EOSINOPHILIC GRANULOMA

Unifocal eosinophilic granuloma of bone is the most localized and benign form of the histiocytosis spectrum and is seen most commonly in older children and young adults. Lesions occur most frequently in the skull and have a characteristic punched-out appearance without evidence of marginal sclerosis or periosteal reaction. Long bone lesions begin in the medullary cavity and usually affect the diaphysis (Fig. 11–10). Vertebral lesions can cause collapse of the vertebral body, with a subsequent "pancake" appearance on x-ray. Isolated eosinophilic granulomas can also occur in the lungs,[41] bladder,[5] skin, lymph nodes, vulva, and pituitary gland.[1, 23]

Pathology

The histology of these lesions is virtually similar to that seen in the multifocal variant, and consequently these disorders are now considered as representative of the same basic pathologic process.[26, 37]

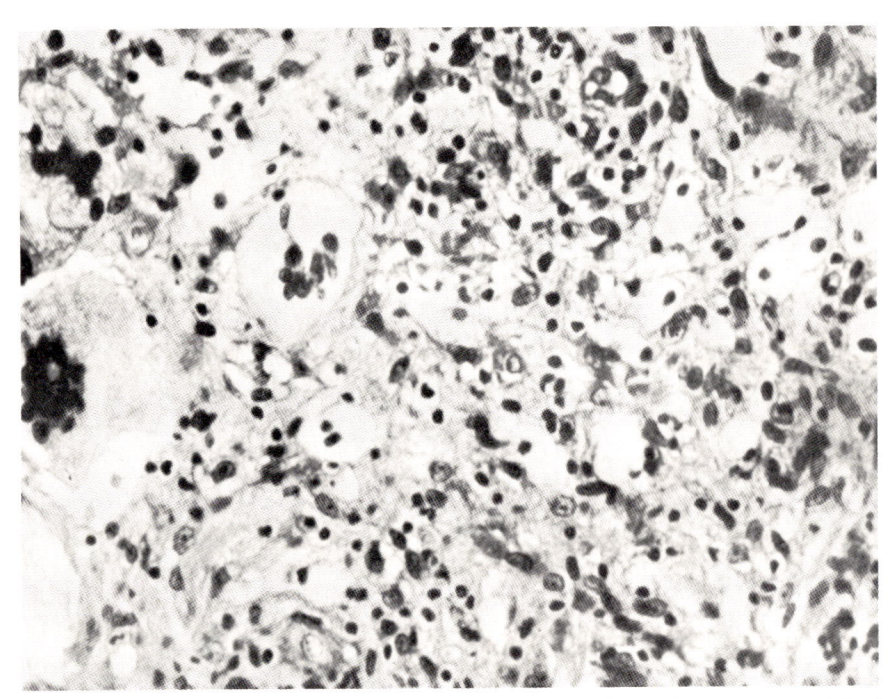

Figure 11–8 Early bone lesion of multifocal eosinophilic granuloma showing eosinophilic leukocytes and histiocytes with oval nuclei and pale, ill-defined cytoplasm. (H & E, ×350) (From Daneshbod, K., and Kissane, J. M.: Am. J. Clin. Pathol. 65:601, 1976.)

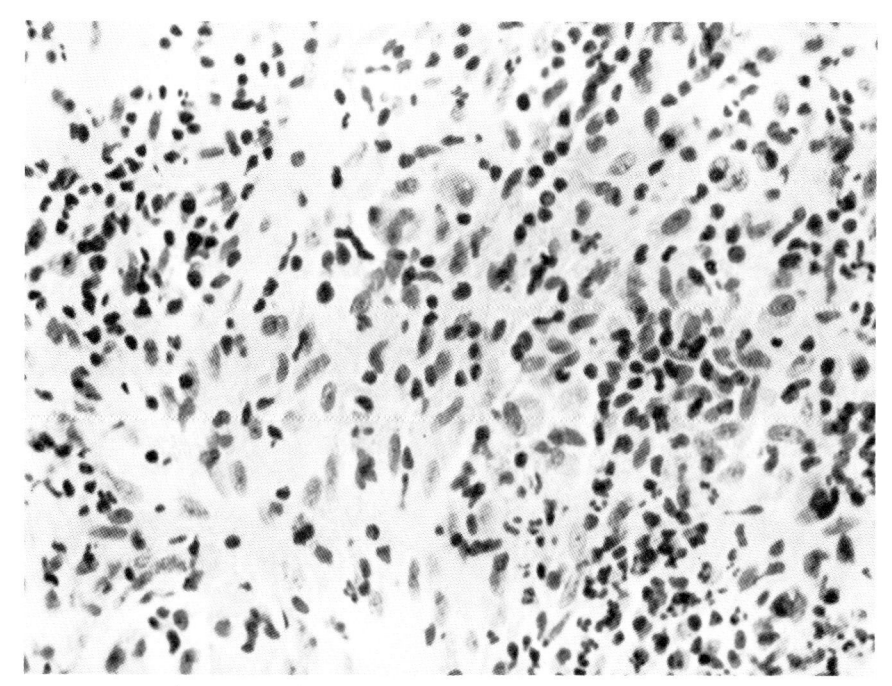

Figure 11-9 Bone lesion of multifocal eosinophilic granuloma of about 2 years' duration showing lipid-filled histiocytes, giant cells full of lipid, fibroblasts, lymphocytes, and cholesterol accumulation in the stroma (H & E, ×350). (From Daneshbod, K., and Kissane, J. M.: Am. J. Clin. Pathol. 65:601, 1976.)

IMMUNOLOGIC FUNCTION IN HISTIOCYTOSIS X PATIENTS

Immunologic studies in children with histiocytosis X have indicated that most have normal delayed hypersensitivity reactions, lymphocyte blastogenesis to mitogens and allogeneic cells, and bactericidal activity; in the few patients who demonstrated impaired delayed hypersensitivity reactions and subnormal lymphocyte blastogenesis, the immunologic dysfunction was considered to be not primary but secondary to the malignancy.[34]

However, another group of patients who presented with a typical Letterer-Siwe type clinical picture as well as peripheral eosinophilia were subsequently found to have the characteristic immunologic and histologic findings of the severe combined immunodeficiency syndrome—i.e., thymic dysplasia and poorly differentiated lymphocyte-depleted peripheral lymphoid tissue.[2, 8, 49, 50] Since most of these patients had not received chemotherapy, these findings could not be attributed to the immunosuppressive effects of these drugs. In many instances these cases exhibited a familial pattern with autosomal recessive inheritance.[2, 49, 50] Indeed, most children with combined immunodeficiency have had varying degrees of histiocytic reaction in the liver, spleen, and lymph nodes,[20] and, in some cases, histiocytic infiltration of the skin has been a transient but impressive manifestation.[19]

The discovery of a subgroup of patients with a histiocytosis-like illness and combined immunodeficiency is indeed intriguing, particularly since a similar clinical syndrome has been described with the "runting" syndrome associated with acquired graft-versus-host disease induced by trans-

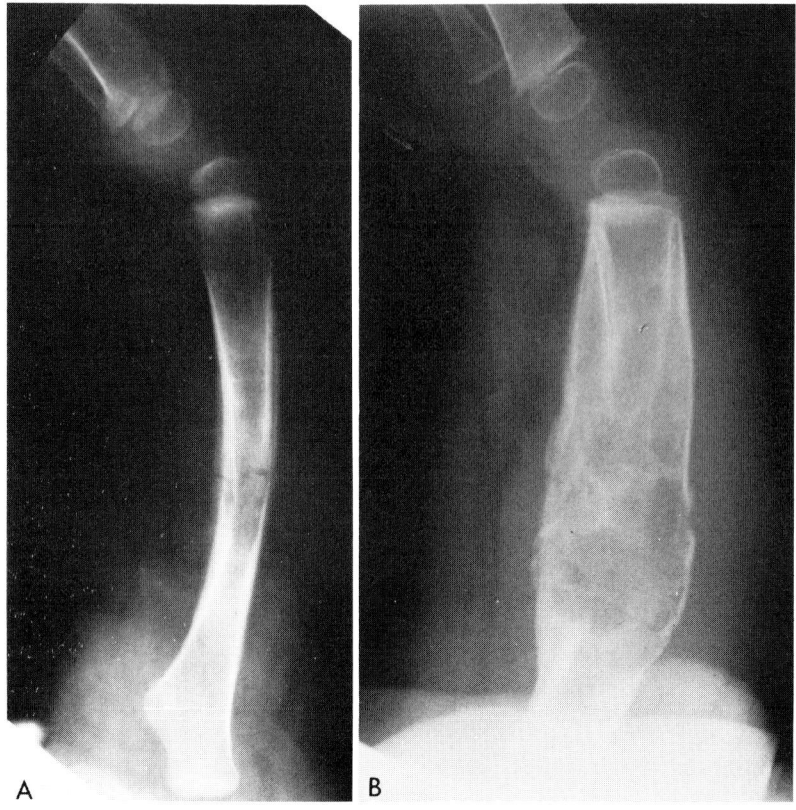

Figure 11–10 X-rays of the femur of a child with eosinophilic granuloma. Patient initially presented with pathologic fracture of the femur (*A*), which then developed massive periosteal reaction and irregularity about the midportion of the bone (*B*).

fusions of fresh blood or bone marrow into patients who lack immunocompetence.[44] It is possible that patients with combined immunodeficiency who present in early infancy with a histiocytosis-like clinical picture have congenital graft-versus-host disease induced by intrauterine transfusion of maternal blood.[2, 49] However, the direct evidence for this hypothesis will depend on documentation of dividing maternal lymphocytes in the patient's peripheral blood or bone marrow.[20]

It would thus appear that histiocytosis X is a heterogeneous disease and that one subgroup of patients may have underlying combined immunodeficiency. This possibility should be considered in all infants with Letterer-Siwe disease, in particular when it is of a familial nature.[8, 50, 58] It has thus been recommended that all infants with Letterer-Siwe syndrome undergo a thorough immunologic evaluation and that unirradiated blood products, live attenuated vaccines, steroids, and immunosuppressive chemotherapy not be used until immunocompetence has been demonstrated.[8]

PROGNOSIS

In general, the prognosis in histiocytosis X depends on the following factors:[30, 32] (1) age at onset, (2) extent of the disease, (3) dysfunction of certain key organs (lung, liver, bone marrow), and (4) histology ("benign" versus "malignant") (Table 11–2).

The worst prognosis is in infants less than 6 months of age,[30] whereas death

Table 11-2 Factors Associated With Poor Prognosis in Histiocytosis X Patients

1. Age of onset less than 3 years old (especially poor if under 6 months).
2. Multifocal disease.
3. Functional derangement of visceral organs (particularly lung, liver, and bone marrow).
4. "Malignant" histology.

rarely occurs in patients over 3 years of age.[30, 32] Multifocal disease has a worse prognosis than unifocal disease,[13] particularly when visceral organs are involved. Functional derangement of these organs has greater significance than mere histologic involvement. Of the visceral organs, dysfunction of lung, liver, or bone marrow appears to have the strongest correlation with poor prognosis—in a recent study comparing three different treatment regimens, good responses were seen in 66 per cent of patients without dysfunction of these organs, while only 33 per cent of those with dysfunction had good responses.[31] In patients without organ dysfunction, the histologic pattern is usually "benign," the response to therapy is good, and there are few deaths. Those patients with liver, lung, or marrow dysfunction usually have "malignant" histology, respond poorly to therapy, and often succumb to the disease.[32]

TREATMENT

A number of single agents or drug combinations have shown activity against disseminated histiocytosis X. Comparative therapeutic trials have indicated that single drugs such as vincristine, vinblastine, or cyclophosphamide,[60] and combinations such as prednisone and vinblastine,[25] prednisone and methotrexate,[25] and prednisone and 6-mercaptopurine[31] produce complete or good partial remissions in about 45 to 65 per cent of patients (Table 11-3). These treatment regimens have reduced the high mortality rate in infants under 6 months of age from 70 per cent[30] to 37 per cent.[31]

In treating patients with disseminated histiocytosis, it is important to realize that response to therapy may be slow and new foci of disease may arise while others are healing. These exacerbations should not be considered to indicate failure of the drug unless there is progressive systemic deterioration or rapid multifocal progression of the disease.

QUALITY OF SURVIVAL

Now that more patients with disseminated histiocytosis X are becoming long-term survivors, attention is being focused on the chronic disabilities which these patients develop (frequently due to fibrosis of the healing

Table 11-3 Response to Therapy for Histiocytosis X in Children Under 2 Years of Age

REGIMEN	COMPLETE AND GOOD REMISSIONS (PER CENT)	MORTALITY (PER CENT)
Vinblastine[31]	56	38
Prednisone + Vinblastine[31]	67	25
Prednisone + 6-mercaptopurine[31]	48	33
Prednisone + Methotrexate[25]	46	46
Prednisone + Vincristine[25]	57	43

histiocytic lesions). Diabetes insipidus is seen in 20 per cent of survivors.[21] In addition, among patients who have survived after having bone and visceral involvement, 63 to 69 per cent had significant disabilities other than diabetes insipidus:[28, 31] growth retardation (due to scoliosis, vertebral collapse, and possibly growth hormone deficiency), neurologic disease, intellectual impairment, emotional disorders, chronic pulmonary disease, hearing impairment (due to mastoiditis, chronic otitis, or cholesteatoma formation), and orthopedic disease. Some patients also develop hepatic cirrhosis with a characteristic macronodular periportal pattern;[21] this appears to result from healing by fibrosis of hepatic histiocytic involvement and may present as portal hypertension (with splenomegaly and bleeding esophageal varices), jaundice, ascites, hypoalbuminemia and prolonged prothrombin time. Portosystemic shunt procedures have relieved the threat of potentially fatal variceal hemorrhage and improved the opportunity for long-term survival.[21]

REFERENCES

1. Anderson, A. E., Jr., and Foraker, A. G.: Eosinophilic granuloma of lung, clinical features and connective disease patterns. Arch. Intern. Med. 103:966, 1959.
2. Barth, R. F., Vergara, O. G., Khurana, S. K., et al.: Rapidly fatal histiocytosis associated with eosinophilia and primary immunological deficiency. Lancet 2:503, 1972.
3. Basset, F., Nezelof, C., Mallet, R., and Turiaf, J.: Nouvelle mise en évidence, par la microscopie électronique de particules d'allure virale dans une seconde cas clinique de l'histiocytose X, le granulome éosinophile de l'os. C.R. Acad. Sci. 261: 5719, 1965.
4. Breathnach, A. S., and Wyllie, L. M.: Electron microscopy of melanocytes and Langerhans cells in human fetal epidermis at fourteen weeks. J. Invest. Derm. 44:51, 1965.
5. Brown, E. W.: Eosinophilic granuloma of the bladder. J. Urol. 83:665, 1960.
6. Byrne, G. E., Jr., and Rappaport, H.: Malignant histiocytosis. Gann. Monogr. Cancer Res. 15:145, 1972.
7. Cancilla, P. A., Lahey, M. E., and Carnes, W. H.: Cutaneous lesions of Letterer-Siwe disease. Electron microscopic study. Cancer 20:1986, 1967.
8. Cederbaum, S., Niwayama, G., Stiehm, E. R., et al.: Combined immunodeficiency presenting as the Letterer-Siwe syndrome. J. Pediatr. 85:466, 1974.
9. Cline, M. J., and Golde, D. W.: A review and reevaluation of the histiocytic disorders Am. J. Med. 55:49, 1973.
10. Daneshbod, K., and Kissane, J. M.: Histiocytosis. The prognosis of polyostotic eosinophilic granuloma. Am. J. Clin. Pathol. 65:601, 1976.
11. Davidson, R. I., and Shillito, J.: Eosinophilic granuloma of the cervical spine in children. Pediatrics 45:746, 1970.
12. Duffy, T. P., Knights, E. B., and Eggleston, J. C.: Elevated muramidase levels in histiocytic medullary reticulosis. N. Engl. J. Med. 294:167, 1976.
13. Ekert, H., and Campbell, P. E.: Histiocytosis X: A review of experience at the Royal Children's Hospital, Melbourne, 1948–1963. Aust. Paediatr. J. 3:139, 1966.
14. Falletta, J. M., Fernbach, D. J., Singer, D. B., et al.: A fatal X-linked recessive reticuloendothelial syndrome with hyperglobulinemia; X-linked recessive reticuloendotheliosis. J. Pediatr. 83:549, 1973.
15. Farquhar, J. W., and Claireaux, A. E.: Familial haemophagic reticulosis. Arch. Dis. Child. 27:519, 1952.
16. Feinberg, S. B., and Langes, L. O.: Roentgen findings of increased intracranial pressure and communicating hydrocephalus in insidious manifestations of chronic histiocytosis-X. Am. J. Roentgenol. 95:41, 1965.
17. Fullerton, P., Ekert, H., Hosking, C., and Tauro, G. P.: Hemophagocytic reticulosis. A case report with investigations of immune and white cell function. Cancer 36:441, 1975.
18. Goodall, H. B., Guthrie, W., and Buist, N. R. M.: Familial haemophagic reticulosis. Scott. Med. J. 10:425, 1965.
19. Gotoff, S. P., Esterly, N. B., Gottbrath, E., et al.: Granulomatous reaction in an infant with combined immunodeficiency disease and short limbed dwarfism. J. Pediatr. 80:1010, 1972.
20. Gotoff, S. P., and Esterly, N. B.: "Histiocytosis." J. Pediatr. 85:592, 1974.
21. Grosfeld, J. L., Fitzgerald, J. F., Wagner, V. M., et al.: Portal hypertension in infants and children with histiocytosis-X. Am. J. Surg. 131:108, 1976.
22. Hurwitz, S.: Histiocytosis in children. Mod. Probl. Paediat. 17:204, 1975.
23. Isitman, A. T., Lorge, H. J., and MacGillivray, W.: Pulmonary eosinophilic granuloma. Report of a case with complete spontaneous remission. Dis. Chest. 52:264, 1967.

24. Jaffe, E. S., Shevach, E. M., Sussman, E. H., et al.: Membrane receptor sites for the identification of lymphoreticular cells in benign and malignant conditions. Brit. J. Cancer 31(Suppl. II):107, 1975.
25. Jones, B., Kung, F., Chevalier, L., et al.: Chemotherapy of reticuloendotheliosis. Comparison of methotrexate plus prednisone vs. vincristine plus prednisone. Cancer 34:1011, 1974.
26. Kaufman, A., Bukberg, P. R., Werlin, S., and Young, I. S.: Multifocal eosinophilic granuloma ("Hand-Schüller-Christian disease"). Am. J. Med. 60:541, 1976.
27. Keats, T. E., and Crane, J. F.: Cystic changes of the lungs in histiocytosis. Am. J. Dis. Child. 88:764, 1954.
28. Komp, D., El-Mahdi, A., Starling, K., et al.: Quality of survival in histiocytosis-X. Pediatr. Res. 10: Abstr. 922, 1976.
29. Koto, A., Morecki, R., and Santorineou, M.: Congenital hemophagocytic reticulosis. Am. J. Clin. Pathol. 65:495, 1976.
30. Lahey, M. E.: Prognosis in reticuloendotheliosis in children. J. Pediatr. 60:664, 1962.
31. Lahey, M. E.: Histiocytosis-X—comparison of three treatment regimens. J. Pediatr. 87:179, 1975.
32. Lahey, M. E.: Histiocytosis-X—an analysis of prognostic factors. J. Pediatr. 87:184, 1975.
33. Latorre, H., Kenney, F. M., Lahey, M. E., and Drash, A.: Short stature and growth hormone deficiency in histiocytosis-X. J. Pediatr. 85:813, 1974.
34. Leikin, S., Puruganan, G., Frankel, A., et al.: Immunologic parameters in histiocytosis-X. Cancer 32:796, 1973.
35. Lichtenstein, L.: Histiocytosis-X. Integration of eosinophilic granuloma of bone, "Letterer-Siwe disease," and Schüller-Christian disease as related manifestations of a single nosologic entity. Arch. Pathol. 56:84, 1953.
36. Lichtenstein, L.: Histiocytosis-X (eosinophilic granuloma of bone, Letterer-Siwe disease, and Schüller-Christian disease). J. Bone Joint Surg. 46A:76, 1964.
37. Lieberman, P. H., Jones, C. R., Dargeon, H. W. K., and Begg, C. F.: A reappraisal of eosinophilic granuloma of bone, Hand-Schüller-Christian syndrome, and Letterer-Siwe syndrome. Medicine 48:375, 1969.
38. Lucaya, J.: Histiocytosis-X. Am. J. Dis. Child. 121:289, 1971.
39. MacMahon, H. E., Bedizel, M., and Ellis, C. A.: Familial erythrophagocytic lymphohistiocytosis. Pediatrics 32:868, 1963.
40. Mauer, A. M., Lampkin, B., and McWilliams, N. B.: The leukemias and reticuloendothelioses. In Nathan, D. G., and Oski, F. A. (eds.): Hematology of Infancy and Childhood. Philadelphia, W. B. Saunders Company, 1974.
41. Mazzitello, W. F.: Eosinophilic granuloma of the lung. N. Engl. J. Med. 250:804, 1954.
42. McClure, P. D., Strachan, P., and Saunders, E. F.: Hypofibrinogenemia and thrombocytopenia in familial hemophagocytic reticulosis. J. Pediatr. 85:67, 1974.
43. Miller, D. R.: Familial reticuloendotheliosis—concurrence of disease in five siblings. Pediatrics 38:986, 1966.
44. Miller, M. E.: Thymic dysplasia ("Swiss agammaglobulinemia"). I. Graft versus host reaction following bone-marrow transfusion. J. Pediatr. 70:730, 1967.
45. Mishima, Y.: Melanosomes in phagocytic vacuoles in Langerhans cells—electron microscopy of keratin-stripped human epidermis. J. Cell Biol. 30:417, 1966.
46. Newton, W. A., Jr., and Hamoudi, A. B.: Histiocytosis—a histologic classification with clinical correlation. In Rosenberg, H. S., and Bolande, R. P. (eds.): Perspectives in Pediatric Pathology. Vol. 1. Chicago, Year Book Medical Publishers, Inc., 1973.
47. Oberman, H. A.: Idiopathic histiocytosis. A clinicopathologic study of 40 cases and review of the literature on eosinophilic granuloma of bone, Hand-Schüller-Christian disease, and Letterer-Siwe disease. Pediatrics 28:307, 1961.
48. O'Brien, R. T., Schwartz, A. D., Pearson, H. A., and Spencer, R. P.: Reticuloendothelial failure in familial erythrophagocytic lymphohistiocytosis. J. Pediatr. 81:543, 1972.
49. Ochs, H. O., Davis, S. D., Mickelson, E., et al.: Combined immunodeficiency and reticuloendotheliosis with eosinophilia. J. Pediatr. 85:463, 1974.
50. Omenn, G. S.: Familial reticuloendotheliosis with eosinophila. N. Engl. J. Med. 273:427, 1965.
51. Perry, M. C., Harrison, E. G., Jr., Burgert, E. O., Jr., and Gilchrist, G. S.: Familial erythrophagocytic lymphohistiocytosis: Report of two cases and clinicopathologic review. Cancer 38:209, 1976.
52. Piñol-Aguadé, J., Ferrando, J., Tomas, J. M., et al.: Necropsy and ultrastructural findings in histiocytic medullary reticulosis. Brit. J. Dermatol. 95:35, 1976.
53. Rappaport, H.: Tumors of the hematopoietic system. In Atlas of Tumor Pathology. Washington, D.C., Armed Forces Institute of Pathology, 1966.
54. Rosenstock, H. A., Sandor, I. M., and Hoenecke, H.: Acute histiocytic medullary reticulosis in a pubescent girl. Tex. Med. 65:56, 1969.
55. Rubé, J., De LaPava, S., and Pickren, J. W.: Histiocytosis X with involvement of brain. Cancer 20:486, 1967.

56. Saba, T. M.: Physiology and physiopathology of the reticuloendothelial system. Arch. Intern. Med. 126:1031, 1970.
57. Scott, R. B., and Robb-Smith, A. H. T.: Histiocytic medullary reticulosis. Lancet 2:194, 1939.
58. Shapiro, M.: Familial autohemolytic anemia and runting syndrome with Rh-specific autoantibody. Transfusion 7:281, 1967.
59. Shelley, W. B., and Juhlin, L.: Langerhans cells form a reticuloepithelial trap for external contact antigens. Nature 261:46, 1976.
60. Starling, K. A., Donaldson, M. H., Haggard, M. E., et al.: Therapy of histiocytosis X with vincristine, vinblastine, and cyclophosphamide. Am. J. Dis. Child. 123:105, 1972.
61. Starling, K. A., and Fernbach, D. J.: Histiocytosis. In Sutow, W. W., Vietti, T. J., and Fernbach, D. J. (eds.): Clinical Pediatric Oncology. St. Louis, C. V. Mosby Company, 1973.
62. Stein, R. S., Moran, E. M., and Byrne, G. E., Jr.: Malignant histiocytosis: complete remission with combination chemotherapy. Cancer 38:1083, 1976.
63. Turiaf, J., and Basset, F.: Un cas d'histiocytose X pulmonaire avec présence de particules de nature probablement virale dans les lésions granulomateuses pulmonaires examinées au microscope électronique. Bull. Soc. Med. Hôp. Paris 116:1197, 1965.
64. Vawter, G. F.: Does Letterer-Siwe disease exist? Or who's not afraid of infantile histiocytes. In Vuksanovic, M. M. (ed.): Clinical Pediatric Oncology. Research, Diagnosis, Treatment, and Prognosis of Malignant Tumors of Childhood. Mt. Kisco, N.Y., Futura Publishing Co., 1972.
65. Warnke, R. A., Kim, H., and Dorfman, R. F.: Malignant histiocytosis (histiocytic medullary reticulosis). I. Clinicopathologic study of 29 cases Cancer 35:215, 1975.
66. Weinberg, A. G., and Rogers, L. E.: Clinical-Pathological Conference: Hepatosplenomegaly, pancytopenia, and fever. J. Pediatr. 82:879, 1973.
67. Yabsley, R. H., and Harris, W. R.: Solitary eosinophilic granuloma of a vertebral body causing paraplegia. J. Bone Joint Surg. 48A:1570, 1966.
68. Yamaguchi, K., Yokoyama, T., and Morimatsu, M.: Involvement of the central nervous system in Hand-Schüller-Christian disease—report of a case and discussion on the entity of the disease. Acta Pathol. Jap. 22:363, 1972.
69. Zak, F. G., and Rubin, E.: Histiocytic medullary reticulosis. Am. J. Med. 31:813, 1961.
70. Zinkham, W. H.: Multifocal eosinophilic granuloma. Natural history, etiology, and management. Am. J. Med. 60:457, 1976.

Chapter Twelve

TUMORS OF THE CENTRAL AND PERIPHERAL NERVOUS SYSTEM

Maria Gumbinas and Allen D. Schwartz

BRAIN TUMORS

Primary brain tumors are the most frequent group of solid tumors occurring in children, and are second only to leukemia as a cause of death from cancer during the childhood years. Young and Miller reported an annual incidence of 23.9 malignant central nervous system tumors per million children under 15 years of age in the United States during the years 1969 to 1971, which includes fatal as well as nonfatal cases.[123] The incidence was identical for white and black children.

Pathogenesis

Little is known about the etiology of tumors of the central nervous system. Tumors such as teratomas, dermoid and epidermoid cysts, and craniopharyngiomas are probably related to embryonic maldevelopment. Congenital brain tumors appearing in the newborn are very rare, but gliomas, teratomas, medulloblastomas, sarcomas, and a variety of other histologic types have been reported in the neonate.[24, 67, 96] It has been postulated that a number of childhood brain tumors are the result of cells "misplaced" during early embryonic development, which retain their ability to proliferate but never mature, only to grow during later childhood.[22]

Exogenous agents have rarely been implicated as a cause of brain tumors in the human, although tumors have been induced in the animal model by radiation, oncogenic viruses, and other carcinogens. Meningiomas have been reported to occur following trauma.[29] Modan and associates[83] presented evidence that ionizing radiation may play an etiologic role in the development of human brain tumors. Of 11,000 children who received radiation of the scalp for tinea capitis, 17 developed either benign or malignant brain tumors during a follow-up period of 12 to 23 years, an incidence significantly higher than that found in two matched control groups. Rarely, spinal cord tumors have been reported years following viral infections of the nervous system, such as poliomyelitis,[86] but most of these tumors have been epidermoid cysts and have presumably been the result of iatrogenic introduction of the patient's own tissue into the subarachnoid space by the spinal needle during the diagnostic lumbar puncture.[106] Lymphoreticular tumors of the brain have been reported in a number of renal-transplant recipients who have undergone immunosuppression[105] and in children with hereditary immunodeficiency syndromes.[2, 108]

Intracranial neoplasms appear to occur with increased incidence in some families with no obvious disorders of the immune system,[3] and siblings of patients appear to be at increased risk of developing brain tumors.[80] Medulloblastomas have occurred in identical twins.[9, 26, 65] Nervous system tumors occur with increased frequency in patients with hereditary neurocutaneous disorders, such as neurofibromatosis, tuberous sclerosis,[52] and von Hippel-Lindau angiomatosis.[49] Those with the basal-cell nevus syndrome, a genetic disorder characterized by multiple basal cell carcinomas, cysts of the jaw, pitting of the skin on the palms and soles, and skeletal anomalies, have an increased incidence of medulloblastomas, which may appear as the first manifestation of the disease.[22, 45] Other disorders associated with an increased incidence of neurogenic tumors are the familial glioma polyposis syndrome[8] and possibly Turner's syndrome.[90, 118] In addition, brain tumors have been found in children with other primary neoplasms, including adrenocortical tumors, adenocarcinoma of the colon, acute leukemia, hepatocellular carcinoma,[36, 97] and in members of cancer-prone families afflicted with a variety of seemingly unrelated malignant diseases.[68] There is also evidence that brain tumors and congenital defects of the central nervous system aggregate in families.[114] Despite the numerous reports of associations with brain tumors, in the majority of young children with these tumors there is no apparent related event, underlying disorder, or familial disease which predisposes them to the development of a malignant disease.

A scarcity of primary brain tumors in blacks has been noted in several reports from Africa,[28, 120] an observation that is not believed to be due to underdiagnosis. These differences in the frequency of brain tumors in United States black children as compared to Nigerian and Ugandan blacks suggests the existence of undetermined environmental factors.

HISTOLOGY, AGE, AND TUMOR LOCATION

A major problem in comparing and compiling data from various reported series of central nervous system tumors is the lack of a uniform pathologic nomenclature. An effort will be made to use a description based on both anatomic site and the more commonly used histologic diagnoses to provide a simple and clinically useful classification system (see Table 12–1). For detailed pathologic descriptions and classifications, the reader is referred to the excellent textbook by Russell and Rubinstein.[101] The histologic classification of 565 intracranial neoplasms reported by Matson is shown in Table 12–2.[74]

Tumors in infancy and childhood tend to occur in the posterior fossa and in the midline. About 60 to 70 per cent of intracranial tumors in those under

Table 12–1 Estimated Occurrence Rate of Common Primary Intracranial Tumors of Childhood[115]

TUMOR TYPE	PERCENTAGE
Infratentorial Tumors	66
Cerebellar astrocytoma	20
Medulloblastoma	18
Brain stem astrocytoma (glioma)	10
Ependymoma	8
Miscellaneous tumors	10
Supratentorial Tumors	33
Astrocytoma	8
Ependymoma	6
Malignant glioma	6
Craniopharyngioma	5
Miscellaneous tumors	8

Table 12-2   Histologic Types of 565 Intracranial Tumors[74] (Site Not Always Indicated)

Astrocytoma	156
Medulloblastoma	107
Brain stem glioma	58
Ependymoma	57
Glioblastoma multiforme and mixed gliomas	41
Craniopharyngioma	39
Optic chiasm glioma	24
Choroid plexus papilloma	18
Dermoid cyst	11
Hemangioma	9
Hamartoma	8
Teratoma	7
Other	30

15 years of age are infratentorial in location, whereas the great majority of tumors in the adult are supratentorial. Tumor location, however, not only differs in adults and children, but also varies in children of different ages. The majority of tumors diagnosed during the first year of life are located supratentorially,[31] but in patients between the ages of about 2 to 12 years, infratentorial tumors account for over 85 per cent of tumors and are mainly cerebellar astrocytomas, medulloblastomas, and brain stem gliomas. During the teenage years, supratentorial tumors again begin to increase in frequency. The astrocytoma, for example, is usually infratentorial in location until adolescence, after which it appears more frequently above the tentorium. At puberty there is also a sharp decline in the incidence of medulloblastomas, and craniopharyngiomas become more common.

A study of death certificates of children who died of cancer between 1960 and 1968 in the United States revealed age and race differences among different brain tumor types.[81] Among white children there is a sharp peak soon after birth in the incidence of ependymoma, a broader and later peak for medulloblastoma, and a progressive increase in astrocytoma with age. These findings are not as dramatic in nonwhite children with ependymoma. Ependymoma and medulloblastoma are more frequently the cause of death in whites, while glioma is more often the cause of death in non-whites. Boys are more prone than girls to many of the more common tumor types. This is especially true of the medulloblastoma.

CLINICAL SIGNS AND SYMPTOMS

Obstruction of the cerebrospinal fluid circulation with resultant increased intracranial pressure is a common early manifestation of childhood tumors because of their anatomic location in the posterior fossa or along the midline. Signs and symptoms of increased intracranial pressure are often the initial and sometimes the only evidence of the neoplasm. Symptoms include headache, irritability, and vomiting. Headache is an uncommon complaint in the very young child and should suggest organic disease. Morning headache should be more suspect than headache that occurs only at the end of the day or after school. An irritable, restless young child who does not wish to be touched or held probably has the same symptoms but is unable to verbally express his complaints. Vomiting, especially upon arising, is also a frequent symptom, and often it is not associated with nausea. Other symptoms due to raised intracranial pressure are increasing lethargy and drowsiness or abnormalities of behavior which may initially be interpreted as functional. Symptoms may be intermittent, particularly in those young enough to develop separation of their cranial sutures and transiently relieve the increased intracranial pressure.

Physical examination may reveal macrocephaly during the early years of life when cranial sutures are more easily separated. The infant may have an enlarged head and a bulging fontanelle as the only sign of raised intracranial pressure. Other nonspecific findings indicative of increased pressure include papilledema and sixth cranial nerve paralysis. The former, when chronic, may lead to optic atrophy, and the latter often causes a compensatory head tilt. Complaints of double vision are rare in the young child. Third nerve paralysis with resultant unilateral ptosis and pupillary dilatation occurs less commonly and is an ominous sign. In addition to the signs and symptoms of increased intracranial pressure, specific localizing findings may be present due to the anatomic location of the tumor. These findings will be discussed in more detail later in this chapter. Most brain tumors can be diagnosed by a careful history and good neurologic examination.

DIAGNOSTIC STUDIES

Plain skull films often demonstrate the effects of chronic increased intracranial pressure with separation of cranial sutures (Fig. 12–1) and, more rarely, demineralization of the dorsum of the sella turcica. A localized area of bony erosion may indicate an underlying tumor mass. The presence of increased convolutional markings on the inner table of the skull is often difficult to evaluate in the growing child and is not a reliable index of increased intracranial pressure. Intrasellar or suprasellar calcifications are present in the great majority of children with craniopharyngiomas. Calcifications occasionally occur in posterior fossa gliomas, but more often are seen in cerebral hemisphere gliomas, in ependymomas and in oligodendrogliomas (Fig. 12–2). It is important to realize that many children with brain tumors have normal skull roentgenograms.[46]

The *electroencephalogram* often localizes tumors of the cerebral hemispheres, but is usually of little value in localizing infratentorial tumors. In-

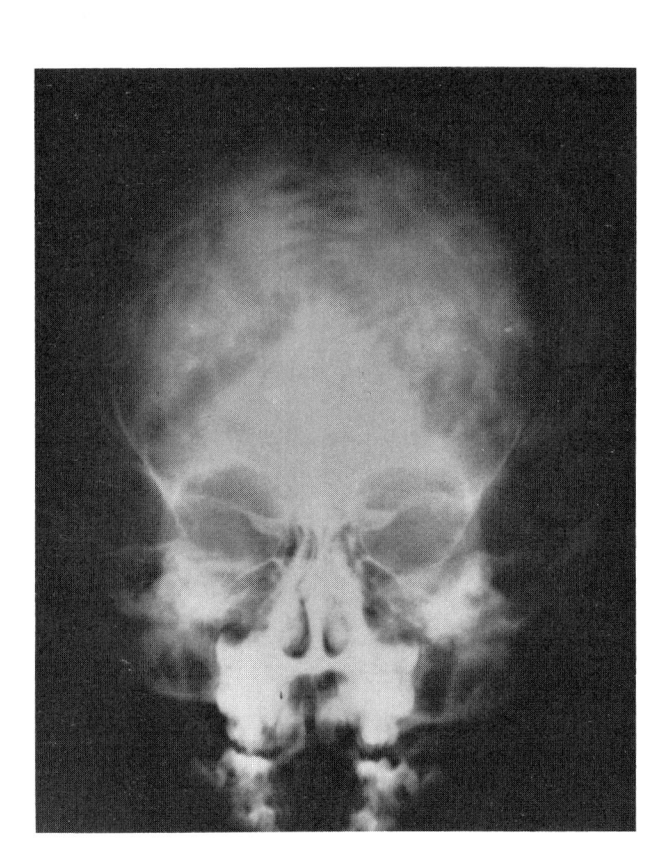

Figure 12–1 Skull roentgenogram demonstrating diastasis of the cranial sutures and increase of the convolutional markings indicating increased intracranial pressure. (Courtesy of Dr. Krishna Rao, University of Maryland Hospital.)

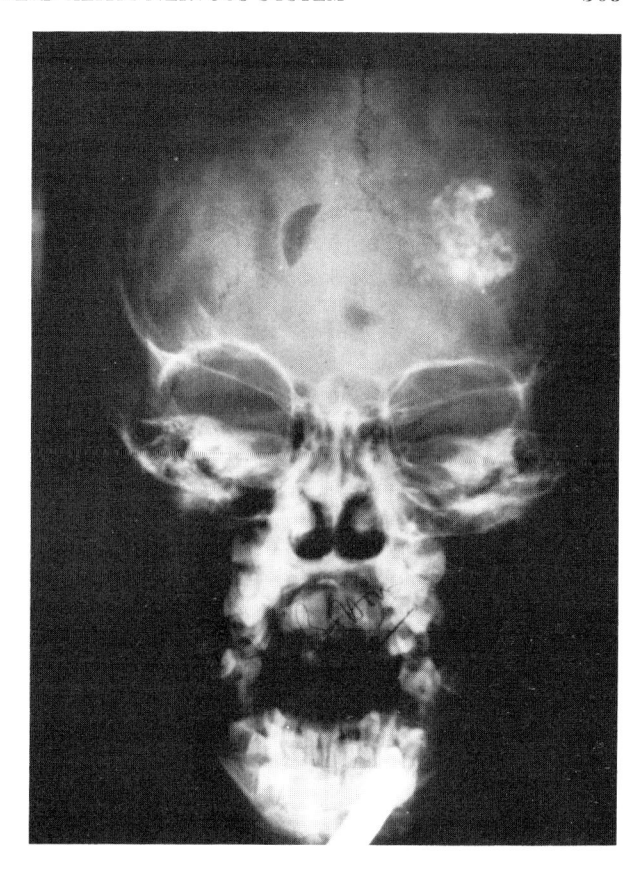

Figure 12–2 Calcifications in an oligodendroglioma. (Courtesy of Dr. Krishna Rao, University of Maryland Hospital.)

creased intracranial pressure may cause nonspecific diffuse slowing without localization. A normal EEG has been noted in 24 per cent of patients with posterior fossa tumors,[73] and the EEG usually shows no abnormality in patients with brain stem tumors.

Radionuclide brain scanning is of particular value in localizing supratentorial lesions. [99m]Technetium as the pertechnetate is the most useful isotope available at present because of its short half-life and exposure of the patient to minimal doses of radiation. Posterior fossa tumors are more difficult to visualize, especially if they lie deep in the brain stem. With meticulous positioning, however, the expert in nuclear medicine experienced in dealing with children can often detect the presence of posterior fossa tumors. The scan also often can determine whether or not the tumor is cystic in nature.[39, 40]

Computerized axial tomography (CAT) of the head has now become one of the most useful single diagnostic laboratory procedures available to the neurologist and neurosurgeon.[48, 50] This ingenious technique, devised by Ambrose and Hounsfield and reported in 1973, uses a digital computer to measure variations in x-ray absorption and has been able to achieve sectional tomograms of the brain substance to a degree of clarity not achieved by other radiologic methods.[1] The major advantage of the procedure is the fact that it is noninvasive. It can be used in the older, cooperative pediatric patient on an outpatient basis, providing the clinician with a means of periodically following the course of disease with little discomfort to the child (Fig. 12–3). It is not only of value in

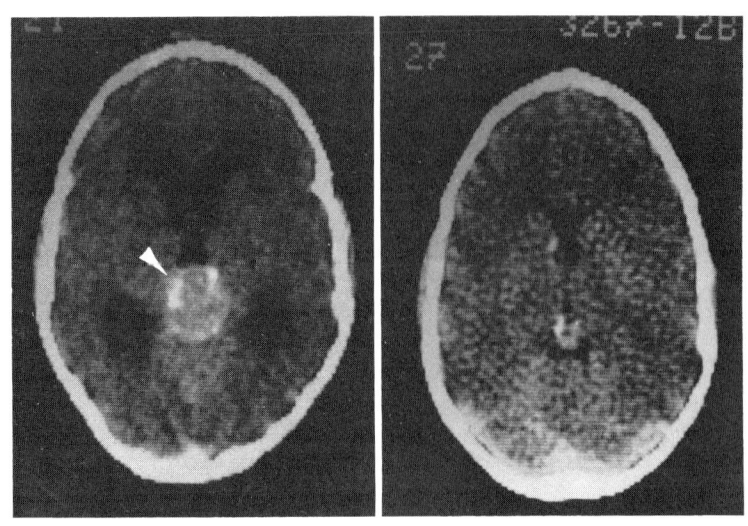

Figure 12-3 Computerized axial tomography scan of a 13 year old boy with the signs and symptoms of increased intracranial pressure. The scan demonstrates a tumor in the pineal area (arrow) and moderately dilated ventricles. A repeat scan (right) four weeks following completion of radiation therapy shows a dramatic decrease in tumor mass and resolution of the hydrocephalus.

localizing intracranial lesions, but also demonstrates the shape and size of the ventricles. If abnormal findings such as enlarged ventricles are found in the patient suspected of having a tumor, but no definite mass lesion is demonstrated, contrast enhanced computerized tomography will usually delineate the lesion. Characteristics of the tumor, such as presence of a cystic component, its vascularity, and the occurrence of calcifications not visualized on standard roentgenograms also can be demonstrated. The study may not be successful in detecting smaller lesions in or near the sella and the third ventricle. Still, it is the most accurate and useful initial diagnostic procedure available at the present time.

Intraventricular and paraventricular tumors can be well delineated by *pneumoencephalography*. Small pineal tumors, optic gliomas, and tumors of the hypothalamus are best demonstrated by this study (Fig. 12-4). If there is evidence of increased intracranial pressure, air ventriculography is probably a safer procedure. Air encephalography had been the most widely employed diagnostic test in the diagnosis of posterior fossa tumors, but with the wider use of angiography and the more recent availability of computerized axial tomography the indications for air studies appear to be changing. These invasive procedures should now only be used in instances where there is a high index of suspicion of the presence of tumor, and other diagnostic studies have been inconclusive.

With the development of selective catheterization studies, *cerebral angiography* is a precise diagnostic tool. Even in the small child these studies are usually safe when performed by the skilled neuroradiologist. Angiography not only demonstrates the displacement of normal vessels by a mass lesion but in addition supplies useful information regarding blood supply to the tumor. It is the study of choice in demonstrating arteriovenous malformations and aneurysms.

A *lumbar puncture* is contraindicated when a mass lesion of the brain is suspected. In the rare instance when the possibility of an infectious process exists but the presence of a mass lesion

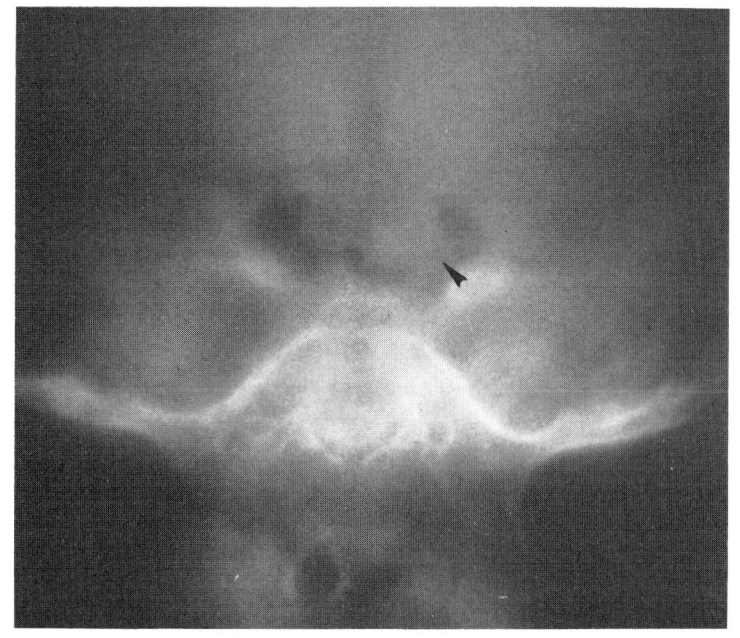

Figure 12–4 Pneumoencephalogram demonstrating an enlarged right optic nerve (arrow). (Courtesy of Dr. Krishna Rao, University of Maryland Hospital.)

is suspected, a lumbar puncture should be carefully performed with a small needle, removing only enough fluid required for analysis. This should be done only by or in the presence of a neurosurgeon, with the patient prepared for immediate surgery if necessary. In such instances, the physician should not only perform routine studies on the cerebrospinal fluid, but should also carefully examine it for the presence of malignant cells. This can best be done with the use of the Millipore filter or cytocentrifuge to concentrate any tumor cells that may be present.

Infratentorial Tumors

The cerebellum is the most common site of brain tumors in children. Signs and symptoms of increased intracranial pressure are common early phenomena, owing to obstruction of the flow of ventricular fluid by blockage at the aqueduct of Sylvius, in the fourth ventricle, or at the foramina of Luschka and Magendie. Flow may also be blocked in the subarachnoid space by herniation of the cerebellum downward through the foramen magnum. This frequently results in head tilt and nuchal rigidity.

Localizing signs in patients with cerebellar tumors depend upon the area of the cerebellum involved.[17] Posterior midline tumors may present with truncal ataxia and nystagmus in all directions of gaze. The more common tumors in this location are the medulloblastoma and ependymoma, two malignant tumors that are rarely resectable. Occasionally a cyst or benign tumor is found in this area. Tumors in the anterior midline are very rare, and often cause the patient to present with a wide-based, stiff-legged gait without nystagmus. Tumors of the cerebellar hemispheres result in limb ataxia on the same side of the body as the tumor and coarse nystagmus when the patient looks toward the lesion. The majority of neoplasms of the cerebellar hemispheres are astrocytomas of low-grade malignancy, which can often be resected surgically.

Medulloblastoma. The medulloblastoma is a highly malignant, rapidly growing tumor that is found almost exclusively in children. It occurs most commonly in males in nearly all series reported, with 2 to 4 males recorded for every female. The tumor is thought to arise from the posterior medullary velum, and extends into the fourth ventricle, cerebellar vermis, or hemispheres. It often seeds throughout the central nervous system by way of the cerebrospinal fluid. Rarely, the initial manifestations are due to spinal metastases, with the symptoms being those of spinal cord compression or pain from sensory nerve root invasion. Metastatic implants over the meninges also may occur. Occasionally, metastases occur outside of the nervous system, even in the absence of a ventriculo-atrial shunt.[60] These metastases are usually to the skeletal system.[11,13] Malignant cells also may disseminate into the abdominal cavity through a ventriculoperitoneal shunt[54] or to the pleura through a ventriculopleural shunt.[18] Although metastatic disease involving different parts of the central nervous system is often present in fatal cases, the reason for therapeutic failure and death is usually tumor recurrence in the posterior fossa.[13,78]

One rarely, if ever, cures the patient with medulloblastoma by surgery alone. Cushing believed the prognosis to be "ultimately hopeless," although a number of his patients experienced temporary symptomatic relief following surgery.[26] Despite transient improvement, patients treated with surgery alone generally survive less than 6 months. The major objective of the surgical procedure is to reestablish normal cerebrospinal fluid circulation and to remove enough tumor to establish a histologic diagnosis. Shunting procedures should be avoided, if possible, to avoid tumor dissemination via the shunt tube to other parts of the body.[54] Extracranial shunting procedures to relieve hydrocephalus may at times be unavoidable when relief of pressure is not afforded by surgical excision, decompression, or radiation therapy. Currently, many neurosurgeons try to remove as much of the tumor as possible without jeopardizing the life of the patient or causing serious neurological disability. In many series it has now been shown that surgical decompression followed by radiation therapy has resulted in a significant improvement in the length of survival and rate of cure. There is some evidence that the survival rate is greater in those who experienced grossly complete tumor excision compared to those who had less radical resections when both groups were treated with radiation therapy following surgery.[13] Some investigators, however, have advocated treatment by radiation alone, without benefit of major surgery. Their patients have had histologically diagnosed medulloblastoma from tissue obtained by a brain needle biopsy through a drill hole.[16,93] Although their series was small, results compared favorably with a larger group of patients treated with surgery and radiation.

In their review of the literature, McFarland and associates[78] reported that 33 per cent of 430 patients developed metastases within the central nervous system. Ninety-four per cent of the metastases were in the spine and 6 per cent were supratentorial. This common pattern of tumor dissemination indicates that irradiation of the entire cerebrospinal axis is required. Radiation therapy should be directed to the entire brain and spine, with an added increment given to the posterior fossa. There is at present no agreement on the optimum dose of radiation needed to provide maximum tumor control with minimum complications. Bloom and Walsh[14] recommend 5000 to 5500 rads directed to the posterior fossa given in 7 to 8 weeks for children 3 years of age or more using supervoltage equipment. The dose to the region of the third ventricle is 4000 to

4500 rads, and the prophylactic dose to the remainder of the central nervous system is 3000 to 3500 rads. This dose is higher than that recommended previously by these investigators.[13] Sheline[107] has recommended 5500 rads in 7 to 8 weeks to the posterior fossa and upper cervical cord, 4500 rads to the remainder of the brain, and 4000 rads to the spinal cord. During the course of treatment to the spine with doses in this range, bone marrow suppression and leukopenia usually occur, and decreased stature is a common late complication.

The survival rates of patients with medulloblastoma treated in a number of institutions with a variety of radiation therapy regimens is shown in Table 12–3. In most large series, a 30 to 35 per cent 5-year survival and 15 to 25 per cent 10-year survival has been reported. The aggressive treatment regimen used by Sheline[107] in one small series appears to give unusually good results. Reirradiation of intracranial and spinal recurrences often achieves good palliative results and may occasionally permit long-term survival.[110]

A number of children who have developed recurrence of medulloblastoma have responded to a variety of chemotherapeutic agents, frequently with dramatic initial improvement. Drugs which have been effective in treating recurrent medulloblastoma have included vincristine sulfate,[23, 59, 62, 63] intrathecal methotrexate,[84, 85, 121] procarbazine,[58] the lipid-soluble alkylating agents BCNU[32] and CCNU,[117] and PTG,[109] a semisynthetic podophyllotoxin derivative. In addition, a number of patients with recurrent disease have been treated with combination chemotherapy with good response.[23, 47] The combination of procarbazine, CCNU, and vincristine was reported to exert a significant antitumor effect on all 5 of 5 patients in one series, with a median duration of response of 10 months.[47] Unfortunately, even those patients who respond to chemotherapy following recurrence of tumor usually die of their disease. At present, many centers are now treating patients with medulloblastoma prophylactically immediately after surgery and radiation therapy. If the experience with this form of treatment is similar to that found with a number of other childhood solid tumors, a significant improvement in the cure rate of medulloblastoma may occur. Only long-term follow-up data from these recently initiated studies will determine whether prophylactic chemotherapy will improve survival rates.

Cerebellar Astrocytoma. This tumor is found almost exclusively in childhood and early adolescence. It is usually well differentiated histologically, grows slowly, and does not spread in the subarachnoid pathways. Children with cerebellar astrocytoma often have a longer duration of symptoms prior to diagnosis than do patients with other posterior fossa tumors. The history has usually been of over several months' duration, and not uncommonly as long as several years. The tumor often has a solitary cystic portion containing a neoplastic mural nodule, or there may be multiple small cysts within a mass of solid

Table 12–3 Survival Rates of Patients With Medulloblastoma Following Treatment With Radiation Therapy

AUTHOR(S)	PER CENT 5-YEAR	PER CENT 10-YEAR
Aron[4]	35	26
Bloom et al.[13]	32	26
Bouchard[16]°	40	
Faust et al.[30]°	38	
Kramer[56]°	50	
McFarland et al.[78]	30	14
Patterson and Farr[88]	29	
Sheline[107]°	84	
Smith et al.[111]	28	
Tice[113]	26	

° Fewer than 15 patients in series.

tumor. The cystic portion may become very large and occupy a good portion of one cerebellar hemisphere. Even when the tumor appears solid, it usually contains multiple microcysts. The cysts contain a highly proteinaceous yellow or amber-colored material.

The cerebellar astrocytoma has the most favorable prognosis of the intracranial tumors of childhood. It often can be totally removed surgically, resulting in cure in the majority of patients. Total removal is not possible, however, in about one third of the cases.[38, 43] Even incomplete removal often is followed by years of normal life, and recurrence of symptoms may again respond to surgery because of the tumor's tendency to maintain its benign character for long periods of time.[20] It is estimated that at least 90 per cent of children with benign cerebellar astrocytoma survive years to decades following surgical treatment.[38] The role of radiation therapy is still unclear, but may be of value in treating the patient in whom there has been incomplete tumor excision, especially if the neoplasm is locally invasive and of the solid variety.[72] Those tumors with a higher grade of malignancy which cannot be totally excised should be treated with radiation therapy. The value of chemotherapy in this group of more malignant cerebellar astrocytomas has not been determined.

Brain Stem Gliomas. The gliomas of the pons, medulla, and midbrain are much more common in children and adolescents than in adults. They rarely occur under the age of 3 years,[61] but patients have been diagnosed during very early life, and a rare case of congenital pontine glioma has been reported.[70] The usual clinical findings are localized multiple cranial nerve deficits, ataxia, and pyramidal tract signs in the absence of signs and symptoms of increased intracranial pressure. It is not unusual for children to eventually die of brain stem involvement by the tumor or intercurrent infection without ever developing increased intracranial pressure. Spinal fluid findings are usually normal. The diagnosis is usually made on the basis of clinical findings and the demonstration by air contrast studies of a characteristic enlargement of the pons, with displacement of the aqueduct and fourth ventricle posteriorly (Fig. 12–5). Computerized axial tomography is also of value in localizing the lesion. Many patients are treated on the basis of the physical and neuroradiologic findings without confirmation of the diagnosis by tissue examination. Surgery is not usually performed because the location of the tumor makes removal impossible.

Histologically, brain stem gliomas show a wide variety of tissue types, ranging from low grade astrocytoma to the highly malignant glioblastoma multiforme.[44, 61] Buckley histologically classified 25 cases of pontine glioma as glioblastoma multiforme (10 cases), astrocytoma (9 cases), spongioblastoma unipolare (5 cases) and unclassified (1 case), and emphasized the cystic nature of these tumors.[19] The observation of the presence of cysts, the isolated case reports of long-term survival following aspiration of brain stem cysts,[89, 95] and the poor prognosis in this group of patients prompted Lassiter and co-workers[64] to analyze the value of surgical exploration in 37 patients with brain stem gliomas. In 5 cases, a surgically significant cyst in the neoplasm could be aspirated, which resulted in neurologic improvement and contributed to long-term survival in four cases. Although there is some disagreement over whether or not surgical exploration is indicated in every case, all agree that exploration should be performed if there is any doubt about the location and nature of the neoplasm. The ability of computerized axial tomography to demonstrate the cystic nature of a neoplasm may be of value in determining which patient might benefit from surgery.

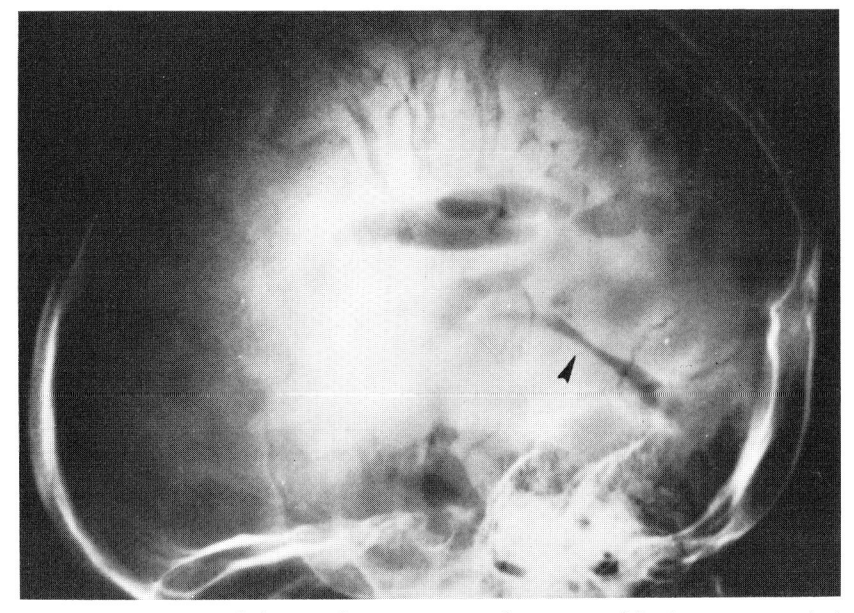

Figure 12–5 Pneumoencephalogram demonstrating enlargement of the brain stem with displacement of the aqueduct and fourth ventricle posteriorly (arrow). (Courtesy of Dr. Krishna Rao, University of Maryland Hospital.)

The prognosis for patients with brain stem gliomas is usually poor, but radiation therapy has been effective in prolonging the mean survival time. Better results have been documented in those receiving 4000 rads or more than in those who receive less,[119] and doses varying from 5000 to 6000 rads have been recommended.[87, 107] Since survivors have seldom had histologic confirmation of their tumor, it is generally believed that few survivors had high-grade gliomas. The entity of transient brain stem encephalitis with radiographic evidence of medullary enlargement may so closely resemble the picture of a brain stem glioma that it has been suggested that radiotherapy or surgical exploration be deferred for a period of time to avoid an incorrect diagnosis of malignancy.[104]

There is little published data on the use of chemotherapy in the managemet of brain stem gliomas, although there is some evidence that a number of chemotherapeutic agents have been of value in the treatment of high-grade gliomas located in other portions of the brain. Agents that have been shown to be effective against brain stem gliomas have included procarbazine,[58] BCNU,[116] CCNU,[99] intrathecal methotrexate,[84] and high-dose intravenous methotrexate followed by citrovorum rescue.[98] To date, most publications regarding the effects of chemotherapeutic agents have been preliminary reports, have included only small numbers of patients, and have provided little long-term follow-up information.

Infratentorial Ependymomas. Ependymomas account for about 8 to 10 per cent of posterior fossa tumors in children. The tumor commonly arises from the floor of the fourth ventricle, extends into and fills the fourth ventricle, and grows into the cervical area or the aqueduct (Fig. 12–6). It may be difficult to differentiate grossly from other tumors that occur within the fourth ventricle. The child presents with the signs and symptoms of increased intracranial pressure. The tumor occasionally arises in the lateral recess of the fourth

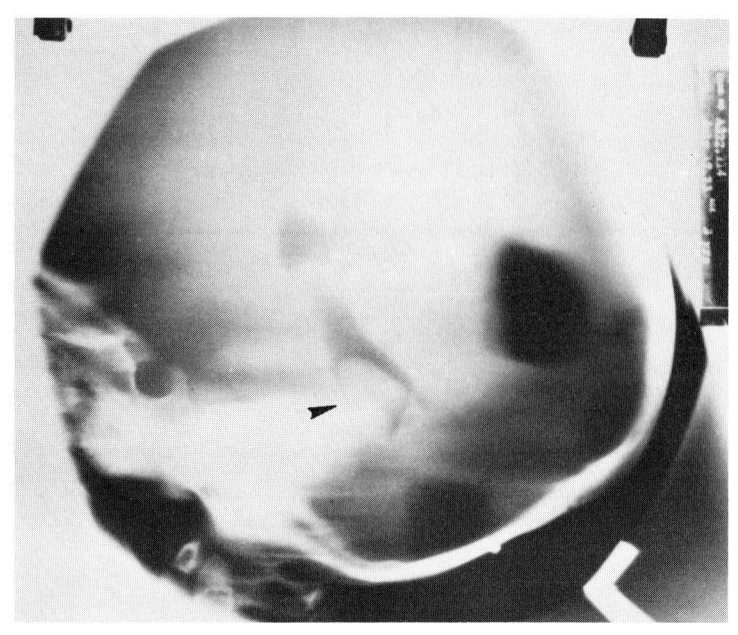

Figure 12-6 Ventriculogram demonstrating a tumor mass arising from the floor of the fourth ventricle (arrow). An ependymoma was found at surgery. (Courtesy of Dr. Krishna Rao, University of Maryland Hospital.)

ventricle and extends into the cerebellopontine angle.

Ependymomas are generally well-circumscribed, solid, nodular neoplasms. They have been classified into various histologic subgroups, depending upon their degree of malignancy, and a number of grading systems have been proposed.[53, 69] Most of the tumors are mixtures of more than one histologic type, and transition from one type into another can often be demonstrated.[69] Those in the posterior fossa tend to be histologically more benign, but malignant forms do occur and, like the medulloblastoma, may seed along the neuraxis. There is evidence that the histologic appearance reflects the biological behavior,[69] but even the more benign appearing tumors have been known to spread through the subarachnoid space.[34]

Treatment of the posterior fossa ependymoma is surgical resection followed by radiation therapy. Complete removal is seldom possible, but the tumor is radiosensitive, and radiation therapy to the posterior fossa has been reported to result in up to 70 to 80 per cent 10-year survival for those with a low-grade malignancy.[107] Doses greater than 4500 rads give the best results.[92] Because of the increased risk of spinal seeding with the most malignant tumors, radiation therapy to the entire neuraxis should probably be given if the tumor has a more malignant histology. The prognosis remains poor in this group, however, despite the more aggressive treatment.[107] There has been little experience with chemotherapy in the treatment of ependymomas, but a few cases have been reported to respond to the nitrosureas[32, 99] and PTG.[109]

Supratentorial Tumors

Cerebral Hemisphere Astrocytomas. Astrocytomas of the cerebral hemispheres occur much less commonly in children than in adults. They vary in their degree of malignancy from the more benign low-grade astrocytoma to the highly malignant glioblastoma multiforme (Grade IV astrocytoma). When located in the cerebrum the astrocytoma carries a poorer prognosis than when located infratentorially, usually because it is more often of a higher degree of malignancy. The tumor may grow to a massive size before a diagnosis is made.

Of the 20 cases of relatively benign cerebral astrocytomas in children reported by Gol,[42] the most common complaints were of headache (16 cases), vomiting (11 cases), and convulsive disorders (8 cases). This group of patients did exceedingly well, with the only deaths in the series being operative mortalities. Gol concluded that the mortality rate from a direct surgical attack on the tumors of the third ventricle was very high, and that a shunting procedure followed by radiotherapy was preferable for treating the tumors located in this area.

Radiotherapy appears to be of value in the treatment of both low-grade[42, 66] and high-grade cerebral astrocytomas.[14, 107] The prognosis for children with both low- and high-grade tumors treated with radiation may be better than that for adults with tumors of the same degree of malignancy.[42, 91] Penman and Smith[91] reported a 50 per cent 3-year survival rate for those under age 14, but only 7 per cent survival rate for those over age 40. Sheline, however, reported all six of the children with glioblastoma multiforme treated in his series to have died of disease.[107]

There has been little experience with chemotherapy in children who have high-grade cerebral astrocytomas. Because of the accumulating evidence that a number of agents have been effective against adult grades III and IV cerebral astrocytomas, and because of the poor prognosis in these children, more vigorous chemotherapeutic regimens should probably be evaluated in the future. The rarity of these tumors during the childhood years makes single institution studies nearly impossible, and most of our future information will probably come from adult or multi-institutional pediatric studies.

Supratentorial Ependymomas. Cerebral hemisphere ependymomas arise from the ependyma of the ventricles. Ependymomas occur less commonly supratentorially than in the posterior fossa.[69, 102] They are radiosensitive tumors and should be treated in a manner similar to infratentorial ependymomas.

Craniopharyngiomas. The craniopharyngioma is a developmental tumor that arises from squamous cell remnants of Rathke's pouch. The tissues are not usually malignant but, in some cases, there is marked cellular proliferation and invasion of the base of the brain. The tumor is usually suprasellar in location, is slow-growing, and exerts its symptoms by blocking cerebrospinal fluid circulation, causing increased intracranial pressure, and by inducing visual defects. Of 67 children reviewed by Banna and associates,[6] presenting symptoms were those of increased intracranial pressure in 78 per cent, visual disturbances in 22 per cent, small stature in 7 per cent, diabetes insipidus in 7 per cent, and limb weakness in 4 per cent. In most instances roentgenograms of the skull are characteristic, with either evidence of calcifications in the suprasellar region or deformity of the sella turcica, or both (Fig. 12–7). In one series of 71 patients, only 4 cases had neither of these abnormalities on plain skull roentgenograms.[6]

Despite the benign histologic nature of this neoplasm, it is usually difficult, if not impossible, to remove the entire tumor surgically. Surgical treatment alone and meticulous postoperative management of endocrine problems have achieved successful long-term results in up to 75 per cent of patients when performed by a skilled and experienced surgical team.[75] Results of subtotal resections, however, are often unsatisfactory because the tumor tends to recur, and the morbidity and mor-

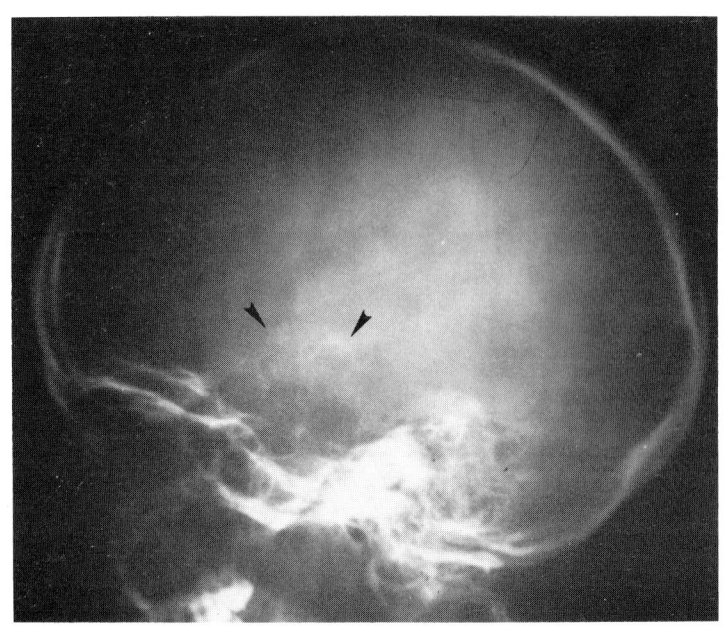

Figure 12-7 Lateral skull roentgenogram demonstrating suprasellar calcifications in a craniopharyngioma. (From the teaching collection of the Division of Pediatric Radiology, Johns Hopkins Hospital.)

tality rates associated with a second operation are great. Aspiration of the cystic portion of the tumor (which commonly is present) and conservative tumor excision without endangering the patient often yield good results if followed by radiation therapy. Kramer and co-workers[57] reported a more conservative approach, using aspiration and radiation therapy in 9 patients and radiation alone in one. Nine of the patients were alive and well over 6 years following treatment, with the only death occurring from a myocardial infarction in an adult. Bloom[12] reported an 85 per cent 5-year survival and 72 per cent 10-year survival in patients treated by aspiration or biopsy followed by radical radiation therapy. Thus, the present outlook for survival in the majority of patients is good, but long-term follow-up is necessary, since tumor recurrence has been reported 20 years following radical surgery.[7]

Optic Nerve Gliomas. Gliomas of the optic nerve are usually slow-growing, nonmetastasizing neoplasms that most often present during the first decade of life. The peak incidence of diagnosis is between the ages of 2 and 6 years.[21] The majority of tumors have the histologic appearance of low-grade astrocytomas. From 20 to 60 per cent of the patients have been noted to have neurofibromatosis,[21,51,71] but some children have been found to have optic gliomas before the appearance of their café-au-lait spots,[10] suggesting that the incidence of neurofibromatosis may be higher than reported in some series.

The presenting symptoms of patients with optic glioma include diminished visual acuity, exophthalmos, evidence of increased intracranial pressure, nystagmus, and strabismus. Examination often reveals a visual field deficit and pallor or blurring of the optic discs. The tumor may involve nerve, chiasm, or tract. Most neoplasms occur intracranially and involve the chiasm; the minority are localized to the optic nerve. Progressive and fatal hydrocephalus is uncommon, but may occur in patients with extensive intracranial tumors.[51]

Controversy exists regarding the

natural course and therapy of the optic glioma. Many advise against operation except for diagnosis or relief of obstructive hydrocephalus, with a possible exception being the case of a tumor confined to one optic nerve which can be completely removed. Radiation therapy has been reported to cause considerable improvement in those who cannot be successfully treated with surgery.[21, 71, 112] Some believe, however, that these are congenital, non-neoplastic tumors with self-limited growth, and advocate excision only for relief of severe proptosis of a blind eye. Over prolonged periods of follow-up in one large series, untreated patients fared as well as those who received radiation, and spontaneous tumor regression was noted in some untreated patients.[41]

Pineal Area Tumors. The majority of patients with this rare group of tumors are older children, teenagers, and young adults, with the marked preponderance of tumors occurring in males.[82, 103] Children with tumors arising in the area of the pineal gland usually present with symptoms of increased intracranial pressure and few other neurologic findings. Occasionally, a characteristic localizing sign, known as Parinaud's syndrome, is seen. This consists of paralysis of conjugate upward gaze accompanied by absent pupillary reaction to light and retraction nystagmus.

Multiple histologic types of pineal area tumors have been described. Numerous germinal varieties have included seminomas, choriocarcinomas, endodermal sinus tumors, and a variety of teratomas.[79] True pinealomas arising from pineal parenchyma originate within the pineal gland and are of neural origin. Also arising in this area are tumors of glial tissue origin and dermoid cysts.

Pineal area tumors are sometimes associated with precocious puberty or, more commonly, with evidence of hypogonadism. Precocious puberty can be explained by a decrease in the normal gonadoinhibitory action of the pineal gland because its cells are destroyed by nonparenchymal pineal tumors, especially teratomas.[103] Delayed puberty is believed to be due to an increased secretion of melatonin-like substances by neoplastic cells of pineal tissue origin, which are known to have an inhibitory effect on gonadal development.[55]

Ectopic pineal tumors located in the hypothalamic area without apparent tumor in the pineal region are called ectopic pinealomas. These tumors often present with the triad of diabetes insipidus, bitemporal hemianopsia, and hypopituitarism,[100] and, rarely, have been reported to produce melatonin-like substances and be associated with delayed puberty.[122] Some studies have found ectopic pineal tissue tumors to be more frequent in children than true pinealomas arising in the pineal gland.[103] Many believe the majority of ectopic pinealomas to be germinomas.[100]

Efforts to excise tumors of the pineal gland have resulted in a high operative morbidity and mortality. Dandy has stated that these tumors are "perhaps the most dangerous of all intracranial tumors to attack surgically."[27] Most patients with these neoplasms are therefore treated with shunting procedures for the increased intracranial pressure, followed by radiotherapy. Most true pineal tissue tumors, pineal germinomas, and ectopic pinealomas are radiosensitive neoplasms.[25, 82, 94, 100, 107] In most reported series, the histologic tumor types were not recorded because no surgical procedure was performed. Despite the lack of pathologic confirmation of pineal region tumors, the great majority have responded to radiation therapy, and 5-year disease-free survivals of up to 60 to 70 per cent have been reported.[25, 107] Because of reports of seeding of the neuraxis in a small number of patients, some have advocated radiating the entire cerebrospinal axis,[35] but this complication probably occurs in fewer than 10 per cent of patients.[82]

Hematogenous spread of pineal germinomas is very rare and has usually followed intracranial surgery. Long-term survival in such patients has been reported following the use of aggressive radiation therapy and combination chemotherapy.[15]

Hypothalamic Tumors. Tumors of either the hypothalamus or the optic nerve that invade the hypothalamus result in a variety of abnormalities. Infants or young children may present with profound emaciation and a marked loss of subcutaneous fat despite a normal or increased caloric intake, the so-called "diencephalic syndrome."[5, 37] Children with this disorder are often alert, hyperactive, and euphoric. Often, no other signs or symptoms are present, but pallor, vomiting, nystagmus, excessive perspiration, hypothermia, and hypotension may occur. Elevated growth hormone levels, hypoglycemia, and eosinophilia may be present, and cerebrospinal fluid protein levels are often increased. Most cases have been due to low-grade astrocytomas arising from the anterior hypothalmus or involvement of this region by optic nerve tumors. Because of the tumor location, surgery has been of little value in treatment, and the prognosis has generally been considered to be poor. A few cases, however, have responded to radiation therapy.[5]

Hypothalamic neoplasms may occasionally result in hyperphagia and obesity, problems with body temperature regulation, hypersomnia and placidity, loss of thirst, diabetes insipidus, hypogonadism, or precocious puberty. Not uncommonly, the child with the diencephalic syndrome may develop obesity and lose previous hyperactivity as the size of his tumor increases.[33, 37]

Miscellaneous Tumors. A variety of other childhood brain tumors have been described, which are very rare, including cerebral oligodendrogliomas, sarcomas, hemangiomas, meningiomas, choroid plexus papillomas, and primary tumors of the pituitary gland. Most symptoms are related to the anatomic location of these lesions rather than to the tissue type, and may result in blockage of cerebrospinal fluid flow, neuroendocrine abnormalities, or focal neurologic signs and symptoms. Intracranial metastases from distant tumors also are uncommon in children, and seldom present as the first manifestation of disease. In contrast, cerebral symptoms due to metastases are common presenting findings of malignant tumors in adults.

INTRASPINAL TUMORS

Tumors of the spinal cord occur about one fifth as frequently as do intracranial tumors in childhood. About 50 per cent of 115 cases reported by Matson and Tachdjian[77] were discovered during the first 4 years of life and were usually tumors of developmental origin or intraspinal extensions of neuroblastomas. Erroneous initial diagnoses are extremely common, especially with benign or slowly growing lesions. A number of children are initially thought to have torticollis, scoliosis, kyphosis, poliomyelitis, and enuresis. An incorrect initial diagnosis was made in over two thirds of the cases in one large series.[77]

The most common type of intramedullary spinal cord tumor is the low-grade astrocytoma. These are usually located in the cervical or upper thoracic region and tend to be more benign than spinal cord gliomas in adults. The initial complaint is usually of motor weakness involving an extremity. The tumors usually are fusiform, extend over several segments of the cord, and occasionally have a cystic component. Most of these tumors cannot be surgically removed because of their infiltrative nature. They usually respond poorly to radiation therapy.

Ependymomas are the second most common intrinsic spinal cord malignant tumors. They more commonly involve the lumbar region, arise from the filum terminale around the roots of the cauda equina and often grow to a very large size. Although they are usually histologically more malignant than the astrocytomas, they are less infiltrative and more amenable to surgical excision. Usually only partial removal is achieved, but the tumor is more responsive to radiation therapy than is the astrocytoma. Ependymomas of the spinal cord may also arise as metastatic lesions from a primary neoplasm in the posterior fossa.

Benign congenital tumors constitute about 10 per cent of intraspinal tumors found in children, and include dermoid cysts, teratomas, and lipomas. They occur most commonly in the lumbosacral region and are frequently associated with dermal or osseous abnormalities. A dimple or tuft of hair over this area is often a clue to the diagnosis. There may be a dermal sinus connection from the subarachnoid space to the skin and, in some instances, the diagnosis is made following repeated episodes of bacterial meningitis.[76] Occasional cases of autotransplanted tissue carried into the subarachnoid space by lumbar puncture have resulted in the growth of benign tumors.[106] Initial complaints of benign tumors are usually increasing radicular symptoms of stiff back, problems with bladder control, or leg weakness. These neoplasms can often be completely excised, but residual disability from benign intraspinal lesions has been reported to be disappointingly high. This is usually the result of a delay in establishing a correct diagnosis rather than an effect of surgery.[77]

Some tumors, such as lymphomas, neuroblastomas, and ganglioneuromas arise outside the spine, grow through the intervertebral foramina, and result in spinal cord compression. Bloodborne metastases from distant primary tumors, such as a lymphoma, Ewing's tumor, and leukemia, may cause signs of spinal cord and root compression, as may subarachnoid metastases from primary brain tumors. The child with a diagnosed malignant disease that is known to be radiosensitive who develops evidence of intraspinal involvement can often be treated with radiotherapy rather than decompressive laminectomy, especially if the child is a poor surgical candidate. Delayed surgical decompression, however, in the presence of rapidly progressive cord compression by a potentially curable lesion, has led to permanent paraplegia in patients later cured of their tumors.

TUMORS OF THE PERIPHERAL NERVES

Benign tumors of the peripheral nerves can be divided into two groups, the schwannomas and the neurofibromas. Although the cell of origin of these tumors has long been debated, both are now believed to arise from Schwann cells.[101] They are both capable of undergoing malignant transformation although this is an uncommon occurrence, especially in children.

Schwannomas are usually solitary neoplasms and may arise within cranial nerves, spinal roots, or peripheral nerves. The acoustic neuroma is a schwannoma arising from the eighth cranial nerve. Although multiple schwannomas may be found in patients with von Recklinghausen's disease, this type of tumor more commonly occurs as a single tumor in patients without this genetic disorder. They are well-encapsulated, readily amenable to surgical resection, and seldom recur. Rarely do they exhibit malignant potential.

Neurofibromas are generally nonencapsulated, multiple tumors which are usually found in patients with von

Recklinghausen's disease. An isolated tumor may occur in an otherwise normal individual. The neoplasms may occur as dermal nodules or as plexiform tumors of the peripheral nerves. Complete excision of these lesions is often difficult, and local tumor recurrence is common. The frequency of malignant transformation of these tumors in patients with von Recklinghausen's disease is difficult to assess, but in some series an incidence as high as 17 per cent has been reported.[48a] This usually occurs in the adult patient.

REFERENCES

1. Ambrose, J., and Hounsfield, G. N.: Computerized axial transverse tomography. Brit. J. Radiol. 46:148, 1973.
2. Amiet, V. A.: Aldrich-Syndrom: Blobachtung zweier fälle. Ann. Paediatr. 201:315, 1963.
3. Armstrong, R. M., and Hanson, C. W.: Familial gliomas. Neurology 19:1061, 1969.
4. Aron, B. S.: Twenty years' experience with radiation therapy of medulloblastoma. Am. J. Roentgenol. Radium Ther. Nucl. Med. 55:37, 1969.
5. Bain, H. W., Darte, J. M. M., Keith, W. S., et al.: The diencephalic syndrome of early infancy due to silent brain tumor: with special reference to treatment. Pediatrics 38:473, 1966.
6. Banna, M., Hoare, R. D., Stanley, P., et al.: Craniopharyngioma in children. J. Pediatr. 83:781, 1973.
7. Bartlett, J. R.: Craniopharyngiomas: an analysis of some aspects of symptomatology, radiology, and histology. Brain 94:725, 1971.
8. Baughman, F. A., Jr., List, C. F., Williams, J. R., et al.: The glioma-polyposis syndrome. N. Engl. J. Med. 281:1345, 1969.
9. Belameric, J., and Chau, A. S.: Medulloblastoma in newborn sisters. J. Neurosurg. 30:76, 1969.
10. Beller, A. J., and Tiberin, P.: Glioma of the optic nerve: its relationship to von Recklinghausen's disease. Harefuah 59:195, 1960.
11. Black, S. P. W., and Keats, T. E.: Generalized osteosclerosis secondary to metastatic medulloblastoma of the cerebellum. Radiology 82:395, 1964.
12. Bloom, H. J. G.: Combined modality therapy for intracranial tumors. Cancer 35:111, 1975.
13. Bloom, H. J. G., Wallace, E. N. K., and Henk, J. M.: The treatment and prognosis of medulloblastoma in children: a study of 82 verified cases. Am. J. Roentgenol. Radium Ther. Nucl. Med. 105:43, 1969.
14. Bloom, H. J. G., and Walsh, L. S.: Tumors of the central nervous system. In Bloom, H. J. G., Lemerle, J., Neidhardt, M. K., et al. (eds.): Cancer in Children: Clinical Management. New York, Springer-Verlag, 1975, p. 93.
15. Borden, S., Weber, A. L., Toch, R., et al.: Pineal germinoma: long-term survival despite hematogenous metastases. Am. J. Dis. Child. 126:214, 1973.
16. Bouchard, J.: Radiation Therapy of Tumors and Diseases of the Nervous System. Philadelphia, Lea & Febiger, 1966.
17. Brown, J. R.: Cerebellar tumors in children. Mayo Clin. Proc. 42:511, 1967.
18. Brust, J. C. M., Moill, R. H., and Rosenberg, R. N.: Glial tumor metastases through a ventriculopleural shunt. Arch. Neurol. 18:649, 1968.
19. Buckley, R. C.: Pontile gliomas: a pathologic study and classification of twentyfive cases. Arch. Path. 9:779, 1930.
20. Bucy, P. C., and Thieman, P. W.: Astrocytomas of the cerebellum: a study of a series of patients operated upon over twenty-eight years ago. Arch. Neurol. 18:14, 1968.
21. Chutorian, A. M., Schwartz, J. F., Evans, R. A., et al.: Optic gliomas in children. Neurology 14:83, 1964.
22. Cohnheim, J.: Vorlesungen über allemeine Pathologie. Berlin, A. Hischwald, 1877.
23. Crist, W. M., Ragab, A. H., Vietti, T., et al.: Chemotherapy of childhood medulloblastoma. Am. J. Dis. Child. 130:639, 1976.
24. Crosley, C. J., Mishkin, M., and Rorke, L. B.: Congenital sarcoma of the brain. Am. J. Dis. Child. 128:523, 1974.
25. Cummins, F. M., Taveras, J. M., and Schlesinger, E. B.: Treatment of gliomas of the third ventricle and pinealomas: with special reference to the value of radiotherapy. Neurology 10:1031, 1960.
26. Cushing, H.: Experiences with cerebellar medulloblastoma—critical review. Acta Pathol. Microbiol. Scand. 7:1, 1930.
27. Dandy, W. E.: In Walters, W. (ed.): Lewis' Practice of Surgery. Hagerstown, Md., W. F. Prior Co., 1945. Vol 12, p. 590.
28. Davies, J. N. P.: Childhood tumours. In A. C. Templeton: Tumours in a Tropical Country: A Survey of Uganda 1964–1968. New York, Springer-Verlag, 1973.
29. Editorial: Trauma and tumour. Lancet 2:545, 1973.

30. Faust, D. S., Tatem, H. R., Brady, L. W., et al.: Radiation therapy in the management of medulloblastoma. Neurology 20:519, 1970.
31. Fessard, C.: Cerebral tumors in infancy. Am. J. Dis. Child. 115:302, 1968.
32. Fewer, D., Wilson, C. B., Boldrey, E. B., et al.: The chemotherapy of brain tumors: clinical experience with carmustine (BCNU) and vincristine. J.A.M.A. 222:549, 1972.
33. Fishman, M. A., and Peake, G. T.: Paradoxical growth in a patient with the diencephalic syndrome. Pediatrics 45:973, 1970.
34. Fokes, E. C., Jr., and Earle, K. M.: Ependymomas: clinical and pathological aspects. J. Neurosurg. 30:385, 1969.
35. Fowler, F. D., Alexander, E., and Davis, C. H.: Pinealoma with metastases in the central nervous system. J. Neurosurg. 13:271, 1956.
36. Fraumeni, J. F., Jr., and Miller, R. W.: Adrenocortical neoplasms with hemihypertrophy, brain tumors, and other disorders. J. Pediatr. 70:129, 1967.
37. Gamstorp, I., Kjellman, B., and Palmgren, B.: Diencephalic syndromes of infancy. J. Pediatr. 70:383, 1967.
38. Geissinger, J. D., and Bucy, P. C.: Astrocytomas of the cerebellum in children. Arch. Neurol. 24:125, 1971.
39. Gilday, D. L., and Ash, J. M.: Accuracy of brain scanning in pediatric craniocerebral neoplasms. Radiology 117:93, 1975.
40. Gilday, D. L., and Harwood-Nash, D. C.: Coordinated investigation of cystic astrocytomas by nuclear medicine and neurological techniques. Child's Brain 1:34, 1975.
41. Glaser, J. S., Hoyt, W. F., and Corbett, J.: Visual morbidity with chiasmal glioma: long-term studies of visual fields in untreated and irradiated cases. Arch. Ophthalmol. 85:3, 1971.
42. Gol, A.: Cerebral astrocytomas in childhood: a clinical study. J. Neurosurg. 19:577, 1962.
43. Gol, A., and McKissock, W.: The cerebellar astrocytomas: a report on 98 verified cases. J. Neurosurg. 16:287, 1959.
44. Golden, G. S., Ghatak, N. R., Hirano, A., et al.: Malignant glioma of the brainstem: a clinicopathological analysis of 13 cases. J. Neurol. Neurosurg. Psych. 35:732, 1972.
45. Gorlin, R. J., Vickers, R. A., Kellen, E., et al.: The multiple basal-cell nevi syndrome. An analysis of a syndrome consisting of multiple nevoid basal-cell carcinoma, jaw cysts, skeletal anomalies, medulloblastoma, and hyporesponsiveness to parathormone. Cancer 18:89, 1965.
46. Grossman, H., Winchester, P. H., Deck, M., et al.: Brain tumors in children with normal skull roentgenograms. Am. J. Roentgenol. Radium Ther. Nucl. Med. 112:329, 1971.
47. Gutin, P. H., Wilson, C. B., Kumar, A. R. V., et al.: Phase II study of procarbazine, CCNU, and vincristine combination chemotherapy in the treatment of malignant brain tumors. Cancer 35:1398, 1975.
48. Harwood-Nash, D. C., Fitz, C. R., and Reilly, B. J.: Cranial computed tomography in infants and children. Canad. Med. Assoc. J. 113:546, 1975.
48a. Heard, G.: Malignant disease in von Recklinghausen's neurofibromatosis. Proc. Roy. Soc. Med. 56:502, 1963.
49. Hoff, J. T., and Ray, B. S.: Cerebral hemangioblastoma occurring in a patient with von Hippel-Lindau disease. J. Neurosurg. 28:365, 1968.
50. Houser, O. W., Smith, J. B., Gomez, M. R., et al.: Evaluation of intracranial disorders in children by computerized transaxial tomography: a preliminary report. Neurology 25:607, 1975.
51. Hoyt, W. F., and Baghdassarian, S. A.: Optic glioma of childhood: natural history and rationale for conservative management. Brit. J. Ophthalmol. 53:793, 1969.
52. Kapp, J. P., Paulson, G. W., and Odom, G. L.: Brain tumors with tuberous sclerosis. J. Neurosurg. 26:191, 1967.
53. Kernohan, J. W., and Fletcher-Kernohan, E.: The ependymomas: a study of 109 cases. Proc. Assoc. Res. Nerv. Ment. Dis. 16:182, 1937.
54. Kessler, L. A., Dugan, P., and Concannon, J. P.: Systemic metastases of medulloblastomas promoted by shunting. Surg. Neurol. 3:147, 1975.
55. Kitay, J. I.: Pineal lesions and precocious puberty: A review. J. Clin. Endocr. Metab. 14:622, 1954.
56. Kramer, S.: Radiation therapy in the management of brain tumors in children. Ann. N.Y. Acad. Sci. 159:571, 1969.
57. Kramer, S., McKissock, W., and Concannon, J. P.: Craniopharyngiomas: treatment by combined surgery and radiation therapy. J. Neurosurg. 18:217, 1961.
58. Kumar, A. R. V., Renaudin, J., Wilson, C. B., et al.: Procarbazine hydrochloride in the treatment of brain tumors: phase 2 study. J. Neurosurg. 40:365, 1974.
59. Lampkin, B. C., Mauer, A. M., and McBride, B. H.: Response of medulloblastoma to vincristine sulfate: a case report. Pediatrics 39:761, 1967.
60. Lassman, L. P.: Diagnosis and management of skeletal metastases from cerebellar medulloblastoma. Child's Brain 2:38, 1976.
61. Lassman, L. P., and Arjona, V. E.: Pontine

gliomas in childhood. Lancet 1:913, 1967.
62. Lassman, L. P., Pearce, G. W., Banna, M., et al.: Vincristine sulfate in the treatment of skeletal metastases from cerebellar medulloblastoma. J. Neurosurg. 30:42, 1969.
63. Lassman, L. P., Pearce, G. W., and Gang, J.: Sensitivity of intracranial gliomas to vincristine sulfate. Lancet 1:296, 1965.
64. Lassiter, K. R. L., Alexander, E., Jr., Davis, C. H., Jr., et al.: Surgical treatment of brain stem gliomas. J. Neurosurg. 34:719, 1971.
65. Leavitt, F. H.: Cerebellar tumors occurring in identical twins. Arch. Neurol. Psychiat. 19:617, 1928.
66. Leibel, S. A., Sheline, G. E., Wara, W. M., et al.: The role of radiation therapy in the treatment of astrocytomas. Cancer 35:1551, 1975.
67. Leibner, W.: Brain tumors in infancy. Pediatrics 1:346, 1948.
68. Li, F. P., Tucker, M. A., and Fraumeni, J. F.: Childhood cancer in sibs. J. Pediatr. 88:419, 1976.
69. Liu, H. M., Boggs, J., and Kidd, J.: Ependymomas of childhood. I. Histological survey and clinicopathological correlation. Child's Brain 2:92, 1976.
70. Luse, S. A., and Teitelbaum, S.: Congenital glioma of brain stem. Arch. Neurol. 18:196, 1968.
71. MacCarty, C. S., Boyd, A. S., Jr., and Childs, D. S., Jr.: Tumors of the optic nerve and optic chiasm. J. Neurosurg. 33:439, 1970.
72. Marsa, G. W., Probert, J. C., Rubinstein, L. J., et al.: Radiation therapy in the treatment of childhood astrocytic gliomas. Cancer 32:646, 1973.
73. Martinius, J., Matthes, A., and Lombroso, C. T.: Electroencephalographic features in posterior fossa tumors in children. Electroencephalogr. Clin. Neurophysiol. 25:128, 1968.
74. Matson, D. D.: Intracranial tumors. In Farmer, T. W. (Ed.): Pediatric Neurology. New York, Harper & Row, 1964.
75. Matson, D. D., and Crigler, J. F., Jr.: Management of craniopharyngioma in childhood. J. Neurosurg. 30:377, 1969.
76. Matson, D. D., and Ingraham, F. D.: Intracranial complications of dermal sinuses. Pediatrics 8:463, 1951.
77. Matson, D. D., and Tachdjian, M. O.: Intraspinal tumors in infants and children: review of 115 cases. Postgrad. Med. 34:279, 1963.
78. McFarland, D. R., Horwitz, H., Saenger, E. L., et al.: Medulloblastoma: a review of prognosis and survival. Brit. J. Radiol. 42:198, 1969.
79. McGovern, V. J.: Tumours of the epiphysis cerebri. J. Pathol. Bact. 61:1, 1949.

80. Miller, R. W.: Deaths from childhood leukemia and solid tumors among twins and other sibs in the United States, 1960–67. J. Natl. Cancer Inst. 46:203, 1971.
81. Miller, R. W., and Dalager, N. A.: U.S. childhood cancer deaths by cell type, 1960–68. J. Pediatr. 85:664, 1974.
82. Mincer, F., Meltzer, J., and Botstein, C.: Pinealoma: a report of twelve irradiated cases. Cancer 37:2713, 1976.
83. Modan, B., Baidatz, D., Mart, H., et al.: Radiation-induced head and neck tumours. Lancet 1:277, 1974.
84. Newton, W. A., Jr., Sayers, M. P., and Samuels, L. D.: Intrathecal methotrexate (NSC-740) therapy for brain tumors in children. Cancer Chemother. Rep. 52:257, 1968.
85. Norrell, H., and Wilson, C.: Brain tumor chemotherapy with methotrexate given intrathecally. J.A.M.A. 201:15, 1967.
86. Ohry, A., and Rozin, R.: Late neoplasm after poliomyelitis. Lancet 2:823, 1975.
87. Panitch, H. S., and Berg, B. O.: Brain stem tumors of childhood and adolescence. Am. J. Dis. Child. 119:465, 1970.
88. Patterson, E., and Farr, R. F.: Cerebellar medulloblastoma: treatment by irradiation of the whole central nervous system. Acta Radiol. 39:323, 1953.
89. Patton, W. B., and Craig, W. W.: Glioma of the pons: report of a case. Proc. Staff Meet. Mayo Clin. 15:506, 1940.
90. Pendergrass, T. W., and Fraumeni, J. F., Jr.: Brain tumors in sibs, one with the Turner syndrome. J. Pediatr. 85:875, 1974.
91. Penman, J., and Smith, H. C.: Intracranial gliomata. Medical Research Council Special Report No. 284. London, Her Majesty's Stationary Office, 1954.
92. Phillips, T. L., Sheline, G. E., and Boldrey, E.: Therapeutic considerations in tumours affecting the central nervous system: ependymomas. Radiology 83:98, 1964.
93. Pierce, C. B., Cone, W. V., Bouchard, J., et al.: Medulloblastoma: nonoperative management with roentgen therapy after aspiration biopsy. Radiology 52:621, 1949.
94. Pinealoma: Case reports. Cancer Bull. 23:95, 1971.
95. Pool, J. L.: Gliomas in the region of the brain stem. J. Neurosurg. 29:164, 1968.
96. Raskin, R., and Beigel, F.: Brain tumors in early infancy—probably congenital in origin. J. Pediatr. 65:727, 1964.
97. Regelson, W., Bross, I. D. J., Hananian, J., et al.: Incidence of second primary tumors in children with cancer and leukemia. A seven-year survey of 150 consecutive autopsied cases. Cancer 18:58, 1965.

98. Rosen, G., Ghavimi, F., Vanucci, R., et al.: Pontine glioma: high-dose methotrexate and leucovorin rescue. J.A.M.A. 230:1149, 1974.
99. Rosenblum, M. L., Reynolds, A. F., Jr., Smith, K. A., et al.: Chloroethyl-cyclohexylnitrosurea (CCNU) in the treatment of malignant brain tumors. J. Neurosurg. 39:306, 1973.
100. Rubin, P., and Kramer, S.: Ectopic pinealoma: a radiocurable neuroendocrinologic entity. Radiology 85:512, 1965.
101. Russell, D. S., and Rubinstein, L. J.: Pathology of tumors of the nervous system. 3rd Ed. Baltimore, Williams & Wilkins Co., 1971.
102. Salazar, O. M., Rubin, P., Bassano, D., et al.: Improved survival of patients with intracranial ependymomas by irradiation: dose selection and field extension. Cancer 35:1563, 1975.
103. Sano, K.: Pinealoma in children. Child's Brain 2:67, 1976.
104. Schain, R. J., and Wilson, G.: Brainstem encephalitis with radiographic evidence of medullary enlargement. Neurology 21:537, 1971.
105. Schenck, S. A., and Penn, I.: De novo brain tumours in renal-transplant recipients. Lancet 1:983, 1971.
106. Shaywitz, B. A.: Epidermoid spinal cord tumors and previous lumbar punctures. J. Pediatr. 80:638, 1972.
107. Sheline, G. E.: Radiation therapy of tumors of the central nervous system in childhood. Cancer 35:957, 1975.
108. Shuster, J., Hart, Z., Stimson, C. W., et al.: Ataxia telangiectasia with cerebellar tumor. Pediatrics 37:776, 1966.
109. Skalansky, B. D., Mann-Kaplan, R. S., Reynolds, A. F., Jr., et al.: 4'-demethylepipodophyllotoxin-B-D-thenylidene-glucoside (PTG) in the treatment of malignant intracranial neoplasms. Cancer 33:460, 1974.
110. Smith, C. E., Long, D. M., Jones, T. K., Jr., et al.: Medulloblastoma: an analysis of time-dose relationships and recurrence patterns. Cancer 32:722, 1973.
111. Smith, R. A., Lampe, I., and Kahn, E. A.: The prognosis of medulloblastoma in children. J. Neurosurg. 18:91, 1961.
112. Taveras, J. M., Mount, L. A., and Wood, E. H.: The value of radiation therapy in the management of glioma of the optic nerves and chiasm. Radiology 66:518, 1956.
113. Tice, G. M.: Treatment and prognosis of medulloblastoma. J.A.M.A. 182:629, 1962.
114. Van der Wiel, H. J.: Inheritance of glioma. The genetic aspects of cerebral glioma and its relation to status dysraphicus. Amsterdam, Elsevier Publishing Co., 1960.
115. Walker, M. D.: Diagnosis and treatment of brain tumors. Pediatr. Clin. North Am. 23:131, 1976.
116. Walker, M. D., and Hurwitz, B. S.: BCNU (1,3-bis[2-chloroethyl]-1-nitrosurea; NSC-409962) in the treatment of malignant brain tumor—a preliminary report. Cancer Chemother. Rep. 54:263, 1970.
117. Ward, H. W. C.: CCNU in treatment of recurrent medulloblastoma. Brit. Med. J. 1:642, 1974.
118. Wertelecki, W., Fraumeni, J. F., Jr., and Mulvihill, J. J.: Nongonadal neoplasia in Turner's syndrome. Cancer 26:485, 1970.
119. Whyte, T. R., Colby, M. Y., and Layton, D. D., Jr.: Radiation therapy of brain stem tumors. Radiology 93:413, 1969.
120. Williams, A. O.: Tumors of childhood in Ibadan, Nigeria. Cancer 36:370, 1975.
121. Wilson, C. B., and Norrell, H. A., Jr.: Brain cancer chemotherapy with intrathecal methotrexate. Cancer 23:1038, 1969.
122. Wurtman, R. J., and Krammer, J.: Melatonin synthesis by an ectopic pinealoma. N. Engl. J. Med. 274:1233, 1966.
123. Young, J. L., and Miller, R. W.: Incidence of malignant tumors in U.S. children. J. Pediatr. 86:254, 1975.

Chapter Thirteen

TUMORS OF THE SYMPATHETIC NERVOUS SYSTEM

Neuroblastoma

Neuroblastomas originate from neural crest cells that normally give rise to the adrenal medulla and the sympathetic ganglia. They are believed to be congenital in origin.[100] They are the most common malignant tumors in infancy, and, during the first decade of life, are exceeded in incidence only by tumors of the central nervous system. The tumors occur in approximately 9.6 white children and 7 black children per million in the United States each year.[149] Many series have shown a higher incidence in males.[20, 106, 129, 146] The majority of neuroblastomas are diagnosed prior to 5 years of age, with a peak incidence occurring at age 2 years. Many cases have been diagnosed at birth.[121, 142] The tumors seldom occur in adults, but a number of cases have been reported in elderly individuals up to 72 years of age.[74, 93]

ETIOLOGY

Unlike a number of other childhood malignancies, neuroblastoma does not appear to occur more commonly in children with immunodeficiency syndromes or congenital defects,[99] although occasional cases associated with congenital heart disease and skull or brain defects have been noted.[100, 111] Two children with the fetal hydantoin syndrome, a pattern of abnormalities noted in the infants of women receiving hydantoin anticonvulsants during pregnancy, have been found to have neuroblastoma.[105, 114] The hydantoins have been reported to be both oncogenic and teratogenic, but an etiologic relationship to neuroblastoma has not been proved. Rarely, neuroblastoma has been found in patients with von Recklinghausen's disease.[76, 147] There is a significant decreased incidence of this tumor in black children in tropical Africa as compared to American black children,[18, 145] an observation that suggests the presence of exogenous influences on the etiology.

Various cytogenetic abnormalities have been demonstrated in a number of children with neuroblastoma.[141, 143] One of two siblings with this tumor was noted to have the classic physical and chromosomal findings of trisomy 21.[33] One family has been reported in which the neoplasm occurred in a child whose parents each had a child

TUMORS OF THE SYMPATHETIC NERVOUS SYSTEM 329

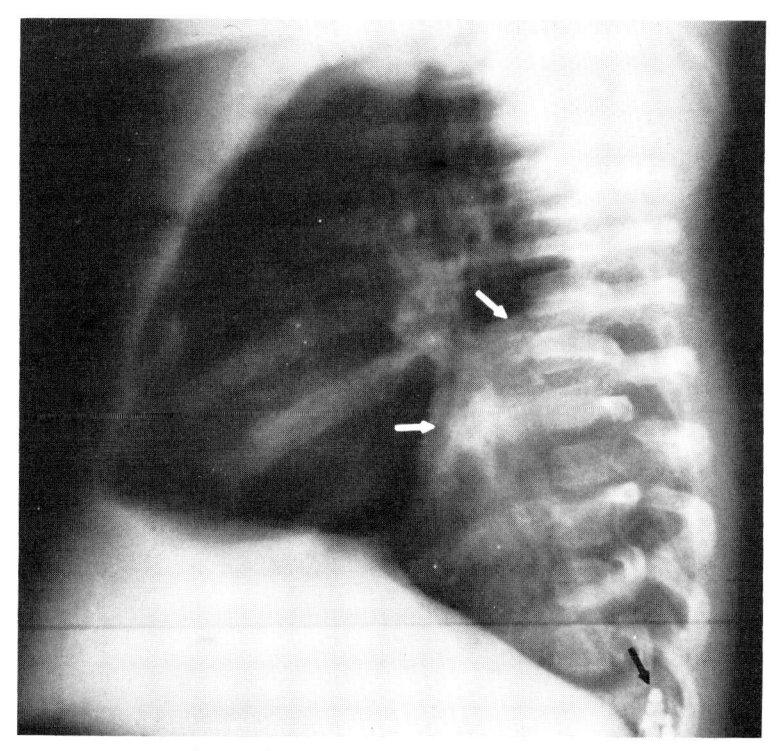

Figure 13-2 Posterior mediastinal neuroblastoma (white arrows) in a child who presented with the signs and symptoms of spinal cord compression. Note the complete block demonstrated by myelography (black arrow).

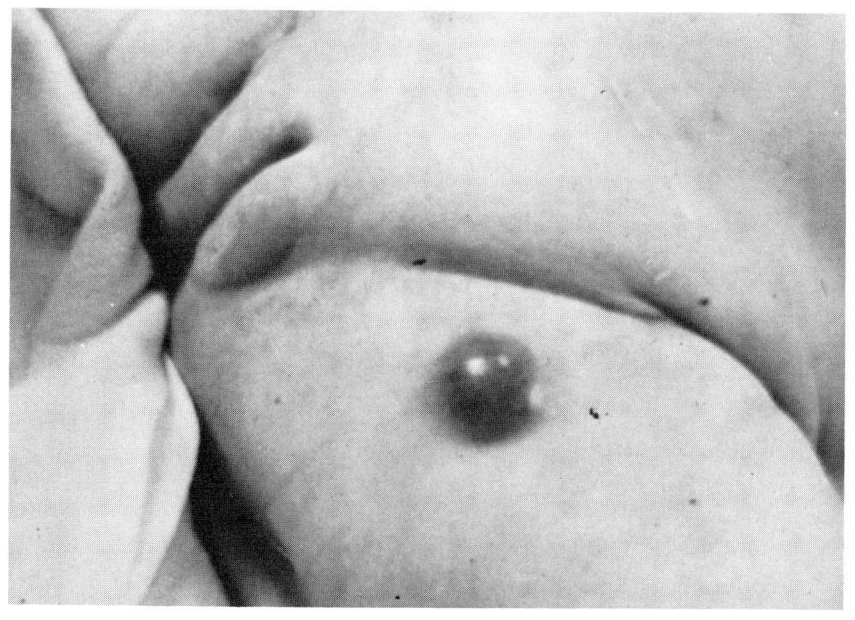

Figure 13-3 Subcutaneous tumor nodule in a neonate with neuroblastoma. (Courtesy of Dr. Howard Pearson, Yale–New Haven Hospital).

blanch, presumably as a result to vasoconstriction from release of catecholamines from the tumor cells. This finding may be a diagnostic sign of subcutaneous neuroblastoma.[56]

The liver often bears the brunt of metastatic dissemination, especially in the infant, with the tumor presenting as a rapidly growing hepatic neoplasm (Fig. 13-4). Rarely, stippled calcification occurs within the liver metastases.[117] Hagstrom[52] reported a fetus that could not be delivered intact because the abdomen contained a nodular 700 g liver. The abdomen had to be opened and much of the liver cut away piecemeal before delivery could be accomplished. The right adrenal gland was entirely replaced by a neuroblastoma. An infant reported by Larimer[86] was delivered easily, but severe respiratory difficulty and cyanosis apparently due to abdominal distention were noted at birth. The child lived only 9 hours. Autopsy showed a huge 425 g liver filled with bulging spherical nodules, a right adrenal gland weighing 83 g and filled with neuroblastoma, and metastatic involvement of mesenteric lymph nodes and the left adrenal gland.

Often the first signs of illness are symptoms of skeletal system involvement. The skull and the tubular bones are most frequently involved. The metastatic lesions appear on x-ray as small, lytic defects with irregular margins and some periosteal reaction. In the tubular bones they usually occur in the diaphysis and are bilaterally symmetrical. The lesions often cause bone pain that may be confused with inflammatory conditions, such as rheumatoid arthritis. Although roentgenographic examination may reveal osteolytic lesions, bone pain may occur before skeletal changes are demonstrable. Extensive involvement may produce a pathologic fracture. Occasionally the bony lesions may be confused with primary bone tumors, histiocytosis, lymphoreticular malignancies, or an infectious process. Retrobulbar soft tissue involvement may cause periorbital edema and proptosis. A "raccoon-like" appearance due to periorbital ecchymosis in a child with an abdominal mass should suggest metastatic neuroblastoma (Fig. 13-5). Intracranial metastatic involvement commonly involves the meninges, but intracerebral metastases are unusual.

Over half the children with neuroblastoma have bone marrow involvement,[37] even in the absence of roentgenographic changes in the bones. The tumor cells are usually distinguishable from leukemic infiltration because they appear in small clusters (Fig. 13-6), but the differentiation may

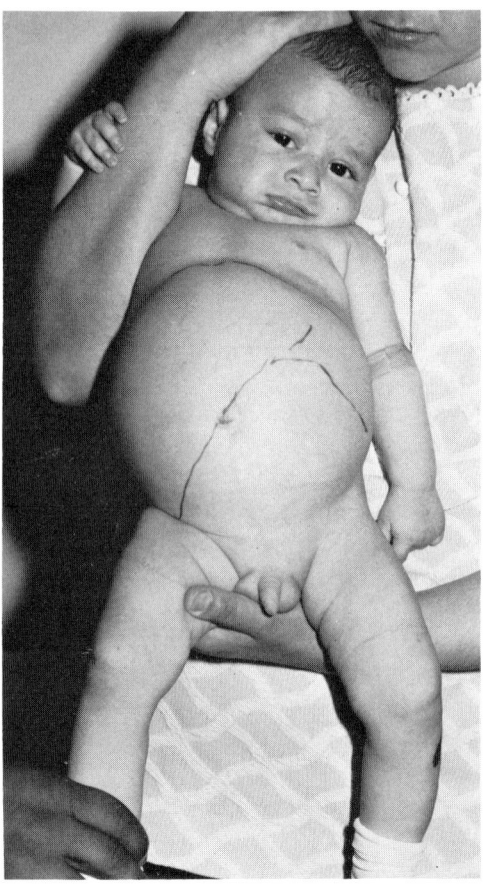

Figure 13-4 Massive liver involvement by metastatic neuroblastoma. The child's initial manifestation of disease was hepatomegaly.

TUMORS OF THE SYMPATHETIC NERVOUS SYSTEM

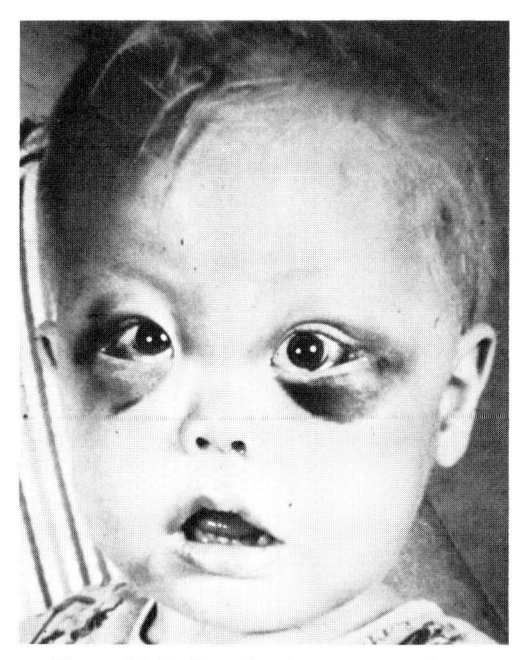

Figure 13-5 Periorbital metastatic disease in a child with a suprarenal neuroblastoma. Note the right sixth cranial nerve paresis secondary to increased intracranial pressure from meningeal metastases. (Courtesy of Dr. Howard Pearson, Yale-New Haven Hospital).

be difficult when there is extensive marrow replacement. The cell arrangement in rosettes and the presence of neurofibrils, although characteristic of neuroblastoma, are usually absent, and one must rely on means other than marrow morphology to distinguish neuroblastoma from other malignancies that invade the bone marrow.

In many cases the first signs and symptoms are manifestations of widespread disease, with weight loss, irritability, fever, and evidence of anemia. Lymphadenopathy from metastatic disease is usually not an early sign except for cervical or supraclavicular node involvement, but node involvement may occasionally mimic infectious lymphadenitis. The history of persistent or progressive lymphadenopathy should be suspect, especially if the node is firm and painless. A child with an enlarged left supraclavicular (Virchow's) node should always be evaluated for the presence of malignancy.

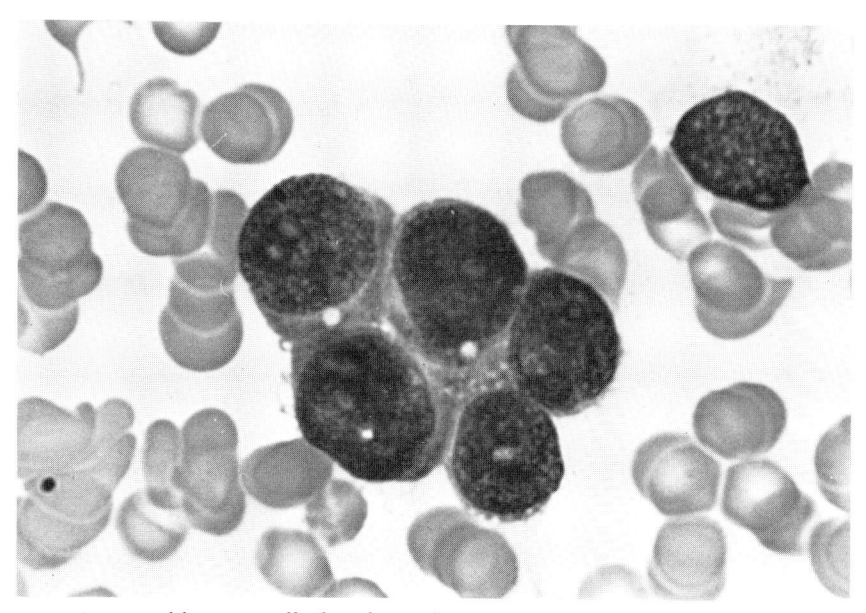

Figure 13-6 Neuroblastoma cells found in a bone marrow aspiration. Despite the fact that the individual cells may resemble lymphoblasts, the sharing of cytoplasm by a cluster of cells indicates that the malignant cells are extramedullary in origin.

Several children with neuroblastoma have been reported whose sole presenting symptom was persistent, intractable diarrhea. Two patients described by Green and associates[48] with chronic diarrhea were discovered to have chest masses and a third had a tumor in the region of the left adrenal gland that contained stippled calcifications. The children were thought to have had either cystic fibrosis or celiac syndrome before the roentgenographic discoveries were made. Their symptoms abated dramatically following surgical removal of their tumors. It had been believed that such symptoms were due to excessive secretion by the tumor of one or more catecholamines or their metabolic end products, but diarrhea is an infrequent complication, although most patients excrete elevated urinary levels of catecholamines. It has recently been proposed that the intractable diarrhea is due to the excretion of a newly discovered enterohormone, vasoactive intestinal peptide, by the tumor, the levels of which have been demonstrated to be elevated in the plasma and the tumor of a number of patients.[69a, 101, 132]

The association of acute myoclonic encephalopathy and neuroblastoma has been described by numerous authors.[11, 97, 102, 124] The neurologic disorder usually consists of rapid multidirectional eye movements (opsoclonus), myoclonus, and truncal ataxia in the absence of increased intracranial pressure. One case has been reported in which the opsomyoclonus did not occur, leading the authors to suggest that neuroblastoma be considered in any child with unexplained or atypical cerebellar signs.[115] In many instances, neurologic improvement occurred once the tumor had been removed. Despite the fact that it has been suggested that the encephalopathy is due to toxic neurologic effects of catecholamine catabolites, at least one child has been described who developed neurologic symptoms 7 months following removal of the tumor and return to normal of the previously elevated levels of urinary catecholamines.[19] It has been proposed that an autoimmune factor, possibly an antibody directed against a neuroblastoma antigen, could cross-react with a common antigen in the cerebellar cells, resulting in cerebellar damage.[11] The excellent prognosis for survival in patients with opsomyoclonus lends credence to such a mechanism.[3]

Occasionally a newborn infant with congenital neuroblastoma may be thought to have erythroblastosis. One infant developed severe jaundice and, because of hepatosplenomegaly, was mistakenly thought for a time to have hemolytic disease of the newborn.[32] An increased number of nucleated red cells was noted in the child's blood. Two newborn infants with congenital neuroblastoma that had metastasized to the liver and placenta were thought to have hydrops fetalis.[4] In one of them the diagnosis was established by histologic examination of the placenta.

Voûte and co-workers[139] have reported six women with sweating, pallor, headaches, palpitations, hypertension, and tingling in the hands and feet during the eighth and ninth months of pregnancy. All the women delivered infants who were diagnosed as having neuroblastoma during the first few months of life. Because the mothers' symptoms disappeared postpartum, the authors proposed that they were caused by fetal catecholamines entering the maternal circulation. It is not known how commonly this syndrome occurs.

BIOCHEMICAL FEATURES

Catecholamines. In 1957, Mason and colleagues[98] reported an increased excretion of pressor amines in the urine of an infant with neuroblastoma. Subsequent studies in children with neuroblastoma have shown elevated levels of norepinephrine, its biochemical precursors, and their metabolites in the urine, including dopa, dopamine, normetanephrine, homovanillic acid (HVA), and vanillylmandelic acid (VMA).[137] According to Williams and Greer, 95 per cent of patients will have an elevated urinary excretion of VMA, HVA, or both.[144] Occasionally however, a patient may show no elevation of catecholamines.[138] It is therefore important to measure urinary catecholamines in a child prior to surgical removal of a neuroblastoma or initiation of therapy in order to determine whether or not it is a catecholamine-producing tumor. There is no correlation between the pattern of excretion of catecholamines and the symptomatology, histologic pattern, or age of the patients.[51] However, this unique property of the neoplasm not only can be used as an aid in diagnosis but also is a useful means of assessing the response to therapy or detection of recurrence of tumor. LaBrosse and associates[84] have shown that periodic assay of the urinary excretion of VMA and HVA during the course of the disease is of prognostic value, with 80 to 90 per cent reliability (Table 13–1). By contrast, when only the excretion in the initial urine specimens is considered, the survival rate is the same for patients with normal and with elevated values.

The use of a spot test to determine elevated levels of urinary VMA has been advocated as an aid in the diagnosis and periodic evaluation of patients with neuroblastoma.[25, 83] The reagents for this test have also been used to produce a dipstick.[91] However, some investigators have pointed out the limitations of these VMA screening tests, which may give false positive and false negative results.[58, 70, 103]

It is of interest that hypertension seldom occurs in patients with neuroblastoma, even in the presence of elevated catecholamines.

Cystathionine. Urinary excretion of cystathionine is detectable in most children with neuroblastoma[42, 60, 136] and may be found in patients with normal excretion of VMA.[60] This intermediary metabolite in the conversion of methionine to cysteine is not normally found in urine. It occurs in the rare patient with congenital cystathioninuria, and has been noted in association with various forms of liver disease, thyroxine therapy, pyridoxine deficiency, and galactosemia.[90] It has also been reported in patients with hepatoblastoma[46] and other childhood neoplasms.[60] This lack of specificity limits its use diagnostically.

Carcinoembryonic Antigen. Plasma carcinoembryonic antigen (CEA) levels are elevated in a number of malignant and clinically active nonmalignant diseases. Most investigators believe that determining CEA levels is of little value diagnostically, but is useful in monitoring response of malignant disease to therapy. Reynoso and associates[113] reported elevated CEA levels in six of six patients they studied with neuroblastoma and normal levels in one patient evaluated years after remission. Three of the six patients were treated successfully and the CEA levels returned to normal. Frens and co-workers[40] found elevated levels in eight of 12 patients before treatment and noted a relationship between initial and sequential titers and the patient's outcome. Children with slight but definite CEA elevations had long-term survival without evidence of tumor recurrence and CEA levels that returned to normal. Those with initially higher levels and persistent elevations died with progressive disease.

Table 13–1 Survival and Urinary Excretion of VMA and HVA in Serial Specimens from Patients with Neuroblastoma[84]

	PER CENT VMA SURVIVED	PER CENT HVA SURVIVED
Normal → Normal	31	71
Normal → Elevated	8	0
Elevated → Normal	82	80
Elevated → Elevated	4	5

PATHOLOGY

The most primitive histologic subgroup of this tumor, the neuroblastoma, is very cellular and composed of small round cells with scant cytoplasm. The diagnosis by light microscopy is often difficult because of similarities between neuroblasts, lymphocytes, and other small round cell malignancies, such as the lymphomas, embryonal rhabdomyosarcoma, and Ewing's tumor. Rosette formation and neurofibrils indicative of neuroblastoma often are not present. The cells of Ewing's tumor and rhabdomyosarcoma usually contain glycogen, which can be demonstrated with PAS staining, while neuroblastoma cells do not. Occasionally, when a child presents with disseminated disease composed of primitive neuroblasts and no evidence of a primary tumor, the diagnosis can only be made on the basis of elevations of urinary catecholamine metabolites.

The ganglioneuroma, a more benign counterpart, is composed of large, mature ganglion cells with abundant cytoplasm, while the ganglioneuroblastoma is intermediate in the degree of cellular differentiation. However, the histologic appearance of an individual tumor may show various degrees of cellular maturation. Although attempts have been made to correlate prognosis with the degree of tumor maturation,[96] there appears to be a much better correlation between prognosis and both clinical staging of the disease and the patient's age at the time of diagnosis. Thus, most oncologists have not used the finer points of histologic grading as a major factor in influencing therapy. Lauder and Aherne[87] believe that the prognosis is related not to maturation but to the degree of lymphocytic infiltration within the tumor, a finding not substantiated by Hughes and co-workers.[64]

The ultrastructure of neuroblastoma cells appears to be distinctive. Electron microscopy has been used to differentiate the neuroblastoma from tumors which may resemble it when examined by light microscopy.[93] The neuroblastoma has typical peripheral dendritic processes that contain longitudinally oriented microtubules. One notable feature is the presence of small, spherical, membrane-bound granules with electron-dense cores. The granules represent cytoplasmic accumulations of catecholamines. Electron microscopy can also be helpful in the positive identification of neuroblastoma cells in the bone marrow.[94]

STAGING AND PROGNOSIS

It has long been known that the chance of survival of a patient with neuroblastoma is inversely correlated with the age of the child at the time of diagnosis.[131] Breslow and McCann[12] noted a 74 per cent survival rate for children diagnosed between 0 and 11 months of age, a 26 per cent survival rate for those diagnosed between 12 and 23 months, and only a 12 per cent survival rate in those diagnosed at age 2 years and over. Although infants more commonly have localized disease, the infant with widespread disease still has a better chance of survival than the older child with a lesser degree of tumor dissemination. The site of origin also is a factor influencing survival. A more favorable prognosis has been observed in children whose primary tumor is in the mediastinum, even when there is involvement of the regional lymph nodes, a Horner's syndrome, erosion of ribs and thoracic vertebrae, or thoracic cord compression from tumor extension through the intervertebral foramina.[34] The major reason, however, that those with primary tumors arising above the diaphragm have a better chance for survival is because the disease is usually less disseminated.[23]

Other factors which appear to be correlated with a good prognosis are increased numbers of bone marrow lymphoblasts[30] and the presence of opsomyoclonus.[3] Some investigators have found a better prognosis in children with increased numbers of peripheral lymphocytes,[7] whereas others have found no obvious influence of the initial total lymphocyte count on survival.[23] There is no significant difference between black and white children with regard to median duration of survival or percentage of long-term survivors,[21] in contrast to the reports of a poorer survival in black children as compared to white children with acute lymphocytic leukemia.

An evaluation by Evans and co-workers[27] of 100 cases led them to propose a clinical staging for children with neuroblastoma, which appears to be helpful in predicting the ultimate prognosis:

Stage I   Tumors confined to the organ or structure of origin.
Stage II Tumors extending in continuity beyond the organ or structure of origin but not crossing the midline. Regional lymph nodes on the ipsilateral side may be involved.
Stage III Tumors extending in continuity beyond the midline. Regional lymph nodes may be involved bilaterally.
Stage IV Remote disease involving the skeleton, organs, soft tissues, or distant lymph node groups.

For tumors arising in midline structures, such as the organs of Zuckerkandl, the sympathetic tissue at the origin of the inferior mesenteric artery, penetration beyond the capsule and involvement of lymph nodes on the same side is considered Stage II disease. Bilateral extension of any sort is considered Stage III. Those with a greater degree of spread tend to have a poorer prognosis, and in Stage IV disease the malignancy is usually fatal. The few long-term survivors who have skeletal metastases are usually under 1 year of age at the time of diagnosis.[110]

One unique group of patients with disseminated disease has such a good prognosis, however, that a separate category called Stage IV-S was proposed to distinguish them from other patients with widespread involvement. This special group of children have remote spread of tumor involving the liver, skin, or bone marrow but do not have roentgenographic evidence of bone metastases on complete skeletal survey. This pattern appears to occur most commonly in infancy. Eighteen of 20 infants under the age of 1 year with Stage IV-S disease reported by D'Angio and associates[17] were cured of their disease. The 2-year survival of all of those with Stage IV-S disease was 84 per cent compared to 5 per cent survival in those with Stage IV disease. This association between age at the time of diagnosis, clinical staging, and survival is shown in Table 13–2. A number of other clinical staging systems have been used,[68, 108, 133] but the one proposed by Evans and co-workers is probably the one most commonly used at the present time.

A number of children have been reported to have experienced spontaneous regression of their tumors. The diagnosis of neuroblastoma was made before the age of 6 months in 21 of 29

Table 13–2   Two-Year Survival of 234 Children With Neuroblastoma[17]

AGE (MONTHS)	I	II	III	IV	IV-S	TOTAL
<12	10/11	14/15	2/4	4/17	18/20	48/67
12–23	4/5	5/8	3/7	0/26	1/1	13/47
24+	2/3	4/12	3/13	3/88	2/4	14/120
Total	16/19	23/35	8/24	7/131	21/25	75/234

patients, collected by Everson and Cole,[31] in whom spontaneous regression occurred. The remaining cases were diagnosed between 6 and 24 months of age. This relationship of spontaneous regression to age has also been noted by Evans and associates,[28] who found that the majority of those with tumor regression were under 6 months of age and were usually those with Stage II or IV-S disease. Spontaneous regression of tumor in patients with Stage I disease could not be evaluated because the tumor was usually completely resected.

In other instances malignant neuroblastomas have apparently undergone transformation into benign ganglioneuromas.[16, 49] Of 170 patients with neuroblastoma or ganglioneuroblastoma at Babies Hospital in New York, five had tumors that matured to ganglioneuroma.[127] One of these patients, 2 months of age at the time of diagnosis, showed tumor maturation and survival in spite of initial exacerbation of the neoplastic disease and widespread bony metastases. However, tumor progression and death have been known to occur despite large areas of maturation of the tumor.[2]

The incidence of spontaneous regression of neuroblastoma may be more common than is clinically evident. Beckwith and Perrin[6] detected the presence of microscopic clusters of neuroblastoma cells, termed neuroblastoma in situ, in the adrenal glands of a significant number of infants under the age of 3 months with no clinical evidence of tumor upon whom postmortem examinations were performed. They estimated the incidence of neuroblastoma in situ to be about 40 times greater than the number of cases of clinically diagnosed disease. Based upon their findings, they proposed that the great majority of these tumors either degenerated or underwent differentiation to normal tissue. Turkel and Itabashi,[135] however, believe that such neuroblastic nodules represent normal changes in the developing adrenal gland and noted their presence in 100 per cent of 169 fetal adrenal glands they examined. Whether or not neuroblastoma in situ is a true neoplasm, it completely disappears after 3 months of life under normal circumstances.

Most reviews indicate that a 2-year survival in a child with neuroblastoma without evidence of disease is equivalent to cure.[20, 50] However, rare fatal recurrences have been reported to occur beyond this period[79] and have led to death more than 10 years after the initial diagnosis and apparent complete regression.[66, 114]

TREATMENT

The unpredictable course of neuroblastoma with its occasional spontaneous maturation or regression not only makes the tumor unusual but also causes difficulty in evaluating therapy. The impressive collection of cases reported by Bodian[9] suggested that massive doses of vitamin B_{12} led to cure, but subsequent evaluation of the collected experience of others failed to confirm these observations.[85, 119] One likely explanation for Bodian's successful results is that his series was heavily weighted with young patients who experienced spontaneous remission. Reports that surgical assault on the primary tumor may influence regression of distant metastases[81] must also be interpreted with caution in view of the natural history of the disease.

Complete surgical removal of the tumor may be accomplished in patients with Stages I and II disease, but is often hazardous and may not be possible in those with Stage III disease. If complete tumor removal cannot be accomplished without endangering the life of the patient, residual tumor should be outlined with metal clips to guide the radiation therapist if this form of therapy is later chosen.

Infants with Stage IV-S disease and

hepatic involvement often develop respiratory difficulties and vascular compression because of increasing hepatomegaly. The creation of a ventral hernia with a Silastic patch has been shown to be a useful means of temporarily relieving the problems caused by the intraabdominal pressure.[120] Closure can easily be accomplished once the liver has returned to normal size.

The neuroblastoma is generally regarded as a radiosensitive tumor, but the role of radiation therapy remains to be defined. This form of treatment has been successful in shrinking large tumor masses and in treating lesions causing spinal cord compression in the patient who is a poor candidate for surgery, and is of unquestionable value in relieving bone pain. Some have advocated aggressive radiation therapy, even in the presence of distant metastases.[106] Although it is common practice to irradiate the tumor bed following surgery, such treatment may not always be indicated. In one series, 12 of 14 children with Stage I disease survived following resection without other therapy.[80] There is also evidence that the addition of radiation therapy does not improve survival in Stage II patients, whether the tumor is completely resected or whether an appreciable amount remains.[82] However, irradiation appears to be of significant benefit to patients with Stage III disease in whom gross residual tumor remains following surgery.[82]

The initial response of neuroblastoma to a number of chemotherapeutic agents is often dramatic, especially in the younger patients. The two drugs most extensively evaluated have been vincristine sulfate[146] and cyclophosphamide,[134] used singly or in combination.[29, 108, 129] Despite the numerous reports of objective tumor regression, Sutow and associates[130] found no significant increase in the median duration of survival or the overall survival among children treated in 1962 compared to those treated in 1956, despite the increased use of chemotherapy. Leikin and co-workers[89] compared the earlier data with survival statistics obtained from the Children's Cancer Study Group with Stages III and IV disease treated with both vincristine and cyclophosphamide and confirmed the lack of improvement in survival, although there was an increase in the median survival time in those patients who initially responded. Evans and co-workers[24] reported no increased rate of survival in children with Stages I, II, or III disease treated with intermittent oral cyclophosphamide compared to those who received no chemotherapy.

Newer chemotherapeutic agents have been reported to be active against neuroblastoma including daunomycin,[118] Adriamycin,[109] dimethyltriazenoimidazole-carboxamide (DTIC),[36] and chloroethyltriazeno-imidazole-carboxamide (TIC mustard).[78] A number of agents have been shown to be effective in the murine neuroblastoma system,[38] suggesting that they may be of value in treating humans. Reports of improvement in the response rate and median duration of response in children with disseminated disease treated with combination chemotherapy[35, 41, 61] have been encouraging, but at present no specific treatment regimen has been shown to significantly increase the survival rate.

It has been suggested that the infant with the special pattern of metastases classed as Stage IV-S disease be observed for a period of time before the decision is made to initiate therapy, because the high cure rate in this group may be the result of spontaneous tumor regression, and therapeutic agents are not without risk.[26, 123] This conservative approach is not universally accepted.[47]

Numerous observations suggest that the host's immune response may play a major role in the cure of neuroblastoma. The commonly observed spontaneous regressions, the frequent occurrence of neuroblastoma in situ which presumably normally regresses in the fetus and young infant, and the reports of a better prognosis in patients with lymphocytic tumor infiltration,[87] increased bone marrow lymphoblasts,[30] and higher peripheral blood lymphocyte counts[7] support this hypothesis. It has been proposed that the association of a good prognosis with opsomyoclonus may be due to antibody formation to the neuroblastoma, which cross-reacts with a common neural tissue antigen in the cerebellar cells, causing damage to the cerebellum.[3] There is also laboratory evidence of a role played by the host's immune response. Lymphocytes from children with neuroblastoma inhibit the in vitro growth of neuroblastoma cells but do not affect the growth of normal fibroblasts or cells from other tumors. These lymphocytes are cytotoxic to cultures of neuroblastoma cells from different patients. This cytotoxicity is also demonstrated by the lymphocytes of siblings and parents of patients. The lymphocytes from those with progressive neuroblastoma and those free of disease are both cytotoxic, but the serum from children with progressive disease can block the cell-mediated activity in vitro.[57] This evidence of a role for host responses suggests that forms of immunotherapy might prove to be of value in future treatment programs.

Pheochromocytoma

Pheochromocytomas arise from cells of the neural crest, but unlike neuroblastomas are of chromaffin tissue origin. The tumors are uncommon in all age groups and are especially rare in children. Most cases are diagnosed during the fifth decade of life.[112] Of 178 patients seen at the Mayo Clinic from 1926 to 1975, only four were 15 years of age or younger.[44] Before adolescence, the tumor is more common in males, but there are no apparent sex differences following puberty. The neoplasm is most commonly seen in girls soon after the onset of puberty.[128]

Pheochromocytomas have been reported in association with neurofibromatosis[13] and renal artery stenosis.[116] There also is an association with medullary carcinoma of the thyroid (Sipple's syndrome), an autosomal dominant disorder with a high degree of penetrance.[126] The association of medullary carcinoma of the thyroid, parathyroid adenoma, pheochromocytoma, and neurofibromatosis has also been described.[9a, 73] The pheochromocytomas in persons with these syndromes are similar to tumors which occur sporadically except that they more often are bilateral and often are unresponsive to provocative diagnostic tests.[73] Other findings associated with pheochromocytoma and medullary thyroid carcinoma include multiple mucosal neuromas of the tongue, lips, and eyelids and a Marfan-like body habitus.[39, 92] These relationships may be due to a maldevelopment of the neural crest or its derivatives.[9a] An autosomal dominant inheritance of pheochromocytoma has been reported in some families in which there were no other stigmata.[44, 128]

Children with pheochromocytoma usually have sustained hypertension, with superimposed episodes of excessive hypertension. There is usually a history of episodic headaches, profuse sweating, palpitations, and anxiety. Weight loss and an increased basal metabolic rate may be present. The more common signs and symptoms are shown in Table 13–3. The systemic symptoms rather than the presence of a mass lesion usually bring the tumor to the physician's attention. A mass was palpated in only six of 100 children reviewed in one large series.[128] If the

Table 13-3 Signs and Symptoms of 95 Children with Pheochromocytomas

	PER CENT
Hypertension	100
Sustained	88
Intermittent	12
Headache	75
Sweating	67
Nausea and vomiting	48
Weight loss	38
Visual disturbances	37
Abdominal pain	32
Polyuria and polydipsia	31
Convulsions	22
Acrocyanosis	22

*Based on the data collected by Stackpole and colleagues.[128]

tumor remains undiagnosed, the hypertension may be followed by congestive heart failure, encephalopathy, and death.

Most of the tumors arise in the adrenal medulla, but they may occur in extra-adrenal sites, such as the organs of Zuckerkandl, or in the retroperitoneal area. Occasionally the tumor may arise in the thorax or the wall of the urinary bladder.[128] The proportion of tumors in extra-adrenal sites appears to be greater in children than in adults. Stackpole and colleagues reported the incidence of extra-adrenal pheochromocytomas to be 32 per cent in children[128] compared with 10 per cent in most large series composed mainly of adults.[112] Children also have a higher incidence of multiple tumors than adults. Stackpole and associates[128] noted multiple tumors in 32 of 100 children, and Hume[65] reported 39 per cent of 76 cases in children to have bilateral adrenal involvement. In contrast, the large series reported by Remine and co-workers,[112] composed mainly of adult patients, had only 7 per cent with multiple tumors and 4.8 per cent with both adrenal glands involved.

Determinations of urinary catecholamines and their metabolites are the procedures of choice for screening patients with a suspected diagnosis of pheochromocytoma. These studies have replaced the pharmacologic tests used in the past based on alterations in blood pressure following challenge with Regitine (phentolamine), or histamine. Pharmacologic testing is now reserved for the rare case in which biochemical results are equivocal. In patients studied at the Mayo Clinic, the most accurate biochemical test was measurement of the 24 hour urinary excretion of metanephrine.[112] Urinary catecholamines and VMA gave 21 per cent and 29 per cent false negative findings, respectively, while false negative results were obtained in only 4 per cent with metanephrine.

Elevated plasma renin activity has been found in over 70 per cent of patients with pheochromocytoma.[95] This finding may lead to an incorrect diagnosis of renal artery stenosis in a child with hypertension due to pheochromocytoma.[63]

Once the diagnosis is suspected on the basis of clinical signs and symptoms, and urinary catecholamines and their metabolites are demonstrated to be elevated, the site of the tumor must be found. The neoplasm is highly vascular and usually can be demonstrated by angiography. Aortography may be used to visualize the tumor (Fig. 13-7), and venography may be of particular value in localizing the lesion when combined with plasma catecholamine assays on serial blood samples removed along the vena cava. This technique is especially useful in locating tumors which are extra-adrenal.

An intravenous pyelogram (IVP) is often negative, even in tumors located in the adrenal gland, and is generally considered to be an unreliable test because of the high incidence of false negative findings.[8] However, a suprarenal mass can sometimes be demonstrated by IVP.

Remine and co-workers[112] have reported nephrotomography to be of value in localizing these tumors. From 1966 through 1970, in 25 of 34 patients with pheochromocytomas reported by

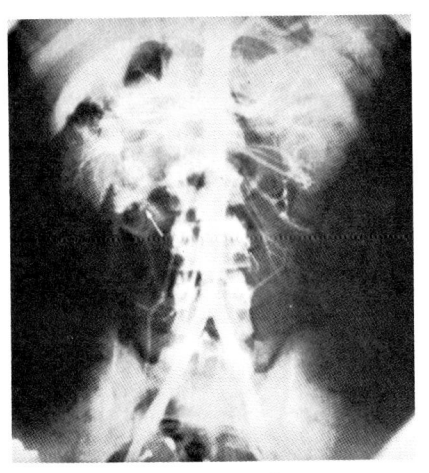

Figure 13-7 Aortogram demonstrating a right pararenal mass in a 15 year old boy with a 6 month history of palpitations, nausea, diaphoresis, and hypertension. A large right extraadrenal pheochromocytoma was found at laparotomy. (From Bloom, D. A., and Fonkalsrud, E. W.: J. Pediatr. Surg. 9:179, 1974.)

these investigators the neoplasms were demonstrated by nephrotomograms. No tumor smaller than 2.5 cm, however, could be demonstrated by this study.

Prior to surgery the patient should have his hypertension controlled by α-adrenergic blocking agents such as phenoxybenzamine or phentolamine. Some have advocated adding propranolol, a β-blocking agent, to the preoperative drug regimen to decrease the incidence of cardiac arrhythmias during surgery.[44, 112] Vasodilatation and adequate correction of the hypovolemic state have decreased the earlier hazards and high mortality rate experienced following tumor removal. Very high mortality rates have been reported when an unsuspected pheochromocytoma is discovered during surgery and is removed without adequate preoperative preparation. Certain anesthetic agents, such as halothane, have been reported to produce cardiac arrhythmias, and it has been recommended that these be avoided.[122]

A transabdominal surgical incision is usually preferred because it allows a thorough abdominal exploration for extra-adrenal or bilateral disease. Because multiple tumors are not uncommon, the contralateral adrenal gland and the abdominal sympathetic chain, including the organs of Zuckerkandl, should be examined. A total adrenalectomy should be performed for a single adrenal tumor. If the contralateral gland is involved, subtotal resection should be done. It has been suggested that a biopsy be considered on the contralateral gland even though it appears normal at operation because of the high incidence of bilateral tumors in children.[8] In a number of series, the operative mortality for primary pheochromocytoma has been less than 5 per cent.[65, 112]

Malignant pheochromocytomas are exceedingly rare in childhood. A recent review revealed that malignant pheochromocytomas in children arise from extra-adrenal sites.[107] Histologic features are not reliable indicators as to whether the tumor is malignant or benign. Elevated homovanillic acid excretion, indicative of malignant pheochromocytoma in adults, does not appear to differentiate malignant from benign neoplasms in children.[45] The diagnosis of malignancy can be made by the demonstration of tumor spread to nonchromaffin tissues, such as lymph nodes. The neoplasm may metastasize to bone, lung, or liver.

Metastatic tumors are generally functional, and treatment is directed toward control of clinical symptoms. Surgical removal of all accessible metastases may be of value in ameliorating systemic symptoms. The tumor does not appear to respond to most therapeutic modalities, although palliation with cyclophosphamide[71] and with radiation therapy[69] has been reported. Current medical treatment to alleviate inoperable tumors usually requires the use of α- and β-adrenergic blocking agents and inhibition of catecholamine synthesis.[107] Patients with malignant disease may sometimes live for long periods of time. Survival with disease present has been reported as long as 20 years following the initial diagnosis.[112] Pheochromocytomas recurring after apparent surgical cure of the original neoplasm may not always be due to malignant disease, but may also result from multiple benign primary tumors which were not initially apparent and caused no symptoms for months to years following the first operation.[54] Patients should therefore be carefully followed with periodic biochemical evaluation of urine and for the recurrence of clinical signs and symptoms of disease.

REFERENCES

1. Albert, D. M., Rubenstein, R. A., and Scheie, H. G.: Tumor metastasis to the eye. Am. J. Ophthalmol. 63:727, 1967.
2. Alterman, K., and Schueller, E. F.: Maturation of neuroblastoma to ganglioneuroma. Am. J. Dis. Child. 120:217, 1970.
3. Altman, A. J., and Baehner, R. L.: Favorable prognosis for survival in children with coincident opso-myoclonus and neuroblastoma. Cancer 37:846, 1976.
4. Anders, D., Kindermann, G., and Pfeifer, U.: Metastasizing fetal neuroblastoma with involvement of the placenta simulating fetal erythroblastosis. J. Pediatr. 82:50, 1973.
5. Arenson, E. B., Hutter, J. J., Jr., Restuccia, R. D., and Holton, C. P.: Neuroblastoma in father and son. J.A.M.A. 235:727, 1976.
6. Beckwith, J. B., and Perrin, E. V.: In situ neuroblastoma: A contribution to the natural history of neural crest tumors. Am. J. Pathol. 43:1089, 1963.
7. Bill, A. H., and Morgan, A.: Evidence for immune reactions to neuroblastoma and future possibilities for investgiation. J. Pediatr. Surg. 5:111, 1970.
8. Bloom, D. A., and Fonkalsrud, E. W.: Surgical management of pheochromocytoma in children. J. Pediatr. Surg. 9:179, 1974.
9. Bodian, M.: Neuroblastoma: An evaluation of its natural history and the effects of therapy, with particular reference to treatment by massive doses of vitamin B_{12}. Arch. Dis. Child. 38:606, 1963.
9a. Bolande, R. P.: The neurocristopathies: a unifying concept of disease arising in neural crest maldevelopment. Hum. Pathol. 5:409, 1974.
10. Bond, J. V.: Familial neuroblastoma and ganglioneuroma. J.A.M.A. 236:561, 1976.
11. Bray, P. F., Ziter, F. A., Lahey, M. E., et al.: The coincidence of neuroblastoma and acute cerebellar encephalopathy. J. Pediatr. 76:983, 1969.
12. Breslow, N., and McCann, B.: Statistical estimation of prognosis for children with neuroblastoma. Cancer Res. 31:2098, 1971.
13. Chapman, R. C., Kemp, V. E., and Taliaferro, I.: Pheochromocytoma associated with multiple neurofibromatosis and intracranial hemangioma. Am. J. Med. 26:883, 1959.
14. Chatten, J., and Voorhess, M. L.: Familial neuroblastoma. Report of a kindred with multiple disorders, including neuroblastomas in four siblings. N. Engl. J. Med. 277:1230, 1967.
15. Cochran, W.: Neuroblastoma (sympathicoblastoma) in Northern Ireland: A review over a ten-year period. Ulster Med. J. 32:82, 1963.
16. Cushing, H., and Wolbach, S. B.: The transformation of a malignant paravertebral sympathicoblastoma into a benign ganglioneuroma. Am. J. Pathol. 3:203, 1927.
17. D'Angio, G. J., Evans, A. E., and Koop, C. E.: Special pattern of widespread neuroblastoma with a favorable prognosis. Lancet 1:1046, 1971.
18. Davies, J. N. P.: Childhood tumours. In Templeton, A. C.: Tumours in a Tropical Country: A Survey of Uganda 1964–1968. New York, Springer-Verlag, 1973.
19. Delalieux, C., Ebinger, G., Maurus, R., et al.: Myoclonic encephalopathy and neuroblastoma. N. Engl. J. Med. 292:46, 1975.
20. deLorimier, A. A., Bragg, K. V., and Linden, G.: Neuroblastoma in childhood. Am. J. Dis. Child. 118:441, 1969.
21. DiNicola, W., Movassaghi, N., and Leikin, S.: Prognosis in black children with neuroblastoma. Cancer 36:1151, 1975.
22. Dodge, H. J., and Brenner, M. C.: Neuroblastoma of the adrenal medulla in siblings. Rocky Mt. Med. J. 42:35, 1945.
23. Evans, A. E., Albo, V., D'Angio, G. J., et al.: Factors influencing survival of children with nonmetastatic neuroblastoma. Cancer 38:661, 1976.
24. Evans, A. E., Albo, V., D'Angio, G. J., et al.: Cyclophosphamide treatment of patients with localized and regional neuroblastoma. Cancer 38:660, 1976.
25. Evans, A. E., Blore, J., Hadley, R., et al.: The LaBrosse spot test: A practical aid in the diagnosis and management of children with neuroblastoma. Pediatrics 47:913, 1971.
26. Evans, A. E., D'Angio, G. J., and Koop, C. E.: Diagnosis and treatment of neuroblastoma. Pediatr. Clin. North Am. 23:161, 1976.

27. Evans, A. E., D'Angio, G. J., and Randolph, J.: A proposed staging for children with neuroblastoma. Cancer 27:374, 1971.
28. Evans, A. E., Gerson, J., and Schnaufer, L.: Spontaneous regression of neuroblastoma. Natl. Cancer Inst. Monogr. 44:49, 1976.
29. Evans, A. E., Heyn, R. M., Newton, W. A., Jr., et al.: Vincristine sulfate and cyclophosphamide for children with neuroblastoma. J.A.M.A. 207:1325, 1969.
30. Evans, A. E., and Hummeler, K.: The significance of primitive cells in marrow aspirates of children with neuroblastoma. Cancer 32:906, 1973.
31. Everson, T. C., and Cole, W. H.: Spontaneous regression of cancer: A study and abstract of reports in the world medical literature and of personal communications concerning spontaneous regression of malignant disease. Philadelphia, W. B. Saunders Company, 1966, pp. 88–163.
32. Falkinburg, L. W., and Kay, M. N.: A case of congenital sympathogonioma (neuroblastoma) of the right adrenal simulating erythroblastosis fetalis. J. Pediatr. 42:462, 1953.
33. Feingold, M., Gheradi, G., and Simons, C.: Familial neuroblastoma and trisomy 21. Am. J. Dis. Child. 121:451, 1971.
34. Filler, R. M., Traggis, D. G., Jaffe, N., et al.: Favorable outlook for children with mediastinal neuroblastoma. J. Pediatr. Surg. 7:136, 1972.
35. Finklestein, J., Leiken, S., Evans, A. E., et al.: Combination chemotherapy for metastatic neuroblastoma (Abstr.). Proc. Am. Ass. Cancer Res. 15:44, 1974.
36. Finklestein, J. Z., Albo, V., Ertel, I., et al.: 5-(3,3-Dimethyl-l-triazeno) imidazole-4-carboxamide (NSC-45388) in the treatment of solid tumors in children. Cancer Chemother. Rep. 59:351, 1975.
37. Finklestein, J. Z., Ekert, H., Isaacs, H., Jr., et al.: Bone marrow metastases in children with solid tumors. Am. J. Dis. Child. 119:49, 1970.
38. Finklestein, J. Z., Tittle, K., Meshnik, R., et al.: Murine neuroblastoma: Further evaluation of the C1300 model with single antitumor agents. Cancer Chemother. Rep. 59:975, 1975.
39. Forsman, P. J., and Jenkins, M. E.: Medullary carcinoma of the thyroid with Marfan-like body habitus. Pediatrics 52:188, 1973.
40. Frens, D. B., Bray, P. F., Wu, J. T., et al.: The carcinoembryonic antigen assay: Prognostic value in neural crest tumors. J. Pediatr. 88:591, 1976.
41. Gasparini, M., Bellani, F. F., Musumeci, R., et al.: Response and survival of patients with metastatic neuroblastoma after combination chemotherapy with Adriamycin (NSC-123127), cyclophosphamide (NSC-25271), and vincristine (NSC-67574). Cancer Chemother. Rep. 58:365, 1974.
42. Geiser, C. F., and Efron, M. L.: Cystathioninuria in patients with neuroblastoma or ganlioneuroblastoma. Cancer 22:856, 1968.
43. Gerson, J. M., Chatten, J., and Eisman, S.: Familial neuroblastoma – a follow-up. N. Engl. J. Med. 290:1487, 1974.
44. Gibbs, M. K., Carney, J. A., Hayles, A. B., et al.: Simultaneous adrenal and cervical pheochromocytomas in childhood. Ann. Surg. 185:273, 1977.
45. Gitlow, S. E., Bertani, L. M., Greenwood, S. M., et al.: Benign pheochromocytoma associated with elevated excretion of homovanillic acid. J. Pediatr. 81:1112, 1972.
46. Gjessing, L. R., and Mauritzen, K.: Cystathioninuria in hepatoblastoma. Scand. J. Clin. Lab. Invest. 17:513, 1965.
47. Green, A. A., and Hayes, F. A.: Neuroblastoma in infants under a year of age: The value of therapy (Abstr.). Pediatr. Res. 10:454, 1976.
48. Green, M., Cooke, R. E., and Lattanzi, W.: Occurrence of chronic diarrhea in three patients with ganglioneuromas. Pediatrics 23:951, 1959.
49. Griffin, M. E., and Bolande, R. P.: Familial neuroblastoma with regression and maturation to ganglioneurofibroma. Pediatrics 43:377, 1969.
50. Gross, R. E., Farber, S., and Martin, L. W.: Neuroblastoma sympathicum: A study and report of 217 cases. Pediatrics 23:1179, 1959.
51. Gutierrez Moyano, M. B.: Bergadá, C., and Becú, L.: Catecholamine excretion in forty children with sympathoblastoma. J. Pediatr. 77:239, 1970.
52. Hagstrom, H. T.: Fetal dystocia due to metastatic neuroblastoma of the liver. Am. J. Obstet. Gynec. 19:673, 1930.
53. Hardy, P. C., and Nesbit, M. E.: Familial neuroblastoma: Report of a kindred with a high incidence of infantile tumors. J. Pediatr. 80:74, 1972.
54. Harrison, T. S., Freier, D. T., and Cohen, E. L.: Recurrent pheochromocytoma. Arch. Surg. 108:450, 1974.
55. Hart, M. N., and Earle, K. M.: Primitive neuroectodermal tumors of the brain in children. Cancer 32:890, 1973.
56. Hawthorne, H. C., Nelson, J. S., Witzleben, C. L., et al.: Blanching subcutaneous nodules in neonatal neuroblastoma. J. Pediatr. 77:297, 1970.
57. Hellström, K. E., and Hellström, I.: Immunity to neuroblastoma and melanomas. Ann. Rev. Med. 23:19, 1972.
58. Helson, L., Bethune, V., and Schwartz, M. K.: Clinical evaluation of the VMA test strip. Pediatrics 51:153, 1973.

59. Helson, L., Blasco, P., and Murphy, M. L.: Familial neuroblastoma. Clin. Res. 17:614, 1969.
60. Helson, L., Fleisher, M., Bethune, V., et al.: Urinary cystathionine, catecholamine, and metabolites in patients with neuroblastoma. Clin. Chem. 18:613, 1972.
61. Helson, L., Vanichayangkul, P., Tan, C. C., et al.: Combination intermittent chemotherapy for patients with disseminated neuroblastoma. Cancer Chemother. Rep. 56:499, 1972.
62. Hepler, A. B.: Presacral sympathicoblastoma in an infant causing urinary obstruction. J. Urol. 49:777, 1943.
63. Hiner, L. B., Gruskin, A. B., Baluarte, H. J., et al.: Plasma renin activity and intrarenal blood flow distribution in a child with a pheochromocytoma. J. Pediatr. 89:950, 1976.
64. Hughes, M., Marsden, H. B., and Palmer, M. K.: Histologic patterns of neuroblastoma related to prognosis and clinical staging. Cancer 34:1706, 1974.
65. Hume, D. M.: Pheochromocytoma in the adult and child. J. Surg. 99:458, 1960.
66. Jaffe, N.: Late death from neuroblastoma. J. Pediatr. 82:1094, 1973.
67. Jaffe, N., Cassady, R., Filler, R. M., et al.: Heterochromia and Horner syndrome associated with cervical and mediastinal neuroblastoma. J. Pediatr. 87:75, 1975.
68. James, D. H., Jr.: Proposed classification of neuroblastoma. J. Pediatr. 71:764, 1967.
69. James, R. E., Baker, H. L., Jr., and Scanlon, P. W.: The roentgenologic aspects of metastatic pheochromocytoma. Amer. J. Roentgenol. Radium Ther. Nucl. Med. 115:783, 1972.
69a. Jansen-Goemans, A. and Engelhardt, J.: Intractable diarrhea in a boy with vasoactive intestinal peptide-producing ganglioneuroblastoma. Pediatrics 59:710, 1977.
70. Johnsonbaugh, R. E., and Cahill, R.: Screening procedures for neuroblastoma: false-negative results. Pediatrics 56:267, 1975.
71. Joseph, L.: Malignant phaeochromocytoma of the organ of Zuckerkandl with functioning metastases. Brit. J. Urol. 39:221, 1967.
72. Kadish, S., Goodman, M., and Wang, C. C.: Olfactory neuroblastoma. A clinical analysis of 17 cases. Cancer 37:1571, 1976.
73. Keiser, H. R., Beaven, M. A., Doppman, J., et al.: Sipple's syndrome: medullary thyroid carcinoma, pheochromocytoma, and parathyroid disease. Ann. Intern. Med. 78:561, 1973.
74. Kilton, L. J., Aschenbrener, C., and Burns, C. P.: Ganglioneuroblastoma in adults. Cancer 37:974, 1976.
75. King, D., Goodman, J., Hawk, T., et al.: Dumbbell neuroblastomas in children. Arch. Surg. 110:888, 1975.
76. Knudson, A. G., and Amromin, G. D.: Neuroblastoma and ganglioneuroma in a child with multiple neurofibromatosis. Cancer 19:1032, 1966.
77. Knudson, A. G., Jr., and Strong, L. C.: Mutation and cancer: neuroblastoma and pheochromocytoma. Amer. J. Hum. Genet. 24:514, 1972.
78. Komp, D. M., Land, V. J., Nitshke, R., et al.: 5-[3,3-Bis(2-chloroethyl)-1-triazeno] imidazole-4-carboxamide (NSC-82196) in the treatment of childhood malignancy. Cancer Chemother. Rep. 59:371, 1975.
79. Konrad, P. N., Singher, L. J., and Neerhout, R. C.: Late death from neuroblastoma. J. Pediatr. 82:80, 1973.
80. Koop, C. E., and Johnson, D. G.: Neuroblastoma: An assessment of therapy in reference to staging. J. Pediatr. Surg. 6:595, 1971.
81. Koop, C. E., Kiesewetter, W. B., and Horn, R. C.: Neuroblastoma in childhood. Survival after major surgical insult to the tumor. Surgery 38:272, 1955.
82. Koop, C. E., and Schnaufer, L.: The management of abdominal neuroblastoma. Cancer 35:905, 1975.
83. LaBrosse, E. H.: Biochemical diagnosis of neuroblastoma: Use of a urine spot test. Proc. Amer. Ass. Cancer Res. 9:39, 1968.
84. LaBrosse, E. H., Comoy, E., Bohuon, C., et al.: Catecholamine metabolism in neuroblastoma. J. Natl. Cancer Inst. 57:633, 1976.
85. Langman, M. J. S.: Treatment of neuroblastoma with vitamin B_{12}. Arch. Dis. Child. 45:385, 1970.
86. Larimer, R. C.: Neuroblastoma (sympathogonioma) of the adrenal in the newborn infant. J. Pediatr. 34:365, 1949.
87. Lauder, I., and Aherne, W.: The significance of lymphocytic infiltration in neuroblastoma. Brit. J. Cancer 26:321, 1972.
88. Lee, C. M., Jr.: The surgical significance of tumors in identical twins: A short review of the literature and a report of sympathico-blastoma occurring in monozygotic twins. Am. Surg. 19:803, 1953.
89. Leikin, S., Evans, A., Heyn, R., et al.: The impact of chemotherapy on advanced neuroblastoma. Survival of patients diagnosed in 1956, 1962, and 1966–68 in Children's Cancer Study Group A. J. Pediatr. 84:131, 1974.
90. Leiberman, E., Shaw, K. N. F., and Donnell, G. N.: Cystathioninuria in galactosemia and certain types of liver disease. Pediatrics 40:828, 1967.
91. Leonard, A. S., Robach, S. A., Nesbit, M. E., Jr., et al.: The VMA test strip: a new tool

for mass screening, diagnosis and management of catecholamine-secreting tumors. J. Pediatr. Surg. 7:528, 1972.
92. Levin, D. L., Perlia, C., and Tashjian, A. H., Jr.: Medullary carcinoma of the thyroid gland: The complete syndrome in a child. Pediatrics 52:192, 1973.
93. MacKay, B., Luna, M. A., and Butler, J. J.: Adult neuroblastoma: electron microscopic observations in nine cases. Cancer 37:1334, 1976.
94. MacKay, B., Masse, S. R., King, O. Y., et al.: Diagnosis of neuroblastoma by electron microscopy of bone marrow aspirates. Pediatrics 56:1045, 1975.
95. Maebashi, J., Miura, Y., and Yoshinaga, K.: Plasma renin activity in pheochromocytoma. Jap. Circul. 32:1427, 1968.
96. Makinen, J.: Microscopic patterns as a guide to prognosis of neuroblastoma in childhood. Cancer 29:1637, 1972.
97. Martin, E. S., and Griffith, J. F.: Myoclonic encephalopathy and neuroblastoma. Am. J. Dis. Child. 122:257, 1971.
98. Mason, G. A., Hart-Mercer, J., Millar, E. J., et al.: Adrenaline-secreting neuroblastoma in an infant. Lancet 2:322, 1957.
99. Miller, R. W.: Relation between cancer and congenital defects: an epidemiologic evaluation. J. Natl. Cancer Inst. 40:1079, 1968.
100. Miller, R. W., Fraumeni, J. F., Jr., and Hill, J. A.: Neuroblastoma: epidemiologic approach to its origin. Am. J. Dis. Child. 115:253, 1968.
101. Mitchell, C. H., Sinatra, F. R., Crast, F. W., et al.: Intractable watery diarrhea, ganglioneuroblastoma and vasoconstrictive intestinal peptide. J. Pediatr. 89:593, 1976.
102. Moe, P. G., and Nellhaus, G.: Infantile polymyoclonia-opsoclonus syndrome and neural crest tumors. Neurology 20:756, 1970.
103. Ong, M., and Dupont, C. L.: The LaBrosse VMA spot test revisited. J. Pediatr. 86:238, 1975.
104. Pegelow, C. H., Ebbin, A. J., Powars, D., et al.: Familial neuroblastoma. J. Pediatr. 87:763, 1975.
105. Pendergrass, T. W., and Hanson, J. W.: Fetal hydantoin syndrome and neuroblastoma. Lancet 2:150, 1976.
106. Perez, C. A., Vietti, T. J., Ackerman, L. V., et al.: Treatment of malignant sympathetic tumors in children: clinicopathological correlation. Pediatrics 41:452, 1968.
107. Phillips, A. F., McMurtry, R. J., and Taubman, J.: Malignant pheochromocytoma in childhood. Am. J. Dis. Child. 130:1252, 1976.
108. Pinkel, D., Pratt, C., Holton, C., et al.: Survival of children with neuroblastoma treated with combination chemotherapy. J. Pediatr. 73:928, 1968.
109. Ragab, A. H., Sutow, W. W., Komp, D., et al.: Adriamycin in the treatment of childhood solid tumors. Cancer 36:1572, 1975.
110. Reilly, D., Nesbit, M. E., and Krivit, W.: Cure of three patients who had skeletal metastases in disseminated neuroblastoma. Pediatrics 41:47, 1968.
111. Reisman, M., Goldenberg, E. D., and Gordon, J.: Congenital neuroblastoma and heart disease. Am. J. Dis. Child. 111:308, 1966.
112. Remine, W. H., Chong, G. C., van Heerden, J. A., et al.: Current management of pheochromocytoma. Ann. Surg. 179:740, 1974.
113. Reynoso, G., Chu, T. M., Holyoke, D., et al.: Carcinoembryonic antigen in patients with different cancers. J.A.M.A. 220:361, 1972.
114. Richards, M. J. S., Joo, P., and Gilbert, E. F.: The rare problem of late recurrence in neuroblastoma. Cancer 38:1847, 1976.
115. Roberts, K. B., and Freeman, J. M.: Cerebellar ataxia and "occult neuroblastoma" without opsomyoclonus. Pediatrics 56:464, 1975.
116. Robinson, M. J., Kent, M., and Stocks, J.: Phaeochromocytoma in childhood. Arch. Dis. Child. 48:137, 1973.
117. Ross, P.: Calcification in liver metastases from neuroblastoma. Radiology 85:1074, 1965.
118. Samuels, L. D., Newton, W. A., Heyn, R., et al.: Daunomycin therapy in advanced neuroblastoma. Cancer 27:831, 1971.
119. Sawitsky, A., and Desposito, F.: A survey of American experience with vitamin B_{12} therapy of neuroblastoma. J. Pediatr. 67:99, 1965.
120. Schnaufer, L., and Koop, C. E.: Silastic abdominal patch for temporary hepatomegaly in stage IV-S neuroblastoma. J. Pediatr. Surg. 10:73, 1975.
121. Schneider, K. M., Becker, J. M., and Krasna, I. H.: Neonatal neuroblastoma. Pediatrics 36:359, 1965.
122. Schnelle, N., Carney, F. M. T., Didier, E. P., et al.: Anesthesia for surgical treatment of pheochromocytoma. Surg. Clin. North Am. 45:991, 1965.
123. Schwartz, A. D., Dadash-Zadeh, M., Lee, H., et al.: Spontaneous regression of disseminated neuroblastoma. J. Pediatr. 85:760, 1974.
124. Senelick, R. C., Bray, P. F., Lahey, M. E., et al.: Neuroblastomas and myoclonic encephalopathy: two cases and a review of the literature. J. Pediatr. Surg. 8:623, 1973.
125. Sherman, S., and Roizen, N.: Fetal hydan-

toin syndrome and neuroblastoma. Lancet 2:517, 1976.
126. Sipple, J. H.: The association of pheochromocytoma with carcinoma of the thyroid gland. Am. J. Med. 31:163, 1961.
127. Sitarz, A., Santulli, T. V., Wigger, H. J., et al.: Complete maturation of neuroblastoma with bone metastases in documented stages. J. Pediatr. Surg. 10:533, 1975.
128. Stackpole, R. H., Melicow, M. M., and Uson, A. C.: Pheochromocytoma in children. J. Pediatr. 63:315, 1963.
129. Sullivan, M. P., Nora, A. H., Kulapongs, P., et al.: Evaluation of vincristine sulfate and cyclophosphamide chemotherapy for metastatic neuroblastoma. Pediatrics 44:685, 1969.
130. Sutow, W., Gehan, E., Heyn, R., et al.: Comparison of survival courses, 1956 versus 1962 in children with Wilms' tumor and neuroblastoma. Pediatrics 45:800, 1970.
131. Sutow, W. W.: Prognosis in neuroblastoma of childhood. Am. J. Dis. Child. 96:299, 1958.
132. Swift, P. G. F., Bloom, S. R., and Harris, F.: Watery diarrhea and ganglioneuroma with secretion of vasoactive intestinal peptide. Arch. Dis. Child. 50:896, 1975.
133. Thurman, W. G., and Donaldson, M. H.: Current concepts in the management of neuroblastoma. In Neoplasia of Childhood. Chicago, Year Book Medical Publishers, Inc., 1967, p. 175.
134. Thurman, W. G., Fernbach, D. J., Sullivan, M. P., et al.: Cyclophosphamide therapy in childhood neuroblastoma. N. Engl. J. Med. 270:1336, 1964.
135. Turkel, S. B., and Itabashi, H. H.: The natural history of neuroblastic cells in the fetal adrenal gland. Am. J. Pathol. 76:225, 1974.
136. von Studnitz, W.: Cystathioninuria in children with neuroblastoma with and without metastasis. Acta Paediatr. Scand. 59:80, 1970.
137. von Studnitz, W., Käser, H., and Sjoerdsma, A.: Spectrum of catechol amine biochemistry in patients with neuroblastoma. N. Engl. J. Med. 269:232, 1963.
138. Voorhess, M. L.: Neuroblastoma with normal urinary catecholamine excretion. J. Pediatr. 78:680, 1971.
139. Voûte, P. A., Jr., Wadman, S. K., and van Putten, W. J.: Congenital neuroblastoma: symptoms of the mother during pregnancy. Clin. Pediatr. 9:206, 1970.
140. Wagget, J., Aherne, G., and Aherne, W.: Familial neuroblastoma. Report of two sib pairs. Arch. Dis. Child. 48:63, 1973.
141. Wakonig-Vaartaja, T., Helson, L., Baren, A., et al.: Cytogenetic observations in children with neuroblastoma. Pediatrics 47:839, 1971.
142. Wells, H. G.: Occurrence and significance of congenital malignant neoplasms. Arch. Path. 30:535, 1940.
143. Whang-Peng, J., and Bennett, J. M.: Cytogenic studies in metastatic neuroblastoma. Am. J. Dis. Child. 115:703, 1968.
144. Williams, C., and Greer, M.: Homovanillic acid and vanilmandelic acid in diagnosis of neuroblastoma. J.A.M.A. 183:836, 1963.
145. Williams, A. O.: Tumors of childhood in Ibadan, Nigeria. Cancer 36:370, 1975.
146. Windmiller, J., Berry, D. H., Haddy, T. B., et al.: Vincristine sulfate in the treatment of neuroblastoma in children. Am. J. Dis. Child. 111:75, 1966.
147. Witzleben, C. L., and Landy, R. A.: Disseminated neuroblastoma in a child with von Recklinghausen's disease. Cancer 34:785, 1974.
148. Wong, K., Hanenson, I. B., and Lampkin, B. C.: Familial neuroblastoma. Am. J. Dis. Child. 121:415, 1971.
149. Young, J. L., and Miller, R. W.: Incidence of malignant tumors in U. S. children. J. Pediatr. 86:254, 1975.
150. Zimmerman, N. J.: Ganglioneuroblastoma als erbliche Systemerkränkung des Sympathicus. Beitr. Pathol. Anat. 111:355, 1951.

Chapter Fourteen

RETINOBLASTOMA

Retinoblastomas are congenital malignant neoplasms which arise from the nuclear layers of the retina. Recent evidence indicates that these tumors are of neuronal tissue origin.[47] They are the most common ocular malignancies in childhood and are of special importance because early diagnosis followed by appropriate therapy can be life-saving and can often successfully prevent loss of vision in the majority of survivors. They may begin in single or multiple foci, and both eyes are often involved. Retinoblastomas are responsible for about 5 per cent of childhood blindness but less than 1 per cent of cancer deaths during infancy.[8]

INCIDENCE

The retinoblastoma is an uncommon tumor which has been reported to occur in about one in 23,000 live births in the United States.[24] It is believed to occur in most countries with a similar frequency.[7, 12] However, an unusually large number of patients with retinoblastoma have been reported in Nigeria, where it is second only to Burkitt's lymphoma as a form of childhood cancer.[52] In contrast, retinoblastoma is the eighth most common malignant childhood tumor in the United States, with no major difference in incidence occurring between black and white children.[55] Despite the similar incidence, the mortality rate is 2½ times greater in black than in white children in this country.[27] It has been suggested that this may be due to a delay in diagnosis and initiation of therapy in black children,[28] but the possibility exists that this tumor may be more aggressive and resistant to therapy in the black population than in the white.

GENETICS

Retinoblastoma has long been known to be inherited as an autosomal dominant disease, but the majority of cases appear sporadically, presumably because of mutation. All patients with bilateral involvement, including familial and sporadic cases, are considered to have the hereditary form, and each offspring of these affected individuals has a 50 per cent chance of developing the disease. However, the transmission of the disease by survivors with unilateral eye involvement occurs much less frequently. This is especially true of the survivor of unilateral retinoblastoma with no family history of the disease. In addition, about 5 per cent of obligate carriers have no clinical evidence of disease, and can pass the disease on to 50 per cent of their offspring.[19] Thus, both hereditary and nonhereditary forms of retinoblastoma appear to exist. An estimated 35 to 45 per cent of cases are hereditary and 55 to 65 per cent are nonhereditary. Of the hereditary form, 25 to 40 per cent are unilateral and 60 to 75 per cent are bilateral.

Knudson has proposed that this cancer is caused by two mutational events.[18,19] In the hereditary form, the first mutation is inherited in the germ cells and the second occurs in somatic cells. In the nonhereditary form, both mutations occur in the somatic cells. The hereditary form, due to a dominant gene, produces a mean number of three retinoblastoma foci per gene carrier, and it is a matter of chance whether the individual develops bilateral disease, unilateral disease, or no disease at all. Children who develop the disease sporadically and do not carry the gene virtually never have bilateral involvement. Therefore, all bilateral cases should be considered heritable regardless of the family history. Only 10 to 15 per cent of unilateral cases are heritable, and this subgroup can only be identified in the presence of a positive family history. Recently, data on 899 cases of retinoblastoma revealed some findings that appeared to differ from the expected results if Knudson's hypothesis were correct. Alternative explanations proposed were the importance of the sequence in which the mutations occur, and the possibility that three mutational events might be required rather than two.[3]

In clinical practice, the following guidelines are proposed for the purposes of family counseling:

1. Unaffected parents with one affected child run a 5 to 6 per cent risk of having another affected child, but siblings should receive regular examinations by an ophthalmologist despite this low risk.

2. There is a 50 per cent chance of each child's developing retinoblastoma if one parent was a survivor of known hereditary retinoblastoma, or a survivor of sporadic bilateral retinoblastoma.

3. If more than one sibling is affected, the risk of each subsequent offspring developing the disease is 50 per cent, even if both parents are unaffected, because one of the parents is probably a silent carrier of the disease.

4. About 10 to 15 per cent of survivors of unilateral disease appear to have the inherited form of retinoblastoma despite the lack of a positive family history.

5. Unaffected persons who come from documented retinoblastoma families can carry the gene, since about 5 per cent of carriers are clinically free of disease. One affected offspring from such an individual would reveal him to be a silent carrier, and each subsequent child would have a 50 per cent chance of developing the disease.

Associated Abnormalities

In an epidemiologic study of the hospital records of 1623 children with retinoblastoma, Jensen and Miller[17] found an increased incidence of severe mental retardation. Mental retardation was about three times more common in children with retinoblastoma than in those with other childhood tumors. Two smaller studies also have indicated an increased incidence of severe mental retardation in retinoblastoma patients.[10,42] It has been suggested that those with mental retardation in association with retinoblastoma may represent a variant of the D-deletion syndrome,[17] a disorder characterized by eczema, microcephaly, colobomata, malformed ears, cleft and high arched palate, and multiple skeletal anomalies. Children with this condition manifest a deletion of the long arm of chromosome 13 and have a high incidence of retinoblastoma, which is often bilateral.[30,53] In at least three cases, children with mental retardation and retinoblastoma but no congenital anomalies were found to have a deletion of chromosome 13.[19a] Patients with retinoblastoma who have no congenital defects generally have normal karyotypes.[20]

Second primary cancers, usually in the head and neck area, have been reported in patients with retinoblastoma, and have usually been attributed to the radiation therapy the patient received for his primary tumor.[33] These tumors have included fibrosarcomas, squamous cell carcinomas of the skin, thyroid carcinomas, embryonal sarcomas, and, in particular, osteogenic sarcomas. However, second malignancies distant to the irradiated area also have been reported, and it appears that children with retinoblastoma may be unusually susceptible to the development of osteogenic sarcomas.[17,36] In addition, at least two children with retinoblastoma have developed leukemia despite the fact that neither received radiotherapy.[14,17] Recent reports suggest that members of the immediate family of retinoblastoma patients may be at increased risk for developing other malignancies.[13,36]

PATHOLOGY

When the retinoblastoma arises in the internal nuclear layers of the retina, the tumor mass extends into the vitreous cavity (Fig. 14-1). This endophytic type of retinoblastoma is the most common and can often be seen with the ophthalmoscope. A tumor arising in the external nuclear layers, termed an exophytic type, may grow in the subretinal space and detach the retina (Fig. 14-2). Because this tumor type cannot be seen directly, it leads to greater problems in diagnosis. One unusual clinical variant, the diffuse infiltrating retinoblastoma, replaces the entire retina by tumor cells with little evidence of a mass lesion.[37]

Retinoblastomas characteristically arise in multiple foci in the involved retina.[9] This is probably due to a multicentric origin, but it is also possible that tumor spreads in the potential subretinal space. Although there are

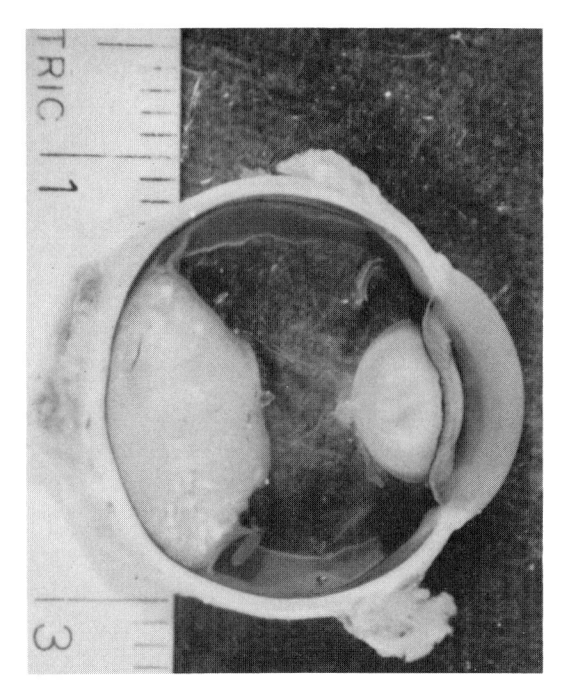

Figure 14-1 Cross section of an enucleated eye with a large endophytic type of retinoblastoma extending into the vitreous cavity. (Courtesy of Drs. James Kelly and Richard Green, Wilmer Ophthalmological Institute, Baltimore.)

RETINOBLASTOMA

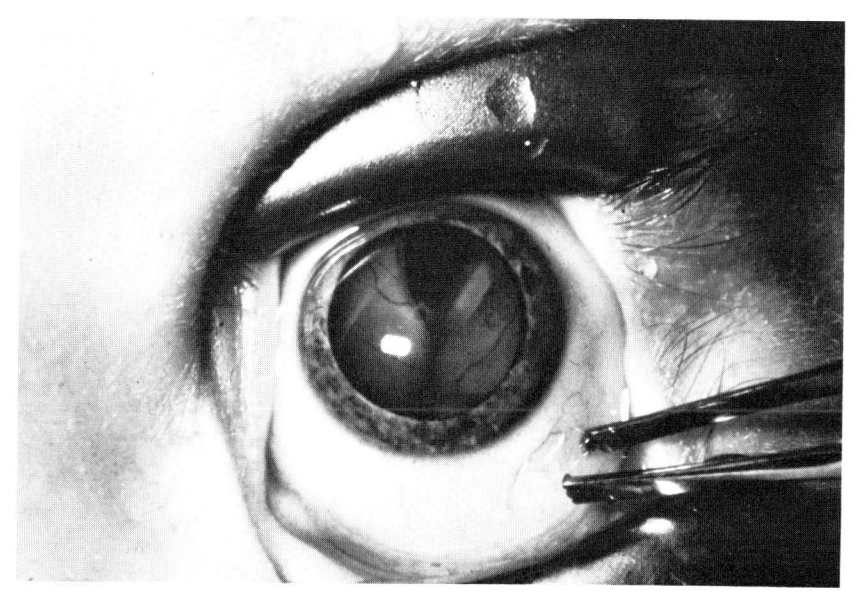

Figure 14–2 Retinal detachment due to a retinoblastoma growing in the subretinal space. (Courtesy of Dr. Richard Green, Wilmer Ophthalmological Institute, Baltimore.)

rare cases in which the tumor spreads from one eye to the other via the optic nerve across the chiasm to the other optic nerve, most bilateral tumors are of true multicentric origin.

The cell most commonly present in the retinoblastoma is a uniform small, round or polygonal cell with scant cytoplasm. The tumor characteristically shows rosette and pseudorosette formation (Fig. 14–3). There is some evidence that the tumors which show

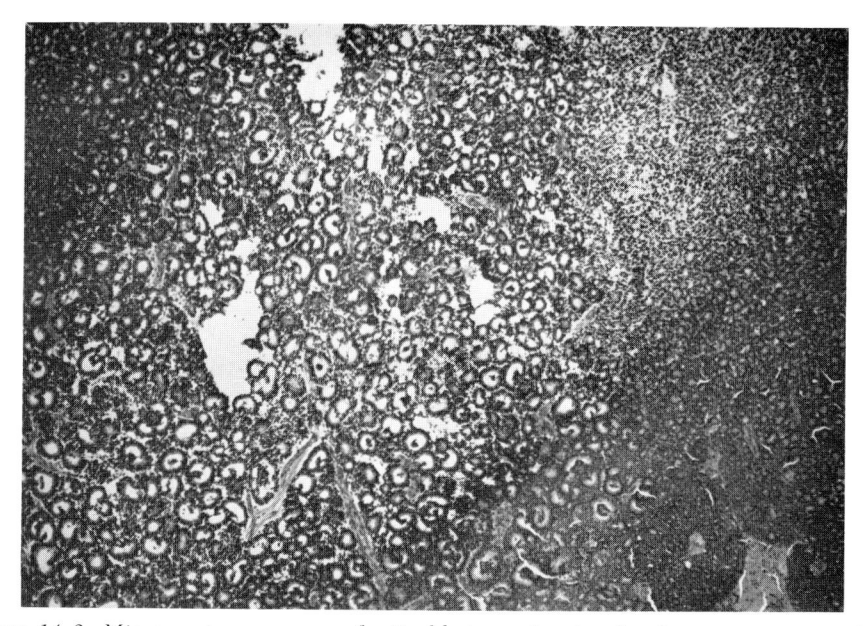

Figure 14–3 Microscopic appearance of retinoblastoma showing the characteristic rosette formation. (Courtesy of Drs. James Kelly and Richard Green, Wilmer Ophthalmological Institute, Baltimore.)

more differentiation are less radiosensitive.[50] Ts'o and his colleagues have presented evidence that one factor that causes radioresistance is photoreceptor-cell differentiation of the tumor.[48, 49] These cells have relatively abundant cytoplasm and an eosinophilic intranuclear matrix.[47]

Histologically, there are many similarities between the retinoblastoma, neuroblastoma, and medulloblastoma, three highly malignant and relatively radiosensitive malignancies of neural tissue origin that occur in young children and are believed to be congenital in origin.

CLINICAL PRESENTATION

Age

In the majority of United States white children with retinoblastoma the condition is diagnosed within the first two years of life, and over 80 per cent are diagnosed before age 3 years. In contrast, fewer black children have their disease diagnosed during the first year of life, and more diagnoses are made in blacks after the age of 2 years than in whites (Table 14–1).[17] This delay in diagnosis may explain the higher mortality rate in blacks.[27] Occasionally adults have been diagnosed as having retinoblastoma, sometimes as late as the fifth or sixth decade of life.[25, 32] In one interesting case, a woman reported by Ellsworth[9] was diagnosed at 34 years of age as having bilateral disease. She apparently experienced spontaneous tumor regressions in both eyes. Although no pathologic diagnosis was mentioned in the proband, the woman produced children with retinoblastoma by two different husbands. One other case of regression of bilateral disease has been recorded.[34] The rare reports of spontaneous regression and of the development of disease in late adulthood suggests that the silent obligate carrier may have had undiagnosed tumor that regressed or may eventually develop disease later in life.

Signs and Symptoms

The most common initial sign of retinoblastoma is an abnormal white pupil (leukokoria). This so-called "amaurotic cat's eye" is usually noted by a parent. When the neoplasm arises in the macular region, the white pupil may be noted when the tumor is still small and is seen when the child looks directly at the observer. When the tumor arises in the periphery of the retina, it grows to a large size before the abnormality is noted. If the parent has noted a white pupil, the diagnosis may still be missed by the physician trying to examine a struggling, uncooperative infant. Examination of the entire fundus of both eyes with dilated pupils is essential when retinoblastoma is suspected, and often must be performed by an experienced ophthalmologist with the child under anesthesia (Fig. 14–4).

The second most common presenting sign is a squint, which is often misdiagnosed as a "weak muscle." When the tumor arises in the macula, strabismus may be a very early sign, but, in many cases, it is seen only after the disease has reached an advanced stage.

Poor vision is most commonly found in infants with massive bilateral tumors which have resulted in extreme loss of vision. The parent usually

Table 14–1 Distribution According to Age at Diagnosis of 1396 White and 167 Black Children With Retinoblastoma[17]

AGE (YEARS)	(PER CENT) WHITES	(PER CENT) BLACKS
<1	31.8	20.4
1	26.3	27.5
2	23.0	25.1
3	10.4	15.0
4	3.4	6.0
5–14	5.1	6.0

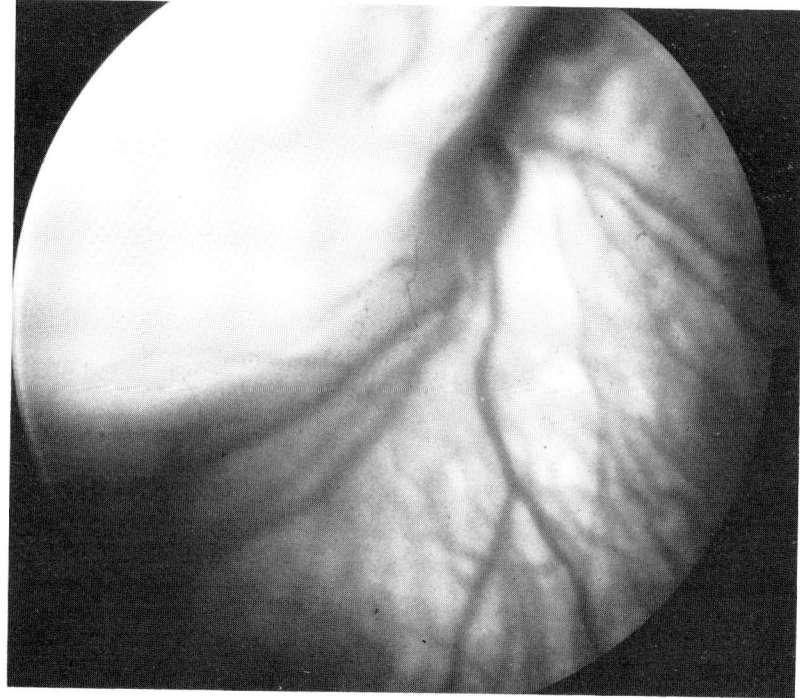

Figure 14-4 Funduscopic appearance of an eye involved with retinoblastoma producing a white membrane in the retina. (Courtesy of Dr. Richard Green, Wilmer Ophthalmological Institute, Baltimore.)

suspects that the child has a visual problem and therefore brings him to the physician. Less commonly, a slow-growing tumor increases in size over a period of years, ultimately involves the macula, and the patient himself complains of poor vision. Occasionally a child with a red, painful eye, often with glaucoma, may be treated for inflammatory disease before the correct diagnosis is made. These symptoms may be secondary to uveitis following spontaneous tumor necrosis or may be related to glaucoma.[1] Other, less common signs and symptoms include unilateral mydriasis, spontaneous hyphema, and a difference noted in the iris color in which the involved iris is darker than normal owing to previous bleeding or inflammation. The most common initial signs and symptoms are listed in Table 14-2.

Table 14-2 Presenting Signs or Symptoms in 235 Patients with Retinoblastoma[16]

	PER CENT
White pupillary reflex	61
Strabismus	22
Decreased vision	5
Routine ocular examination (family history)	2
Routine ocular examination (no family history)	2
Orbital inflammation and proptosis	2
Red, painful eye due to secondary glaucoma	2
Unilateral dilated pupil	1
Spontaneous hyphema	0.5
Heterochromia iridis	0.5
Not recorded	2

DIFFERENTIAL DIAGNOSIS

A number of disorders involving the eye may mimic retinoblastoma. Many children with visceral larva migrans infection have been mistakenly diagnosed as having a tumor. These toddlers ingest the ova of Toxocara organisms, usually by eating dirt or sand soiled with the feces of dogs or cats. The ova hatch and the larvae migrate through the intestinal wall to invade a variety of human tissues, including the eye. A clinical picture very closely resembling retinoblastoma may result, sometimes with no manifestations of visceral larva migrans infection in other organs. Although a striking eosinophilia often accompanies this parasitic infection, it is often absent when the eye is involved.[56] The presenting complaint is usually of strabismus, and ophthalmologic examination often reveals a white pupil. The clinical picture so closely resembles that of retinoblastoma that the eye is often enucleated.[51, 56]

A number of other, less common disorders, including granulomatous uveitis, infections, congenital defects, and severe retrolental fibroplasia, may closely resemble retinoblastoma, and are discussed in detail in the excellent review by Ellsworth.[9] The two features that are almost pathognomonic of retinoblastoma and seldom occur in other disorders are the presence of a typical pattern of fluffy calcifications, and the presence of vitreous seeding by tumor cells. Calcium can be observed with the ophthalmoscope in over 50 per cent of cases and has been reported to be present in 75 per cent of properly obtained roentgenograms.[31] Both these findings, however, may be absent in the child with retinoblastoma. When marked orbital involvement with proptosis occurs, the tumor may be confused with orbital rhabdomyosarcoma, metastatic neuroblastoma, optic nerve glioma, histiocytosis X, lymphoma, hemangioma, or orbital cellulitis.

EVALUATION OF THE PATIENT

Once the diagnosis of retinoblastoma is considered in a child, examination of both eyes should be conducted under general anesthesia, and a detailed record of all abnormalities should be carefully made. A staging system of 5 groups is commonly used, which is based on the size, location, and number of tumors in each eye. Bedford and associates[2] have added a sixth group to this staging system to include patients with residual and metastatic disease (Table 14–3).

Vitreous seeding by tumor fragments is generally associated with large neoplasms and often is an ominous sign. However the presence of vitreous seeding does not invariably carry a poor prognosis.[2] The vitreous can keep these tumor seeds viable for a long period of time. They may then settle

Table 14–3 Staging System for Retinoblastoma[2, 9]

Group I
a. Solitary tumor, less than 4 disc diameters in size, at or behind the equator*
b. Multiple tumors, none over 4 disc diameters in size, all at or behind the equator

Group II
a. Solitary tumor, 4 to 10 disc diameters in size, at or behind the equator
b. Multiple tumors, 4 to 10 disc diameters in size, behind the equator

Group III
a. Any lesion anterior to the equator
b. Solitary tumors larger than 10 disc diameters behind the equator

Group IV
a. Multiple tumors, some larger than 10 disc diameters
b. Any lesion extending anteriorly to the ora serrata †

Group V
a. Massive tumors invading over half the retina
b. Vitreous seeding

Group VI
a. Residual orbital disease
b. Optic nerve involvement and extrascleral extension

*Equator: the midplane of the eye.
†Ora serrata: junction of the retina and ciliary body.

on other areas of the retina, obtain a good blood supply, and establish secondary growths.

Extension of the retinoblastoma into the choroid, the highly vascular layer between the retina and sclera, increases the risk of hematogenous metastases. However, blood-borne metastases do not appear to occur commonly, since choroidal extension is often present in Group IV or V tumors, yet the majority of these patients still survive. When hematogenous metastases do occur, the bone marrow, long bones, lymph nodes, and liver may become involved. For unknown reasons, the lung is seldom the site of metastatic disease.

Tumor extension into the sclera and involvement beyond the globe into the orbit are poor prognostic findings. Long-standing cases with such marked local growth seldom occur in most countries, but in some areas of the world, massive tumor growth at the time of presentation is not uncommon.[29] Direct extension of tumor into the optic nerve may also occur. As the tumor grows further back into the nerve, it may eventually involve the subarachnoid space, disseminate tumor cells into the spinal fluid, and seed along the base of the brain.[35] About half of the deaths from retinoblastoma are due to extension via the optic nerve to the meninges, and the remainder are due to widespread hematogenous metastases.

Prior to surgery, evaluation should include roentgenograms of the skull with orbital views. Many retinoblastomas will show calcifications, but erosion of the bony walls of the orbit and involvement of the optic foramina are uncommon radiologic findings. By the time the tumor has enlarged the optic canal, there is essentially a 100 per cent chance of orbital, cranial, and distant metastases, with little hope for cure.[9] A skeletal survey, bone marrow aspiration, and examination of spinal fluid for malignant cells should also be performed, because evidence of distant disease usually significantly changes the plans for surgery. When distant disease is present, treatment is palliative.

Urinary levels of homovanillic acid (HVA) and vanillylmandelic acid (VMA) have been reported to be elevated in a small percentage of children with retinoblastoma.[4] The levels decreased after the lesions were treated with radiation. The measurement of these substances, however, has usually not been of clinical value, nor have quantitative measurements proved to be an index of metastatic involvement.[9] Urinary VMA levels have been normal in the few patients upon whom we have done determinations, including one child with disseminated disease.

Plasma carcinoembryonic antigen (CEA) and alpha fetoprotein (AFP) levels were noted to be elevated in 4 of 5 patients reported by Michaelson and colleagues.[26] The one child with a normal CEA level had elevated AFP values and the only one with a normal AFP level had elevated CEA values. The levels of these tumor-associated antigens were significantly lowered following enucleation and radiation therapy. These investigators have also noted elevated CEA levels in unaffected close relatives of 9 of 17 patients with sporadic retinoblastoma,[11] but the significance of this finding remains to be determined.

THERAPY

Retinoblastoma is usually a curable tumor when diagnosed early, and vision need not be sacrificed to cure the patient, even in the child with bilateral disease. Optimal results can be achieved only if the patient receives prompt evaluation by an experienced ophthalmologist and is treated by those with expertise in the management of this tumor. Taktikos has shown that the prognosis is directly related to the interval between the discovery of clinical signs and the initiation of proper treatment.[13] Since few children receive routine ophthalmologic examinations and the disease usually presents during the early years of life, a knowledge of the presenting findings and a high degree of suspicion by the pediatrician or general practitioner are essential so that appropriate consultation can be made.

Surgery

Not many years ago the initial treatment recommended for all children with unilateral retinoblastoma was prompt enucleation of the involved eye.[6, 21] Those with bilateral involvement usually underwent enucleation of the most involved eye, and radiation therapy was given to the remaining eye. Fortunately, asymmetrical bilateral involvement is the rule; the one eye that brought the disease to the attention of the physician is involved to a greater extent than the other eye, which may be found to be involved only after careful examination under anesthesia. A less aggressive surgical approach is now advocated at a number of treatment centers, but the indications for enucleation still differ among various institutions. Ellsworth[9] has advocated prompt enucleation in unilateral cases when the tumor is classified as either Group IV or Group V disease. Radiation therapy is used as the primary treatment for those with Group I, II, or III disease. However, the tumor is usually extensive at the time of diagnosis, and only the child in a family with a history of retinoblastoma or one presenting with squint because of early macular involvement usually falls into the group who receives radiation therapy. In the patient with bilateral tumor in whom both eyes are extensively involved, an attempt is made to salvage the least involved eye unless disease is so severe that no hope of retaining vision exists. Bedford and coworkers[2] have used optic nerve involvement as their indication for enucleation, and have performed this surgery on only 31 of 139 cases. They reported excellent results using radiation as the major form of therapy, and achieved an overall survival rate of 92 per cent.

When enucleation is performed, removal of as long a segment of the optic nerve as possible is essential. It is not uncommon to find tumor extending for only a few millimeters behind the lamina cribrosa, and removal of a long portion of optic nerve often totally removes a tumor that might otherwise eventually have involved the subarachnoid space.

Radiation Therapy

Retinoblastomas are considered to be relatively radiosensitive neoplasms, and radiation therapy is the major treatment modality used to destroy tumor and preserve useful vision. The temporal field x-ray beam technique advocated by a number of radiation therapists in this country delivers a tumor dose to the posterior retina of 3500 rads in nine fractions over a 3-week period.[44] This technique attempts to avoid radiation-induced cataracts by sparing the lens from high-dose radiation, but leaves much of the retina anterior to the equator untreated. It is therefore unsuitable for lesions arising or extending anterior to the equator or for tumors with vitreous seeding. It is most suited for those with Groups I and II disease, and for some patients with Group III disease. Some recommend this method of treatment only for localized tumors at the posterior pole if one eye has already been enucleated.[2] Those with large tumors and lesions involving the area anterior to the equator can be treated using a direct anterior field, which should treat all parts of the retina and vitreous.[39] The normal ocular structures and the brain receive radiation using this method, and a cataract develops within 2 years of therapy.[23] This complication can usually be corrected surgically.

Radioactive [60]cobalt surface applicators have been developed which can be sutured to the outer scleral surface of the globe over the base of the tumor.[41] They are designed to deliver a continuous dose of radiation in the range of 25,000 to 30,000 rads to the tumor base and 4000 rads to the tumor apex over a 7-day period, after which time they are removed. They have the advantage of delivering little radiation to surrounding ocular structures, but may cause nerve fiber damage at the site of treatment and hemorrhage from large retinal vessels if placed near the optic disc.[2, 23] Therefore, tumors near the macula or optic disc should not be treated with applicators but are best treated by external beam radiation. The indications for the use of surface applicators vary among institutions. The presence of multiple tumors would lead to radiation overdose of the retina if applicators were used for all lesions. Some believe that the incidence of new tumors appearing in an untreated portion of the retina is too high to use this as a primary form of therapy,[45] whereas others use it as the initial means of therapy for single tumors less than 13 mm in diameter or 2 separate tumors or groups of tumors requiring no more than one 10 mm plaque each, provided the lesions are not near the macula or optic disc.[2]

Light Coagulation

Light coagulation is a method of destroying small retinal tumors by obliterating their nutrient vessels with the use of a powerful light beam.[15] Some have used it as a primary form of focal therapy to treat tumors that are 4 mm or less in diameter if they are posteriorly located and not near the macula or temporal edge of the disc.[2] The major use of this method has been to treat small recurrences after external beam or cobalt applicator therapy.[2, 45]

Cryotherapy

In most centers, cryotherapy is seldom used. It has been reported to be of value in the treatment of small peripheral tumors under certain circumstances.[46]

Chemotherapy

A number of chemotherapeutic agents have been used in the treatment of extensive localized and metastatic retinoblastoma. Cyclophosphamide alone[22] or with vincristine,[45] a combination of actinomycin D, chlorambucil and methotrexate,[38] and a combination of actinomycin D, cyclophosphamide, and methotrexate[54] have been reported to result in a transient response in a number of patients with widespread extracranial disease. We have had one patient with disseminated disease, including bone marrow involvement, who experienced a dramatic but transient response following Adriamycin therapy. Those with central nervous system involvement often respond for varying periods of time to intrathecal methotrexate, radiation therapy, or a combination of the two. Despite an initial response to radiation or chemotherapy in those with central nervous system or distant disease, such therapy is palliative with the agents in use at the present time. Radiation therapy has been of value in controlling bone pain.

The use of chemotherapy for local disease control is not well defined. There is some evidence that triethylene melamine (TEM) given intramuscularly or intra-arterially probably does little to improve survival rates when used with radiation therapy in the treatment of patients with Groups I to V disease.[5] However, some still advocate its use intra-arterially in patients with Group IV or Group V disease, and in those with residual or recurrent orbital disease.[9, 45] The effect of any drug on the survival rate of patients with extensive localized disease has yet to be determined.

THERAPEUTIC RESULTS

The prognosis of patients with retinoblastoma that has not spread beyond

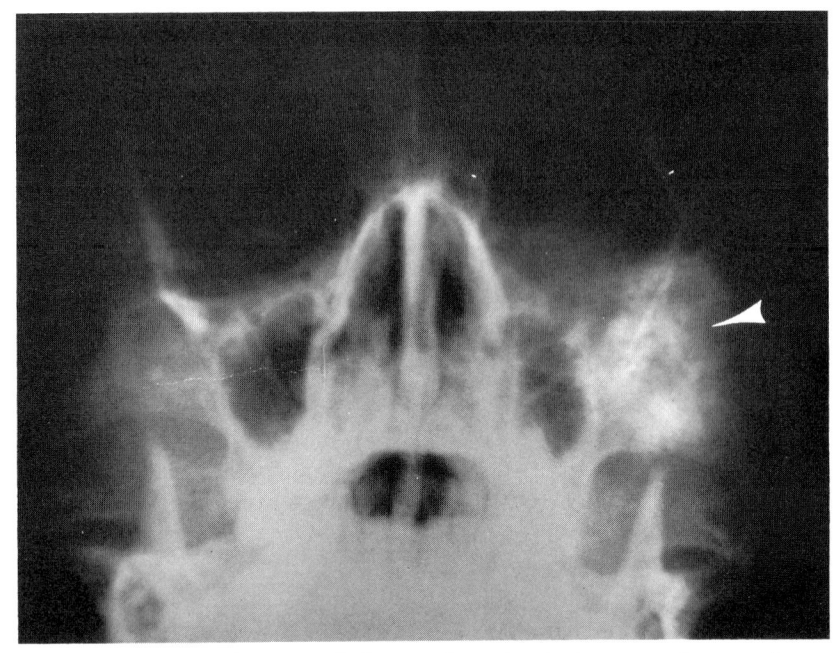

Figure 14-5 Tumor mass showing calcification (arrow), which appeared years after cure of a retinoblastoma treated with radiation therapy. Biopsy of the maxillary lesion revealed it to be an osteogenic sarcoma. (From the teaching collection of the Division of Pediatric Radiology, Johns Hopkins Hospital.)

the globe is generally very good. The highest rate of cure and preservation of vision is achieved in those with less extensive disease. Mortality rates from 10 to 20 per cent due to metastatic disease or intracranial extension have been reported in most large series.[2, 9, 17] In general, a 3-year disease-free period indicates cure, but occasional long-term recurrences have occurred. A large number of patients in whom local tumor recurrence develops may still be cured. One cause of mortality long after cure of the retinoblastoma has been the development of osteogenic sarcoma, which usually occurs in the field of radiation[33] (Fig. 14-5).

Table 14-4 shows the results reported by Ellsworth[9] of a series of 192

Table 14-4 Results of Treatment of 192 Cases of Retinoblastoma With Minimum Follow-up of 3 Years[9]

GROUP	NUMBER OF CASES	CURE RATE* PER CENT
I	20	95
II	32	87
III	24	67
IV	32	69
V	74	34
Orbital tumor	10	30

*Cure = preservation of useful vision.

Table 14-5 Results of Treatment of 139 Cases of Retinoblastoma[2]

GROUP	CURE RATE* PER CENT
I	100
II	100
III	86
IV	75
V	75

*Cure = preservation of useful vision. (Follow-up of 2 years or more in 66 per cent and of more than 1 year in 81 per cent).

patients treated between 1960 and 1965 who had an average follow-up of 5 years and minimum follow-up of 3 years. The overall mortality was 18 per cent despite the fact that the largest number of patients had Group V disease. A more recent report by Bedford and associates[2] of a series of 132 patients is also very encouraging (Table 14–5), although the follow-up has been for less than 2 years in 34 per cent of patients and less than 1 year in 19 per cent. It is clear that prognosis for life and useful vision is excellent when retinoblastoma is diagnosed early and treated properly.

RETINOBLASTOMA

1. Andrew, J. M., and Smith, D. R.: Unsuspected retinoblastoma. Am. J. Ophthalmol. 60:536, 1965.
2. Bedford, M. A., Bedotto, C., and MacFaul, P. A.: Retinoblastoma: a study of 139 cases. Brit. J. Ophthalmol. 55:19, 1971.
3. Bonaïti-Pelli, C., Briard-Guillemot, M. L., Feingold, J., et al.: Mutation theory of carcinogenesis in retinoblastoma. J. Natl. Cancer Inst. 57:269, 1976.
4. Brown, D. H.: The urinary excretion of vanillylmandelic acid (VMA) and homovanillic acid (HVA) in children with retinoblastoma. Am. J. Ophthalmol. 62:239, 1966.
5. Cassady, J. R., Sagerman, R. H., Tretter, P., et al.: Radiation therapy in retinoblastoma: an analysis of 230 cases. Radiology 93:405, 1969.
6. Chapman, R. B., and Toch, R.: Retinoblastoma. Clin. Pediatr. 5:86, 1966.
7. Davies, J. N. P.: Childhood tumors. In Templeton, A. C. (ed.): Tumours in a Tropical Country: A Survey of Uganda 1964–1968. New York, Springer-Verlag, 1973.
8. Editorial: The changing pattern of retinoblastoma. Lancet 2:1016, 1971.
9. Ellsworth, R. M.: The practical management of retinoblastoma. Trans. Am. Ophthalmol. Soc. 67:462, 1969.
10. Falls, H. F., and Neel, J. V.: Genetics of retinoblastoma. Arch. Ophthalmol. 46:367, 1951.
11. Felberg, N. T., Michaelson, J. B., and Shields, J. A.: CEA family syndrome: abnormal carcinoembryonic antigen (CEA) levels in asymptomatic retinoblastoma family members. Cancer 37:1397, 1976.
12. François, J., and Matton-Von Leuven, M. T.: Recent data on the heredity of retinoblastoma. In Boniuk, M. (ed.): Ocular and Adnexal Tumors. St. Louis, C. V. Mosby Co., 1964.
13. Gordon, H.: Family studies in retinoblastoma. In Bergsma, D. (ed.): Medical Genetics Today. Baltimore, Johns Hopkins Press, 1974.
14. Hoefnagel, D., McIntyre, O. R., Storrs, R. C., et al.: Retinoblastoma followed by acute lymphoblastic leukemia. Lancet 1:725, 1973.
15. Höpping, W., and Meyer-Schwickerath, G.: Light coagulation treatment in retinoblastoma. In Boniuk, M. (ed.): Ocular and Adnexal Tumors. St. Louis, C. V. Mosby Co., 1964.
16. Howard, G. M., and Ellsworth, R. M.: Differential diagnosis of retinoblastoma. Statistical survey of 500 children. II. Factors relating to diagnosis of retinoblastoma. Am. J. Ophthalmol. 60:618, 1965.
17. Jensen, R. D., and Miller, R. W.: Retinoblastoma: Epidemiologic characteristics. N. Engl. J. Med. 285:307, 1971.
18. Knudson, A. G.: Genetics and the etiology of childhood cancer. Pediatr. Res. 10:513, 1976.
19. Knudson, A. G.: Mutation and cancer: Statistical study of retinoblastoma. Proc. Natl. Acad. Sci. U.S.A. 68:820, 1971.
19a. Knudson, A. G., Jr., Meadows, A. T., Nichols, W. W., et al.: Chromosomal deletion and retinoblastoma. N. Engl. J. Med. 295:1120, 1976.
20. Ladda, R., Atkins, L., Littlefield, J., et al.: Retinoblastoma: chromosome banding in patients with heritable tumour. Lancet 2:506, 1973.
21. Leelawongs, N., and Regan, C. D. J.: Retinoblastoma: a review of ten years. Am. J. Ophthalmol. 66:1050, 1968.
22. Lonsdale, D., Berry, D. H., Holcomb, T. M., et al.: Chemotherapeutic trials in patients with metastatic retinoblastoma. Cancer Chemother. Rep. 52:631, 1968.
23. MacFaul, P. A., and Bedford, M. A.: Ocular complications after therapeutic irradiation. Brit. J. Ophthalmol. 54:237, 1970.
24. Macklin, M. T.: A study of retinoblastoma in Ohio. Am. J. Hum. Genet. 12:1, 1960.
25. Makley, T. A., Jr.: Retinoblastoma in a 52 year old man. A.M.A. Arch. Ophthalmol. 69:325, 1963.
26. Michelson, J. B., Felberg, N. T., and Shields, J. A.: Fetal antigens in retinoblastoma. Cancer 37:719, 1976.
27. Miller, R. W., and Dalager, N. A.: U.S. childhood cancer deaths by cell type, 1960–68. J. Pediatr. 85:664, 1974.
28. Newell, G. R., Roberts, J. D., and Baranovsky, A.: Retinoblastoma: presentation

and survival in Negro children compared with whites. J. Natl. Cancer Inst. 49:989, 1972.
29. Olurin, O., and Williams, A. O.: Orbito-ocular tumors in Nigeria. Cancer 30:580, 1972.
30. Orye, E., Delbeke, M. J., and Vandenabeele, B.: Retinoblastoma and long arm deletion of chromosome 13: attempts to define the deleted segment. Clin. Genet. 5:457, 1974.
31. Pfeiffer, R. L.: Roentgenographic diagnosis of retinoblastoma. A.M.A. Arch. Ophthalmol. 15:811, 1936.
32. Rasmussen, K.: Retinoblastoma in a man aged 48 years. Acta Ophthalmol. 21:210, 1944.
33. Sagerman, R. H., Cassady, J. R., Tretter, P., et al.: Radiation-induced neoplasia following external beam therapy for children with retinoblastoma. Amer. J. Roentgenol. Radium Ther. Nucl. Med. 105:529, 1969.
34. Sakic, D.: A case of retrogressed bilateral glioma retinae. Ber. Deutsch. Ophthalmol. Gesellsch. 62:300, 1959.
35. Sato, K., Fujikura, T., Kawi, S., et al.: Retinoblastoma with intracranial extension: an autopsy case with light and electron microscope. Acta Pathol. Jap. 19:103, 1969.
36. Schimke, R. N., Lowman, J. T., and Cowan, G. A. B.: Retinoblastoma and osteogenic sarcoma in siblings. Cancer 34:2077, 1974.
37. Schofield, P. B.: Diffuse infiltrating retinoblastoma. Brit. J. Ophthalmol. 44:35, 1960.
38. Sitarz, A. L., Heyn, R., Murphy, M. L., et al.: Triple drug therapy with actinomycin D (NCS-3053), chlorambucil (NCS-3088, and methotrexate (NSC-740) in metastatic solid tumors in children. Cancer Chemother. Rep. 45:45, 1965.
39. Skeggs, D. B. L., and Williams, I. G.: The treatment of advanced retinoblastoma by means of external irradiation combined with chemotherapy. Clin. Radiol. 17:169, 1966.
40. Sorsby, A.: Bilateral retinoblastoma: a dominantly inherited affliction. Brit. Med. J. 2:580, 1972.
41. Stallard, H. B.: The conservative treatment of retinoblastoma. In Boniuk, M. (ed.): Ocular and Adnexal Tumors. St. Louis, C. V. Mosby Co., 1964.
42. Taktikos, A.: Association of retinoblastoma with mental defect and other pathological manifestations. Brit. J. Ophthalmol. 48:495, 1964.
43. Taktikos, A.: Investigation of retinoblastoma with special references to histology and prognosis. Brit. J. Ophthalmol. 50:225, 1966.
44. Tapley, N. duV.: The treatment of bilateral retinoblastoma with radiation and chemotherapy. In Boniuk, M. (ed.): Ocular and Adnexal Tumors. St. Louis, C. V. Mosby Co., 1964.
45. Tapley, N. duV., and Tretter, P.: Retinoblastoma. In Sutow, W. W., Vietti, T. J., and Fernbach, D. J. (eds.): Clinical Pediatric Oncology. St. Louis, C. V. Mosby Co., 1973.
46. Tolentino, F. I., Jr., and Tablante, R. T.: Cryotherapy of retinoblastoma. Arch. Ophthalmol. 87:52, 1972.
47. Ts'o, M. O. M., Fine, B. S., and Zimmerman, L. E.: The nature of retinoblastoma. II. Photoreceptor differentiation: an electron microscopic study. Am. J. Ophthalmol. 69:350, 1970.
48. Ts'o, M. O. M., Zimmerman, L. E., and Fine, B. S.: The nature of retinoblastoma. I. Photoreception differentiation: a clinical and histopathologic study. Am. J. Ophthalmol. 69:339, 1970.
49. Ts'o, M. O. M., Zimmerman, L. E., Fine, B. S., et al.: A cause of radioresistance in retinoblastoma: photoreceptor differentiation. Trans. Amer. Acad. Ophthalmol. Otolaryngol. 74:959, 1970.
50. Tsukahara, I.: A histopathological study on the prognosis and radiosensitivity of retinoblastoma. A.M.A. Arch. Ophthalmol. 63:1005, 1960.
51. Wilder, H.: Nematode endophthalmitis. Trans. Amer. Acad. Ophthalmol. Otolaryngol. 55:99, 1950.
52. Williams, A. O.: Tumors of childhood in Ibadan, Nigeria. Cancer 36:370, 1975.
53. Wilson, M. G., Melnyk, J., and Towner, J. W.: Retinoblastoma and deletion D (14) syndrome. J. Med. Genet. 6:322, 1969.
54. Wolff, J. A., Pratt, C. B., and Sitarz, A. L.: Chemotherapy of metastatic retinoblastoma. Cancer Chemother. Rep. 16:435, 1962.
55. Young, J. L., Jr., and Miller, R. W.: Incidence of malignant tumors in U.S. children. J. Pediatr. 86:254, 1975.
56. Zinkham, W. H.: Visceral larva migrans due to Toxocara as a cause of eosinophilia. Johns Hopkins Hosp. Med. J. 123:41, 1968.

Chapter Fifteen

RENAL TUMORS

Wilms' tumor or congenital nephroblastoma is the most common intrarenal malignant tumor of childhood. It was first recognized as a clinical entity in 1899 by the German surgeon Marx Wilms.[139] The first case, however, was described by Gairdner[40] 71 years prior to Wilms' report. The increasing rate of cure of this neoplasm as a result of therapy has been one of the dramatic success stories in the field of oncology. At present, Wilms' tumor has the best prognosis for long-term survival of any of the common malignant disorders found in children.

AGE

The majority of children with Wilms' tumor are diagnosed between 1 and 5 years of age, with the peak incidence occurring at 3 to 4 years. Occasional cases have been reported in adolescents[78] and adults.[57,93a] The tumor is seldom discovered at birth or during the neonatal period; however, these tumors have been found in newborns and occasionally have been so large as to have caused dystocia during delivery. Wells[136] reported five certain cases and 11 probable ones presenting during the early weeks of life. In addition to those reported by Wells, Hartenstein[50] found seven cases diagnosed in the neonatal period and added one of his own. Goldschmidt and Bachman[46] reviewed 113 cases of children who were discovered to have Wilms' tumor at birth or within the first 2 weeks of life. However, only one of 77 children treated at the M. D. Anderson Hospital and Tumor Institute over a period of 18 years was diagnosed during the first month of life,[119] and, although the tumor occurs in the very young, most children are over 1 year of age when the diagnosis is made. It is possible that a number of neonatal tumors described prior to Bolande's description of the benign renal tumors of infancy in 1967[11] were erroneously diagnosed as Wilms' tumors.

INCIDENCE

Wilms' tumor occurs in about 7.8 children per million per year in the United States.[144] It occurs in all parts of the world with a remarkably stable and constant incidence, and does not appear to be affected by race, climate, or environment. This has allowed the Wilms' tumor to be used as a yardstick for estimating cancer underreporting in various parts of the world.[90]

Clinical Manifestations

In the majority of children with Wilms' tumor the presenting symptom is increasing size of the abdomen or an abdominal mass. Abdominal pain, vomiting, or fever are other common presenting features. The mass is often discovered by a parent, who calls it to the attention of the physician. The tumor lies deep in the flank, arising from the kidney, and is usually firm and smooth. It sometimes extends beyond the midline and may cause deviation of the inferior vena cava. Occasionally it may extend downward beyond the iliac crest. In most reports, the left kidney is more frequently involved than the right.

Tumors involving both kidneys occur in 4 to 13 per cent of children in most large series. Bilateral involvement is noted in the majority of these children at the time of initial diagnosis, but may be discovered much later during a routine examination or roentgenographic study.[13] A few rare cases of extrarenal Wilms' tumor have been reported.[29, 126]

Gross hematuria is an uncommon presenting symptom, but microscopic hematuria is found in approximately one quarter of the cases. Some investigators have considered this an unfavorable sign,[47, 118] but others have not found it to be the poor prognostic finding that it is in adults with hypernephroma.[119]

Hypertension, first reported in association with Wilms' tumor in 1938,[16] has not been a common finding in most series. In fact, it has not even been mentioned as a finding in a number of reports of large series. However, in one report of 81 children, initial blood pressure measurements were recorded in 36 patients. In 10 (28 per cent), both the systolic and diastolic levels were elevated above normal.[5] This finding suggests that hypertension may often be overlooked, because blood pressure measurements are not routinely performed in children. The hypertension found in these children is probably caused by increased renin secretion. The tumor tissue has been shown to contain high concentrations of renin,[82] and elevated levels have been measured in the venous drainage of the involved kidney.[72]

Rare cases of Wilms' tumor associated with polycythemia have been reported. This appears to be secondary to an increased production of erythropoietin by the neoplasm.[112, 127] The demonstration of elevated plasma erythropoietin levels in five of eight non-polycythemic children with Wilms' tumor studied preoperatively led one group of investigators to suggest that this finding might be useful in the diagnosis and the evaluation of response to therapy.[89]

Wilms' tumor has occasionally been found in association with the nephrotic syndrome.[69, 145] Since both disorders are not uncommon, their association may be coincidental. It has been proposed, however, that both conditions may be a result of an embryonic renal insult, and the relationship may not be due to chance alone.[28]

Intrarenal arteriovenous fistulae in Wilms' tumor are an extremely rare cause of congestive heart failure in childhood. Two such cases have been recorded.[109, 117]

Associated Congenital Anomalies

Children with Wilms' tumor have an increased incidence of congenital abnormalities. Lemerle and associates[66] noted congenital defects in 13 per cent of 248 patients treated at the Gustave-Roussy Institute in Paris, and Pendergrass[96] recorded a 15 per cent incidence of anomalies in his survey of the records of 547 patients registered in the National Wilms' Tumor Study (Table 15–1). A large number of cases have been reported in association with genitourinary abnormalities, including cryptorchidism, hypospadias, duplications of the collecting system, and renal anomalies. At least 20 cases have

Table 15-1 Anomalies in 547 Patients With Wilms' Tumor[96]

Hamartomas	43
Genitourinary anomalies	24
Hemihypertrophy	16
Musculoskeletal anomalies	16
CNS anomalies	12
Aniridia	6
Other eye anomalies	9
Heart anomalies	7
Other anomalies	7

occurred in fused ectopic (horseshoe) kidneys.[9, 113]

The association of sporadic aniridia (congenital absence of the iris) and Wilms' tumor was first reported in 1964,[81] and has now been documented by numerous investigators. The relationship is relatively common; aniridia affects about 1 in 70 children with Wilms' tumor but occurs in only about 1 in 50,000 live births.[79] It is usually inherited as an autosomal dominant anomaly. The child with aniridia who has Wilms' tumor does not have this usual inheritance pattern but has sporadic congenital aniridia. In the combined series of 35 patients with sporadic aniridia reported by Fraumeni[37] and Pilling,[99] 12 patients were eventually discovered to have Wilms' tumor, giving an incidence of 34 per cent. There appears to be a distinct syndrome of Wilms' tumor diagnosed before 3 years of age that is associated with congenital aniridia, secondary cataracts, microcephaly, mental retardation, a folding-over of the upper pinna, genitourinary tract anomalies, and a variety of other congenital defects.[49]

Children born with congenital hemihypertrophy have an increased incidence of Wilms' tumor.[36, 79, 81, 96] Sixteen of 547 patients registered in the National Wilms' Tumor Study since 1969 have had this anomaly.[96] The hypertrophy may involve an entire side of the body, may be segmental, with only a limb, the face, or the tongue involved, or may be crossed, with a leg involved on one side and an arm involved on the other. The tumor does not necessarily occur on the same side of the body as the hypertrophy (Fig. 15-1). The hemihypertrophy may occasionally develop following the diagnosis and removal of the tumor.[13, 50a] The pathology and biological behavior of the tumor is no different from when it is not associated with this anomaly. Congenital hemihypertrophy has also been recorded in association with adrenocortical[38] and hepatic tumors,[39] hamartomas,[106] and the visceral cytomegaly syndrome described by Beckwith. One child with the Klippel-Trenaunay syndrome, a disorder of embryonic development characterized by hemangiomas and limb hypertrophy, has been reported with bilateral Wilms' tumor.[71] Hamartomas occur excessively in patients with Wilms' tumor[81] and adrenocortical neoplasms.[38] One child has been reported with both hepatoblastoma and Wilms' tumor;[39] another with congenital hemihypertrophy had an adrenocortical adenoma and years later developed a Wilms' tumor.[105] The Beckwith syndrome has been reported in association with Wilms' tumor, hepatoblastoma, adrenocortical carcinoma, and gonadoblastoma.[103] Of interest is the fact that Beckwith's visceral cytomegaly syndrome affects the kidney, adrenal cortex, and liver, the same organs which develop the malignancies that are associated with hemihypertrophy.

Aniridia and congenital hemihypertrophy are both associated with genitourinary anomalies but do not appear to be associated with one another. However, a number of children with the Wilms' tumor–aniridia syndrome have had hamartomas.[49] These fascinating relationships between congenital anomalies, hemihypertrophy, hamartomas, and malignant neoplasms have been reviewed by Miller.[79]

A number of children with pseudohermaphroditism, nephron disorders, and Wilms' tumor have been reported.[6, 26, 28, 116] It has been proposed

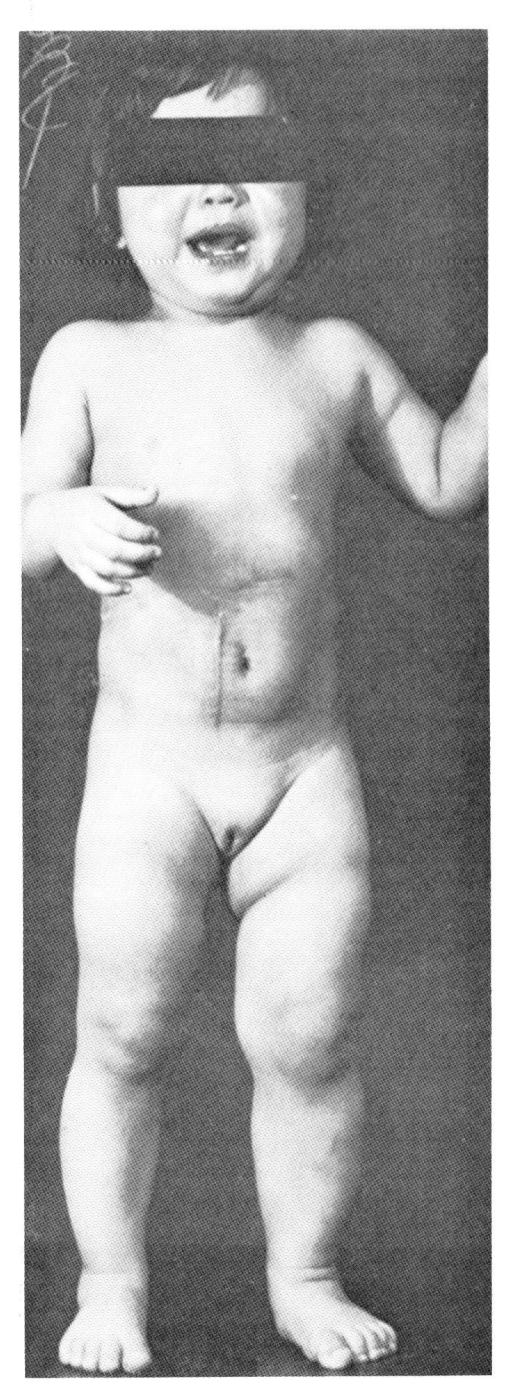

Figure 15-1 Eighteen month old child showing hemihypertrophy of left leg. A Wilms' tumor of the right kidney had been previously removed. (From Fraumeni, J. F., Jr., Geiser, C. F., and Manning, M. D.: Pediatrics 40:893, 1967.)

that this unusual association of disorders may be the result of an embryogenic event which occurred prior to the differentiation of renal and genital structures, and therefore affected both.[28]

The striking association of Wilms' tumor and other childhood neoplasms with a number of congenital abnormalities and disorders of growth control strongly suggests that there is a close relationship between oncogenesis and teratogenesis.

GENETICS

Familial cases of Wilms' tumor have been reported, but are uncommon. Cochran and Froggatt[20] estimated that there was less than a 1 per cent incidence of familial disease in their review of 1926 cases. There have been occasional reports of the tumor occurring in cousins,[81] siblings,[20, 74, 81] identical twins,[42, 81] and successive generations.[17, 56] The neoplasm has been noted in one of a pair of monozygous twins and in their younger brother.[54] When the disease does occur in siblings there is a higher incidence of bilateral involvement, and the patients tend to be younger than the usual child with Wilms' tumor.[20] It has been estimated that if two siblings are affected, the chance of another sibling's having the tumor is 20 per cent.[20]

Occasionally, some members of a family may have a congenital anomaly that has been associated with Wilms' tumor, whereas others have the neoplasm. Meadows and co-workers[77] reported one family in which a mother had congenital hemihypertrophy, three of her children had Wilms' tumor, and a fourth had a urinary tract anomaly. There are two reports of aniridia in monozygous twins in which only one member of each pair developed Wilms' tumor.[80] A familial syndrome lethal in the perinatal period in five siblings born of a consanguinous marriage has been described. The main features of the disorder were bilateral renal hamartomas with or without nephroblastomatosis, somatic gigantism, and unusual facies.[98]

Chromosomal abnormalities have been demonstrated in some children with Wilms' tumor, including trisomy 18,[45] trisomy 8,[92] pseudohermaphroditism with XX/XY mosaicism,[26] B-C translocation,[44] and translocation of part of chromosome 11 to chromosome 8, with a deletion of the latter.[64]

It has been proposed that two groups of patients with Wilms' tumor exist, an autosomal dominant form and a nonhereditary form, the relationship between the two groups being similar to that found in retinoblastoma.[60] If such is the case, more examples of vertical transmission should occur as more patients are cured and survive to reproduce.

PATHOLOGY

Wilms' tumor arises from renal parenchyma and usually is separated from normal kidney tissue by a fibrous pseudocapsule (Fig. 15-2). It often has many areas of necrosis and hemorrhage, and fluid or blood-filled cysts, probably the result of necrosis, may be present. The neoplasm often infiltrates through the renal capsule into the perinephric tissues and can invade the renal pelvis and ureter. It may invade the renal vein, and sometimes extends into the inferior vena cava. Renal vein involvement has been reported in 12 to 40 per cent of cases.[59, 75] Rarely, the tumor has extended up the inferior vena cava into the heart,[3, 88] or a tumor embolus traveling from the inferior vena cava into the heart or lung has caused sudden death.[95] The tumor often becomes very large and extends directly into the liver or colon. Although it metastasizes mainly by the hematogenous route, hilar lymph nodes are commonly involved. Sometimes multiple tumor nodules occur within the kidney.

Microscopically, the neoplasm resembles developing embryonic renal tissue, with mesenchymal and epithelial elements. There is often evidence of an abortive attempt of the epithelial elements to form tubules or glomeruli.

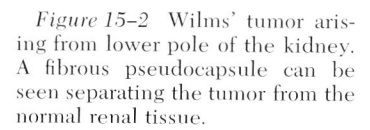

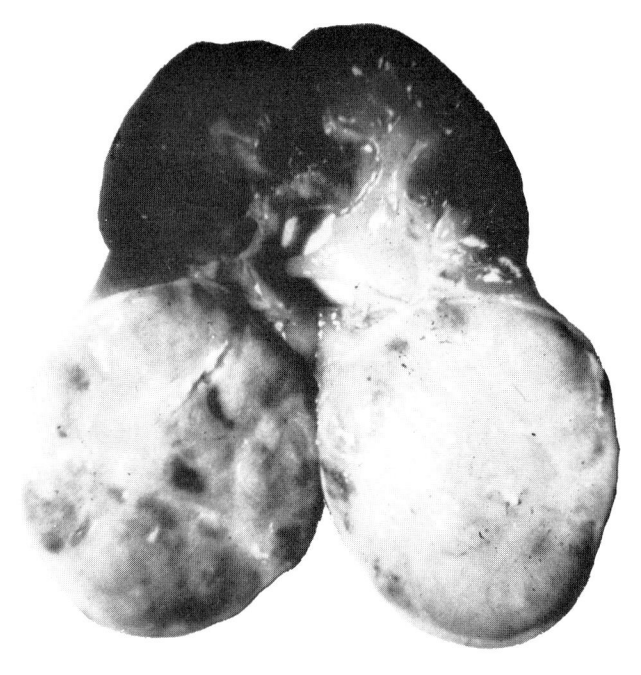

Figure 15-2 Wilms' tumor arising from lower pole of the kidney. A fibrous pseudocapsule can be seen separating the tumor from the normal renal tissue.

There are variable amounts of the mesenchymal element, which sometimes shows differentiation into striated muscle, cartilage, and bone. Some tumors are composed mainly of sheets of anaplastic cells, with little evidence of differentiation.

PROGNOSTIC FACTORS

The three factors that appear to be related to the prognosis for the child with Wilms' tumor are the histologic pattern of the neoplasm, the age of the patient at the time of diagnosis, and the extent of the disease. Some investigators have noted a poor prognosis in patients who present with the symptom of abdominal pain.[66, 119] Larger tumors have been associated with a greater chance of recurrence in some reports,[41, 66] but tumor size has had no prognostic significance in others.[18, 97]

Histology

A good prognosis appears to be correlated with a high degree of differentiation of the epithelial elements of the tumor.[52, 65, 66, 97] Jereb and Sandstedt[52] found the histologic type to be the main prognostic factor when considering 2-year survival rate, and second only to the extent of disease when considering cure rate. The degree of tubular formation was reported by Lawler and co-workers[65] to be the most important prognostic feature, the presence of glomerular structures appearing to be of little importance (Table 15–2). In contrast, Lemerle and associates[66] found that the abundance of differentiated tissue in the tumor was not of prognostic value in itself, but the number of different epithelial types of differentiation were significant; the more varieties there were the more favorable the outcome was (Table 15–3). Kenny and associates[58] noted a more favorable prognosis in patients whose tumors had no sarcomatous elements. The presence of multiple foci of tumor in the kidney has been linked to a poorer outcome.[66, 119]

Age at Diagnosis

Younger patients appear to have a more favorable outcome, even when those infants with congenital mesoblastic nephroma are excluded. In most reports this appears to be due to the fact that the disease is usually less extensive in the younger child; thus, the clinical staging appears to be more important than age.[35, 66, 97] Some investigators have found age and histology to be independent variables,[65] while others have found them to be closely correlated.[66]

Table 15–2 Histologic Tubule Classification Related to Per Cent Survivors (For 3 or More Years)*

HISTOLOGIC TYPE	PER CENT SURVIVAL
Large number of tubules	83
Moderate tubule formation	46
Definite tubules, but scanty	20
No definite tubules	17

*Based on the data of Lawler and associates.[65]

Table 15–3 Number of Different Epithelial Components Versus Outcome*

	CASES (PER CENT)	PER CENT 2-YEAR RELAPSE FREE SURVIVAL	PER CENT 5-YEAR SURVIVAL
No epithelial component	25	34	43
1 or 2 types of differentiation	63	54	61
3 types of differentiation	12	90	90

*Based on the data of Lemerle and associates.[66]

Table 15-4 Clinical Staging According to the National Wilms' Tumor Study[141]

Group I. Tumor limited to the kidney and completely resected.
Group II. Tumor extending beyond the kidney, but completely resected.
Group III. Residual nonhematogenous tumor confined to the abdomen.
Group IV. Hematogenous metastases.
Group V. Bilateral renal involvement either initially or subsequently.

Extent of Disease

The most significant factor in determining the patient's chance for survival appears to be the extent of tumor involvement at the time of diagnosis. A number of staging systems have been proposed to document the extent of disease.[34, 35, 41] The classification proposed by the National Wilms' Tumor Study is the one most commonly used in the United States[141] and has also been adopted by the International Society of Pediatric Oncology (Table 15-4).[66a] In general, those with more extensive spread of disease have a poorer prognosis. It is of interest, however, that in a number of reports, there is a better long-term survival rate in patients with Group IV or V disease than in those with Group III disease.[5, 14, 97]

A retrospective analysis of 52 patients treated at St. Jude Children's Research Hospital revealed that local tumor recurrence was more common when the neoplasm had extended or ruptured through the capsule at the time of nephrectomy, and systemic metastases were most frequent in those with gross or microscopic renal vascular or lymphatic invasion (Table 15-5). The investigators who reported these findings proposed that both capsular and vascular invasion be included as a part of future staging systems.[63]

EVALUATION OF THE PATIENT

The older view that Wilms' tumor be treated as a surigcal emergency is no longer accepted. Although the preoperative evaluation should be carried out with as little delay as possible, it is more important that the appropriate studies be completed and that the child be in good condition for surgery than that he be immediately rushed to the operating room. An aspiration needle biopsy, advocated a number of years ago, is contraindicated, since tumor can seed the needle tract or spill into the peritoneal cavity.

The preliminary investigation of a child with an abdominal mass should include abdominal roentgenograms and an intravenous pyelogram. These studies often differentiate between hydronephrosis, multicystic kidney, Wilms' tumor, or neuroblastoma. If neuroblastoma is suspected, urine should be collected for determination of catecholamine levels before the tumor is removed. The intravenous pyelogram will usually demonstrate an intrarenal mass with distorted calyces if a Wilms' tumor is present (Fig. 15-3), but similar findings may occur in the presence of a hypernephroma, mesoblastic nephroma, or renal ab-

Table 15-5 Effect of Capsular and Vascular Tumor Invasion on Prognosis

	PATIENTS	LOCAL RECURRENCE	METASTASES	DEATHS
Capsular	17	6	4	8
Vascular	9	0	6	6
Both	17	3	7	5
Neither	9	0	1	0

Based on the data of Kumar and associates.[63]

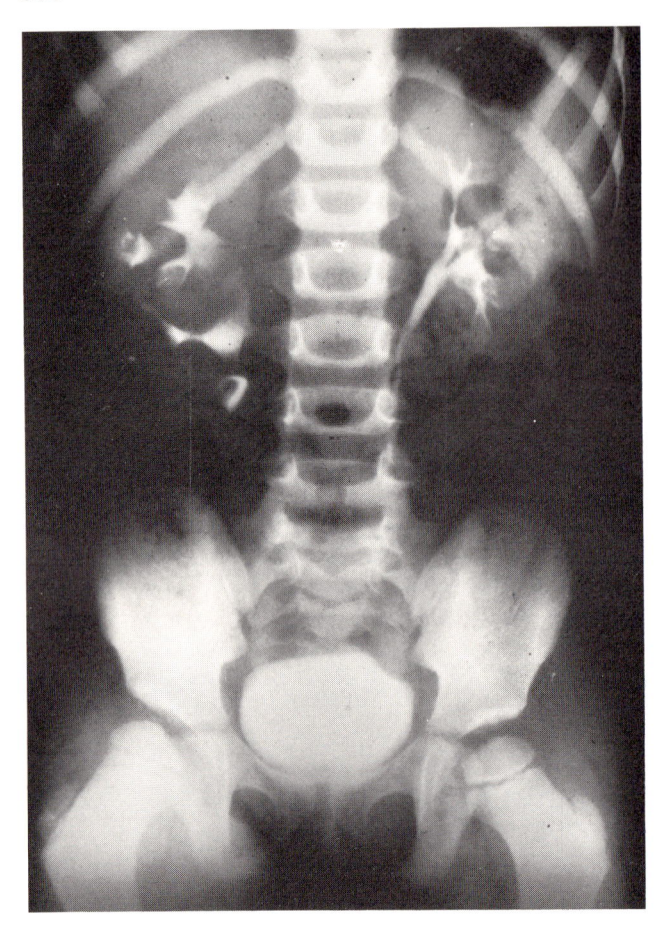

Figure 15-3 Intravenous pyelogram in a patient with a flank mass demonstrating distortion of the right calyceal system. At surgery, a Wilms' tumor arising from the right lower renal pole was found. (Courtesy of Dr. J. O. Salik, Radiologist-in-Chief, Sinai Hospital of Baltimore.)

scess.[114] It is not unusual for the involved kidney not to be visualized if the renal function is severely impaired. Important information regarding the function and possible involvement of the contralateral kidney may significantly influence the surgical procedure, since renal anomalies, such as congenital absence of the contralateral kidney, are sometimes associated with Wilms' tumor. Some have advocated the routine use of an inferior venacavogram followed by the excretory urogram to help determine the size of the tumor and possible extension into the renal vein or vena cava.[61] Chest roentgenograms should be obtained, because hematogenous metastases in children with Wilms' tumor are most frequently discovered in the lung (Fig. 15–4). A liver-spleen scan may help detect the presence of hepatic metastases.

There is presently no laboratory test specific for Wilms' tumor, but some cases have been reported to have a mucinous substance in the peripheral blood and urine,[86, 101] and others have been demonstrated to have a glycoprotein antigen in the blood.[132]

INITIAL TREATMENT

Surgery

Surgery should be performed as soon as initial evaluation has been completed and any underlying problems, such as anemia, electrolyte imbalance, or hypertension, have been corrected. Some physicians have used preoperative irradiation or chemotherapy in an effort to shrink the tumor

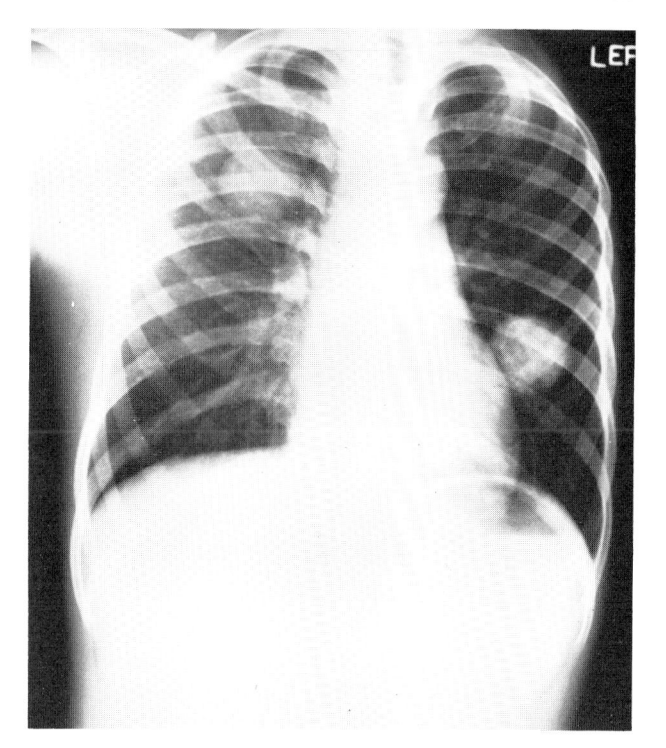

Figure 15-4 Chest roentgenogram of a child with an abdominal mass found at surgery to be a Wilms' tumor. Two metastatic pulmonary lesions are present.

mass to make surgical removal simpler and decrease the possibility of rupture of a large tumor. A dramatic reduction in size can usually be achieved by either of these means.[111, 120, 130] At the present time, preoperative treatment is seldom used in most centers in the United States unless the tumor is massive.

There is at present no evidence that preoperative radiation therapy[66a] or preoperative vincristine treatment[22a] significantly influences survival. However, results from the clinical trial conducted by the International Society of Pediatric Oncology indicate a significant decrease in the incidence of tumor rupture during surgery in those who received preoperative radiation therapy.[66a]

The tumor should be approached through a large transabdominal incision, and the vessels of the renal pedicle of the involved kidney should be examined to determine if they are involved with tumor. If free of tumor, the vessels should be ligated before mobilizing the kidney and tumor mass. If there is tumor extension into renal vein and inferior vena cava, it must be removed prior to vessel ligation to prevent tumor embolization. The kidney and tumor should then be excised along with adjacent perirenal tissue and adjacent lymph nodes. The surgeon should examine the abdominal contents, including the liver and contralateral kidney, and biopsy any suspicious areas. Suspected or obviously involved lymph nodes should be removed. However, there is often a poor correlation between the gross appearance and microscopic involvement of lymph nodes.[73] Some have advocated para-aortic node dissection,[5, 73] but this is not routinely performed, since there are no data to indicate that it is of benefit when used along with current methods of therapy. Following surgical resection, the tumor bed and any residual tumor should be outlined with metallic clips to guide the radiation therapist if this mode of therapy is later used.

Radiation Therapy

Wilms' tumor is generally a radiosensitive neoplasm. Radiation therapy can usually be safely begun 2 to 3 days following surgery. In the past, children with tumors classified as Group I or II received radiation to the tumor bed. The doses recommended in the National Wilms' Tumor Study (NWTS) are listed in Table 15-6; however, lower doses in the range of 2500 rads given in 20 fractions have been reported to be adequate.[51] The entire width of the vertebral bodies should be included in the field to minimize late asymmetric growth deformities. Data collected by the NWTS show a 2-year actuarial survival rate for Group I patients under 2 years of age to be 97 per cent for those treated with radiation therapy and actinomycin D and 94 per cent for those treated with actinomycin D alone, suggesting that radiation adds little therapeutic benefit to the young child with Group I tumor.[22a, 141] However, not enough data is yet available to determine whether or not the child over the age of 2 years with Group I disease requires tumor bed irradiation to decrease the chances of flank recurrence. For these older children, 2 year relapse-free survival rates in the radiated and nonirradiated groups were 77 per cent and 58 per cent, respectively, but the percentage of patients alive at 2 years were 97 per cent and 91 per cent. The statistical analysis suggests an increased rate of abdominal recurrence in the nonirradiated group.[22a] Few deaths have occurred, even among the patients with relapse, and the observed difference between the two treatment regimens could be due to chance.[22a] The second NWTS does not include radiation therapy in the treatment of children with Group I tumors, but combination chemotherapy with vincristine and actinomycin D is advocated. At present, patients in all other groups receive radiation to the tumor bed.

All Group III patients were initially believed to require whole abdominal irradiation. However, it appears that localized irradiation to the involved renal fossa is sufficient, even for cases with tumor spillage at surgery, if the spill is localized to the tumor bed.[124] Children who have diffuse peritoneal contamination, however, should receive whole abdominal irradiation.

Pulmonary involvement at the time of diagnosis should not delay surgery unless the lung involvement is significant enough to increase the anesthetic risk. Initial roentgenographic evidence of lung metastases is not usually associated with any significant decrease in pulmonary function. Following surgery, both lungs should be irradiated during the time radiation is being delivered to the abdomen if there is any evidence of pulmonary involvement.

Hepatic metastases which are not surgically resectable at the initial operation should be treated with radiation. However, severe chronic hepatic impairment has been reported to occur following a major hepatic resection if radiation and chemotherapy are used during the time of liver regeneration.[32] It has been suggested that a large hepatic resection be avoided during the initial operation because it would delay initiating therapy, and that resection be considered later if the liver involvement does not respond to radiation and chemotherapy.[51]

Table 15-6 Recommended Doses of Radiation Therapy to Tumor Bed (NWTS)

AGE	RECOMMENDED DOSE (RADS)
0–18 months	1800–2400
19–30 months	2400–3000
31–40 months	3000–3500
41 months or older	3500–4000

Chemotherapy

The dramatic effect of actinomycin D on Wilms' tumor was documented by Farber in 1966, who reported an 89 per cent survival rate in children with no evidence of metastatic disease at the time of diagnosis who were followed for at least 2 years, and a 53 per cent survival rate in those who presented with evidence of metastatic disease.[31] The drug therapy appeared to prevent clinical hematogenous metastases from occurring following surgical removal and radiation to the tumor bed, presumably by destroying nondetectable microscopic tumor foci, especially in the lungs. Multiple courses of actinomycin D have been shown to be more effective than a single course in preventing pulmonary metastases in patients with Groups I and II disease. Eighty-six per cent of subjects receiving maintenance chemotherapy had no recurrence, compared with 48 per cent without recurrence in the group given a single course of actinomycin D.[143] However, there was no significant difference in long-term survival between the two groups.[142] Multiple courses of therapy with actinomycin D are still preferred, because fewer relapses require fewer additional control measures; thus, there is less morbidity from both disease and treatment.[142] A course of actinomycin D consists of five consecutive days of intravenous therapy in a dose of 15 μg/kg/day, with no single injection exceeding 500 μg.

Vincristine sulfate has also been found to be an effective drug in the treatment of Wilms' tumor.[120, 129] This agent has been shown to produce a response in patients who have had prior therapy with actinomycin D.[121] Vincristine appears to be as effective as actinomycin D, but the combination of the two is more effective than either drug alone. The combined 2-year actuarial survival in children with Groups II and III disease has been reported to be 67 per cent for those receiving actinomycin D alone, 72 per cent for those treated with vincristine alone, and 86 per cent for patients given both drugs.[22a] Clinical trials have demonstrated that Adriamycin[133] also has activity against Wilms' tumor and may further improve the response in those with more advanced disease when used in combination with other agents. However, the cardiotoxicity induced by this drug may be further potentiated by radiation therapy to the chest. This complication has been fatal in a child with Wilms' tumor treated with thoracic radiation for pulmonary metastases.[43] Cyclophosphamide also has been found to have some effect against this neoplasm.[33]

Metastatic Recurrence of Disease

The lungs are the most common site of tumor recurrence. Therefore, chest roentgenograms should be obtained routinely every 1 to 2 months during the first year of therapy and periodically thereafter. Whenever a pulmonary lesion is noted, tomographic examination of the lungs should be performed, since the lesions are often multiple. A number of patients with pulmonary metastases have been cured by irradiation to both lungs, chemotherapy, and, in selected cases, surgical excision.[1, 135, 137]

The liver is the second most common organ involved with metastatic disease. Apparent cures have been reported following surgical removal of localized hepatic metastases by partial or complete hepatic lobectomy followed by radiation and chemotherapy.[115, 135] The dangers of initiating therapy soon after hepatic resection have been mentioned previously.[32]

Rarely, Wilms' tumor has metastasized to brain, bone, bone marrow, salivary glands, tonsils, and other unusual sites[87] (Fig. 15–5). The tumor cells in the marrow are morphologically different from neuroblastoma cells.[87, 94] Occasionally patients with cerebral metastases have survived following radiation and chemotherapy, with or without surgical removal of the metastatic lesions.[83a, 85, 128]

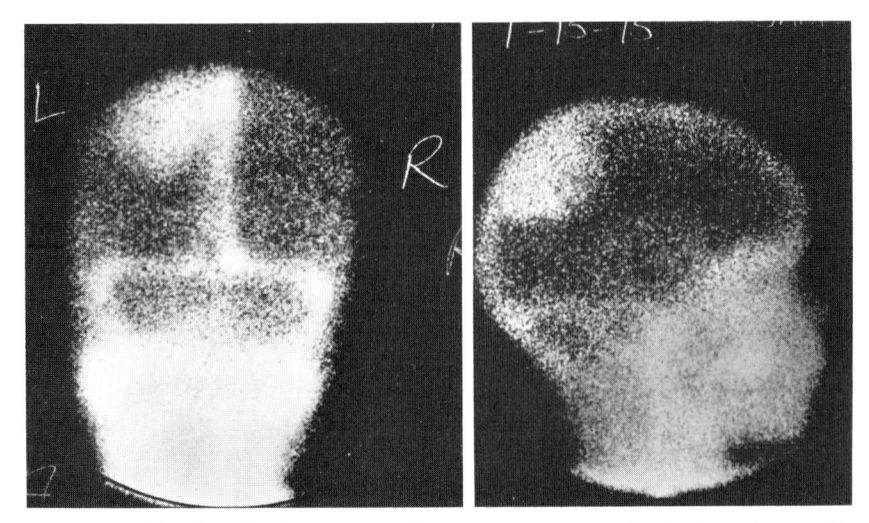

Figure 15–5 Child with Wilms' tumor and pulmonary metastases who developed generalized convulsions. Brain scan revealed a left parietal lesion. The mass lesion and all neurological symptoms disappeared following radiation therapy.

BILATERAL WILMS' TUMOR

Children with bilateral Wilms' tumor may present with neoplasms in both kidneys initially (Fig. 15–6), or be found to have tumor in the second kidney later, sometimes as long as 10 years after the initial diagnosis.[107] It is generally believed that these are usually separate primary tumors rather than the result of metastatic disease. This hypothesis is supported by the observation that remote metastases from Wilms' tumors usually first appear in the lung, but the lungs are seldom involved in patients with bilateral renal involvement.[22a] The children with simultaneously occurring bilateral tumors usually have multifocal tumors in both kidneys, are younger than the average patient with Wilms' tumor, and have 10 times the incidence of associated congenital anomalies than those with unilateral disease.[12,13] The maternal age at the time of the child's birth is usually older than average.[13]

Treatment of children with bilateral renal involvement must be highly individualized. Approaches have included heminephrectomy of the least involved kidney and nephrectomy of the other, extensive bilateral partial nephrectomy, unilateral nephrectomy followed by radiation therapy to the remaining kidney, medical treatment without surgery, and bilateral nephrectomy followed by renal transplantation.[8,25,102,122] Radiation therapy to the one remaining kidney must be judiciously used in an effort to avoid radiation nephritis and possible renal failure. The outlook in these patients is far from hopeless. A survival rate of approximately 50 per cent has been reported in most series.[5,13,97] A high incidence of late metastases has been noted in this group of children, suggesting that chemotherapy may have to be continued for a longer period than for other groups.[5]

PROGNOSIS

Improvement in survival has occurred in patients with all stages of Wilms' tumor and appears to be the result of therapeutic advances rather than earlier detection.[30] The addition of radiation therapy to surgery increased the survival rate to between 40 and 50 per cent, and the use of chemotherapeutic agents continues to

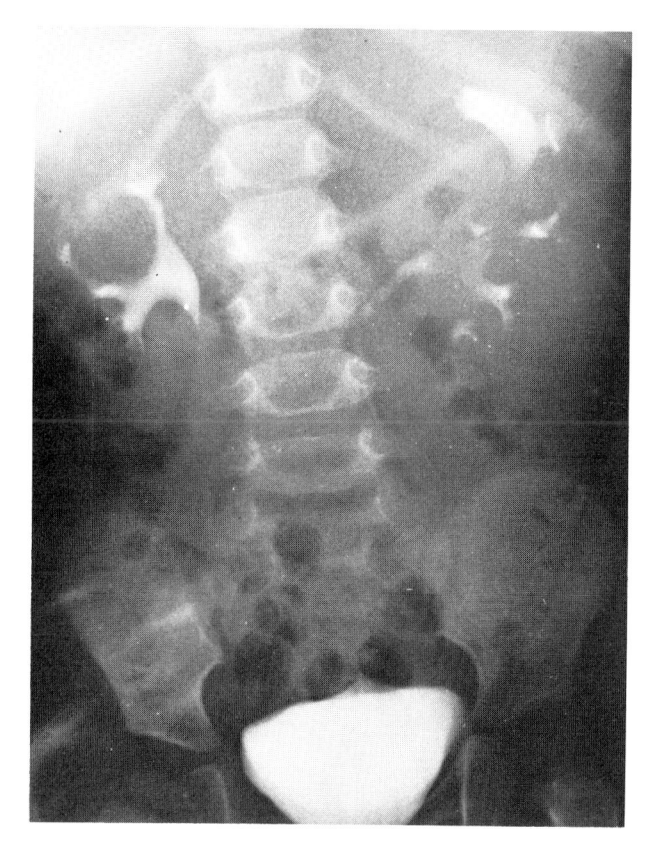

Figure 15-6 Child with bilateral flank masses which were both found to be Wilms' tumors. Both calyceal systems reveal evidence of intrarenal lesions on the intravenous pyelogram.

improve the survival rate. The chances of a patient's experiencing long-term survival has more than doubled between 1940–1949 (26 per cent) and 1965–1969 (61 per cent).[30] Initial results of the National Wilms' Tumor Study, begun in 1969, reveal a 2-year actuarial survival rate of over 95 per cent in patients with Group I tumors treated with actinomycin D with or without radiation, and 92 per cent in those with Group II or III tumors treated with radiation, vincristine, and actinomycin D. At the present time, the survival rate is greater than 80 per cent in patients with localized tumor, and about 50 per cent in those with metastatic disease.[141]

COMPLICATIONS OF THERAPY

Hematologic, neurologic, and gastrointestinal complications often occur in patients with malignant disorders treated with chemotherapeutic agents and are discussed elsewhere. However, a number of potentially life-threatening side effects commonly seen following the treatment of Wilms' tumor appear to be due mainly to radiation therapy and are often potentiated by the addition of chemotherapy. Of 14 deaths occurring among 140 patients who survived for 36 months after diagnosis, Li and coworkers[67] reported that 9 died in remission as a result of treatment-associated disorders. Four died of second neoplasms in irradiated sites, and five had either renal or pulmonary failure following treatment of these organs with surgery, irradiation, and actinomycin D.

Gastrointestinal Problems

Vomiting and diarrhea may become severe during the postoperative period when actinomycin D and radiation therapy are being administered. This occasionally necessitates interrupting treatment. The symptoms are usually worse in the younger child and the patient who requires total abdominal radiation. A number of children have developed a delayed intestinal syndrome of radiation enteritis within 2 months of completion of radiotherapy, with an acute onset of vomiting and diarrhea, and a distended abdomen.[27] A special diet free of gluten, lactose, and bovine protein, with limited amounts of fat and residue, has been reported to be of value in treating children with radiation enteritis and malabsorption.[27] The child may also develop small bowel obstruction due to adhesions, fibrosis, or intussusception.[48, 62]

Hepatic Damage

Severe hepatic damage can occur following radiation to the liver. This complication most commonly occurs in children with right-sided tumors when the radiation field includes a portion of the right lobe of the liver, or when total abdominal radiation is used. There may be transient hepatic enlargement, a decrease in blood counts, and abnormalities in liver function.[76, 108] Liver-spleen scanning often reveals lack of hepatic reticuloendothelial uptake of Tc-99m sulfur colloid in the irradiated area. The symptoms may reappear during subsequent courses of actinomycin D therapy.[125] The hepatic enlargement and a filling defect on scan may sometimes be mistaken for liver involvement with tumor. Occasionally, severe portal hypertension may gradually develop.[135]

Renal Problems

Acute radiation nephritis may occur a few months following radiation to the remaining kidney. Significant amounts of radiation are given to a single kidney when the entire abdomen is treated, when a Wilms' tumor is present in a unilateral kidney, or when there is bilateral renal involvement and the most involved kidney is removed, with the remaining kidney being treated with radiotherapy. Chemotherapeutic agents appear to make the kidney more susceptible to radiation nephritis.[4] The patient may develop edema, microscopic hematuria, azotemia, and other evidence of impaired renal function.

Chronic nephritis has been known to occur long after radiation exposure. Fatal renal failure has been reported as late as 18 years following treatment of 1400 rads to the remaining kidney of a 3 month old child.[93] The course of chronic nephritis is usually slow and progressive, and may occur despite the absence of a history of acute nephritis. It appears that normal renal function can be preserved in children after unilateral nephrectomy, irradiation, and administration of chemotherapy provided that irradiation to the remaining kidney is kept below 1200 rads.[83]

Pulmonary Complications

Therapeutic irradiation to the lungs may result in an acute interstitial pneumonitis 1 to 3 months following radiotherapy. This may be asymptomatic or cause mild cough, fever, and respiratory discomfort. Symptoms usually disappear in less than one month. The development of radiation pneumonitis is influenced by the dose of radiation, the fractionation of the volume of lung treated, infection, and the use of drugs such as actinomycin D.[134] The acute reaction may subside or progress to an irreversible fibrosis. Long-term effects of therapeutic pulmonary irradiation given during a period of lung growth include a decrease in the subsequent size of both the lung and chest wall.[140] Although abnormal pulmonary function studies have been demonstrated in patients years following whole lung irradiation, the changes are not generally severe if appropriate doses were initially given by an experienced radiotherapist.[70]

Orthopedic Sequelae

Significant orthopedic deformities commonly occur years following radiation therapy to the growing child. The changes are more severe in children treated before the age of 2 years and in those who received higher doses of radiation.[91] The skeletal sequelae observed by Katzman and co-workers[55] on 28 patients followed 3 to 24 years after treatment included changes in the vertebral bodies, scoliosis, hypoplasia of the ilium and rib cage, osteocartilaginous exostoses, and epiphyseal destruction with limb-length discrepancy and deformity.

Oncogenic Complications

There have been numerous reports of second neoplastic diseases developing in patients years following completion of therapy and apparent cure of their primary malignancy. Soft tissue sarcomas, bone tumors, hepatomas, thyroid carcinomas, and leukemia have occurred in children who were originally treated for Wilms' tumor.[21, 68, 110] Most second malignancies have been attributed to prior radiotherapy, and the solid tumors have usually appeared within the field of radiation. A number of cases of apparent transformation of the malignant Wilms' tumor to benign rhabdomyoma have been reported following radiation therapy.[137a] One interesting report indicates that the risk of developing secondary neoplasms following radiation therapy is decreased in patients who received actinomycin D.[23]

CONGENITAL MESOBLASTIC NEPHROMA

A unique group of neonatal renal tumors has been confused with the classical Wilms' tumor in the past. These neoplasms, now considered to be a separate group of entities, are termed mesoblastic nephromas or fetal renal hamartomas (Fig. 15–7). They were clearly distinguished from Wilms' tumor in 1967 by Bolande and co-workers,[11] who emphasized their benign nature. It is likely that the

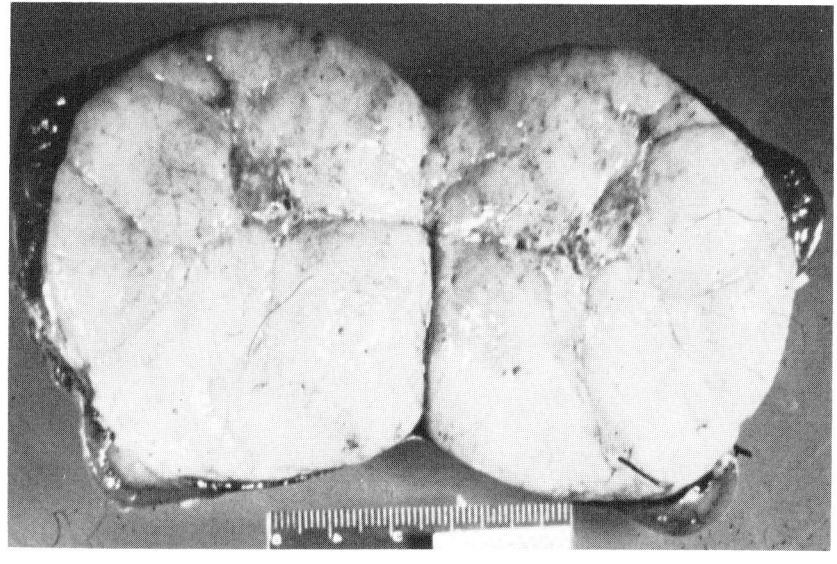

Figure 15–7 Congenital mesoblastic nephroma removed from a neonate. The tumor is compressing and nearly totally replacing the normal kidney.

previous confusion with Wilms' tumor accounts at least in part for the excellent survival rate reported in infants who had what were mistakenly called Group I nephroblastomas.

The involved kidney is usually greatly enlarged and distorted by the tumor, but, unlike Wilms' tumor, there is usually no lobulation, necrosis, hemorrhage, or discrete capsule between the neoplasm and the compressed kidney. Histologically, there is a preponderance of interlacing bundles of spindle-shaped cells within which dysplastic tubules and glomeruli are irregularly scattered.

The vast majority of patients have been cured by nephrectomy alone.[7, 10] There is good evidence that more patients with mesoblastic nephroma have died as a result of aggressive chemotherapy and radiation therapy than from the tumor.[104, 138] In very rare instances, the tumor has been unusually aggressive.[53, 131] Because of the occasional case in which there is tumor recurrence, additional therapy is indicated beyond surgical removal of the involved kidney when the surgical margins are involved or uncertain, or when the typical histologic appearance is not present.[7]

RENAL CELL CARCINOMA

Renal cell carcinoma (hypernephroma, Grawitz tumor, clear cell carcinoma of the kidney) seldom occurs in children. Most children are 5 years or older at the time of diagnosis,[19, 24] but cases presenting during the first year of life have been reported.[19, 100] The patient usually presents with hematuria, pain, or an abdominal mass. Occasionally the child manifests hypertension due to excessive production of renin by the tumor.[84] The appearance of the intravenous pyelogram is similar to that seen in Wilms' tumor, but calcifications are more commonly found in association with the renal cell carcinoma than with Wilms' tumor.[19] The tumor most commonly metastasizes to the lungs, liver, regional lymph nodes, and bones. The presence of renal vascular invasion and the absence of a fibrous pseudocapsule appear to be the most ominous anatomic features.[24]

A review of childhood renal cell carcinoma by Castellanos and associates[19] revealed that the actuarial survival for 2 years was 50 of 84 patients, for 5 years was 47 of 84, and for 10 years was 42 of 84. Thus the overall survival is about 50 per cent.[19, 24] However, there were no survivors of 31 patients with direct vascular invasion or distant metastases.

Nephrectomy appears to be sufficient therapy for those with localized encapsulated tumors. If there is residual tumor, radiation therapy may be of value, but the tumor is not as radiosensitive as is Wilms' tumor, and larger doses are therefore needed. Up to the present time, chemotherapeutic agents[123] or hormonal therapy[2] has been of little value.

REFERENCES

1. Albers, D. D., Bell, A. H., Kalmon, E. H., et al.: Pulmonary excision for solitary metastasis from a Wilms' tumor with apparent cure. J. Urol. 86:43, 1961.
2. Alberto, P., and Senn, H. J.: Hormonal therapy of renal carcinoma alone and in association with cytostatic drugs. Cancer 33:1226, 1974.
3. Anselmi, G., Suárez, J. A., Machado, I., et al.: Wilms' tumour propagated through the inferior vena cava into the right heart cavities. Brit. Heart J. 32:575, 1970.
4. Arneil, G. C., Harris, F., Emmanuel, I. G., et al.: Nephritis in two children after irradiation and chemotherapy for nephroblastoma. Lancet 1:960, 1974.
5. Aron, B. S.: Wilms' tumor—a clinical study of eighty-one patients. Cancer 33:637, 1974.
6. Barakat, A. Y., Papadoupoulou, Z. L., Chandra, R. S., et al.: Pseudohermaphroditisim, nephron disorder and Wilms' tumor: a unifying concept. Pediatrics 54:366, 1974.
7. Beckwith, J. B.: Mesenchymal renal neoplasms of infancy revisited. J. Pediatr. Surg. 9:803, 1974.

8. Bishop, H. C., and Hope, J. W.: Bilateral Wilms' tumors. J. Pediatr. Surg. *1*:476, 1966.
9. Blackard, C., and Mellinger, G. T.: Cancer in a horse-shoe kidney. Arch. Surg. 97:616, 1968.
10. Bolande, R. P.: Congenital and infantile neoplasia of the kidney. Lancet *2*:1497, 1974.
11. Bolande, R. P., Brough, A. J., and Izant, R. J., Jr.: Congenital mesoblastic nephroma of infancy. A report of eight cases and the relationship to Wilms' tumor. Pediatrics *40*:272, 1967.
12. Bond, J. V.: Bilateral Wilms' tumour and urinary-tract anomalies. Lancet *2*:721, 1975.
13. Bond, J. V.: Bilateral Wilms' tumour. Age at diagnosis, associated congenital anomalies, and possible pattern of inheritance. Lancet *2*:482, 1975.
14. Bond, J. V.: Prognosis and treatment of Wilms' tumor at Great Ormond Street Hospital for Sick Children. Cancer *36*:1202, 1975.
15. Boxer, L. A., and Smith, D. L.: Wilms' tumor prior to onset of hemihypertrophy. Am. J. Dis. Child. *120*:564, 1970.
16. Bradley, J. E., and Pincoffs, M. C.: Association of adeno-myo-sarcoma of the kidney (Wilms' tumor) with arterial hypertension. Ann. Intern. Med. *11*:1613, 1938.
17. Brown, W. T., Puranik, S. R., Altman, D. H., et al.: Wilms' tumor in three successive generations. Surgery *72*:756, 1972.
18. Cassady, J. R., Tefft, M., Filler, R. M., et al.: Considerations in the radiation therapy of Wilms' tumor. Cancer *32*:598, 1973.
19. Castellanos, R. D., Aron, B. S., and Evans, A. T.: Renal adenocarcinoma in children: incidence, therapy, and prognosis. J. Urol. *111*:534, 1974.
20. Cochran, W., and Froggatt, P.: Bilateral nephroblastoma in two sisters. J. Urol. *97*:216, 1967.
21. Cohen, J., and D'Angio, G. J.: Unusual bone tumors after roentgen therapy of children: two case reports. Am. J. Roentgenol. *86*:502, 1961.
22. D'Angio, G. J., Beckwith, J. B., Bishop, H., et al.: The National Wilms' Tumor Study—preliminary results. Proc. Am. Ass. Cancer Res. *15*:68, 1974.
22a. D'Angio, G. J., Evans, A. E., Breslow, N., et al.: The treatment of Wilms' tumor: results of the National Wilms' Tumor Study. Cancer *38*:633, 1976.
23. D'Angio, G. J., Meadows, A., Miké, V., et al.: Decreased risk of radiation-associated second neoplasms in actinomycin-D treated patients. Cancer *37*:1177, 1976.
24. Dehner, L. P., Leestma, J. E., and Price, E. B., Jr.: Renal cell carcinoma in children—a clinicopathologic study of 15 cases and review of the literature. J. Pediatr. *76*:358, 1970.
25. deLorimier, A., Belzer, F. O., Kountz, S. L., et al.: Simultaneous bilateral nephrectomy and renal allotransplantation for bilateral Wilms' tumor. Surgery *64*:850, 1968.
26. Denys, P., Malvaux, P., Van den Berghe, H., et al.: Association d'un syndrome anatomo-pathologique de pseudohermaphrodisme masculin, d'une tumeur de Wilms, d'une nephropathie parenchymateuse et d'un mosaicisme XX/XY. Arch. Franç. Pediatr. *24*:729, 1967.
27. Donaldson, S. S., Jundt, S., Ricour, C., et al.: Radiation enteritis in children. A retrospective review, clinicopathologic correlation, and dietary management. Cancer *35*:1167, 1975.
28. Drash, A., Sherman, F., Hartmann, W. H., et al.: A syndrome of pseudohermaphroditism, Wilms' tumor, hypertension, and degenerative renal disease. J. Pediatr. *76*:585, 1970.
29. Edelstein, G.: Extra-renal Wilms' tumour. Am. J. Surg. *109*:509, 1965.
30. Everson, R. B., and Fraumeni, J. F., Jr.: Declining mortality and improving survival from Wilms' tumor. Med. Pediatr. Oncol. *1*:3, 1975.
31. Farber, S.: Chemotherapy in the treatment of leukemia and Wilms' tumor. J.A.M.A. *198*:826, 1966.
32. Filler, R. M., Tefft, M., Vawter, G. F., et al.: Hepatic lobectomy in childhood: effects of x-ray and chemotherapy. J. Pediatr. Surg. *4*:31, 1969.
33. Finklestein, J. Z., Hittle, R. E., and Hammond, G. D.: Evaluation of a high dose cyclophosphamide regimen in childhood tumors. Cancer *23*:1239, 1969.
34. Fleming, I., and Pinkel, D.: Clinical staging of Wilms' tumor. J. Pediatr. *74*:324, 1969.
35. Fleming, I. D., and Johnson, W. W.: Clinical and pathological staging as a guide in the management of Wilms' tumor. Cancer *26*:660, 1970.
36. Fraumeni, J. F., Jr., Geiser, C. F., and Manning, M. D.: Wilms' tumor and congenital hemihypertrophy: Report of five new cases and review of the literature. Pediatrics *40*:886, 1967.
37. Fraumeni, J. F., Jr.: The aniridia–Wilms' tumor syndrome. Birth Defects *V*:198, 1969.
38. Fraumeni, J. F., Jr., and Miller, R. W.: Adrenocortical neoplasms with hemihypertrophy, brain tumors, and other disorders. J. Pediatr. *70*:129, 1967.
39. Fraumeni, J. F., Jr., Miller, R. W., and Hill, J. A.: Primary carcinoma of the liver in childhood: an epidemiologic study. J. Natl. Cancer Inst. *40*:1087, 1968.
40. Gairdner, E.: Case of fungus haematodes in

the kidneys. Edinburgh Med. Surg. J. 29:312, 1828.
41. Garcia, M., Douglass, C., and Schlosser, J. V.: Classification and prognosis in Wilms' tumor. Radiology 80:574, 1963.
42. Gaulin, E.: Simultaneous Wilms' tumors in identical twins. J. Urol. 66:547, 1951.
43. Gerber, M. A., Gilbert, E. M., and Chung, K. J.: Adriamycin cardiotoxicity in a child with Wilms' tumor: Report of a case and review of the literature. J. Pediatr. 87:629, 1975.
44. Giangiacomo, J., Penchansky, L., Monteleone, P. L., et al.: Bilateral neonatal Wilms' tumor with B-C chromosomal translocation. J. Pediatr. 86:98, 1975.
45. Geiser, C. F., and Schindler, A. M.: Long-term survival in a male with 18-trisomy syndrome and Wilms' tumor. Pediatrics 44:111, 1969.
46. Goldschmidt, H., and Bachman, K. D.: Der Wilms-tumor beim Neugeborenen. Wochenschrift 104:658, 1974.
47. Gross, R. E., and Neuhauser, E. B. D.: Treatment of mixed tumors of the kidneys in childhood. Pediatrcs 6:843, 1950.
48. Guttman, F. M., Ducharme, J. C., and Collin, P. P.: Intussusception after major abdominal operations in children. Can. J. Surg. 13:427, 1970.
49. Haiken, B. N., and Miller, D. R.: Simultaneous occurrence of congenital aniridia, hamartoma, and Wilms' tumor. J. Pediatr. 78:497, 1971.
50. Hartenstein, H.: Wilms' tumor in a newborn infant: report of a case with autopsy studies. J. Pediatr. 35:381, 1949.
50a. Janik, J. S., and Seeler, R. A. Delayed onset of hemihypertrophy in Wilms' tumor. J. Pediatr. Surg. 11:581, 1976.
51. Jenkin, R. D. T.: The treatment of Wilms' tumor. Pediatr. Clin. North Am. 23:147, 1976.
52. Jereb, B., and Sandstedt, B.: Structure and size versus prognosis in nephroblastoma. Cancer 31:1473, 1973.
53. Joshi, V. V., Kay, S., Milsten, R., et al.: Congenital mesoblastic nephroma of infancy: Report of a case with unusual clinical behavior. Am. J. Clin. Pathol. 60:811, 1973.
54. Juberg, R. C., Martin, E. C., and Handley, J. R.: Familial occurrence of Wilms' tumor: Nephroblastoma in one of monozygous twins and in another sibling. Am. J. Hum. Genet. 27:155, 1975.
55. Katzman, H., Waugh, T., and Berdon, W.: Skeletal changes following irradiation of childhood tumors. J. Bone Joint Surg. 51A:825, 1969.
56. Kaufman, R. L., Vietti, T. J., and Wabner, C. I.: Wilms' tumour in father and son. Lancet 1:43, 1973.
57. Kaushik, S., Schdeva, H., and Dutta, B.: Renal embryoma in an adult. Ann. Surg. 38:468, 1972.
58. Kenney, G. M., Webster, J. H., Sinks, L. M., et al.: Results from treatment of Wilms' tumor at Roswell Park, 1927–1968. J. Surg. Oncol. 1:49, 1969.
59. Kinzel, R. C., Miles, S. D., Childs, D. S., Jr., et al.: Wilms' tumor: a review of 47 cases. J.A.M.A. 174:1925, 1960.
60. Knudson, A. G., Jr., and Strong, L. C.: Mutation and cancer: a model for Wilms' tumor of the kidney. J. Natl. Cancer Inst. 48:313, 1972.
61. Koop, C. E., and Kaufman, H. J.: The diagnosis of cancer in children. Semin. Oncol. 1:5, 1974.
62. Kuffer, F., Fortner, J., and Murphy, M. L.: Surgical complications of children undergoing cancer therapy. Ann. Surg. 167:21, 1968.
63. Kumar, A. P. M., Hustu, O., Fleming, I. D., et al.: Capsular and vascular invasion: Important prognostic factors in Wilms' tumor. J. Pediatr. Surg. 10:301, 1975.
64. Ladda, R., Atkins, L., Littlefield, J., et al.: Computer-assisted analysis of chromosomal abnormalities: detection of a deletion in aniridia/Wilms' tumor syndrome. Science 185:784, 1974.
65. Lawler, W., Marsden, H. B., and Palmer, M. K.: Wilms' tumor—histologic variation and prognosis. Cancer 36:1122, 1975.
66. Lemerle, J., Tournade, M., Gerard-Marchant, R., et al.: Wilms' tumor: natural history and prognostic factors. Cancer 37:2557, 1976.
66a. Lemerle, J., Voute, P. A., Tournade, M. F., et al.: Preoperative versus postoperative radiotherapy, single versus multiple courses of actinomycin D, in the treatment of Wilms' tumor. Cancer 38:647, 1976.
67. Li, F. P., Biship, Y., and Katsioules, C.: Survival in Wilms' tumour. Lancet 1:41, 1975.
68. Li, F. P., Cassady, J. R., and Jaffe, N.: Risk of second tumors in survivors of childhood cancer. Cancer 35:1230, 1975.
69. Lines, D. R.: Nephrotic syndrome and nephroblastoma. J. Pediatr. 72:264, 1968.
70. Littman, P., Meadows, A. T., Polgar, G., et al.: Pulmonary function in survivors of Wilms' tumor. Cancer 37:2773, 1976.
71. Mankad, V. N., Gray, G. F., Jr., and Miller, D. R.: Bilateral nephroblastomatosis and Klippel Trenaunay syndrome. Cancer 33:1462, 1974.
72. Marosvári, I., Kontor, E., and Kállay, K.: Renin-secreting Wilms' tumour. Lancet 1:1180, 1972.
73. Martin, L. W., and Reyes, P. M.: An evaluation of 10 years' experience with retroperitoneal lymph node dissection

74. Maslow, L. A.: Wilms' tumor: report of three cases and a possible fourth one in the same family. J. Urol. 43:75, 1940.
75. McDonald, J. R., and Priestly, J. T.: Malignant tumors of the kidney. Surgical and prognostic significance of tumor thrombosis of the renal vein. Surg. Gynec. Obstet. 77:295, 1943.
76. McVeagh, P., and Ekert, H.: Hepatotoxicity of chemotherapy following nephrectomy and radiation therapy for right-sided Wilms' tumor. J. Pediatr. 87:627, 1975.
77. Meadows, A. T., Lichtenfeld, J. L., and Koop, C. E.: Wilms's tumor in three children of a woman with congenital hemihypertrophy. N. Engl. J. Med. 291:23, 1974.
78. Merten, D. F., Yang, S. S., and Bernstein, J.: Wilms' tumor in adolescence. Cancer 37:1532, 1976.
79. Miller, R. W.: Relation between cancer and congenital defects: an epidemiologic evaluation. J. Natl. Cancer Inst. 40:1079, 1968.
80. Miller, R. W.: Wilms' tumor: evidence against Knudson's hypothesis (?). Childhood Cancer Etiology Newsletter No. 15, 1975.
81. Miller, R. W., Fraumeni, J. F., Jr., and Manning, M. D.: Association of Wilms' tumor with aniridia, hemihypertrophy, and other congenital malformations. N. Engl. J. Med. 270:922, 1964.
82. Mitchell, J. D., Baxter, T. J., Blair-West, J. R., et al.: Renin levels in nephroblastoma (Wilms' tumor). Arch. Dis. Child. 45:376, 1970.
83. Mitus, A., Tefft, M., and Fellers, F. X.: Long-term follow-up of renal function of 108 children who underwent nephrectomy for malignant disease. Pediatrics 44:912, 1969.
83a. Mohammad, A. M., Meyer, J., and Hakami, N.: Long-term survival following brain metastasis of Wilms' tumor. J. Pediatr. 90:660, 1977.
84. More, I. A. R., Jackson, A. M., and MacSween, R. N. M.: Renin-secreting tumor associated with hypertension. Cancer 34:2093, 1974.
85. Morgan, S. K., and Buse, M. G.: Survival following brain metastases in Wilms' tumor. Pediatrics 58:130, 1976.
86. Morse, B. S., and Nussbaum, M.: The detection of hyaluronic acid in the serum and urine of a patient with nephroblastoma. Am. J. Med. 42:996, 1967.
87. Movassaghi, N., Leiken, S., and Chandra, R.: Wilms' tumor metastasis to uncommon sites. J. Pediatr. 84:416, 1974.
88. Murphy, D. A., Rabinovitch, H., Chevalier, L., et al.: Wilms' tumor in right atrium. Am. J. Dis. Child. 126:210, 1973.
89. Murphy, G. P., Mirand, E. A., Johnson, G. S., et al.: Erythropoietin release associated with Wilms' tumor. Bull. Johns Hopkins Hosp. 120:26, 1967.
90. Nephroblastoma: an index reference cancer (Editorial). Lancet 2:651, 1973.
91. Neuhauser, E. B. D., Wittenborg, M. H., Berman, C. Z., et al.: Irradiation effects of roentgen therapy on the growing spine. Radiology 59:637, 1952.
92. Niss, R., and Passarge, E.: Trisomy 8 restricted to cultured fibroblasts. J. Med. Genet. 13:229, 1976.
93. O'Malley, B., D'Angio, G. J., and Vawter, G. F.: Late effects of roentgen therapy given in infancy. Am. J. Roentgenol. Radium Ther. Nucl. Med. 89:1067, 1963.
93a. Olsen, B., and Bischoff, A.: Wilms' tumor in an adult. Cancer 25:2, 1970.
94. O'Neill, P., and Pinkel, D.: Wilms' tumor in bone marrow aspirate. J. Pediatr. 72:396, 1968.
95. Osler, W. M.: Two cases of striated myosarcoma of the kidney. J. Anat. Physiol. 14:229, 1879.
96. Pendergrass, T. W.: Congenital anomalies in children with Wilms' tumor: a new survey. Cancer 37:403, 1976.
97. Perez, C. A., Kaiman, H. A., Keith, J., et al.: Treatment of Wilms' tumor and factors affecting prognosis. Cancer 32:609, 1973.
98. Perlman, M., Goldberg, G. M., Bar-Ziv, J., et al.: Renal hamartomas and nephroblastomatosis with fetal gigantism: a familial syndrome. J. Pediatr. 83:414, 1973.
99. Pilling, G. P.: Wilms' tumor in seven children with congenital aniridia. J. Pediatr. Surg. 10:87, 1975.
100. Pochodly, C., Suwansirikul, S., and Penzer, P.: Renal-cell carcinoma with extrarenal manifestations in a 10-month-old-child. Am. J. Dis. Child. 121:528, 1971.
101. Powars, D. R., Allerton, S. E., Brierle, J., et al.: Wilms' tumor: clinical correlation with circulating mucin in three cases. Cancer 29:1597, 1972.
102. Ragab, A. H., Vietti, T. J., Crist, W., et al.: Bilateral Wilms' tumor. A review. Cancer 30:983, 1972.
103. Reddy, J. K., Schimke, R. N., Chang, C. H. J., et al.: Beckwith-Wiedemann syndrome—Wilms' tumor, cardiac hamartoma, persistent visceromegaly, and glomeruloneogenesis in a 2 year old boy. Arch. Pathol. 94:523, 1972.
104. Richmond, H., and Dougall, A. J.: Neonatal renal tumors. J. Pediatr. Surg. 5:413, 1970.
105. Riedel, H. A.: Adrenogenital syndrome in a male child due to adrenocortical tumor; report of a case with hemihypertrophy and subsequent development of embryoma (Wilms' tumor). Pediatrics 10:19, 1952.
106. Ringrose, R. E., Jabbour, J. T., and Keele,

D. K.: Hemihypertrophy. Pediatrics 36: 434, 1965.
107. Ritter, J. A., and Scott, E. S.: Embryoma of contralateral kidney ten years following nephrectomy for Wilms' tumor. J. Pediatr. 34:753, 1959.
108. Samuels, L. D., Grosfeld, J. L., and Kartha, M.: Radiation hepatitis in children. J. Pediatr. 78:68, 1971.
109. Sanyal, S. K., Saldivar, V., Coburn, T. P., et al.: Hyperdynamic heart failure due to A-V fistula associated with Wilms' tumor. Pediatrics 57:564, 1976.
110. Schwartz, A. D., Lee, H., and Baum, E. S.: Leukemia in children with Wilms' tumor. J. Pediatr. 87:374, 1975.
111. Schweisguth, O., Taris, N., Lemerle, J., et al.: Action de la vincristine dans les néphroblastomes. Bull. Cancer 57:93, 1970.
112. Shalet, M. F., Holder, T. M., and Walters, T. R.: Erythropoietin-producing Wilms' tumor. J. Pediatr. 70:615, 1967.
113. Shashikumar, V. L., Somers, L. A., Pilling, G. P., et al.: Wilms' tumor in the horseshoe kidney. J. Pediatr. 9:185, 1974.
114. Simonowitz, D. A., and Reyes, H. M.: Renal abscess mimicking a Wilms' tumor. J. Pediatr. Surg. 11:269, 1976.
115. Smith, W. B., Wara, W. M., Margoli, L. W., et al.: Partial hepatectomy in metastatic Wilms' tumor. J. Pediatr. 84:259, 1974.
116. Spear, G. S., Hyde, T. P., Gruppo, R. A., et al.: Pseudohermaphroditism, glomerulonephritis with the nephrotic syndrome, and Wilms' tumor in infancy. J. Pediatr. 79:677, 1971.
117. Sukarochana, K., Tolentino, W., and Kiesewetter, W. B.: Wilms' tumor and hypertension. J. Pediatr. Surg. 7:573, 1972.
118. Sukarochana, K., and Kiesewetter, W. B.: Wilms' tumor: factors influencing long-term survival. J. Pediatr. 69:747, 1966.
119. Sullivan, M. P., Hussey, D. H., and Ayala, A. G.: Wilms' tumor. In Sutow, W., Vietti, T., and Fernbach, D. (eds.): Clinical Pediatric Oncology. St. Louis, C. V. Mosby Co., 1973, p. 359.
120. Sullivan, M. P., Sutow, W. W., Cangir, A., et al.: Vincristine sulfate in the management of Wilms' tumor. Replacement of preoperative irradiation by chemotherapy. J.A.M.A. 202:381, 1967.
121. Sutow, W. W., Thurman, W. C., and Windmiller, J.: Vincristine (leurocristine) sulfate in the treatment of children with metastatic Wilms' tumor. Pediatrics 32: 880, 1963.
122. Swenson, O., and Brenner, R.: Aggressive approach to the treatment of Wilms' tumor. Ann. Surg. 166:657, 1967.
123. Talley, R. W.: Chemotherapy of adenocarcinoma of the kidney. Cancer 32:1062, 1973.
124. Tefft, M., D'Angio, G. J., and Grant, W.: Postoperative radiation therapy for residual Wilms' tumor: review of Group III patients in the National Wilms' Tumor Study. Cancer 37:2768, 1976.
125. Tefft, M., Mitus, A., and Jaffe, N.: Irradiation of the liver in children: Acute effects enhanced by concomitant chemotherapeutic administration? Am. J. Roentgenol. Radium Ther. Nucl. Med. 111: 165, 1971.
126. Thompson, M. R., Emmanuel, I. G., Campbell, M. S., et al.: Extrarenal Wilms' tumors. J. Pediatr. Surg. 8:37, 1973.
127. Thurman, W. G., Grabstald, H., and Lieberman, P. H.: Elevation of erythropoietin levels in association with Wilms' tumor. Arch. Intern. Med. 117:280, 1966.
128. Traggis, D., Jaffe, N., Tefft, M., et al.: Successful treatment of Wilms' tumor with intracranial metastases. Pediatrics 56:472, 1975.
129. Vietti, T. J., Sullivan, M. P., Haggard, M. E., et al.: Vincristine sulfate and radiation therapy in metastatic Wilms' tumor. Cancer 25:12, 1970.
130. Wagget, J., and Koop, C. E.: Wilms' tumor: Preoperative radiotherapy and chemotherapy in the management of massive tumors. Cancer 26:338, 1970.
131. Walker, D., and Richard, G. A.: Fetal hamartoma of the kidney: recurrence and death of patient. J. Urol. 110:353, 1973.
132. Wallace, A. C., and Nairn, R. C.: Renal tubular antigens in kidney tumors. Cancer 29:977, 1972.
133. Wang, J. J., Cortes, E., Sinks, L. F., et al.: Therapeutic effect and toxicity of Adriamycin in patients with neoplastic disease. Cancer 28:837, 1971.
134. Wara, W. M., Philips, T. L., Margolis, L. W., et al.: Radiation pneumonitis: a new approach to the derivation of time-dose factors. Cancer 32:547, 1973.
135. Wedemeyer, P. P., White, J. G., Nesbit, M. E., et al.: Resection of metastases in Wilms' tumor: a report of three cases cured of pulmonary and hepatic metastases. Pediatrics 41:446, 1968.
136. Wells, H. G.: Occurrence and significance of congenital malignant neoplasms. Arch. Pathol. 30:535, 1940.
137. White, J. G., and Krivit, W.: Surgical excision of pulmonary metastases. Pediatrics 29:927, 1962.
137a. White, J. J., Golladay, E. S., Kaizer, H., et al.: Conservatively aggressive management with bilateral Wilms' tumors. J. Pediatr. Surg. 11:859, 1976.
138. Wigger, H. J.: Fetal hamartoma of kidney. Am. J. Clin. Pathol. 51:323, 1969.
139. Wilms, M.: Die Mischgeschiwülste. Leipzig, A. Georgi, 1899.
140. Wohl, M. E. B., Griscom, N. T., Traggis, D.

G., et al.: Effects of therapeutic irradiation delivered in early childhood upon subsequent lung function. Pediatrics 55:507, 1975.
141. Wolff, J. A.: Advances in the treatment of Wilms' tumor. Cancer 35:901, 1975.
142. Wolff, J. A., D'Angio, G., Hartmann, J., et al.: Long-term evaluation of single versus multiple courses of actinomycin D therapy of Wilms' tumor. N. Engl. J. Med. 290:84, 1974.
143. Wolff, J. A., Krivit, W., Newton, W. A., Jr., et al.: Single versus multiple dose dactinomycin therapy of Wilms' tumor. N. Engl. J. Med. 279:290, 1968.
144. Young, J. L., Jr., and Miller, R. W.: Incidence of malignant tumors in U. S. children. J. Pediatr. 86:254, 1975.
145. Zunin, C., and Soave, F.: Association of nephrotic syndrome and nephroblastoma in siblings. Ann. Pediatr. 203:29, 1964.

Chapter Sixteen

THE SOFT TISSUE SARCOMAS

The soft somatic tissues are located between the epidermis and the visceral organs and consist of peripheral nerves, fibrous and adipose connective tissues, blood vessels, lymphatic structures, smooth and striated muscle, fasciae, and synovial structures. With the exception of the peripheral nerves (which are ectodermally derived), these tissues are all descended from primitive mesenchyme and can give rise to a wide variety of tumors which are classified as sarcomas ("fleshy tumors"). Soft tissue sarcomas account for approximately 6.5 per cent of all malignant neoplasms in U.S. children, with an annual incidence of 0.84/100,000 whites and 0.39/100,000 blacks.[98]

General Features of Soft Tissue Sarcomas

Despite the diversity of their apparent tissue of origin (fat, muscle, blood vessels, connective tissue, etc.), the soft tissue sarcomas share many morphologic and behavioral characteristics as a reflection of their common mesenchymal ancestry. For this reason, concepts relating to sarcomas in general will be covered before discussing the specific entities.

1. Grossly the tumors usually appear as fleshy, ill-defined, soft, primary growths which tend to be hemorrhagic, necrotic, and invasive of surrounding tissues; however, some sarcomas may be quite fibrous and firm or markedly vascular.

2. In some tumors there will be a predominant cell type, such as primitive muscle or fat cells, but many sarcomas are composed of a mixture of the various mesenchymally derived cells; this probably reflects the multipotentiality of undifferentiated mesenchyme.

3. Growth is usually insidious; pain or interference with function are apt to be late problems.

4. Although many lesions appear well encapsulated, in reality they are "pseudoencapsulated" and frequently infiltrate surrounding tissues. Because of this propensity to extend for considerable distances beyond the palpable tumor mass, mere local resection is not adequate for control of the tumor.

5. Prior to the use of adjuvant chemotherapy and radiotherapy, successful treatment usually required radical surgical procedures (e.g., amputation for extremity lesions). However, it is now possible to limit the extent of

surgery in many instances by utilizing high-dose radiotherapy and combination chemotherapy.

6. The success of radiotherapy in local control of primary soft tissue sarcomas depends to a large extent on the size of the tumor and the dose of radiation administered.

7. When distant metastasis occurs, it is primarily via the bloodstream and to the lungs; however, involvement of regional lymph nodes is observed in 5 to 20 per cent of cases.

8. Excision of a soft tissue mass without biopsy is only justified when a tumor is small and so situated that the sacrifice of a wide margin on all sides can be carried out without causing deformity; otherwise, biopsy should be carried out before definitive therapy in order to confirm the presence of malignancy.

Etiology

Although some sarcomas may arise in tissues injured by thermal burns, irradiation, war wounds, or other trauma, these factors cannot be implicated in most sarcomas. Sarcomas can also be produced in laboratory animals by chemical carcinogens (benzpyrene, methylcholanthrene, plastic sheet), but there is no direct evidence for the role of chemical oncogens in humans.

Since 1911, when the Rous sarcoma virus of chickens was described, efforts have been made to implicate viruses in the etiology of human sarcomas. Although there is, as yet, no direct evidence linking viruses etiologically to human sarcoma formation, viruses have been detected in sarcomas of other mammalian species, notably the mouse and cat. These mammalian sarcoma viruses resemble the chicken sarcoma virus by virtue of their ribonucleic acid (RNA) core and characteristic type C morphology.

Indirect evidence implicating similar viruses with human sarcomas has also been accumulated:[49, 50]

1. Type C viral particles which are morphologically similar to avian, murine, and feline sarcoma viruses have been seen in human sarcomas.

2. Human skeletal and soft tissue sarcomas contain a sarcoma-specific antigen to which patients with these neoplasms form antibody, a situation similar to the case of virus-induced animal tumors whereby all neoplasms induced by the same virus contain common virus-specific tumor antigen.

3. Relatives and close associates of sarcoma patients also possess a high incidence of antibody to the sarcoma-specific antigens, suggesting the association of an infectious agent in this neoplasm.

Classification

Stout has proposed a system which classifies soft tissue sarcomas according to their tissue of origin[80] (Fig. 16–1). When classifying tumors according to this system, certain considerations must constantly be borne in mind:

1. The more primitive neoplasms will often be so undifferentiated that their exact histogenesis cannot be determined; these tumors are sometimes classified as undifferentiated or spindle-cell sarcoma.

2. Due to the common mesenchymal ancestry of these tumors, they tend to undergo metaplasia into related tissues. This is especially true of fibroblastic cells, which may proliferate extensively as a response to neoplasia; a close search for the characteristic cell type must be made in order to avoid an erroneous diagnosis of fibrosarcoma.

3. Some sarcomas may contain several different cell types; malignant mesenchymomas, for instance, may contain as many as five different cell types within the same tumor.

RHABDOMYOSARCOMA

Rhabdomyosarcoma is a malignancy which arises from the same embryonal mesenchyme that is destined to give rise to striated skeletal muscle. This

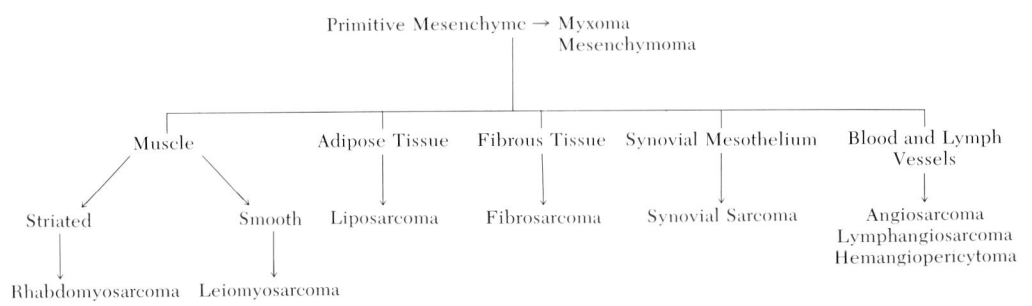

Figure 16-1 A histogenetic classification of soft-tissue sarcomas.

highly malignant tumor accounts for over half of the soft tissue tumors in childhood (Table 16-1). However, because of its ubiquitous distribution and variable pathology, it is probably also the most frequently misdiagnosed tumor of childhood.

Although showing slight predominance in males (male:female ratio, 1.3),[98] there is apparently no racial variance in incidence of this tumor.[58] Most cases do not appear to exhibit a familial tendency; however, five families have been reported in which there was a second child with a soft tissue sarcoma and a high frequency of multiple primary cancers (breast, lung, pancreas, skin) in young adult relatives.[44]

PATHOLOGY

Morphologically, rhabdomyosarcoma is the neoplastic analogue of skeletal muscle embryogenesis. Normally skeletal muscle development progresses by a series of stages from a primitive round cell through a spindle cell to a multinucleated muscle fiber with characteristic transverse and longitudinal striations.[5,56] This process is recapitulated in a highly disorganized manner by the primitive muscle cells (rhabdomyoblasts), which are the characteristic element of all rhabdomyosarcomas.

The cytoplasm of the rhabdomyoblast is acidophilic and generally contains cross-striations (Fig. 16-2), longitudinal myofibrils, or some vague suggestion of their formation. Glycogen granules may also be present in the cytoplasm; sometimes these are peripherally arranged with delicate cytoplasmic strands separating them, giving the cell a "spider web" appearance (Fig. 16-3). The electron microscopic appearance of these cells is highly characteristic, with eccentric nuclei, abundant mitochondria, and large numbers of thin cytoplasmic filaments which tend to form bands; occasionally thick and thin filaments and primitive Z-bands are also seen (Fig. 16-4).[21,58]

Within individual tumors the rhabdomyoblasts may assume various morphologic appearances, among which are: round or spindle-shaped cells, "tadpole" or racquet-shaped cells (with a single nucleus at one expanded rounded end and a tapering body extending outward for a variable distance), and multinucleated giant cells (Fig. 16-3).

Table 16-1 Soft Tissue Sarcomas in U.S. Children[98]

CLASSIFICATION	FREQUENCY (PER CENT)
Rhabdomyosarcoma	51.7
Fibrosarcoma	10.1
Mesenchymoma	5.8
Synovial sarcoma	5.8
Liposarcoma	4.2
Neurofibrosarcoma	2.9
Hemangiopericytoma	2.9
Leiomyosarcoma	2.2
Hemangiosarcoma	2.2
Alveolar soft part sarcoma	1.5
Unspecified	10.7

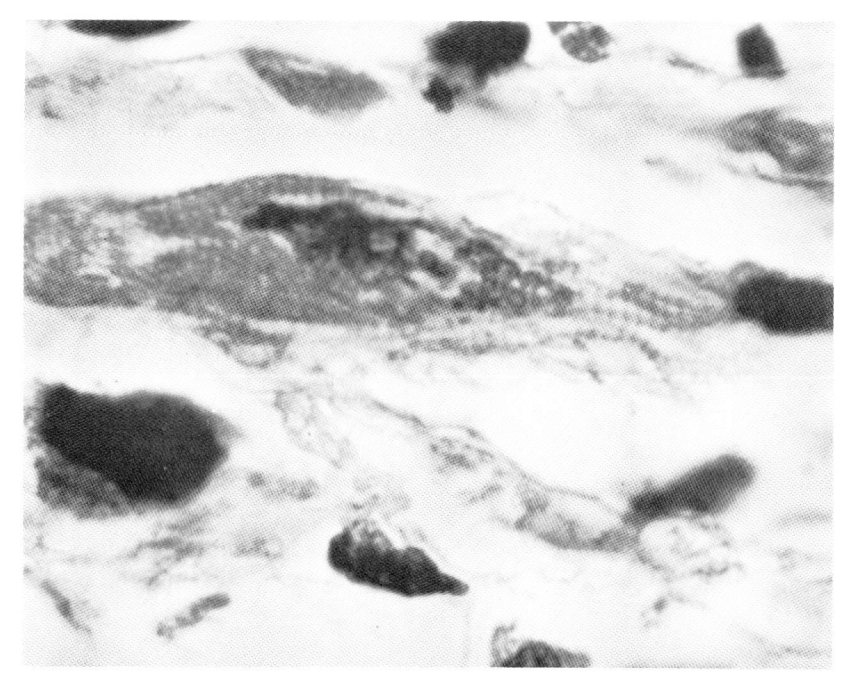

Figure 16–2 Rhabdomyoblast with cross-striations (×1212). (From Delaney, W. C., et al.: The soft tissues. *In* Nealon, T. F., Jr. [ed.]: Management of the Patient with Cancer. 2nd Ed. Philadelphia, W. B. Saunders Co., 1976.)

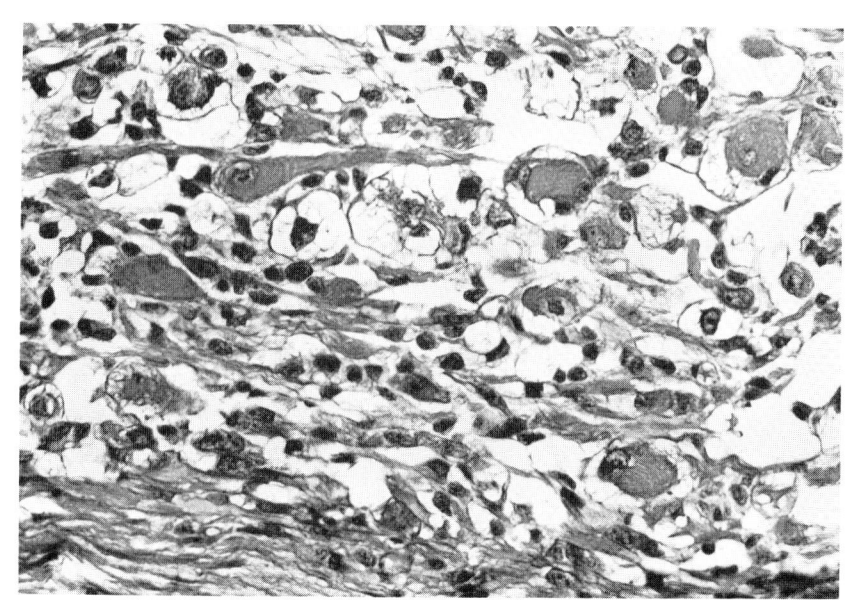

Figure 16–3 Embryonal rhabdomyosarcoma with round and racquet shaped rhabdomyoblasts. "Spider-web" cells are also evident. (Courtesy of Dr. Ronald Maenza.)

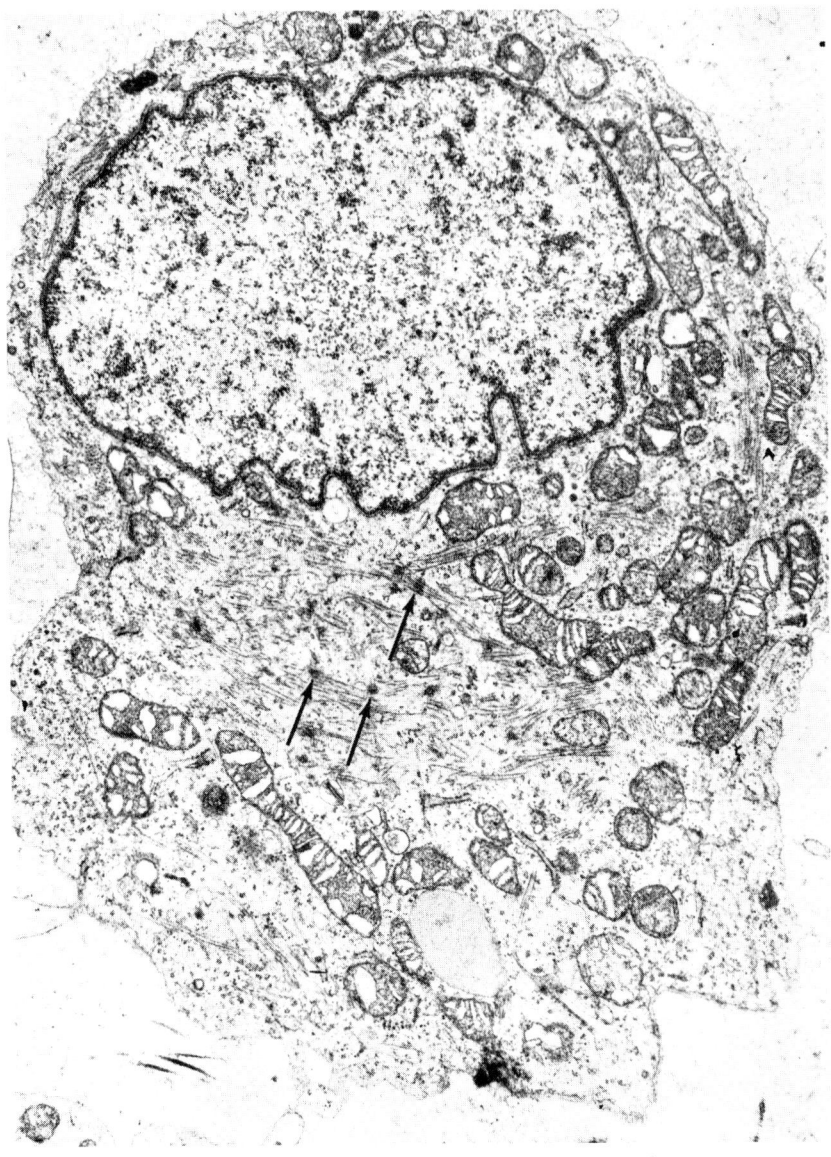

Figure 16–4 Electron photomicrograph (× 8600) of a rhabdomyoblast showing eccentric nucleus, numerous mitochondria, parallel cytoplasmic filaments, and primitive Z-bands (arrows). (From Pinkel, D., and Pratt, C.: Embryonal rhabdomyosarcoma. *In* Holland, J. F., and Frei, E., III [eds.]: Cancer Medicine. Philadelphia, Lea & Febiger, 1973.)

Because of the variable histologic picture of rhabdomyosarcoma, the initial pathologic diagnosis may be incorrect in as many as 50 per cent of patients and range from hemangioma, hemangioendothelioma, myxoma, and fibrosarcoma to neuroblastoma, lymphosarcoma, and reticulum cell sarcoma.[58] The ultrastructure of the rhabdomyosarcoma cell, however, is sufficiently distinctive to be diagnostic. Consequently, if there is any doubt about a tumor's histology it should be processed for electron microscopy by fixation in 2.5 per cent glutaraldehyde.

Rhabdomyosarcoma Variants

Rhabdomyosarcoma has been classified into four pathologic categories: *embryonal, alveolar, pleomorphic,* and *mixed.*[17]

Embryonal Rhabdomyosarcoma. The morphology of this variant closely resembles that of normally developing skeletal muscle in the 7 to 10 week fetus.[55] The predominant cell types are long, slender, and spindle-shaped, or small, round rhabdomyoblasts. Because of the primitive nature of these cells, cross-striations are not readily seen with light microscopy.

When embryonal rhabdomyosarcoma involves the soft tissues it may have a fleshy appearance and vary from firm to cystic in consistency. On the other hand, those tumors which grow in hollow viscera (bladder, vagina, uterus, ear nasopharynx, biliary tree) have a glistening polypoid appearance ("cluster of grapes") known as *sarcoma botryoides* (Fig. 16–5). Histologically sarcoma botryoides tumors have dilated blood vessels and a loose, edematous stroma, as well as a deeper compact zone composed of round and spindle-shaped rhabdomyoblasts.

Alveolar Rhabdomyosarcomas. These tumors bear a close resemblance to the developing skeletal muscle of the 10 to 21 week fetus.[55] They are usually seen in adolescents and young adults and are associated with the deep tissues of the trunk and extremities.[18, 49] Alveolar rhabdomyosarcomas are generally more firm and less myxoid than the embryonal type. Histologically their overall pattern is

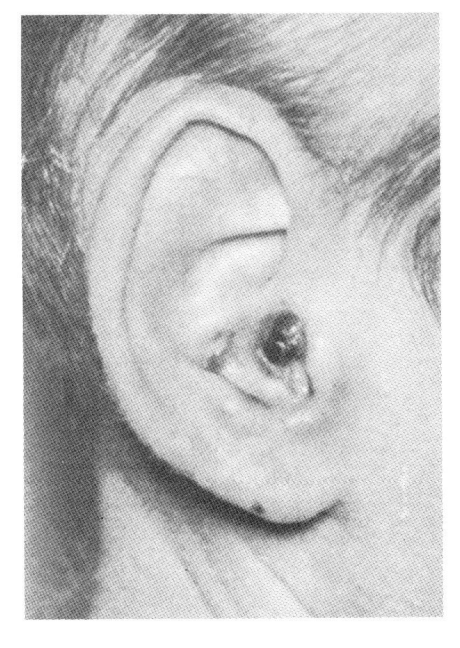

Figure 16–5 Sarcoma botryoides growing from the external auditory canal. (From Moore, O., and Grossi, C.: Cancer *12*:71, 1959.)

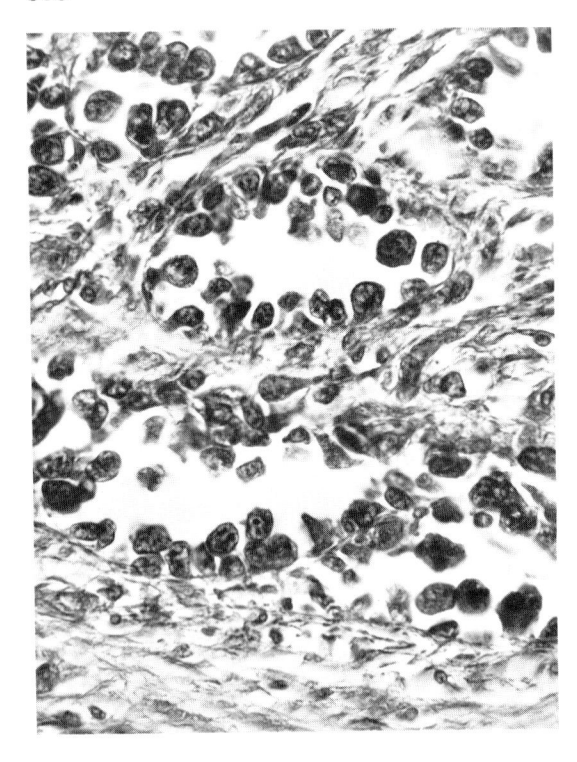

Figure 16-6 Alveolar rhabdomyosarcoma showing gland-like arrangement of rhabdomyosarcoma cells; the intervening septa also contain muscle-like cells (H&E, ×460). (Reprinted from Soule, E. H. et al: Cancer 23:1336, 1969.)

reminiscent of a pulmonary alveolus, with clusters of small, round rhabdomyoblasts separated by bundles of connective tissue or bands of primitive muscle fibers (Fig. 16-6); this pattern appears to be a caricature of the hollow tube stage of fetal muscle development.[55] Glycogen granules and cross-striations can generally be seen in the rhabdomyoblasts; giant multinucleated cells, tadpole, and racquet-shaped cells are also seen.

Pleomorphic Rhabdomyosarcoma. This tumor, seen mainly in adults, does not bear any close resemblance to embryonal muscle and may represent dedifferentiation of mature skeletal muscle.[55] Although seen mainly in older males and occurring mainly on the extremities, it may involve any site. The gross appearance is that of a deep, semifixed, softish mass that may contain areas of hemorrhage and necrosis.

Mixed Rhabdomyosarcoma. These tumors contain more than one of the above histologic types in the same tumor.

CLINICAL MANIFESTATIONS

Rhabdomyosarcoma may occur at any time in the childhood years or even in adulthood; however, the peak incidence is in the 1 to 5 year age group, with 10 per cent of cases occurring in the first year of life.[34, 43]

In the pediatric years, rhabdomyosarcoma is the most common primary malignant tumor of the orbit, bladder, prostate, vagina, uterus, paratesticular area, pelvis, nasopharynx, middle ear, and soft tissues of the trunk and extremities;[39, 67] it can also present in the oropharynx, neck, retroperitoneum, abdominal cavity, and miscellaneous other sites.[29] Table 16-2 shows the relative incidence of rhabdomyosarcoma in these various locations. As might be expected, the presenting signs and symptoms are also variable and reflective mainly of the location of the tumor (Table 16-3).

Table 16-2 Primary Sites of Rhabdomyosarcomas in 84 Patients[29]

SITE	NUMBER	PER CENT OF TOTAL
Head and neck	24	28.6
Nasopharynx	3	
Ear	7	
Larynx	2	
Neck	4	
Other (tongue, cheek, mandible)	8	
Orbit	10	11.9
Extremities	14	16.65
Upper	4	
Lower	10	
Genitourinary	14	16.65
Vagina	3	
Bladder	4	
Testicular or paratesticular	5	
Prostate	2	
Trunk	22	26.2
Chest wall	8	
Abdominal wall	2	
Retroperitoneal	1	
Pelvis	4	
Other (peritoneal cavity, bile ducts, bronchus, buttocks)	7	

CLINICAL COURSE

Rhabdomyosarcoma may spread either by local extension or by metastasis via the venous and lymphatic systems. When metastases develop, 74 per cent will become manifest within 6 months of diagnosis and 83 per cent by 1 year.[29] The most frequent sites involved by metastases are the regional lymph nodes (Fig. 16-7), lungs, liver, bone marrow, bones, and brain. The incidence of lymphatic spread correlates strongly with the anatomic site of origin of the primary tumor. Thus, lymphatic spread is relatively common when the primary rhabdomyosarcoma arises in the genitourinary region (19 per cent) or the extremities (17 per cent), less common in the trunk (10 per cent), rare for head and neck sites (3 per cent), and not seen at all in lesions of the orbit.[43] Cardiac metastases may also develop and these can result in congestive heart failure.[60] Bone marrow metastases are detectable by routine marrow aspiration in approximately 30 per cent of patients; they may appear individually or in clumps as tadpole-shaped and racquet-shaped cells (Fig. 16-8), primitive monoblast-like cells, or multinucleated cells. Indeed, sometimes the marrow may be completely replaced by tumor cells.

Prognostic Factors

The major factors related to prognosis appear to be (1) age, (2) primary site, (3) histologic type, (4) stage of disease at the time of diagnosis, and (5) treatment.

Age. In general, children between the ages of 1 and 7 years have better survival curves than those above or below this age.[14, 26, 85] They have significantly less extensive disease at the time of diagnosis and significantly lower rates of tumor recurrence and metastasis; there is also a higher frequency of the more favorable tumor types in this age group. Children under 1 year of age, on the other hand, appear to have an especially poor prognosis.[14, 26]

Primary Site. The anatomy of the primary site appears to influence both the timing of the onset of symptoms and the opportunities for metastasis: the orbit (which has bony confines and a paucity of lymphatics) will limit both local extension and lymphatic metastasis of a tumor. The relatively small area resulting from these bony confines also results in early recognition due to exophthalmos. Consequently, orbital tumors have a very good prognosis.[12, 14, 85]

The nasal cavity, nasopharynx, and maxillary antrum, on the other hand, have abundant lymphatics and lack of anatomic confines. Tumors arising here can easily extend to neighboring structures and lymphatic channels. Moreover, they usually do not produce

Table 16-3 Signs and Symptoms of Rhabdomyosarcoma According to Location of Tumor

Location	Signs and Symptoms
Head and neck	
Orbit	Exophthalmos, ptosis Eyelid swelling
Middle ear	Bloody aural discharge Facial nerve palsy Polypoid mass in aural canal
Nasopharynx	Airway obstruction Nasal discharge Polypoid mass in nose Serous otitis media
Oropharynx	Dysphagia Painful mastication
Neck	Mass lesion Cervical or brachial plexus palsy
Pelvis	
Prostate	Urinary obstruction
Bladder	Urinary obstruction Hematuria
Vagina and uterus	Vaginal bleeding, "cluster of grapes" extruding through vaginal opening
Scrotum, spermatic cord	Mass lesion
Buttocks	Mass lesion
Extremity	Mass lesion Local pain

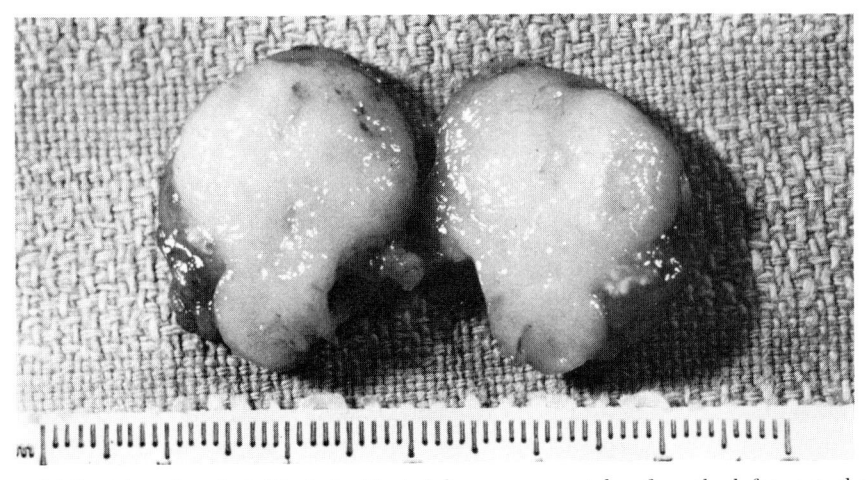

Figure 16-7 A lymph node infiltrated with rhabdomyosarcoma taken from the left inguinal region of a 12-year-old boy; a small primary lesion was subsequently found on the dorsum of the left foot. (Courtesy of Dr. Ronald Maenza.)

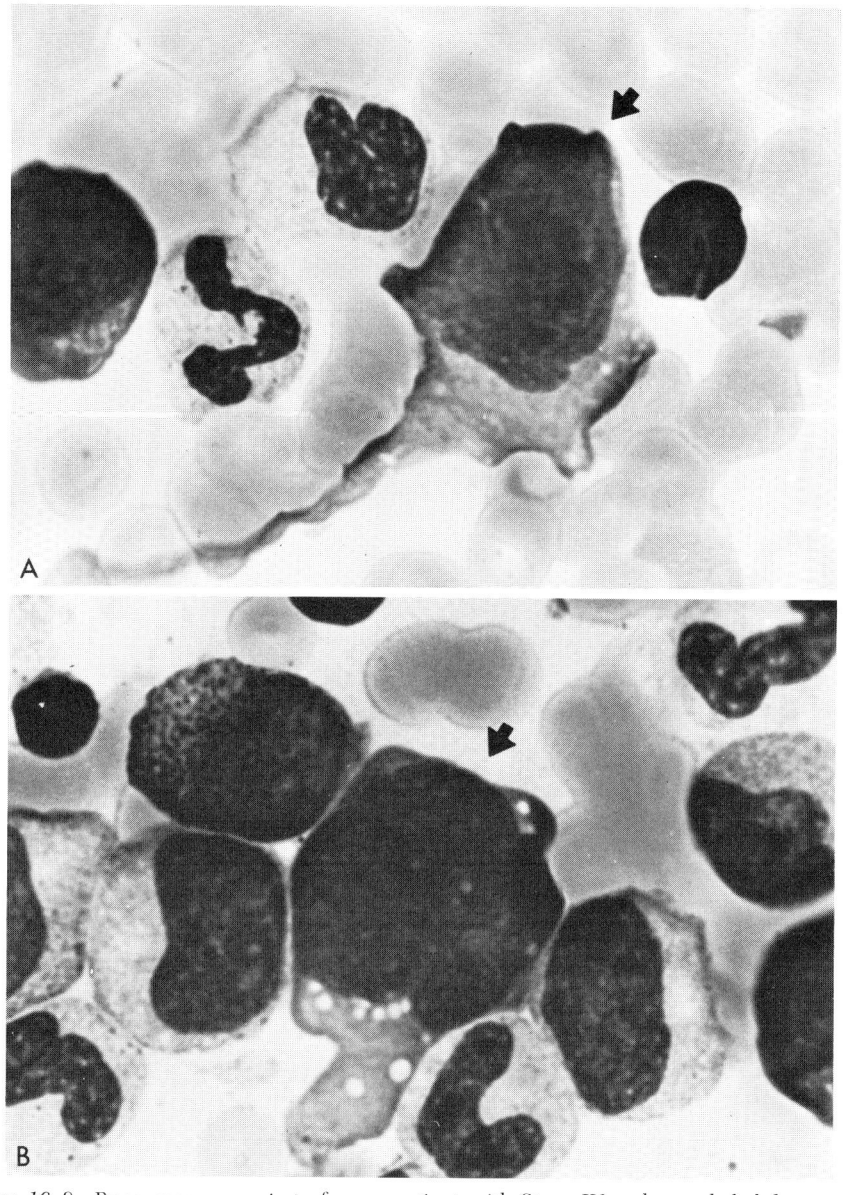

Figure 16–8 Bone marrow aspirate from a patient with Stage IV embryonal rhabdomyosarcoma showing tadpole-shaped (A) and racquet-shaped (B) rhabdomyoblasts.

symptoms until fairly far advanced. Thus, they have a very poor prognosis.[46, 85]

Rhabdomyosarcoma of the ear also is associated with anatomic features which augur a poor prognosis; these lesions exhibit aggressive destructive local growth and metastasis through lymphatic and hematogenous routes. Involvement of the CNS occurs in approximately one third of cases,[58a] usually as a result of direct meningeal invasion.

Extremity and genitourinary tumors have intermediate prognostic significance. Within the genitourinary tract, prostatic lesions have a poorer prognosis than do those of the bladder, probably because prostatic rhabdomyosarcoma disseminates rapidly through tissue planes, with regional node involvement in about 20 per cent of patients and distant metastases in 40 per cent;[88] by contrast, bladder lesions tend to remain superficial, and regional or distant metastases are a late development.

Histologic Type. The best survival rate has occurred with the sarcoma botryoides variant of embryonal rhabdomyosarcoma and the poorest with alveolar rhabdomyosarcoma.[18, 85] These differences could be attributed partly to the more extensive disease present at the time of diagnosis in patients with the alveolar type; however, tumor recurrence and metastatic spread were also significantly more rapid and frequent in the alveolar rhabdomyosarcoma cases.

Stage of Disease. Listed below are the staging criteria used by the Intergroup Rhabdomyosarcoma study group:

Stage I Localized disease, completely resected (regional nodes not involved and margins of resection microscopically free of tumor).

Stage II Grossly resected tumor with microscopic local residual disease (or regional nodes involved, but all disease completely removed).

Stage III Incomplete resection (gross residual disease).

Stage IV Metastatic disease present.

Accurate staging at the time of diagnosis is critically important both as a guide to therapy and as probably the most important determinant of prognosis. Localized (Stage I) and regionally resectable (Stage II) tumors are frequently curable using methods presently available.[59, 93] Aggressive multidisciplinary treatment has recently produced some long-term survivors even among patients with more extensive disease,[91, 92, 93] but the prognosis for these groups still remains guarded.

TREATMENT

In recent years it has become common practice to employ concurrent prophylactic irradiation and combination chemotherapy in the *initial* management of all stages of rhabdomyosarcoma rather than reserve them for delayed palliative management of recurrence and metastasis. The goal of these multidisciplinary programs is cure of the patient by the complete eradication of *all* tumor and, indeed, more than half of all children with rhabdomyosarcoma can now be expected to be alive without disease 5 years after initiation of such therapy.[93] Some groups have even reported long-term* disease-free survival in over 70 per cent of their patients.[8, 12, 29]

The current approach to treatment of rhabdomyosarcoma may be summarized as follows:[91]

Stage I If the primary lesion has been completely resected and the margins of the specimen are free of tumor, therapy is directed towards eradication of possible micrometastases with adjuvant chemotherapy. Preliminary results indicate that chemotherapy is also effective in preventing local recurrence at the resection site, and radiotherapy does not appear to enhance this effect.[48]

Stage II Radiation therapy is used to eradicate local microscopic residual disease; simultaneous chemotherapy is also given to potentiate the radiation effect against the local disease and to treat occult micrometastases.

Stage III Chemotherapy is used to shrink gross residual tumor and to treat occult micrometastases. Radiotherapy may be used simultaneously or after chemotherapy has caused shrinkage of the tumor.

---

*Since 90 per cent of deaths from this tumor occur during the 2-year period following diagnosis, most studies have defined long-term survivors as those living for more than 2 years after diagnosis.[34, 37]

Stage IV Chemotherapy is used to shrink both the primary lesion and manifest metastases; radiotherapy may also be utilized to treat the primary disease or selected metastases.

Specific Modalities of Therapy

Surgery. Surgery remains the most effective mode of therapy for localized rhabdomyosarcoma. Because this tumor infiltrates diffusely into surrounding tissue, evidence of encapsulation must be regarded as misleading, and a wide margin of normal tissue should be resected along with the tumor mass; this should be performed as part of an en bloc resection of the tumor along with the entire group of muscles involving the tumor from their origin to their insertion.[49, 59, 63] In the past, this has sometimes required radical excision or amputation (when an extremity is involved). When feasible, regional lymph nodes draining the affected area are also removed.[58, 59]

Recently the recognition that radiotherapy and chemotherapy are capable of controlling microscopic residual disease has resulted in a less mutilative surgical approach to rhabdomyosarcoma. In some groups, for instance, extremity lesions are no longer treated by amputation, but an en bloc resection is performed whenever possible.[32] Bladder and prostate lesions have been treated by extensive local resection or anterior exenteration, with preservation of acceptable appearing external genitalia;[8] some authors have suggested that preoperative radiotherapy and chemotherapy may not only reduce the necessity for extensive surgery in the pelvic region, but can sometimes even make it unnecessary.[66] Head and neck lesions have been treated with local excision or biopsy only; recent data indicate that as many as 74 per cent of patients with rhabdomyosarcoma of the head and neck may be maintained free of disease for two years or more with radiotherapy and combination chemotherapy following local excision or biopsy.[12, 45]

There are two common indications for postponing an attempt at surgical resection of a rhabdomyosarcoma: (1) when the tumor mass is large and treatment with chemotherapy and radiotherapy will shrink it sufficiently to allow removal with less residual defect (e.g., to preserve a functional limb or avoid pelvic exenteration), (2) when metastatic disease requires immediate treatment with chemotherapy (e.g., large lung lesions, bone marrow metastases).

Radiation Therapy. The major purposes of radiation therapy are to achieve local control of the malignancy by eradicating gross or microscopic tumor, shrink a large tumor to provide a better surgical approach, or treat tumors in unresectable sites (nasopharynx, middle ear).

Early radiotherapists pronounced rhabdomyosarcoma a radioresponsive but not a radiocurable lesion. However, in 1968 Cassady and co-workers[5a] demonstrated that localized orbital rhabdomyosarcoma could be controlled with adequate radiation therapy doses and fields in 90 per cent of cases. Subsequently, Donaldson and co-workers[12] reported a similar local control rate in pediatric head and neck rhabdomyosarcomas treated with surgery, aggressive chemotherapy, and large volume irradiation (5000 to 6000 rads).

Doses in the range of 5000 to 6000 rads over a 5 to 6 week period are required for complete tumor destruction; in children under 3 years the dosage is usually limited to 4000 rads, however.[11, 22] Sometimes, either because of their site of origin or wide extension, some rhabdomyosarcomas cannot be treated with full dosage; consequently, variations in the dose-time relationship may be necessary to minimize injury to normal tissue (therapy should not exceed 1800 rads

Table 16-4 Standard VAC

DRUG	DOSAGE
Vincristine	2 mg/m² intravenously weekly for 12 weeks (max., 2 mg)
Actinomycin D	0.015 mg/kg/day intravenously for 5 days (max., 0.5 mg/day) every 3 months for 5 or 6 courses
Cyclophosphamide (Cytoxan)	2.5 mg/kg/day orally for 2 years

to both lungs, 1500 to 2000 rads to the kidneys, or 3000 rads to the liver).

Chemotherapy. The four most effective drugs against rhabdomyosarcoma (and other soft tissue sarcomas as well) are cyclophosphamide, vincristine, actinomycin D, and Adriamycin;[91, 92, 93] imidazole carboxamide (DTIC) also shows some promise.[25] All of these drugs have been used in varying combinations with very encouraging results.[23, 48, 91, 92, 93]

The use of the combination known as *Standard VAC* for two years (Table 16-4) (in association with surgery and radiotherapy) in previously untreated patients with embryonal rhabdomyosarcoma or undifferentiated sarcoma has resulted in 68 per cent of patients remaining alive and free of disease for a median follow-up period in excess of 5 years[93] (Table 16-5).

A recent modification of the VAC protocol known as *Pulse VAC* (Table 16-6) uses a more intensive dose of cyclophosphamide given simultaneously with actinomycin D and vincristine. Use of this combination in patients with rhabdomyosarcoma and a variety of other soft tissue sarcomas produced responses (usually complete remission) in 19 of the first 20 patients treated.[93] It is too early, however, to determine the long-term survival figures for these patients.

Preliminary results from the Intergroup Rhabdomyosarcoma Study suggest that the combination of modified Pulse VAC with Adriamycin is a highly effective remission induction combination for Stage III or IV disease, producing responses in over 80 per cent of cases.[48] The long-term survival statistics for this group likewise are not yet available.

All of these regimens produce significant toxicity, particularly severe nausea and vomiting and bone marrow suppression. The many risks and potentials for life-threatening complications require the effort of individuals experienced in the treatment of cancer and management of chemotherapy.

FIBROUS TISSUE TUMORS (FIBROMATOSIS, DERMATOFIBROSARCOMA PROTUBERANS, FIBROSARCOMA)

Fibrous tissue tumors have not been easy to identify or classify. Because

Table 16-5 Results of Treatment of Rhabdomyosarcoma and Undifferentiated Sarcoma with Standard VAC[93]

STAGE	NUMBER OF PATIENTS	ALIVE WITHOUT RESIDUAL DISEASE°
I, II	8	8 (100%)
III	16	10 (62.5%)
IV	8	4 (50%)
Total	32	22 (68%)

°Median follow-up period >5 years.

Table 16-6 Pulse VAC

DRUG	DOSAGE
Vincristine	2 mg/m² intravenously weekly for 12 weeks (max., 2 mg)
Actinomycin D	0.015 mg/kg/day intravenously for 5 days (max., 0.5 mg/day) every 3 months for 5 or 6 courses
Cyclophosphamide (Cytoxan)	10 mg/kg/day intravenously or orally for 7 days every 6 weeks

mesenchymal cells of all types may revert to the appearance of fibroblasts under neoplastic conditions, nearly all soft tissue sarcomas contain some fibroblastic elements. Consequently, true fibroblastic tumors are considered to be those whose cells are primary fibroblasts and produce only connective tissue fibers with no other recognizable elements present in the growth.

These tumors may arise from scars, subcutaneous tissue, or from deep connective tissue around tendon or nerve sheaths, muscle fascia, or periosteum. They may occasionally occur in bone,[10] brain,[69] the orbit,[15] lung,[31] and retroperitoneal tissues.[71] Some have apparently been induced by radiotherapy.[68]

Grossly the tumor may be quite firm and the cut surface is pale gray or white in color (Fig. 16-9); the more primitive lesions may be soft, with areas of hemorrhage and necrosis. Although they may appear to be encapsulated, they are actually surrounded by a pseudocapsule consisting of a compression zone of neoplastic cells; tumor cells are often present beyond the limits of this pseudocapsule and may serve as a focus for tumor recurrence if the lesion is merely "shelled out."

The tumors are composed of elongated fusiform or spindle cells arranged in sinuous interweaving bundles; these cells are capable of synthesizing collagen and reticulin (a precursor of collagen) fibers. The consistent arrangement of reticulin fibers surrounding these tumor cells is a characteristic feature. Fibrous tumors may vary in histology from well-differentiated lesions with few mitotic figures and low cellularity (fibromatosis) to highly anaplastic lesions (fibrosarcoma).

THE FIBROMATOSES

The fibromatoses have been defined as a group of nonmetastasizing fibrous tumors which tend to invade locally and recur after surgical excision.[1] These distinctive lesions can be subdivided into two groups: (1) "adult" fibromatoses, which occur predominantly (but not exclusively) in people older than 20 years of age, and (2) "juvenile" fibromatoses, which usually affect patients less than 20 years of age (Table 16-7).

Fibromatoses occur mainly in fasciae and aponeuroses. Some of these growths consist of dense masses of mature fibroblasts and may be histologically so well differentiated that they resemble scar tissue; nonetheless, they may manifest aggressive, infiltrative behavior. Some fibromatoses may be very cellular and difficult to distinguish from fibrosarcoma. However, the location, lack of pseudoencapsulation, and lack of anaplasia are helpful differentiating features.

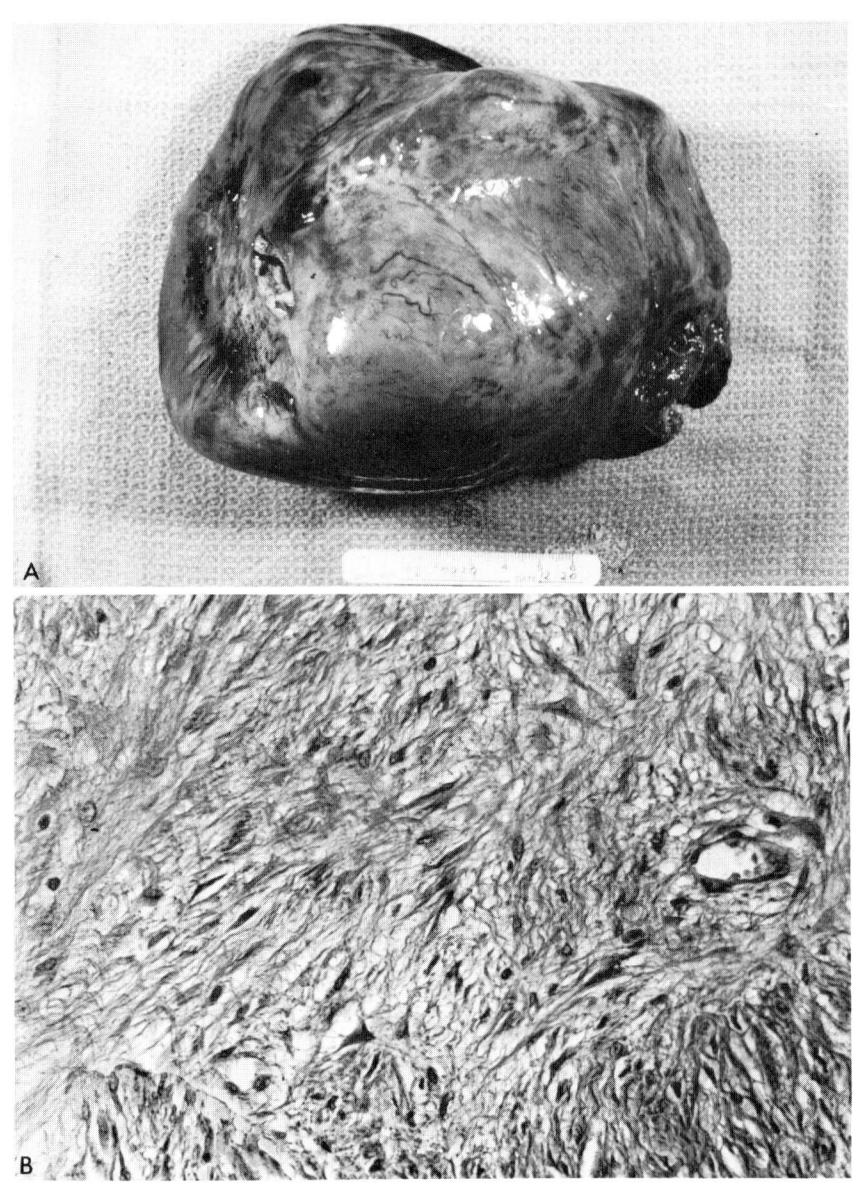

Figure 16-9 Fibrous tumor (fibromatosis) of the chest wall. A, Gross specimen. B, Microscopic section, showing fibroblasts and sinuous collagenous fibers (H&E, ×80). (Courtesy of Dr. Ronald Maenza.)

Table 16-7 The Fibromatoses[1]

"Adult" Fibromatoses
1. Dupuytren type fibromatoses
    Palmar fibromatosis
    Plantar fibromatosis
    Knuckle pads
    Peyronie's disease
    Ectopic locations
2. Desmoid fibromatoses
    Extraabdominal desmoids
    Abdominal wall desmoids
    Intraabdominal desmoids
    Multiple desmoids
    Multiple familial desmoids
    Gardner's syndrome

"Juvenile" Fibromatoses
1. Congenital fibrosarcoma-like fibromatosis
2. Congenital generalized fibromatosis
3. Congenital localized fibromatosis
4. Fibromatosis colli
5. Diffuse infantile fibromatosis
6. Juvenile aponeurotic fibroma
7. Fibrous hamartoma of infancy
8. Recurring digital fibrous tumor of childhood
9. Juvenile nasopharyngeal angiofibroma
10. Hereditary gingival fibromatosis
11. Fibromatosis hyalinica multiplex juvenilis

Juvenile Fibromatoses

These tumors occur most frequently from birth ("congenital fibrosarcoma") to 4 years of age, and although they frequently have a histologically malignant appearance, they rarely develop distant metastases.[2, 61, 82] Local recurrences are common, however. Several cases of massive congenital fibrosarcoma have undergone spontaneous cure.[3, 11]

One form of fibromatosis in early infancy is *Fibromatosis colli* of the sternocleidomastoid muscle (congenital muscular torticollis). In its early stages this lesion is often very cellular and consists of proliferating fibroblasts infiltrating between degenerating skeletal muscle. Eventually, however, replacement of the muscle fibers by fibrous tissue ensues. The muscle involvement may be diffuse, affecting the entire sternocleidomastoid muscle, or it may be localized, producing a rounded, firm mass. Differentiation from more malignant tumors of fibrous tissue is made on the basis of the clinical course (onset at 1 to 2 weeks of age, reaching maximum size at 1 to 2 months of age) and location (the sternomastoid muscle rarely, if ever, is involved by sarcomas).

Among other forms of fibromatosis in childhood are *fibrous hamartoma of infancy, recurrent digital fibrous tumor, juvenile aponeurotic fibromatosis*, and *congenital generalized fibromatosis*. Specific anatomic localization in some cases and a characteristic microscopic appearance in others permit differentiation of these various subgroups.[11] *Fibrous hamartoma of infancy*, for instance, usually is a solitary lesion with a predilection for the axilla and upper extremities; it occurs almost exclusively in the first 2 years of life and its recurrence rate is approximately 16 per cent.[19] *Recurrent digital fibrous tumor*, unlike the other fibromatoses, is primarily a dermal lesion and has a high local recurrence rate. The extensor surface of the fingers or toes are the usual sites of involvement, and the lesion is most commonly seen in a child who is less than two years old. The local recurrence rate following surgical excision is about 60 per cent, but metastatic spread does not occur.[2a]

Treatment of Fibromatosis

The primary treatment for fibrous tumors is surgical. The initial procedure should involve a wide excisional biopsy, with removal of at least 1 cm of tissue beyond the obvious lesion.[28]

Since fibromatoses are not encapsulated or even pseudoencapsulated, but grow by infiltration, the margin of normal tissue included in the excision depends upon the surgeon's judgment.

Recurrence should be treated by wide local excision. Some authors feel that when fibromatoses occur in early infancy, they tend to evolve into more mature forms over a period of time; accordingly, local excision with careful observation for local recurrence has been recommended for such cases.[24] Radiation therapy with doses approximating 5000 rads may be useful in treating large progressive fibromatoses (*desmoids*);[30] unfortunately, this dose of irradiation will cause epiphyseal destruction and subsequent deformities in a young child. More recently, Stein has reported a good response to multiagent chemotherapy in a single patient with a large fibromatosis of the neck.[74]

DERMATOFIBROSARCOMA PROTUBERANS

Dermatofibrosarcoma protuberans develops in the corium and usually produces multiple confluent hard nodules, which elevate the epidermis and often have a reddish hue. Although it is a lesion which truly arises in the skin, it is traditionally classified as a soft tissue sarcoma. The tumor is composed of spindle-shaped fibroblasts arranged about a central area of collagen or a small vascular space; this arrangement gives a cartwheel-like appearance, which is considered to be pathognomonic of the tumor.[87] The history is usually that of a nodule in the skin which may have been present for many years that begins to increase in size and cause pain. These tumors may be locally aggressive but rarely metastasize to distant sites.

FIBROSARCOMA

Fibrosarcoma is generally considered to be a cellular fibroblastic tumor in which the cells are significantly anaplastic, with marked variation in size and shape and frequent mitoses. Multiple sections of the specimen should be examined before the diagnosis of fibrosarcoma is established, since other tumors (e.g., osteogenic sarcoma) may contain broad zones of fibrosarcoma-like cells; therefore, a small biopsy specimen is not adequate.

Although common in adults, this tumor is rare in the pediatric age group. When it does occur in children, it is most commonly found either in the head and neck region or in the lower extremities. Common head and neck locations are the mandible and soft tissues of the cheek, but some arise in the nasopharynx and orbit as well.[86] Lower extremity lesions tend to involve the thigh most frequently in adults, but the ankle and foot are the most frequent sites in infants.[7]

The highly anaplastic fibrosarcomas are rapidly growing and frequently metastasize via the bloodstream to the lungs; regional lymph nodes are involved in 5 to 10 per cent of cases.[49]

Treatment of Fibrosarcoma

If the lesion proves to be a poorly differentiated fibrosarcoma, radical excision of the local area should be carried out with removal of all possible areas of direct spread, without regard to nodal drainage.[22, 28, 36, 65, 86] For superficial lesions, wide excision should include the underlying fascia and frequently requires a split-thickness skin graft for closure, with proper precautions to avoid seeding of tumor in the donor site; for deeper lesions, involved muscle bundles should be removed at their origins and insertions.[65]

Extremities should not be amputated without first exhausting the possibilities of less drastic measures.[20, 65, 82] If recurrence follows radical local excision of fibrosarcoma in an extremity, some authors recommend amputation;[28] others[20] feel it is justifiable to continue repeated local excisions as long as the extremity is functional. Unfortunately, even with this latter approach, which makes every attempt to salvage the extremity, a number of children with fibrosarcoma in an extremity will ultimately require amputation.[29]

A large en bloc resection has been recommended for fibromatosis and fibrosarcoma of the nasal cavity, paranasal sinuses, or nasopharynx (after biopsy confirmation of the diagnosis); this approach appears to result in far fewer recurrences than does the practice of limited local excision.[22] Mandibular lesions may be treated by mandibulectomy with reconstruction, while maxillary sinus or maxillary bone lesions may be treated with subtotal or total maxillectomy.[22, 36]

Radical neck dissection is used for treatment of primary neck lesions, but is not routinely performed when the primary lesion is in the head, since neck metastases are rare in those situations.[36]

Radiation therapy may be of benefit in recurrent disease[20, 28, 69] and in unresectable tumors.[86] The role of chemotherapy has not been well established for this tumor; some regressions have been noted with Adriamycin and imidazole carboxamide.[25]

Prognosis of Fibrosarcoma in Children

In general, the prognosis for fibrosarcoma in children is good, owing to the low incidence of distant metastases; in Stout's series of 54 cases of juvenile fibrosarcoma, only 8 per cent had demonstrable metastases.[82] However, local recurrences are a major problem and may occur as late as 31 years following resection of the primary tumor.[64]

Children in whom the fibrosarcomas arise deep in the thoracic or pelvic cavity do not fare as well as those with more superficial tumors; these patients tend to have distant metastases and to pursue a fatal course.[28] This poor prognosis may reflect the relatively late clinical manifestations and consequent delay in diagnosis of these deep tumors rather than any unique biological properties.

TUMORS OF PRIMITIVE MESENCHYME

MYXOMA

Myxoma is composed of cells and stroma identical to those of primitive mesenchyme; no evidence at all of specialized tissue is present. Although this tumor occurs most commonly in middle-aged adults, as many as 25 to 30 per cent of cases occur in patients under 20 years of age.[79] Myxoma may appear at any site, but heart, skin, and soft tissue, bones, and the genitourinary system are the organs most frequently involved.

In gross appearance, these tumors appear as mucoid, slimy, soft gray growths with a solid, homogeneous interior. Microscopically they are similar in structure to the stroma of the umbilical cord, with scanty numbers of stellate or spindle cells, amorphous ground substance, exceedingly delicate reticulin fibers, and sparse capillaries.[6, 49, 79]

Although these tumors do not metastasize, they infiltrate widely and should be treated by wide local excision.

So-called primary myxomas of the heart are probably a collection of various tumor types (undifferentiated myxomas, rhabdomyomas, mixed tumors). Myxomas of the heart are the only tumors given that name from which metastases have been reported; such metastasizing tumors are probably not true myxomas but sarcomas of another type masquerading as myxoma.[79]

MESENCHYMOMA

Mesenchymoma is a mixed mesenchymal tumor composed of more mature cells than are found in myxoma; in order to establish the diagnosis, two or more malignant mesenchymal elements (exclusive of fibroblasts) not ordinarily associated together must be present. Fibroblastic elements are not counted as a basic cell type in this tumor because mesenchymal cells of all types may revert to the appearance of fibroblasts,[49, 78] and fibrosarcoma elements are commonly found in many sarcomas composed chiefly of a single cell type.[51]

Benign mesenchymomas commonly contain well differentiated mixtures of adipose tissue, blood vessels, nerves, muscle (smooth and skeletal); cartilage, bone, and lymphoid aggregates may also occasionally be seen. *Malignant mesenchymomas* contain mixtures of poorly differentiated rhabdomyoblasts, endothelial cells, leiomyoblasts, lipoblasts, chondroblasts, histiocytes, and synovial elements.

In children, approximately 8 per cent of all malignant mesodermal tumors are mesenchymomas.[51] The tumors can be found not only in the superficial soft tissues, but also in deep soft tissues, the orbit, spinal canal, liver, ileum, and anal canal.

Although grossly these tumors may appear to be encapsulated, microscopically there is evidence of tissue invasion outside the apparent gross limits of the tumor; consequently, an aggressive surgical approach is indicated. Unlike myxoma, these tumors may metastasize to local lymph nodes and distant sites. Long-term survival is approximately 60 per cent, with death more likely to occur if the tumor is larger than 5 cm.[51]

SYNOVIAL SARCOMA

Synovial sarcomas present histologic features characteristic of synovial tissue and arise from the synovial tissue of joints, tendon sheaths, and bursae. They constitute between 8 and 10 per cent of all soft tissue sarcomas in adults[1a, 4] and 2 to 7 per cent of soft tissue sarcomas of children.[9, 65] More than half of the childhood cases occur between the ages of 10 and 14 years,[9] but patients as young as 2 weeks of age have been reported.[63]

Pathology

In gross appearance the synovial sarcoma is firm, pink or grey, with areas of hemorrhage, necrosis, calcification, or cyst formation. The tumor may arise from synovial membranes of joints, tendons, and bursae, or in areas totally devoid of synovial tissue; however, it is almost never directly connected to the joint space. A pseudocapsule composed of compressed contiguous structures may be present, but there is usually microscopic invasion beyond its limits.

Histologically at least two elements are evident—a fibrosarcoma-like stroma and an inner synovial layer resembling epithelium and containing gland-like slits lined by epithelioid cells of columnar or cuboidal shape. The reticulin stain imparts a characteristic and diagnostic pattern consisting of an abundance of reticulin fibers in the fibrosarcomatous stroma and an absence of these fibers in the epithelium-like layers; the mucicarmine stain will be taken up by mucopolysaccharide secretions in the gland-like spaces unless the tumor is poorly differentiated.

Clinical Features

The common sites of involvement are the knee, thigh, foot, and hand (synovial sarcoma is the most common soft tissue sarcoma of the hands and feet).[49] Clinical symptomology includes a painless mass, a tender mass, or pain preceding the development of a mass.[53] The tumors vary greatly in growth rate and some may remain localized for long periods of time without spread, whereas others may demonstrate pulmonary metastases shortly after the initial onset of symptoms.

Metastasis occurs chiefly via the bloodstream; in almost every case in which metastases have been reported the lungs have been involved.[9] Metastasis to regional nodes occurs in 20 to 23 per cent of cases,[4, 49] and bone metastases in 20 per cent.[4] The tumor also spreads locally along fascial and muscle planes for extraordinary distances and is notorious for its high frequency of local recurrence (66 to 77 per cent).[4, 49, 53]

Therapy

The best hope for cure in this condition is total surgical excision before metastasis occurs. The type of excision depends on the extent and location of the neoplasm. A wide local excision requires resection of the entire muscle group in which the tumor is growing—this should be attempted only in those lesions arising from extra-articular synovial tissue tendons or very superficial lesions of the hands and feet.[49] Most tumors arising around joints or involving hands and feet will require amputation.[4, 49, 63] Because of the high incidence of regional node metastasis, regional node resection has also been recommended.[49]

Radiotherapy may have an adjuvant role in local control of this tumor; in Cadman's series the local recurrence rate in patients receiving radiotherapy after local excision was 50 per cent, whereas it was 91 per cent in those treated by local excision only.[4]

Several reviews[4, 4a, 22a] have emphasized the long natural history of this tumor and its propensity to recur after a long latent period. Consequently, 5 year, or even 10 year, disease-free survival may not necessarily represent "cure." In the series of Cameron and Kostuik, for instance, the average survival rate at 5 years was 45 per cent, but fell to 30 per cent at 10 years, and to 10 per cent after 10 years.[4a]

LIPOSARCOMA

Liposarcoma is a malignant tumor of adipose tissue; it may occur in any area where fat is present, but usually develops in deep fat deposits. Common sites are the thigh (Fig. 16–10) and adjacent popliteal space, the inguinal and gluteal regions, and the retroperitoneum; retroperitoneal tumors in particular, may attain tremendous size due to prolonged "silent" growth.

These tumors are relatively rare in children, occurring with increasing frequency as age advances; peak incidence is in the third to six decades of life, when they are probably the most common malignant tumors of the soft tissues.[54] In children there appear to be two age peaks: in infancy and in adolescence.[40]

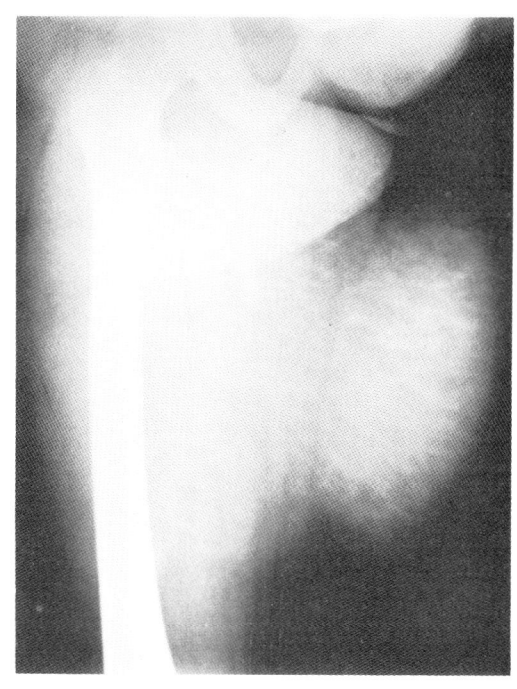

Figure 16–10 Liposarcoma arising in the right thigh of a 9 year old boy. The mass is relatively lucent (due to high fat control content), and denser connective tissue strands are seen running through it. (From Gyepes, M. T., and Smith, L. E.: Pediatric neoplasms. *In* Steckel, R. J., and Kagan, A. R. [eds.]: Diagnosis and Staging of Cancer: A Radiologic Approach. Philadelphia, W. B. Saunders Co., 1976.)

Liposarcomas usually develop de novo rather than in preexisting lipomas, as attested by the great frequency of lipomas and rarity of liposarcomas (120:1);[54, 63] however, rapid growth of a preexisting lipoma or associated pain should suggest the possibility of malignant transformation.

Pathology

The gross appearance of these tumors is multilobed, with a gelatinous mucoid consistency and a partially defined or totally absent capsule. Histologically they vary from poorly differentiated to well differentiated. The well differentiated type (which is the most common type seen in children) resembles embryonal fat with stellate or spindle-shaped cells containing lipoid material; mitoses are rare.[76] The least differentiated form is composed predominantly of lipoblasts — round cells with centrally placed nuclei and voluminous foamy cytoplasm containing vacuoles filled with lipoid material.

The tumor may metastasize to lungs, liver, and bone in adults,[73] but rarely does so in children;[40] local recurrences, on the other hand, are quite common in the pediatric age group.

Therapy

Because of the tendency for local recurrence, surgery should be aggressive. The tumor should be totally excised, with a sufficient rim of normal tissue around it to ensure that no residual microscopic disease remains;[49, 63] amputation may be necessary, particularly if the underlying bone is involved.[63] With the addition of radiation therapy to the tumor bed, the local recurrence rate may be reduced from 73 per cent to 20 per cent.[73]

The role of chemotherapy for this tumor remains unclear. At least one child with massive recurrent intraabdominal liposarcoma has responded well to vincristine and cyclophosphamide,[38] and some patients have responded to Adriamycin and imidazole carboxamide.[25] Pulse VAC chemotherapy (see Table 16–6) may also be effective in controlling the disease.[91] However, in young children, the desire for aggressive therapy must be balanced against the relative unlikelihood that distant metastases or local recurrence will take place.

Because of the tendency of childhood liposarcomas (particularly in infants) to be well differentiated, the prognosis is generally good; in Kaufman and Stout's study, recurrence has occurred in only two of the 11 children for whom follow-up data were obtained.[40] By contrast, survival rate is only 18 per cent for adults with poorly differentiated lipoblastomas and 70 per cent for well differentiated tumors.[19]

LEIOMYOSARCOMA

Leiomyosarcoma is a malignant tumor of smooth (nonstriated) muscle. It is very rarely seen in childhood, but of those that do occur in the pediatric age group, 53 per cent appear within the first 5 years of life.[97] Common locations are the gastrointestinal, genitourinary, and respiratory tracts, and the soft tissues. Metastases occur via the bloodstream and mainly to the lungs; other metastatic sites are liver, peritoneum, and pancreas.[49, 70] Regional nodes may also occasionally be involved.

Presenting signs and symptoms are related mainly to the location of the tumor:

Gastrointestinal: Bleeding, as manifested by hematemesis, melena, hematochezia, or anemia, is the most common symptom, occurring in 88 per cent of cases.[96] Other symptoms include abdominal pain, nausea, vomiting, and weight loss. These tumors rarely, if ever, occur in infants under 2 years of age.

Genitourinary (bladder and prostate): Dysuria and urinary retention, prostatic mass.

Soft Tissue: Mass lesion.

The microscopic appearance of leiomyosarcoma consists of spindle cells with blunt-ended, oval nuclei. The cells are arranged in intertwining bundles or whorls and may contain longitudinal myofibrils. Criteria for malignancy include elevation of the mitotic rate, anaplasia, and bizarre cell forms; however, some leiomyosarcomas do not manifest these criteria and may be mistaken for benign leiomyomas.

Radical surgical excision is usually the treatment of choice for leiomyosarcoma.[49, 63] If metastases are not evident at the time of diagnosis and the tumor can be completely excised, the prognosis may be relatively good. When subgastric resection or more radical therapy was used for treatment of gastric lesions, eight of nine pediatric patients survived 1 year, and four of five of those for whom follow-up information was available were alive at 5 years.[96]

REFERENCES

1. Allen, P. W.: The fibromatoses: A clinicopathologic classification based on 140 cases. Am. J. Surg. Pathol. *1*:255, 1977.
1a. Ariel, I. M., and Pack, G. T.: Synovial sarcoma. N. Engl. J. Med. *268*:1272, 1963.
2. Balsaver, A. M., Butler, J. J., and Martin, R. G.: Congenital fibrosarcoma. Cancer *20*: 1607, 1967.
2a. Beckett, J. H., and Jacobs, A. H.: Recurring digital fibrous tumors of childhood. Pediatrics *59*:401, 1977.
3. Berner, R. E., and Laub, D. L.: The spontaneous cure of massive fibrosarcoma. Plast. Reconst. Surg. *36*:257, 1965.
4. Cadman, S. L., Soule, E. H., and Kelly, P. J.: Synovial sarcoma. An analysis of 134 tumors. Cancer *18*:613, 1965.
4a. Cameron, H. U., and Kostuik, J. P.: A long-term follow-up of synovial sarcoma. J. Bone Joint Surg. *56B*:613, 1974.
5. Cappel, D. F., and Montgomery, C. L.: On rhabdomyoma and myoblastoma. J. Path. Bact. *44*:517, 1937.
5a. Cassady, J. R., Sagerman, R. H., Tretter, P., and Ellsworth, R. W.: Radiation therapy for rhabdomyosarcoma. Radiology *91*:116, 1968.
6. Chaves, E., Nobrega, C., Oliveira, A. M., and Cartaxo, O.: Congenital myxoma in childhood. A Report of Two Cases. Cancer *28*:239, 1971.
7. Chung, E. B., and Enzinger, F. M.: Infantile fibrosarcoma. Cancer *38*:729, 1976.
8. Clatworthy, H. W., Jr., Braren, V., and Smith, J. P.: Surgery of bladder and prostatic neoplasms in children. Cancer *32*:1157, 1973.
9. Crocker, D. W., and Stout, A. P.: Synovial sarcoma in children. Cancer *12*:1123, 1959.
10. Dahlin, D. C., and Ivins, J. C.: Fibrosarcoma of bone: a study of 114 cases. Cancer *23*:35, 1969.
11. Dehner, L. P., and Askin, F. B.: Tumors of fibrous tissue origin in childhood. A clinicopathologic study of cutaneous and soft tissue neoplasms in 66 children. Cancer *38*:888, 1976.
12. Donaldson, S., Castro, J. R., Wilbur, J. R., and Jessee, R. H., Jr.: Rhabdomyosarcoma of head and neck in children. Combination treatment by surgery, irradiation, and chemotherapy. Cancer *31*:26, 1973.
13. Edland, R. W.: Embryonal rhabdomyosarcoma. Am. J. Roentgenol. Radium Ther. Nucl. Med. *93*:671, 1965.
14. Ehrlich, F. E., Haas, J. E., and Kiesewetter, W. B.: Rhabdomyosarcoma in infants and children: factors affecting long-term survival. J. Pediatr. Surg. *6*:571, 1971.
15. Eifrig, D. E., and Foos, R. Y.: Fibrosarcoma of the orbit. Am. J. Ophthal. *67*:244, 1969.
16. Enzinger, F. M.: Fibrous hamartoma of infancy. Cancer *18*:241, 1965.
17. Enzinger, F. M., Lattes, R., Torloni, H.: Histologic typing of soft tissue tumors. Geneva, World Health Organization, 1969.
18. Enzinger, F. M., and Shiraki, M.: Alveolar rhabdomyosarcoma: an analysis of 110 cases. Cancer *24*:18, 1969.
19. Enzinger, F. M., Winslow, D. J.: Liposarcoma; study of 103 cases. Virchows Arch. (Pathol. Anat.) *335*:367, 1962.
20. Exelby, P. R., Knapper, W. H., Huvos, A. G., and Beattie, E. J.: Soft tissue fibrosarcoma in children. J. Pediatr. Surg. *8*:415, 1973.
21. Freeman, A. I., and Johnson, W. W.: A comparative study of childhood rhabdomyosarcoma and virus-induced rhabdomyosarcoma in mice. Cancer Res. *28*:1490, 1968.
22. Fu, Y. S., Perzin, K. H.: Nonepithelial tumors of the nasal cavity, paranasal sinuses, and

nasopharynx. A clinico-pathologic study. VI. Fibrous tissue tumors (fibroma, fibromatosis, fibrosarcoma). Cancer 37:2912, 1976.
22a. Gerner, R. E., and Moore, G. E.: Synovial sarcoma. Ann. Surg. 181:22, 1975.
23. Ghavimi, F., Exelby, P. R., D'Angio, G. J., et al.: Multidisciplinary treatment of embryonal rhabdomyosarcoma in children. Cancer 35:677, 1975.
24. Goslee, L., Clermont, V., Bernstein, J., and Woolley, P. J., Jr.: Superficial connective tissue tumors in early infancy. A study of fibromatosis and lipoblastomatosis. J. Pediatr. 65:378, 1964.
25. Gottlieb, J., Baker, L., Quagliana, J., et al.: Chemotherapy of sarcomas with a combination of Adriamycin and dimethyltriazeno imidazole carboxamide. Cancer 30:1632, 1972.
26. Grosfeld, J. L., Clatworthy, H. W., Jr., and Newton, W. A., Jr.: Combined therapy in childhood rhabdomyosarcomas: an analysis of 42 cases. J. Pediatr. Surg. 4:637, 1969.
27. Grosfeld, J. L., Ballantine, T. V. N., and Baehner, R. L.: Current management of childhood solid tumors. Surg. Clin. North Am. 56:513, 1976.
28. Hays, D. M., Mirabel, V. Q., Karlan, M. S., et al.: Fibrosarcoma in infants and children. J. Pediatr. Surg. 5:176, 1970.
29. Heyn, R. M., Holland, R., Newton, W. A., Jr., et al.: The role of combined chemotherapy in the treatment of rhabdomyosarcoma in children. Cancer 34:2128, 1974.
29a. Heyn, R., Holland, R., Joo, P., et al.: Treatment of rhabdomyosarcoma in children with surgery, radiotherapy and chemotherapy. Med. Pediatr. Oncol. 3:21, 1977.
30. Hill, D. R., Newman, H., and Phillips, T. L.: Radiation therapy of desmoid tumors. Am. J. Roentgenol. 117:84, 1973.
31. Holinger, P. H., Johnston, K. C., Gossweiler, N., and Hirsch, E. C.: Primary fibrosarcoma of bronchus. Dis. Chest. 37:137, 1960.
32. Holton, C. P., Chapman, K. E., Lackey, R., et al.: Extended combination therapy of childhood rhabdomyosarcoma. Cancer 32:1310, 1973.
33. Horn, R. C., and Enterline, H. T.: Rhabdomyosarcoma: a clinicopathological study and classification of 39 cases. Cancer 11:181, 1958.
34. Hornback, N. B., and Shidnia, H.: Rhabdomyosarcoma in the pediatric age group. Am. J. Roentgenol. 126:542, 1976.
35. Horvat, B. L., Caines, M., and Fisher, E. R.: The ultrastructure of rhabdomyosarcoma. Am. J. Clin. Pathol. 53:555, 1970.
36. Jaffe, B. F., and Jaffe, N.: Head and neck tumors in children. Pediatrics 51:731, 1973.
37. Jaffe, N. J., Filler, R. M., Farber, S., et al.: Rhabdomyosarcoma in children. Improved outlook with a multidisciplinary approach. Amer. J. Surg. 125:482, 1973.
38. James, D. H., Johnson, W. W., and Wrenn, E. L.: Effective chemotherapy of an abdominal liposarcoma. J. Pediatr. 68:311, 1966.
39. Jones, I. S., Reese, A. B., and Krout, J.: Orbital rhabdomyosarcoma. An analysis of 62 cases. Trans. Am. Ophthalmol. Soc. 63:223, 1965.
40. Kaufman, S. L., Stout, A. P.: Lipoblastic tumors of children. Cancer 12:912, 1959.
41. Kinne, D. W., Chu, F. C. H., Huros, A. G., et al.: Treatment of primary and recurrent retroperitoneal liposarcoma. Twenty five year experience at Memorial Hospital. Cancer 31:53, 1973.
42. Lawrence, W., Jr., Jegge, G., and Foote, F. W., Jr.: Embryonal rhabdomyosarcoma: A clinicopathological study. Cancer 17:361, 1964.
43. Lawrence, W., Jr., Hays, D. M., and Moon, T. E.: Lymphatic metastasis with childhood rhabdomyosarcoma. Cancer 39:556, 1977.
44. Li, F. P., and Fraumeni, J. F.: Rhabdomyosarcoma in children: epidemiologic study and identification of a familial cancer syndrome. J. Natl. Cancer Inst. 43:1365, 1969.
45. Liebner, E. J.: Embryonal rhabdomyosarcoma of the head and neck in children. Cancer 37:2777, 1976.
46. Lindberg, R. D.: Rhabdomyosarcoma in children. Treatment and results. In M.D. Anderson Hospital and Tumor Institute: Neoplasia in Children. Chicago, Year Book Medical Publishers, Inc., 1969.
47. Mahour, G. H., Soule, E. H., Mills, S. D., and Lynn, H. B.: Rhabdomyosarcoma in infants and children: a clinicopathological study of 75 cases. J. Pediatr. Surg. 2:402, 1967.
48. Maurer, H. M.: Intergroup Rhabdomyosarcoma Study: progress report. Proceedings of the Twelfth Annual Meeting of the American Society of Clinical Oncology, Abstr. C–24, 1976.
49. Morton, D. L.: Soft tissue sarcomas. In Holland, J. F., and Frei, E., III (eds.): Cancer Medicine. Philadelphia, Lea & Febiger, 1973.
50. Morton, D. L., Malmgren, R. A., Hall, W. T., and Schidlovsky, G.: Immunologic and virus studies with human sarcomas. Surgery 66:152, 1969.
51. Nash, A., and Stout, A. P.: Malignant mesenchymomas in children. Cancer 14:524, 1961.
52. Pack, G. T., and Anglem, T. J.: Tumors of the soft somatic tissues in infancy and childhood. J. Pediatr. 15:372, 1939.
53. Pack, G. T., Ariel, I. M.: Tumors of the soft somatic tissues and bone. In Treatment of

Cancer and Allied Disease. 2nd Ed. Vol. 8. New York, Harper & Row, 1964.
54. Pack, G. T., and Pierson, J. C.: Liposarcoma: a study of 105 cases. Surgery 36:687, 1954.
55. Patton, R. B., and Horn, R. C., Jr.: Rhabdomyosarcoma; clinical and pathological features and comparison with human fetal and embryonal skeletal muscle. Surgery 52:572, 1962.
56. Phelan, J. T., and Juardo, J.: Rhabdomyosarcomas. Surgery 52:585, 1962.
57. Pinkel, D., and Pickren, J.: Rhabdomyosarcoma in children. J.A.M.A. 175:293, 1961.
58. Pinkel, D., and Pratt, C.: Embryonal rhabdomyosarcoma. In Holland, J. F., and Frei, E., III (eds.): Cancer Medicine. Philadelphia, Lea & Febiger, 1973.
58a. Prat, J., and Gray, G. F.: Massive neuraxial spread of aural rhabdomyosarcoma. Arch. Otolaryngol. 103:301, 1977.
59. Pratt, C. B.: Childhood rhabdomyosarcoma. Pediatr. Ann. 3:8, 1974.
60. Pratt, C. B., Dugger, D. L., Johnson, W. W., and Ainger, L. E.: Metastatic involvement of the heart in childhood rhabdomyosarcoma. Cancer 31:1492, 1973.
61. Pritchard, D. J., Soule, E. H., Taylor, W. F., and Ivins, J. C.: Fibrosarcoma—a clinicopathological and statistical study of 199 tumors of the soft tissues of the extremities and trunk. Cancer 33:888, 1974.
62. Pullen, D. J., Dyment, P. G., Humphrey, G. B., et al.: Combined chemotherapy in childhood rhabdomyosarcoma. Cancer Chemother. Rep. 59:359, 1975.
63. Ragab, A. H., Vietti, T. J., Perez, C. A., and Berry, D. H.: Malignant tumors of the soft tissues. In Sutow, W. W., Vietti, T. J., and Fernbach, D. J. (eds.): Clinical Pediatric Oncology. St. Louis, C. V. Mosby Co., 1973.
64. Renaud, J., Van Slooten, E. A., and Hampe, J. F.: The treatment of fibrosarcoma of soft tissues; a survey of 39 patients. Arch. Chir. Neerl. 15:187, 1963.
65. Richardson, W. R., and Dewar, J. P.: Problems of managing fibrous tissue tumors in infants and children. Surgery 56:426, 1964.
66. Rivard, G., Ortega, J., Hittle, R., et al.: Intensive chemotherapy as primary treatment for rhabdomyosarcoma of the pelvis. Cancer 36:1593, 1975.
67. Rogers, P. C. J., Howards, S. S., and Komp, D. M.: Urogenital rhabdomyosarcoma in childhood. J. Urol. 115:738, 1976.
68. Schwartz, E. E., and Rothstein, J. D.: Fibrosarcoma following radiation therapy. J.A.M.A. 203:296, 1968.
69. Senyszyn, J. J., and O'Conor, G.: Fibrosarcoma of the brain. A case report describing response of the primary and metastatic tumors to radiotherapy. Oncology 24:431, 1970.
70. Skandalakis, J. E., Gray, S. W., Shepard, D., and Bourne, G. H.: Smooth muscle tumors of the alimentary tract. Springfield, Ill., Charles C Thomas, 1962.
71. Synder, W. H., Jr., Kruse, C. A., Greaney, E. M., and Chaffin, L.: Retroperitoneal tumors in infants and children: a report of 88 cases. Arch. Surg. 63:26, 1951.
72. Soule, E. H., Mahour, G. H., Mills, S. D., and Lynn, H. B.: Soft tissue sarcomas of infants and children. Mayo Clin. Proc. 43:313, 1968.
73. Spittle, M. F., Newton, K. A., and Mackenzie, D. H.: Liposarcoma; a review of 60 cases. Brit. J. Cancer 24:696, 1970.
74. Stein, R.: Chemotherapeutic response in fibromatosis of the neck. J. Pediatr. 90:482, 1977.
75. Stobbe, G. D., and Dargeon, H. W.: Embryonal rhabdomyosarcoma of the head and neck in children and adolescents. Cancer 3:825, 1950.
76. Stout, A. P.: Liposarcoma—the malignant tumor of lipoblasts. Ann. Surg. 119:86, 1944.
77. Stout, A. P.: Rhabdomyosarcoma of the skeletal muscles. Ann. Surg. 123:447, 1946.
78. Stout, A. P.: Mesenchymoma, the mixed tumor of mesenchymal derivatives. Am. Surg. 127:278, 1948.
79. Stout, A. P.: Myxoma, the tumor of primitive mesenchyme. Am. Surg. 127:706, 1948.
80. Stout, A. P.: In Pack, G. T., and Ariel, I. M., (eds.): Tumors of the Soft Somatic Tissues; A Clinical Treatise. New York, Paul B. Hoeber, Inc., 1958.
81. Stout, A. P.: Sarcomas of the soft tissues. CA 11:210, 1961.
82. Stout, A. P.: Fibrosarcoma in infants and children. Cancer 15:1028, 1962.
83. Stowens, D.: Pediatric Pathology. 2nd Ed. Baltimore, Williams & Wilkins, 1966.
84. Suit, H. D., and Russell, W. O.: Radiation therapy of soft tissue sarcomas. Cancer 36:759, 1975.
85. Sutow, W. W., Sullivan, M. P., Reid, H. L., et al.: Prognosis in childhood rhabdomyosarcoma. Cancer 25:1384, 1970.
86. Swain, R. E., Sessions, D. G., and Ogura, J. H.: Fibrosarcoma of the head and neck in children. Laryngoscope 86:113, 1976.
87. Taylor, H. B., and Helwig, E. B.: Dermatofibrosarcoma protuberans; a study of 115 cases. Cancer 15:717, 1962.
88. Tefft, M., and Jaffe, N.: Sarcoma of the bladder and prostate in children: rationale for the role of radiation therapy based on a review of the literature and a report of fourteen additional patients. Cancer 32:1161, 1973.
89. Van der Werf-Messing, B., and Vann Unnik,

J. A. M.: Fibrosarcoma of the soft tissues: a clinicopathologic study. Cancer 18:1113, 1965.
90. Vinik, M., and Altman, D. H.: Congenital malignant tumors. Cancer 19:967, 1966.
91. Wilbur, J. R.: Sarcomas. In Greenspan, E. M. (ed.): Cancer Chemotherapy. New York, Raven Press, 1975.
92. Wilbur, J. R.: Treatment of soft tissue sarcomas. Pediatr. Clin. North Am. 23:171, 1976.
93. Wilbur, J. R., and Sutow, W. W., et al.: Chemotherapy of sarcomas. Cancer 36:765, 1975.
94. Williams, D. J.: Pediatric Urology. New York, Appleton-Century-Crofts, 1968.
95. Wilson, D. A.: Tumors of the subcutaneous tissue and fascia with special reference to fibrosarcoma—clinical study. Surg. Gynec. Obstet. 80:500, 1945.
96. Wurlitzer, F. P., Mares, A. J., Isaacs, H., Jr., et al.: Smooth muscle tumors of the stomach in childhood and adolescence. J. Pediatr. Surg. 8:421, 1973.
97. Yannopoulos, K., and Stout, A. P.: Smooth muscle tumors in children. Cancer 15:958, 1962.
98. Young, J. L., and Miller, R. W.: Incidence of malignant tumors in U.S. children. J. Pediatr. 86:254, 1975.

Chapter Seventeen

PRIMARY BONE CANCERS

INCIDENCE AND AGE

Primary cancers of bone are uncommon malignancies in children. They are, however, the second most common group of solid malignant neoplasms that occur in adolescent children and young adults, exceeded in frequency only by malignant lymphomas. They have been reported to occur in the United States at an annual rate of about 5.6 cases per million white children and 4.8 cases per million black children under 15 years of age.[140] An earlier study of mortality data from this country, which included children over the age of 15 years, reported annual death rates from bone cancer to be 2.87 per million in those under the age of 14 years, with an increase to 11.97 per million in those 15 to 19 years of age.[77]

Mortality rates for the two most common forms of childhood bone cancer, osteogenic sarcoma and Ewing's tumor, rise with age until 15 to 19 years, after which a sharp decline occurs.[78] An analysis of death certificates of children in the United States dying of cancer in the 1960's by Glass and Fraumeni[42] revealed a number of interesting findings regarding these two bone tumors. Deaths from osteogenic sarcoma, rare in early life, increased rapidly in incidence during the teenage years in both sexes. The male death rate became greater than the female rate at age 14, and reached a peak after age 16. Ewing's tumor also showed an increasing rate with age in both sexes, but after age 16, the male rate continued to rise, while the female rate declined. The dramatic increase in incidence of these bone tumors that occurs during adolescence suggests a relationship between increased bone growth and the development of bone cancer.[21, 93] The earlier pubertal growth spurt in girls may account for the earlier onset in females, and the later growth and greater height in boys may be responsible for its later occurrence and overall higher incidence in males. Children with malignant bone tumors have been found to be significantly taller than average.[35, 109] The interesting observation that bone sarcomas in giant dogs such as the Saint Bernard and Great Dane occur nearly 200 times more frequently than in small and medium sized breeds also suggests a link between greater bone growth and bone tumors.[127]

TUMOR TYPES

The review by Dahlin[20] of 3987 cases of bone tumors from the Mayo

Clinic revealed 990 cases of pathologically verified primary bone tumors which were diagnosed during the first two decades of life. Of these tumors, 530 were malignant and 460 were benign. Osteogenic sarcoma was the most common bone cancer and Ewing's tumor was second in frequency during this time of life, findings in agreement with other surveys of childhood malignancies.[78, 140] During the first 10 years of life, however, patients with Ewing's tumor outnumbered those with osteogenic sarcoma (Table 17–1). A variety of benign bone neoplasms and non-neoplastic bone masses exist; their major importance to the oncologist is that they be clearly differentiated from malignant tumors. The histologic types, number, and age of occurrence of the 460 benign tumors reported by Dahlin are recorded in Table 17–2. Detailed descriptions and treatment of these benign lesions appear in a number of orthopedic texts.[20, 67, 126]

ETIOLOGY

Ionizing radiation is at present the only environmental agent known to produce bone tumors in the human. In 1929, Martland and Humphries[74] re-

Table 17–1 Distribution of Malignant Bone Tumors by Histologic Type and Patient Age*

TUMOR TYPE	UNDER 10 YEARS	10–20 YEARS
Osteogenic sarcoma	25	294
Ewing's tumor	45	103
Fibrosarcoma	2	14
Reticulum cell sarcoma	10	17
Chondrosarcoma	1	8
Parosteal osteogenic sarcoma	0	4
Adamantinoma	0	3
Chordoma	1	1
Hemangioendothelioma	1	1
Total	85	445

*Based on the data of Dahlin.[20]

Table 17–2 Distribution of Benign Bone Tumors by Histologic Type and Patient Age*

TUMOR TYPE	UNDER 10 YEARS	10–20 YEARS
Osteochondroma	51	206
Chondroma	11	28
Chondroblastoma	1	14
Chondromyxoid fibroma	3	6
Osteoid osteoma	16	43
Benign osteoblastoma	2	12
Giant cell tumor	0	17
Fibroma	11	34
Hemangioma	2	1
Neurilemmoma	0	2
Total	97	363

*Based on the data of Dahlin.[20]

corded this association in their now-classic report of two painters of luminous watch dials who continually pointed their brushes with their lips, thereby ingesting radium, mesothorium, and phosphorescent zinc sulfide from the paint. These authors concluded that "the incidence of two osteogenic sarcomas in fifteen persons dying as the result of an occupational poisoning by radioactive substances is too high to be mere coincidence." Osteogenic sarcomas, fibrosarcomas, and chondrosarcomas, as well as benign bone tumors, have developed following radiation exposure used for therapeutic purposes.[15, 88, 103, 113] Dahlin[20] recorded 23 osteogenic sarcomas, 18 fibrosarcomas, one chondrosarcoma, and one Ewing's tumor that arose in previously irradiated bone. It is of interest that there does not appear to be an excess of bone cancer among atomic bomb survivors of Hiroshima and Nagasaki.[139]

Bone tumors have also been linked to the use of internal bone-seeking radioisotopes.[68] Osteogenic sarcoma has been reported following Thorotrast administration for visualization of the spleen,[2] and extraskeletal tumors histologically diagnosed as chondrosarcoma[107] and osteogenic sarcoma[46] have occurred in the areas of soft tissue extravasation of this colloidal solution of radioactive thorium dioxide.

A small number of reports have appeared in the literature describing families with multiple members who developed osteogenic sarcoma,[25, 34, 121] Ewing's sarcoma,[50] chondrosarcoma,[106] or medullary fibrosarcoma.[4] The aggregation of cancer cases in families has not always been organ-specific, and some families with a variety of neoplasms, including bone tumors, have been described.[25, 66]

An increased incidence of osteogenic sarcoma occurs in individuals with retinoblastoma and can appear not only within[103] but also outside the field of radiation.[59, 108] The association between retinoblastoma and the later development of osteogenic sarcoma of the lower extremities usually occurs with the bilateral or familial type of retinoblastoma.[42, 59] Gordon described one patient who had two children with retinoblastoma by two different wives. None of the parents had retinoblastoma, but the father developed osteogenic sarcoma,[44] suggesting that he was a carrier for the retinoblastoma gene who did not develop the ocular tumor, but who did not escape a malignancy known to have an increased incidence in those with familial retinoblastoma.

Malignant bone tumors occur excessively in a number of congenital diseases of bone. Multiple exostoses (osteochondromas on the surfaces of growing bone) may be hereditary. A number of patients with this genetic disorder have developed chondrosarcomas, as have patients with Ollier's disease (enchondromatosis) and Maffucci's syndrome (enchondromatosis combined with hemangiomas of the skin).[20, 23, 47] Osteogenic sarcoma has been reported in two patients with osteogenesis imperfecta.[61] Paget's disease, a disorder not found in children, also predisposes to the development of bone cancer,[92] especially osteogenic sarcoma. A small number of patients without obvious underlying disease have been described with multicentric osteogenic sarcoma,[3] suggesting an unusual susceptibility for either environmental or genetic reasons.

An infectious etiology for bone cancer has been suggested by a number of observations. Bone sarcomas have been induced by viruses in animal models,[32] osteosarcomas have occurred in hamsters injected with cell-free extracts of human osteosarcomas,[31] type C virus particles have been seen in thin sections of human and hamster osteosarcomas,[33] and serum antibodies have been observed in a number of patients with osteogenic sarcoma and in their relatives and friends.[80, 95] An infectious agent could explain case clusters in families or unrelated children,[128] but such occurrences are rare.

In 1933 Coley and Higinbotham[16] reported 360 cases of bone sarcoma, of which 181 patients had histories of trauma. The descriptions of the cases, however, were scanty. Evidence that trauma may cause a malignancy remains largely circumstantial, and has not been produced in a laboratory situation.[79] Most investigators believe, as Ewing[27] stated in 1935, that "traumas reveal more malignant tumors than they produce."

DIAGNOSTIC EVALUATION

Clinical Presentation. The two complaints that most commonly cause a patient with a bone tumor to seek a physician are pain and the presence of a mass. Persistent pain, progressive in severity, is characteristic of a malignant tumor. A benign neoplasm is more likely to be painless unless its presence results in a pathologic fracture or causes some mechanical difficulty. Bone tumors often cause referred pain, occasionally leading the inexperienced clinician to miss the diagnosis on examination, or to order roentgenograms that do not include the involved area. In one series, over half of the patients with osteomas involving the femur had referred pain to the hip or knee or in the distribution of the sciatic nerve.[102] Other symptoms depend upon the site of the tumor and may result in weakness, limp, or a reluctance to move a limb.

Roentgenographic Examination. If a neoplasm is suspected, the roentgenographic appearance usually can determine whether the lesion is benign or malignant.[85] The zone of transition, the line of demarcation between tumor and adjacent normal bone, is usually narrow, with a sharp, distinct border between tumor and surrounding normal bone when a lesion is slowly growing and is benign. However, if the zone of transition is wide and the tumor appears to infiltrate surrounding normal bone without clearly defined margins, the neoplasm is usually rapidly growing and malignant. Benign lesions are often surrounded with a thick rind of cortical bone. This shell, or marginal sclerosis, is produced by the normal bone in response to the tumor, and its thickness increases with the chronicity of the tumor. Coarser trabeculation indicates a slowly growing tumor, and fine or absent trabeculation suggests a rapidly expanding lesion. A pathologic fracture through the bone tumor may occur with benign or malignant neoplasms, but extensive cortical breakthrough by the tumor indicates malignancy, especially when tumor extends into the adjacent soft tissues. Periosteal reaction does not always indicate malignancy, but it usually indicates rapid tumor growth. A lamellated "onionskin" periosteal appearance or "sunburst" appearance produced by spicules of new bone is highly indicative of cancer. Although benign bone lesions may occasionally be large, in general the larger the lesion, the more likely it is malignant. The interested reader is referred to a good review of the roentgenographic findings of the various bone tumors by Osborne,[85] written specifically for the nonradiologist.

Histologic Diagnosis. Following the clinical and roentgenographic evaluation, histologic examination of an adequate tissue specimen is required to make the definitive diagnosis. In at least 90 per cent of bone tumors, soft portions can be sectioned and examined for immediate diagnosis.[20] Usually these soft portions yield the best material to make the correct diagnosis. The surgeon can obtain valuable information and advice regarding the biopsy procedure by reviewing the roentgenograms with the radiologist and pathologist. Fresh frozen sections evaluated by an experienced pathologist permit an immediate, accurate diagnosis in the majority of cases of bone tumors. If a definitive diagnosis cannot be made on frozen section, the pathologist can have permanent sections ready for diagnosis in 24 hours in the case of most bone tumors if suitable tissue has been obtained. In some centers, aspiration biopsy has been used in the diagnosis of bone tumors with an accuracy in experienced hands reported to range from 70 to 90 per cent.[45] The hazards of diagnosis by this method are due to sampling errors and scanty material that is often obtained. The oncologist and surgeon should decide prior to surgery whether amputation will be performed immediately following the biopsy if a definitive diagnosis by frozen section examination reveals a malignancy treated best by this means. Appropriate discussions with the patient and his family are mandatory before the operation if such a decision is made. If there is any question regarding the diagnosis or hesitancy on the part of the pathologist to give a definitive diagnosis on the basis of the frozen section, an indicated amputation should be performed at a second operation.

OSTEOGENIC SARCOMA

Osteogenic sarcoma is a malignant neoplasm which arises from bone-

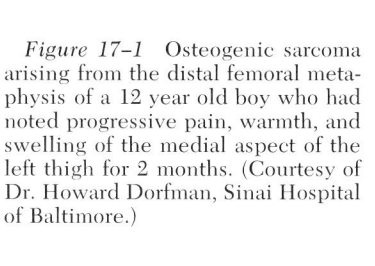

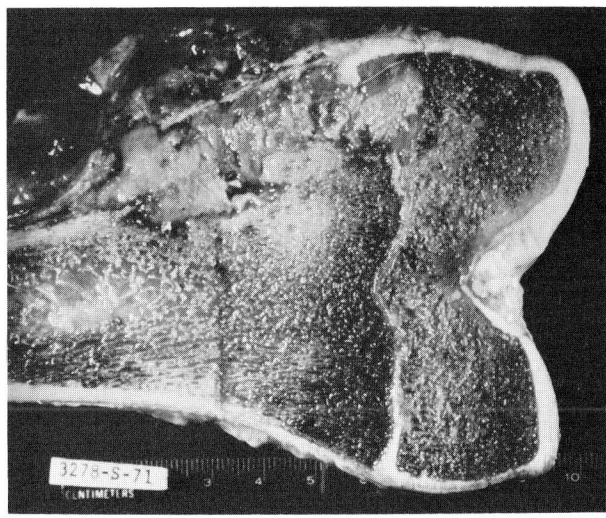

Figure 17-1 Osteogenic sarcoma arising from the distal femoral metaphysis of a 12 year old boy who had noted progressive pain, warmth, and swelling of the medial aspect of the left thigh for 2 months. (Courtesy of Dr. Howard Dorfman, Sinai Hospital of Baltimore.)

producing mesenchymal cells. It is characterized by the production of osteoid substance or bone by malignant stromal cells in some portion of the tumor. Although it most commonly occurs in adolescents and young adults, the tumor has been reported to occur in a child as young as 35 months.[112] Nearly all large series show this to be the most common malignant primary bone tumor of childhood, with about 60 per cent of the patients being male and 40 per cent female. Some series have reported an increased survival rate in females.[109]

Clinical Presentation. A painful swelling is usually apparent on physical examination. Pain usually precedes the development of the mass, which sometimes is very large on initial examination. A pathologic fracture through the lesion may be the presenting condition, but this is very rare.[20] At the time of the initial diagnosis, most patients do not appear to have a systemic illness with weight loss or anemia unless there is evidence of metastatic disease. Enlarged lymph nodes are seldom found.

Osteosarcomas have a predilection for the metaphyseal region of the long, tubular bones, with the extremities being most commonly involved. The majority of tumors occur in the distal femur (Fig. 17-1). The region around the knee accounts for nearly 50 per cent of the cases, and the tumor is uncommonly found distal to the wrist or ankle joints. Facial and cranial bone involvement also occurs in children.[12] Extraosseous osteosarcomas[1, 30] are very rare and must be differentiated from benign heterotopic ossification. Other common sites are the proximal tibia, proximal humerus, and ilium. The anatomic, age, and sex distribution in Dahlin's series of 650 cases are shown in Figure 17-2.

Diagnostic Studies. No laboratory test except for tissue examination is diagnostic for osteogenic sarcoma. Elevated levels of serum alkaline phosphatase have been found in osteoid-producing neoplasms[55] but are not diagnostic, nor are they always in the abnormal range. Significant increases of serum ceruloplasmin levels have been demonstrated in patients with osteogenic sarcoma. Shifrine and Fisher[111] have suggested that ceruloplasmin determinations may be of value in the differential diagnosis in selected patients and in evaluating the efficacy of therapy.

Roentgenograms of the involved bone usually demonstrate destruction with a loss of the normal trabecular pattern, radiolucent defects, and new

Osteogenic Sarcoma

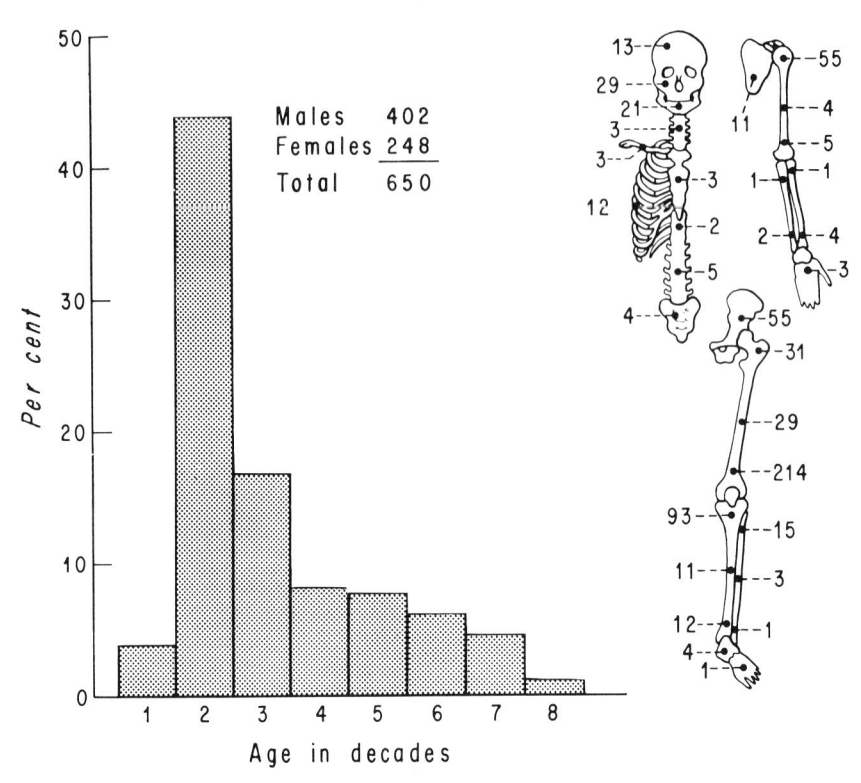

Figure 17-2 Skeletal, age, and sex distribution of osteogenic sarcoma. (From Dahlin, D. C., Bone Tumors, 2nd Ed., 1967. Courtesy of Charles C Thomas, Publisher, Springfield, Illinois.)

bone formation. Occasionally the tumors are completely lytic or sclerotic. Where the tumor encounters the cortex, it penetrates the bone, causing a periosteal reaction, which characteristically has a radial "sunburst" appearance due to spicules of new non-neoplastic bone that are produced (Fig. 17-3). With continued tumor growth, a large soft-tissue mass contiguous to the bone may be seen. The finding of fluffy calcification in the soft tissue mass or within the central lesion is strongly suggestive of osteosarcoma (Fig. 17-4). However, osteoid substance, even if present in large amounts, is not opaque if it is completely uncalcified. Metastases to lung and bone via the bloodstream are frequent. Chest films, including tomography, a skeletal survey, and a bone scan, are indicated to document evidence of dissemination of disease, since the finding of widespread tumor involvement may influence the surgical procedure, especially if amputation is being considered.

The diagnosis ultimately rests on the histologic examination of an adequate tissue specimen. The essential criterion for diagnosis is the presence of frankly sarcomatous stroma with the formation of neoplastic osteoid and bone.[67] However, a great variability in histopathology of osteogenic sarcomas exists and a number of histologic subgroups have been proposed. Osteosarcomas have been subdivided into osteoblastic, chondroblastic, and fibroblastic varieties, depending on the dominating microscopic pattern,[39] or classified on the basis of the quantity of osteoid or bone.[43] Neither method of classification appears to be

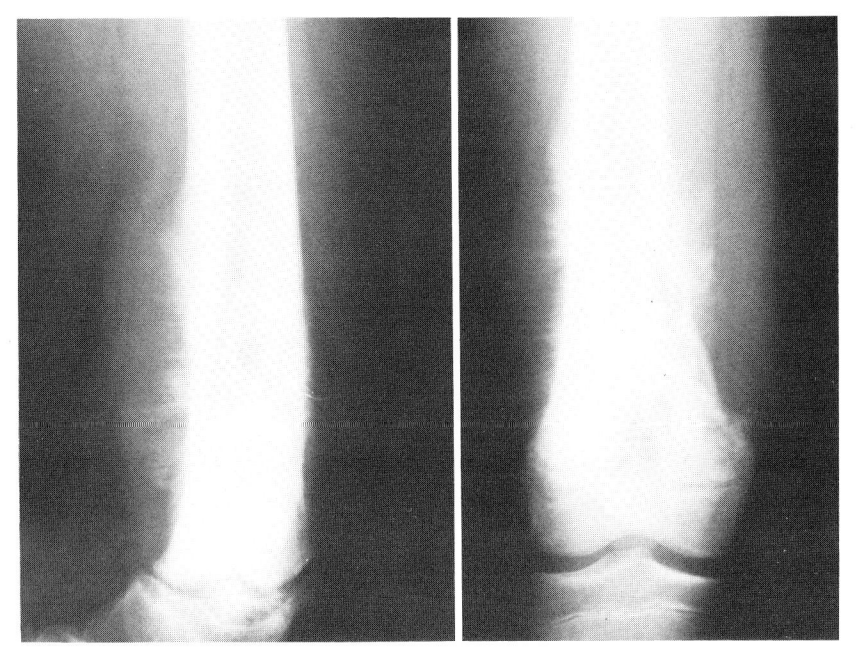

Figure 17-3 Osteogenic sarcoma of the distal femur, demonstrating the "sunburst" appearance on roentgenograms due to spicules of new bone. (Courtesy of Dr. Franklin Angell, Mercy Hospital, Baltimore.)

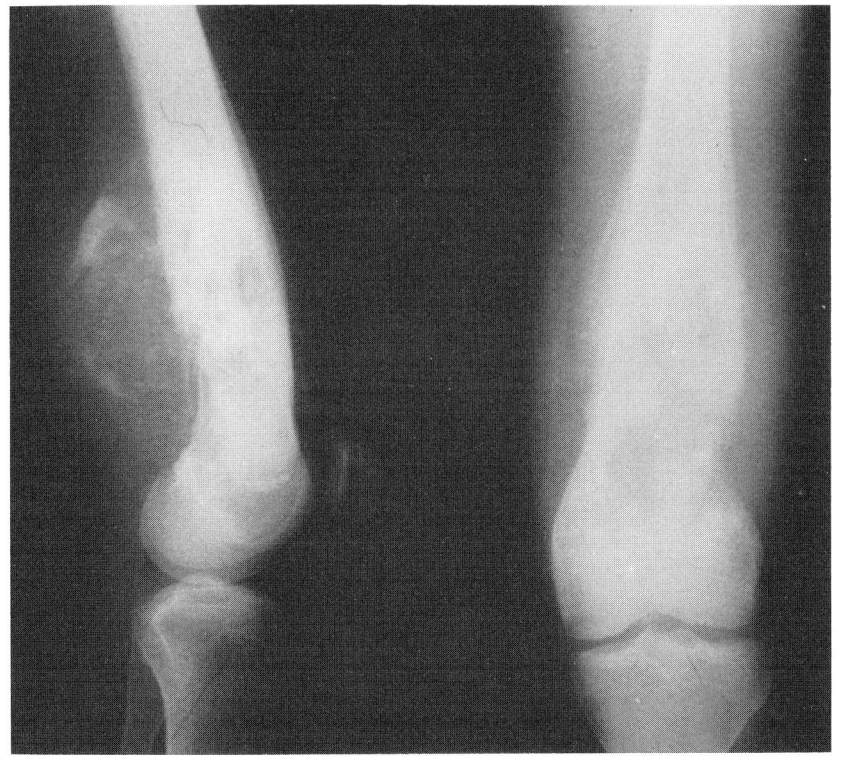

Figure 17-4 Osteogenic sarcoma of the distal femur, showing a large soft-tissue mass containing calcifications contiguous to the bone. (From the teaching files of the Johns Hopkins Hospital, Division of Pediatric Radiology.)

helpful in predicting the chances of survival. O'Hara and associates[83] found no particular pattern to warrant histologic subdivision in their study of 30 patients who survived for 10 years or longer. Scranton and co-workers[109] described six predominant tumor patterns, two of which appeared to have an increased incidence of survival, but their series was small. At the present time, there appears to be no histologic pattern that accurately predicts prognosis or dictates therapy.

Skip areas are secondary, smaller foci of osteosarcoma that are anatomically separate from the primary lesion. They are found either in the same bone or on the opposing side of the adjacent joint. Most studies[20, 65, 132] have found them to be rare, but Enneking and Kagan[24] found such lesions to occur in 10 of 40 cases, only two of which were apparent on the initial roentgenogram.

Clinical Course. Osteosarcoma is a highly malignant tumor which rapidly disseminates via the venous route. Lymphatic spread from the primary tumor to regional nodes occurs infrequently.[10] Lung lesions are usually the first clinical evidence of metastatic disease (Fig. 17-5). Prior to the use of chemotherapy the majority of patients developed pulmonary lesions within a year of amputation. This was often followed by metastases to multiple visceral organs and other portions of the skeleton. Recurrence of tumor meant death within a year.[70] There appears to be an increased incidence of spontaneous pneumothorax in patients with pulmonary metastases compared to patients with other tumors which metastasize to the lung.[115, 122] The reasons for this are not clearly understood. This complication may result in the patient's rapid demise if it is not appropriately treated. If the problem is recognized and properly managed, functional recovery may ensue, as in the case of one patient who, following chest tube drainage, returned to school to play trombone in the band.[115]

Treatment and Prognosis. Patients with disease localized to a limb with no obvious evidence of metastases should be treated by amputation. The majority of oncologists with experience in treating this tumor have advocated entire surgical removal of the involved bone. Since this tumor most commonly presents in the lower extremity in children, a hip disarticula-

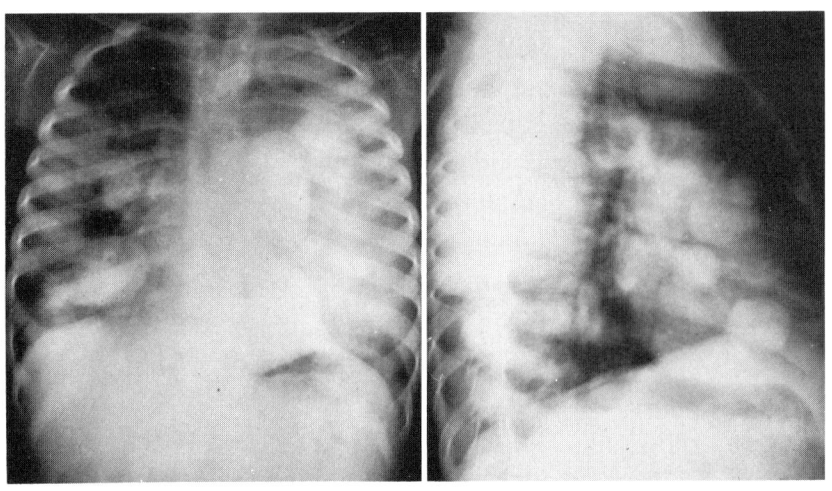

Figure 17-5 Multiple pulmonary metastases in a child with osteogenic sarcoma. (From the teaching files of the Johns Hopkins Hospital, Division of Pediatric Radiology.)

tion for tumors of the femur and above-knee amputation for lesions of the proximal tibia or fibula are the procedures most commonly performed. Such approaches have been recommended because of the possible presence of intramedullary extension[132] or of "skip" metastases which may be found proximal to the primary tumor.[24] Some believe that above-knee transection of the femur should be performed if the lesion is in the distal femur, and that a hip disarticulation is not justified.[48] Lewis and Lotz[65] analyzed 20 amputation specimens and failed to find skip areas. They also found the most proximal extent of the tumor, by preoperative radiographic evaluation, to be within 1 cm of the gross intramedullary extent. In 18 patients, microscopic sections proximal to the gross tumor margin revealed no extension, and in the remaining two cases, although there was tumor within 1 cm, sections 2 cm from the gross tumor margin and beyond showed no tumor. However, a number of localized tumor recurrences at the stump have been reported.[75,123] There is no randomized series available comparing transmedullary amputation with radical amputation at the proximal joint.

Radiation therapy, when used alone, has not usually produced results as good as surgery. The resistance of this neoplasm to radiation is demonstrated by the presence of viable tumor cells in pathologic specimens after receiving up to 10,000 rads.[89] Even when there is evidence of metastatic disease, surgery may be preferred to local radiation therapy to the primary tumor when it is very large. Following radiation therapy, the patient may be left with a painful, nonfunctioning limb with tissue breakdown, which often becomes the site of infection. A decision to avoid "unnecessary" amputation in a patient with metastatic disease sometimes becomes a disservice to the patient, and often is eventually performed despite the original decision.

Preoperative radiation has been used by a number of investigators. Cade[11] utilized preoperative radiation with 6000 to 9000 rads to control local tumor growth and performed amputation only if pulmonary lesions did not appear in the following few months. This was done in an effort to avoid amputation in the patient who already had metastatic disease, which was initially roentgenographically inapparent. This often does not result in palliation or preservation of a functioning limb unless the tumor is small, nor does it improve the chances of survival.[56,124] Radiation therapy followed shortly by amputation has been utilized in an effort to improve the disappointing results achieved by surgery alone. This has been done to avoid possible tumor dissemination at the time of surgery. There is some evidence that such an approach may improve survival,[56,89] but the numbers in most studies are small.

At the present time, a local attack upon the primary tumor by amputation with or without radiation seldom yields survival rates greater than 20 per cent despite the absence of detectable metastases during the initial evaluation. One must therefore assume that the majority of patients with osteogenic sarcoma have disseminated disease at the time of diagnosis. Rab and co-workers,[94] in an effort to prevent the development of pulmonary metastases, treated patients with prophylactic whole lung irradiation following actinomycin D infusions, but found the subsequent occurrence of pulmonary disease to be no different from that of a control group. More encouraging results, however, are now being reported from a number of cancer treatment centers that are using programs of adjuvant chemotherapy immediately following amputation. These treatment programs were devised because of reports of regression of metastatic tumor masses following treatment with Adriamycin[18] or high-dose methotrexate with citrovorum factor rescue.[53] Cortes and associates[17] treated 21 patients without detectable metastases with multiple courses of Adriamycin after surgical amputation of the primary lesion and, using life-table analyses, determined that 71 per cent would be expected to be free of pulmonary metastases at 18 months. Jaffe and associates[54] treated 20 consecutive patients without metastases with vincristine followed by high-dose methotrexate with citrovorum rescue and significantly reduced the incidence of pulmonary metastases to two as opposed to 12.2 expected cases. Sutow and co-workers[120] used a four-drug regimen (cyclophosphamide, vincristine, phenylalanine mustard, and Adriamycin) following surgical amputation. Of 18 children, 10 (55 per cent) were free of disease 24 months or longer from the time of amputation.

Most data indicate that, prior to the use of adjuvant chemotherapy, metastases rarely developed in patients who were disease free for 12 months. The report of four patients who demonstrated late metastases between 16 and 26 months following amputation suggests that the chemotherapy they received may have merely delayed the recurrence of disease.[118] As more patients receive chemotherapy and follow-up data are collected, the long-term influence of antineoplastic drugs on the course of this disease will eventually be established.

Prior to the use of chemotherapy and surgical attacks upon metastatic lesions, the discovery of pulmonary metastases was followed by the patient's death in over 50 per cent of the cases by 4 months and nearly 100 per cent of the cases within a year.[70] A number of reports of surgical excision of a solitary pulmonary metastasis or multiple lesions, if they were not too numerous, indicated that a number of patients derived benefit from such an approach, with prolonged survival.[5, 73, 125] In 1971 Martini and co-workers[73] reported attempts to control multiple pulmonary lesions by surgical excision. In 22 patients, all grossly palpable disease was removed and at the time of the report 10 patients (45 per cent) were alive. A subsequent publication in 1975[6] stated that six of the 22 patients remained alive and free of disease 5 or more years following amputation, representing a 5-year survival of 27 per cent in patients with pulmonary metastases treated by surgical resection.

Numerous investigators have now reported regression of metastatic osteosarcoma lesions following the use of various chemotherapeutic regimens.[18, 53, 96, 98, 99, 136] Rosen and colleagues reported a 54 per cent response rate in children with metastatic disease treated with Adriamycin and high-dose methotrexate with citrovorum factor rescue[98] and increased this to 77 per cent (seven of nine patients) using these drugs with vincristine and cyclophosphamide.[99] The addition of radiation therapy to this latter regimen[100] resulted in a response in 14 of 16 patients with metastatic lesions with a better response in bone lesions than lung lesions, probably because of the ability to use high doses of radiation to bone. Unfortunately, the toxicity from the addition of pulmonary irradiation contributed to the death of two of four patients.

The encouraging results following surgical resections of pulmonary lesions and the reports of chemotherapeutic responses prompted Beattie and co-workers[6] to combine these modalities. All gross tumor was removed surgically in five of 10 patients and three of the five were free of disease at the time of their report. The ultimate impact of this treatment on these and other patients treated with various regimens will only be known after long-term follow up. The dangers of early conclusions based on short-term observations are demonstrated by the data reported by Rosen[96] (Fig. 17–6), which indicates that the natural

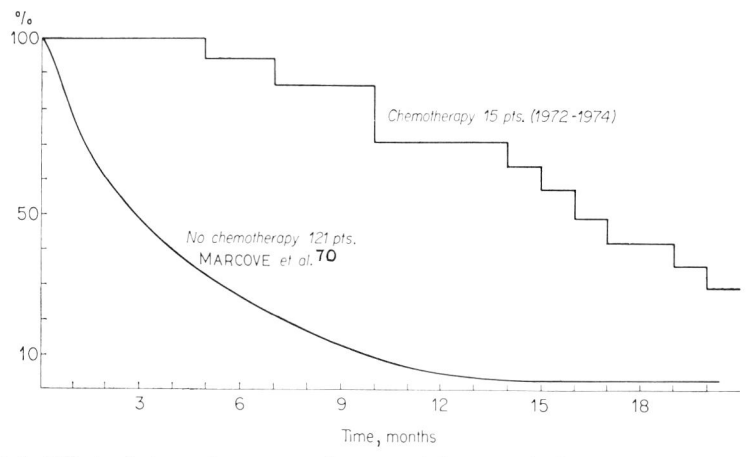

Figure 17-6 Effect of chemotherapy on the natural history of advanced metastatic osteogenic sarcoma. Although the median survival time of 15 patients treated with chemotherapy (upper line) is significantly longer than that of 121 patients in a control group (lower line)—16 months versus 3 months—the continuing late deaths in the chemotherapy group demonstrate the need for caution in interpreting prolonged survival as cure. (From Rosen, G.: Front. Radiat. Ther. Oncol. 10:115, 1975.)

course of the disease may be markedly altered, and death may still occur from tumor recurrence, but at a much later date.

A number of investigators have used various forms of immunotherapy as an adjunct to the surgical management of osteosarcoma because of evidence that osteosarcoma contained tumor-specific antigens and that the cellular and humoral immune mechanisms responded to the presence of this tumor.[14, 72, 138] At the present time, most studies involving the use of immunotherapy have been inconclusive because of small numbers,[38, 114] or the treatment has been ineffective.[81]

Parosteal Osteogenic Sarcoma

The parosteal osteogenic sarcoma was first delineated in 1951 by Geschichkter and Copeland[40] as a variant of osteogenic sarcoma with distinct clinical and pathological features. Unni and associates[131] reviewed a series of 79 patients with this tumor and, unlike the more typical osteogenic sarcoma, found it to be more common in females, an observation also made in another large series.[133] It did not appear in any patient in the first decade of life, was diagnosed in 23 patients in the second decade and 21 each in the third and fourth decades. The most frequent sign was localized painless swelling, and the duration of symptoms generally was long, with 21 having complaints for over 5 years. The posterior aspect of the distal femur was most commonly involved, followed in frequency by involvement of the proximal tibia and proximal humerus. The roentgenographic appearance was that of an extremely dense, lobulated mass arising superficially from the metaphyseal region of the long bone, attached to the cortex by a broad base (Fig. 17-7). The tumor has a tendency to encircle the bone but not become attached to it except at the base. The majority of tumors are heavily ossified, with no tendency for spicule formation. Microscopically they are usually very well differentiated. Medullary involvement is seldom found but when it occurs, the patient has a poorer prognosis.[131] These tumors tend to recur if incompletely removed and occasionally may metastasize.

In Unni and co-workers' series,[131] 27

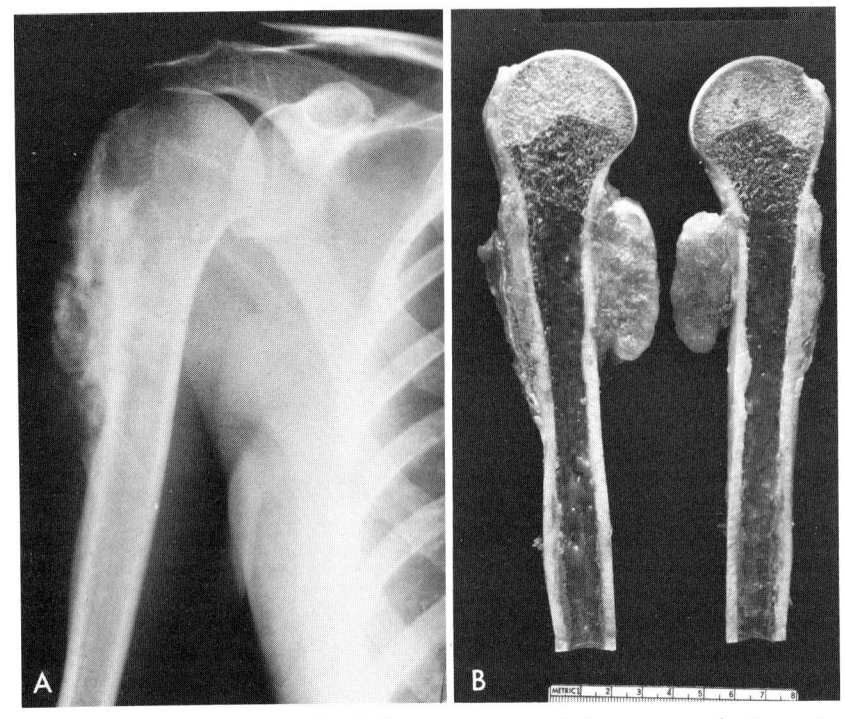

Figure 17-7 Roentgenographic and pathologic appearance of a large parosteal osteogenic sarcoma involving the proximal portion of the humerus. The lesion is opaque and lobulated, with small radiolucent areas. The gross lesion has a broad base on the cortical surface, and there is no invasion of the medulla. (From Unni, K. K., et al.: Cancer 37:2466, 1976.)

of 31 patients who had local excision of the tumor had recurrence. Of 10 who had complete removal of tumor with its surrounding normal tissues, three developed local recurrence. Twenty-seven underwent amputation as primary therapy and four were later documented to have pulmonary metastases. Those who experienced local recurrence often did well following amputation or a second resection. All of the patients who eventually died of metastatic disease lived for more than 5 years. These authors suggest that complete radical surgical removal is the treatment of choice, with resection when the lesions are small, and amputation when large. An analysis of 61 cases by Van der Heul and von Ronnen[133] led them to recommend complete local removal of smaller tumors with a histologically low-grade degree of malignancy that are separated from the neighboring cortex, but amputation or disarticulation when the growths are large and more malignant, or when there is a recurrence. Although the prognosis is much better than that of the more typical osteosarcoma, and the majority of patients survive following surgical treatment, long-term follow-up is necessary because of the slow evolution of this neoplasm.

Recently, another variant of osteogenic sarcoma has been reported which has been termed "periosteal osteogenic sarcoma."[129] These tumors usually involve the proximal tibia and present as small radiolucent lesions on the surface with bone spicules perpendicular to the shaft. They are histologically relatively high-grade in their degree of malignancy but the prognosis appears to be better than that of the usual osteosarcoma.

EWING'S TUMOR

In 1921, James Ewing first described a malignant nonosseous small cell tumor of bone.[26] He believed that the neoplasm arose from the endothelium of blood vessels and therefore called this neoplasm "diffuse endothelioma of bone." Today most investigators believe that Ewing's tumor originates from immature reticulum cells.[37] The tumor is now known to be the second most common bone malignancy that occurs during the first three decades of life. Nearly half the patients are between the ages of 10 and 20 years, and 70 per cent are under the age of 20 (Fig. 17-8). The tumor occurs about 1.5 times more commonly in males than in females. It is extremely rare among black children in the United States in contrast to osteogenic sarcoma, in which no significant racial difference in incidence is found.[36, 58, 140] Ewing's tumor is also rare in black children in Africa.[22, 137]

Clinical Presentation. Pain is the first symptom of Ewing's tumor in the majority of patients. This is usually followed by localized swelling, and is sometimes associated with fever, leukocytosis, and an elevated sedimentation rate, suggesting the presence of an infectious process. Often the patient has had pain for over a month before he seeks medical aid. The average duration of delay in diagnosis in the series of 30 patients reported by Chan and colleagues[13] was 6 months. The tumor most commonly involves the upper end or midshaft of the femur, or arises in the pelvis. The tibia, fibula, humerus, scapula, or ribs are also likely sites of the primary lesion, but

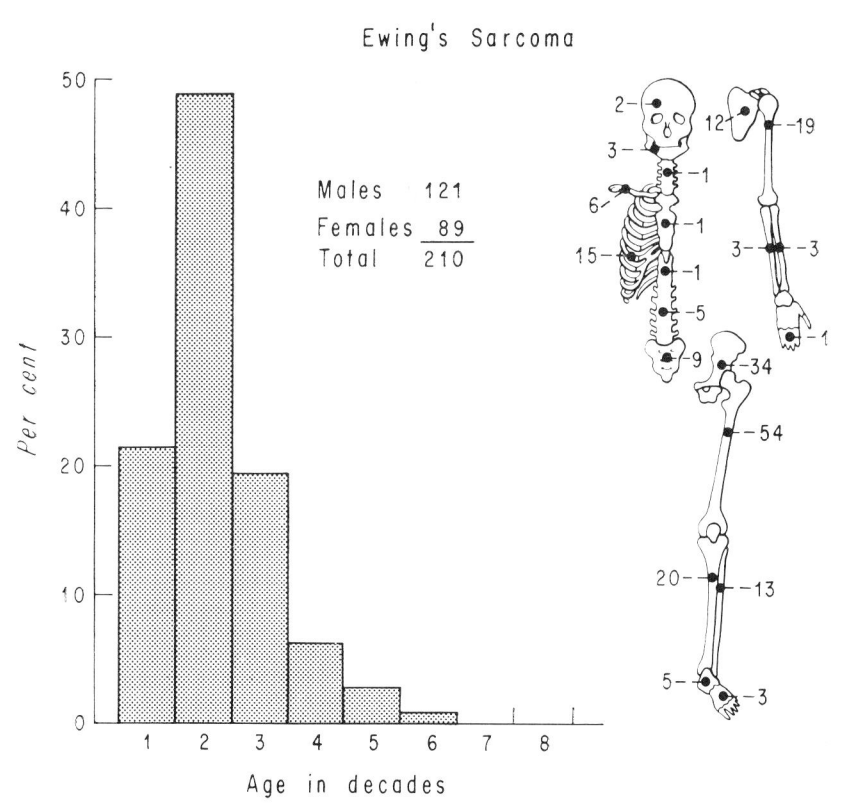

Figure 17-8 Skeletal, age, and sex distribution of Ewing's tumor. (From Dahlin, D. C., Bone Tumors, 2nd Ed., 1967. Courtesy of Charles C Thomas, Publisher, Springfield, Illinois.)

nearly any bone may be involved (Fig. 17–8). When the tumor involves a superficially located bone such as a rib, a large extraosseous mass may be present (Fig. 17–9).

Diagnostic Studies. The roentgenographic appearance that suggests Ewing's tumor usually shows localized, mottled rarefaction due to bone destruction (Fig. 17–10). Although the early lesion may appear small, the actual involvement of the marrow space by the neoplasm is often extensive. This early lesion may resemble infection, histiocytosis, or metastatic neuroblastoma. As the tumor extends through the cortex, it often elevates the periosteum, producing multiple layers of subperiosteal reactive new bone, which gives an "onionskin" appearance. Radiating spicules may also appear, which may cause it to resemble an osteosarcoma roentgenographically. A soft tissue mass overlying the area of bone destruction is frequently seen. No radiologic picture is pathognomonic, and the definitive diagnosis can only be made by biopsy. If one is highly suspicious of the presence of a Ewing's tumor, a skeletal survey, isotopic bone scan, chest roentgenograms and chest tomography may be performed prior to surgery. We have routinely performed a bone marrow

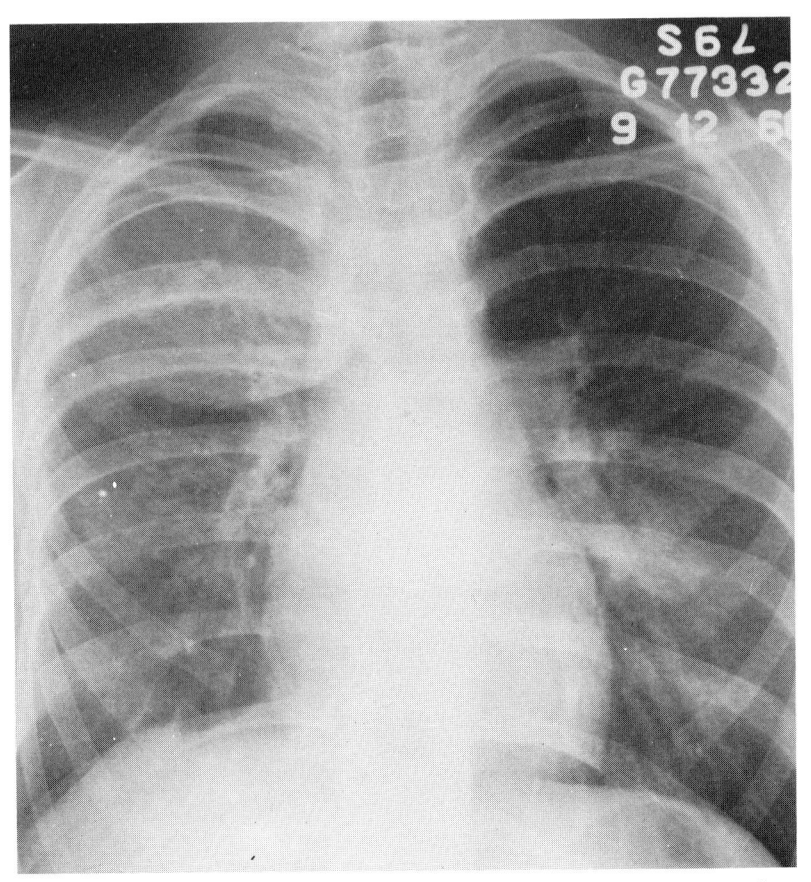

Figure 17–9 Chest roentgenogram of a 10 year old white girl with a chronic, nonproductive cough, anorexia, and weight loss. A large, nonfluctuant mass was palpable to the right of the spine and overlying the fifth rib. The large extraosseous mass represented a Ewing's tumor that originated in the rib. (From Gwinn, J. L.: Amer. J. Dis. Child, *116*:179, August 1968. Copyright 1968, American Medical Association.)

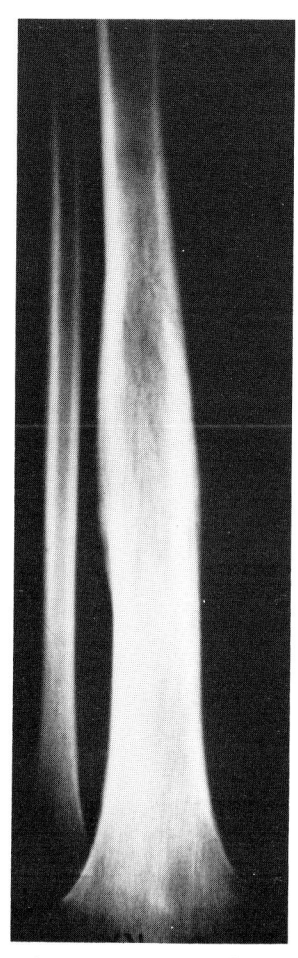

Figure 17-10 Permeative diaphyseal expanding intramedullary lesion of the tibia in an 11 year old white female. The tumor margins are poorly defined and appear to run up and down the shaft of the bone. There are also laminar, thin, periosteal reactive changes over the tumor site. Biopsy revealed Ewing's tumor.

aspiration and biopsy at a site distant from the primary lesion at the time of the surgical procedure on patients with suspected malignancy known to metastasize to bone. If not performed prior to surgery, the evaluation for metastatic disease should be done following a definitive diagnosis because of the tendency of this neoplasm to metastasize early to lungs and bone.

The medullary cavity appears to be the site of origin of most Ewing's tumors. The biopsy should be performed in the soft tissue component and cortical bone removed only in the rare case in which the tumor is confined within the bone. Removal of cortical bone may be detrimental to efforts to obtain good, long-term function of the limb. Histologically, the neoplasm is composed of densely packed, highly anaplastic small, round cells with little variation in size. Sheets of these cells may be separated into aggregates by strands of fibrous tissue. The tumor is often difficult to differentiate microscopically from other small, round-cell tumors, such as neuroblastoma, rhabdomyosarcoma, and non-Hodgkin's lymphoma, all of which may directly invade or metastasize to bone. Ewing's tumor cells often contain granules that contain glycogen, which can be demonstrated by special histochemical staining techniques utilizing the periodic acid–Schiff (PAS) reaction,[105] which often helps in diagnosing the tumor. PAS-positivity was present in 53 of 66 patients reported in one large study.[90] The difficulty of establishing a diagnosis is emphasized by Pomeroy and Johnson,[91] who reported an incorrect diagnosis in 17 of 95 patients suspected of having Ewing's sarcoma who were referred to the National Cancer Institute. Occasionally a definitive diagnosis of a "small round-cell tumor" cannot be made histologically or following an extensive medical evaluation, and the oncologist must decide on a course of therapy based upon judgment and experience.

Clinical Course. Ewing's tumor is one of the most lethal malignancies found in children. The majority of reports of the results of local therapy have demonstrated 5-year survival rates ranging from less than 5 to 20 per cent. A summary by Nesbit[82] of the results of six large series totaling 374 patients revealed that only 36 survived for 5 years. Falk and Albert[28] found the 5-year survival rate in 944 patients to be 8 per cent. Unfortunately, even those alive at 5 years may eventually die of their disease. Dahlin[20] reported deaths in 6 of 20 patients who did survive 5 years, one 12 years after the initial diagnosis.

Approximately 10 to 30 per cent of patients have apparent metastases at the time of diagnosis.[7, 13, 90, 135] The majority of the remainder develop detectable hematogenous metastases within 12 months of diagnosis. The most common sites of early metastases are the lungs and bones, especially the skull. Of 54 children in one series, metastatic disease appeared first in the lungs in 21 patients, first in the bones in 16, and simultaneously in lungs and bone in five.[87] The incidence of central nervous system involvement has been reported to be high in a few series.[64, 76] Later in the patient's course, disseminated disease may appear in numerous organs.

Treatment. The majority of cancer treatment centers currently treat patients with Ewing's tumor with high-dose radiation therapy to the primary lesion combined with intensive multidrug chemotherapy. The "case against surgery" put forth by Boyer and coworkers[9] was based on the fact that the great majority of patients eventually died of disseminated disease and that the survival rates following amputation or radiation therapy were the same.

Most radiation therapists recommend supervoltage radiation therapy and use a tumor dose between 6000 and 7000 rads when an extremity is involved.[13, 116] This is accomplished by delivering 5000 rads to the entire bone and an additional 1500 rads to the main tumor, usually over a period of between 6 to 8 weeks. The entire circumference of the limb should not be irradiated to avoid the complication of constrictive fibrosis and lymphedema. When the tumor dose is less than 4000 rads, local failure is common.[13] When the dose is up to or beyond 7000 rads, a high incidence of complications occur, including pain, edema, and functional impairment. One must remember that concomitant administration of radiation therapy and chemotherapy decreases the tolerance of normal tissues to radiation.

Treatment of lesions in certain anatomic sites such as those in the pelvis, ribs, or vertebrae requires the design of special fields and often a reduction in radiation dose because of the limits set by the tissues in the radiation field. One technique to spare pulmonary tissue from the effects of radiation has been to create a pneumothorax to collapse the lung temporarily during the time of administration of radiation.[19] Some have advocated surgical removal of lesions that may be difficult to treat with radiation therapy if the surgery does not result in a functional defect. Thus, removal of lesions of the rib or removal of an involved fibula may at times be preferred to the use of radiation therapy. It has recently been suggested that Boyer's prechemotherapeutic-era case against surgery may no longer be applicable and that amputation, especially of a weight-bearing limb, may be preferred. This argument is based on the observation that the irradiated limb often does not function normally, local recurrences followed by metastases leading to death have occurred, and chemotherapy has often been stopped prematurely due to reactions in the field of radiation.[97]

Despite the fact that the primary tumor can usually be controlled by local measures, early dissemination detected at the time of diagnosis or shortly thereafter is the rule. There is increasing evidence that the addition of chemotherapy decreases the incidence of early metastases, prolongs the time of survival and appears to be increasing the rate of cure. In 1967, Phillips and Higinbotham[87] reported 13 of 39 children with clinically localized disease to be alive and free of tumor 5 years after diagnosis. These children were treated with 3000 to 4000 rads to the affected bone, accompanied in most cases by various forms of chemotherapy, most notably nitrogen mustard used as a single agent. A number of other agents used singly have also been shown to be effective in treating Ewing's sarcoma, including mithramycin,[62] BCNU,[86] 5-fluorouracil,[63] cyclophosphamide,[104] vincristine,[119] actinomycin D,[110] and Adriamycin.[84]

Combination chemotherapy plus radiotherapy to the primary lesion now appears to give the best results in patients with clinically localized disease. Hustu and colleagues[49] reported 11 of 15 patients surviving with no evidence of disease from 4 to over 91 months after diagnosis following local radiation to the primary tumor and treatment with vincristine and cyclophosphamide. Pomeroy and Johnson[90] reported 64 per cent 2-year and 52 per cent 5-year survival rates in 43 patients without clinically detectable metastases at diagnosis who were treated with local radiation and various chemotherapeutic regimens, two of which included central nervous system prophylactic treatment. Such central nervous system prophylaxis has been advocated by some investigators[76, 90] because of the occasional occurrence of metastatic disease first appearing in the brain or meninges.[71]

The impressive results reported by Rosen and co-workers[101] following the use of local radiation and a four-drug protocol consisting of actinomycin D, Adriamycin, cyclophosphamide, and vincristine showed 12 of 12 children to be free of disease 10 to 37 months following the start of therapy. Three of these patients had evidence of metastatic disease at the time of diagnosis. A more recent follow-up report[97] of this treatment regimen revealed 15 of 19 patients with clinically localized tumor to be free of disease at a median time of 37 months from the start of therapy, but only two of eight who had detectable metastases at diagnosis to be disease-free despite the fact that all eight had initially experienced a complete remission. Although such reports of late recurrence may temper the earlier enthusiasm regarding various treatment regimens, it is clear that chemotherapy has a major impact on the course of this disease by decreasing the incidence of local and early metastatic recurrence, and by prolonging the time of survival.[29, 49, 90, 101] There now appears to be less interest in treatment with total body irradiation,[57] but the benefits of prophylactic pulmonary or central nervous system radiation therapy have yet to be determined and are now being evaluated. The most effective therapy of localized or disseminated disease and the impact on the ultimate cure rate of Ewing's tumor will only be determined with time.

MISCELLANEOUS MALIGNANT BONE TUMORS

Fibrosarcoma

The fibrosarcoma is an uncommon primary malignancy of bone which represents less than 5 per cent of bone cancers in most series.[20, 52] The primary tumor sites do not differ remarkably from those involved by osteosarcoma. The tumor seldom occurs during the first decade of life and is evenly distributed among patients in the second through the sixth decades. Only 11 children under the age of 15 years were in one series of 130 patients.[52] Males and females are equally affected. Many cases occur in the site of previous irradiation or preexisting bone disease. The tumor is characterized by interlacing bundles of collagen fibers and lacks any tendency to form tumor bone, osteoid, or cartilage. The 5-year survival rate following amputation alone is better than that achieved with osteosarcoma, but late recurrence and death is not uncommon, with the tumor often metastasizing to lung and bone. There is some evidence that well-differentiated fibrosarcomas and those arising in a periosteal location have a better prognosis.

Malignant Lymphoma (Reticulum Cell Sarcoma) of Bone

This tumor is uncommon in the very young. When the primary tumor is in the skeleton with no evidence of multifocal disease, it often responds to radiation therapy alone with survival rates reported between 40 to 50 per cent.[8, 134] One must be certain, especially in the child, that the patient does not have a focal infiltrate as a manifestation of acute lymphocytic leukemia that is mistaken for a local disease.

Chondrosarcoma

The chondrosarcoma most commonly occurs during the middle and later years of life. Only one of 334 patients reported by Dahlin[20] with this tumor was under the age of 10 years. Over 75 per cent of these neoplasms arise in the trunk or the proximal ends of the femur or humerus. They may arise in preexisting osteochondromas. The tumors are slow-growing and may recur 5 to 10 years after primary therapy. Radical surgical removal appears to give the best results.

Other primary malignant bone tumors that are very rare include adamantinomas of long bones,[130] malignant vascular tumors,[41] malignant giant cell tumors,[51] and chordomas.[60]

REHABILITATION

Deformity and disability from the absence of a limb can be devastating to the patient, especially the teenager and young adult. The improved chances of survival may initially give little consolation to the adolescent who faces the immediate problem of losing an arm or leg, and the physician is often confronted with a patient who states that he would "rather die" than undergo a mutilating operation. Some have advocated an immediate fitting of a prosthetic device at the time of surgery when an above-knee or transmedullary amputation is performed,[117] mainly for the psychological effect it has on the patient. En bloc resection with prosthetic bone replacement has been utilized in some cases of osteosarcoma,[97, 97a] and a preliminary report of massive resection and allograft transplantation of cadaver bone for the treatment of malignant bone tumors has demonstrated encouraging results.[69] Although the use of newer prosthetic devices and surgical techniques offers more to the patient in terms of physical rehabilitation than ever before, the psychological and social rehabilitation of the patient is often as much, if not more, a challenge to those caring for the child or adolescent than is the treatment of the tumor itself.

REFERENCES

1. Allan, C. J., and Soule, E. H.: Osteogenic sarcoma of the somatic soft tissues. Cancer 27:1121, 1971.
2. Altner, P. C., Simmons, D. J., Lucas, H. F., et al.: Osteogenic sarcoma in a patient injected with Thorotrast. J. Bone Joint Surg. 54-A:670, 1972.
3. Amstutz, H. C.: Multiple osteogenic sarcoma — metastatic or multicentric? Report of two cases and review of the literature. Cancer 24:923, 1969.
4. Arnold, W. H.: Hereditary bone dysplasia with sarcomatous degeneration. Study of a family. Ann. Intern. Med. 78:902, 1973.
5. Ballantine, T. V. N., Wiseman, N. E., and Filler, R. E.: Assessment of pulmonary wedge resection for the treatment of lung metastases. J. Pediatr. Surg. 10:671, 1975.
6. Beattie, E. J., Jr., Martini, N., and Rosen, G.: The management of pulmonary metastases in children with osteogenic sarcoma with surgical resection combined with chemotherapy. Cancer 35:618, 1975.
7. Bhansali, S. K.: Ewing's sarcoma. Observations on 107 cases. J. Bone Joint Surg. 45-A:541, 1963.
8. Boston, H. C., Dahlin, D. C., Ivins, J. C., et al.: Malignant lymphoma (so-called reticulum cell sarcoma) of bone. Cancer 34:1131, 1974.
9. Boyer, C. W., Jr., Brickner, T. J., Jr., and Perry, R. H.: Ewing's sarcoma: case against surgery. Cancer 20:1602, 1967.
10. Caceres, E., Zaharia, M., and Tantalean,

E.: Lymph node metastases in osteogenic sarcoma. Surgery 65:421, 1969.
11. Cade, S.: Osteogenic sarcoma. A study based on 113 patients. J. Roy. Coll. Surg. Edinb. *1*:79, 1955.
12. Caron, A. S., Hajdu, S. I., and Strong, E. W.: Osteogenic sarcoma of the facial and cranial bones. A review of forty-three cases. Am. J. Surg. *122*:719, 1971.
13. Chan, P. Y. M., Gilbert, H. A., Stein, J. J., et al.: The role of early diagnosis and radiation therapy in the management of Ewing's sarcoma. Front. Radiat. Ther. Oncol. *10*:141, 1975.
14. Cohen, A. M., Ketcham, A. S., and Morton, D. L.: Tumor-specific cellular cytotoxicity to human sarcoma: evidence for a cell-mediated host immune response to a common sarcoma cell surface antigen. J. Natl. Cancer Inst. *50*:585, 1973.
15. Cohen, J., and D'Angio, G. J.: Unusual bone tumors after roentgen therapy of children: two case reports. Am. J. Roentgenol. *86*:502, 1961.
16. Coley, W. B., and Higinbotham, N. L.: Injury as a causative factor in the development of malignant tumors. Ann. Surg. *98*:991, 1933.
17. Cortes, E. P., Holland, J. F., Wang, J. J., et al.: Amputation and Adriamycin in primary osteosarcoma. N. Engl. J. Med. *291*:998, 1974.
18. Cortes, E. P., Holland, J. F., Wang, J. J., et al.: Doxorubicin in disseminated osteosarcoma. J.A.M.A. *221*:1132, 1972.
19. D'Angio, G. J.: *In* Kinney, T. R., and Chung, S. M. K.: Advances in the treatment of tumors arising in bone. Semin. Oncol. *1*:47, 1974.
20. Dahlin, D. C.: Bone Tumors. General Aspects and Data on 3987 Cases. 2nd Ed. Springfield, Ill., Charles C Thomas, Publisher, 1967.
21. Ederer, F., Miller, R. W., and Scotto, J.: U.S. childhood cancer mortality patterns, 1950–1959: etiologic implications. J.A.M.A. *192*:593, 1965.
22. Edington, G. M., and Maclean, C. M.: A cancer rate survey in Ibadan. Brit. J. Cancer *19*:471, 1965.
23. Elmore, S. M., and Cantrell, W. C.: Maffucci's syndrome. Case report with a normal karyotype. J. Bone Joint Surg. *48-A*:1607, 1966.
24. Enneking, W. F., and Kagan, A.: "Skip" metastases in osteosarcoma. Cancer *36*:2192, 1975.
25. Epstein, L. I., Bixler, D., and Bennett, J. E.: An incident of familial cancer. Including 3 cases of osteogenic sarcoma. Cancer *25*:889, 1970.
26. Ewing, J.: Diffuse endothelioma of bone. Proc. N.Y. Path. Soc. *21*:17, 1921.
27. Ewing, J.: Modern attitude toward traumatic cancer. Arch. Path. *19*:690, 1935.
28. Falk, S., and Albert, M.: Five year survival of patients with Ewing's sarcoma. Surg. Gynec. Obstet. *124*:319, 1967.
29. Fernandez, C. H., Lindberg, R. D., Sutow, W. W., et al.: Localized Ewing's sarcoma—treatment and results. Cancer *34*:143, 1974.
30. Fine, G., and Stout, A. P.: Osteogenic sarcoma of the extraskeletal soft tissues. Cancer *9*:1027, 1956.
31. Finkel, M. P., Biskis, B. O., and Farrel, C.: Osteosarcomas appearing in Syrian hamsters after treatment with extracts of human osteosarcomas. Proc. Natl. Acad. Sci. *60*:1223, 1968.
32. Finkel, M. P., Biskis, B. O., and Jinkins, P. B.: Virus induction of osteosarcomas in mice. Science *151*:698, 1966.
33. Finkel, M. P., Reilly, C. A., Jr., and Biskis, B. O.: Viral etiology of bone cancer. Front. Radiat. Ther. Oncol. *10*:28, 1975.
34. Fraumeni, J. F., Jr.: Bone cancer: epidemiologic and etiologic considerations. Front. Radiat. Ther. Oncol. *10*:17, 1975.
35. Fraumeni, J. F., Jr.: Stature and malignant tumors of bone in childhood and adolescence. Cancer *20*:967, 1967.
36. Fraumeni, J. F., Jr., and Glass, A. G.: Rarity of Ewing's sarcoma among U.S. Negro children. Lancet *1*:366, 1970.
37. Friedman, B., and Gold, H.: Ultrastructure of Ewing's sarcoma of bone. Cancer *22*:306, 1968.
38. Fudenberg, H. H.: An admittedly biased view of the role of immunology in human bone cancer. Front. Radiat. Ther. Oncol. *10*:63, 1975.
39. Gavanis, M. D., and Whitesides, T. E., Jr.: The unreliability of prognostic criteria in osteosarcoma. Am. J. Clin. Pathol. *53*:15, 1970.
40. Geschickter, C. F., and Copeland, M. M.: Parosteal osteoma of bone: a new entity. Ann. Surg. *133*:790, 1951.
41. Gilbert, E. F., Jones, B., and Majzoub, H. S.: Malignant hemangioendothelioma of bone in childhood. Am. J. Dis. Child. *121*:410, 1971.
42. Glass, A. G., and Fraumeni, J. F., Jr.: Epidemiology of bone cancer in children. J. Natl. Cancer Inst. *44*:187, 1970.
43. Goidanich, I. F., Battaglia, L., Lenzi, L., et al.: Osteogenic sarcoma. Analysis of factors influencing prognosis in 100 cases. Clin. Orthop. *48*:209, 1966.
44. Gordon, H.: Family studies in retinoblastoma. *In* D. Bergsma (ed.): Medical Genetics Today. Baltimore, Johns Hopkins Press, 1974.
45. Hajdu, S. I.: Aspiration biopsy of primary malignant bone tumors. Front. Radiat. Ther. Oncol. *10*:73, 1975.
46. Hasson, J., Hartman, K. S., Milikow, E., et al.: Thorotrast-induced extraskeletal osteosarcoma of the cervical region. Cancer *36*:1827, 1975.
47. Henderson, E. D., and Dahlin, D. C.:

Chondrosarcoma of bone – a study of two hundred and eighty-eight cases. J. Bone Joint Surg. 45-A:1450, 1963.
48. Hill, P.: Local recurrence in primary osteosarcoma of the femur. Brit. J. Surg. 60:41, 1973.
49. Hustu, H. O., Pinkel, D., and Pratt, C.: Treatment of clinically localized Ewing's sarcoma with radiotherapy and combination chemotherapy. Cancer 30:1522, 1972.
50. Hutter, R. V. P., Francis, K. C., and Foote, F. W., Jr.: Ewing's sarcoma in siblings. Report of the second known occurrence. Am. J. Surg. 107:598, 1964.
51. Hutter, R. V. P., Worcester, J. N., Jr., Francis, K. C., et al.: Benign and malignant giant cell tumors of bone. A clinicopathological analysis of the natural history of the disease. Cancer 15:653, 1962.
52. Huvos, A. G., and Higinbotham, N. L.: Primary fibrosarcoma of bone. A clinicopathologic study of 130 patients. Cancer 35:837, 1975.
53. Jaffe, N.: Recent advances in the chemotherapy of metastatic osteogenic sarcoma. Cancer 30:1627, 1972.
54. Jaffe, N., Frei, E., Traggis, D., et al.: Adjuvant methotrexate and citrovorum-factor treatment of osteogenic sarcoma. N. Engl. J. Med. 291:994, 1974.
55. Jeffree, G. M., and Price, C. H. G.: Bone tumors and their enzymes. A study of the phosphatases, non-specific esterases and beta-glucuronidase of osteogenic and cartilaginous tumors, fibroblastic and giant-cell lesions. J. Bone Joint Surg. 47-B:120, 1965.
56. Jenkins, R. D. T., Allt, W. E. C., and Fitzpatrick, P. J.: Osteosarcoma – an assessment of management with particular reference to primary irradiation and selective delayed amputation. Cancer 30:393, 1972.
57. Jenkins, R. D. T., Rider, W. D., and Sonley, M. J.: Ewing's sarcoma – a trial of adjuvant total-body irradiation. Radiology 96:151, 1970.
58. Jensen, R. D., and Drake, R. M.: Rarity of Ewing's tumor in Negroes. Lancet 1:777, 1970.
59. Jensen, R. D., and Miller, R. W.: Retinoblastoma: epidemiologic characteristics. N. Engl. J. Med. 285:307, 1971.
60. Kamrin, R. P., Potanos, J. N., and Pool, J. L.: An evaluation of the diagnosis and treatment of chordoma. J. Neurol. Neurosurg. Psychiat. 27:157, 1964.
61. Klenerman, L., Ockenden, B. G., and Townsend, A. C.: Osteosarcoma occurring in osteogenesis imperfecta. Report of two cases. J. Bone Joint Surg. 49-B:314, 1967.

62. Kofman, S., Perlia, C. P., and Economou, S. G.: Mithramycin in the treatment of metastatic Ewing's sarcoma. Cancer 31:889, 1973.
63. Krivit, W., and Bentley, H. P.: Use of 5-fluorouracil in the management of advanced malignancies in childhood. A.M.A. J. Dis. Child. 100:217, 1960.
64. Kullick, S. A., and Mones, R. J.: The neurological complications of Ewing's sarcoma – incidence of neurological involvement and value of radiation therapy. Mt. Sinai J. Med. N.Y. 37:40, 1970.
65. Lewis, R. S., and Lotz, M. J.: Medullary extension of osteosarcoma – implications for rational therapy. Cancer 33:371, 1974.
66. Li, F. P., Tucker, M. A., and Fraumeni, J. F.: Childhood cancer in sibs. J. Pediatr. 88:419, 1976.
67. Lichtenstein, L.: Bone Tumors. 4th Ed. St. Louis, C. V. Mosby Co., 1972.
68. Loutit, J. F.: Malignancy from radium. Brit. J. Cancer 24:195, 1970.
69. Mankin, H. J., Fogelson, F. S., Thrasher, A. Z., et al.: Massive resection and allograft transplantation in the treatment of malignant bone tumors. N. Engl. J. Med. 294:1247, 1976.
70. Marcove, R. C., Miké, V., Hajek, J. V., et al.: Osteogenic sarcoma under the age of twenty-one. A review of 145 operative cases. J. Bone Joint Surg. 52-A:411, 1970.
71. Marsa, G. W., and Johnson, R. E.: Altered pattern of metastasis following treatment of Ewing's sarcoma with radiotherapy and adjuvant chemotherapy. Cancer 27:1051, 1971.
72. Marsh, B., Flynn, L., and Enneking, W.: Immunologic aspects of osteosarcoma and their application to therapy. J. Bone Joint Surg. 54-A:1367, 1972.
73. Martini, N., Huvos, A. G., Miké, V., et al.: Multiple pulmonary resections in the treatment of osteogenic sarcoma. Ann. Thorac. Surg. 12:271, 1971.
74. Martland, H. S., and Humphries, R. E.: Osteogenic sarcoma in dial painters using luminous paint. Arch. Pathol. 7:406, 1929.
75. McKenna, R. J., Schwinn, C. P., Soong, K. W., et al.: Sarcomata of the osteogenic series. J. Bone Joint Surg. 48-A:1, 1966.
76. Mehta, Y., and Hendrickson, F. R.: CNS involvement in Ewing's sarcoma. Cancer 33:859, 1974.
77. Miller, R. W.: Fifty-two forms of childhood cancer: United States mortality experience, 1960–1966. J. Pediatr. 75:685, 1969.
78. Miller, R. W., and Dalager, N. A.: U.S. childhood cancer deaths by cell type, 1960–68. J. Pediatr. 85:664, 1974.

79. Moritz, A. R., and Helberg, D. S.: Trauma and disease. Brooklyn, N.Y., Central Book Co., Inc., 1959.
80. Morton, D. L., and Malmgren, R. A.: Human osteosarcomas: immunologic evidence suggesting an associated infectious agent. Science 162:1279, 1968.
81. Neff, J. R., and Enneking, W. F.: Adoptive immunotherapy in primary osteosarcoma. J. Bone Joint Surg. 57-A:145, 1975.
82. Nesbit, M. E.: Ewing's sarcoma. CA 26:174, 1976.
83. O'Hara, J., Hutler, R., Fotote, F., et al.: An analysis of thirty patients surviving longer than ten years after treatment for osteogenic sarcoma. J. Bone Joint Surg. 50-A:335, 1968.
84. Oldham, R. K., and Pomeroy, T. C.: Treatment of Ewing's sarcoma with Adriamycin (NSC-123127). Cancer Chemother. Rep. 56:635, 1972.
85. Osborne, R. L.: The differential radiologic diagnosis of bone tumors. CA 24:194, 1974.
86. Palma, J., Gailani, S., Freeman, S., et al.: Treatment of metastatic Ewing's sarcoma with BCNU. Cancer 30:909, 1972.
87. Phillips, R. F., and Higinbotham, N. L.: The curability of Ewing's endothelioma of bone in children. J. Pediatr. 70:391, 1967.
88. Phillips, T. L., and Sheline, G. E.: Bone sarcomas following radiation therapy. Radiology 81:992, 1963.
89. Phillips, T. L., and Sheline, G. E.: Radiation therapy of malignant bone tumors. Radiology 92:1537, 1969.
90. Pomeroy, T. C., and Johnson, R. E.: Combined modality therapy of Ewing's sarcoma. Cancer 35:36, 1975.
91. Pomeroy, T. C., and Johnson, R. E.: Integrated therapy of Ewing's sarcoma. Front. Radiat. Ther. Oncol. 10:152, 1975.
92. Price, C. H. G.: The incidence of osteogenic sarcoma in southwest England and its relationship to Paget's disease of bone. J. Bone Joint Surg. 44-B:366, 1962.
93. Price, C. H. G.: Primary bone-forming tumors and their relationship to skeletal growth. J. Bone Joint Surg. 40-B:574, 1958.
94. Rab, G. T., Ivins, J. C., Childs, D. S., Jr., et al.: Elective whole lung irradiation in the treatment of osteogenic sarcoma. Cancer 38:939, 1976.
95. Reilly, C. A., Pritchard, D. J., Biskis, B. O., et al.: Immunologic evidence suggesting a viral etiology of human osteosarcoma. Cancer 30:603, 1972.
96. Rosen, G.: The development of an adjuvant chemotherapy program for the treatment of osteogenic sarcoma. Front. Radiat. Ther. Oncol. 10:115, 1975.
97. Rosen, G.: Management of malignant bone tumors in children and adolescents. Pediat. Clin. North Am. 23:183, 1976.
97a. Rosen, G., Murphy, M. L., Huvos, A. G., et al.: Chemotherapy, en bloc resection, and prosthetic bone replacement in the treatment of osteogenic sarcoma. Cancer 37:1, 1976.
98. Rosen, G., Suwansirikul, S., Kwon, C., et al.: High-dose methotrexate with citrovorum factor rescue and Adriamycin in childhood osteogenic sarcoma. Cancer 33:1151, 1974.
99. Rosen, G., Tan, C., Sanmaneechai, A., et al.: The rationale for multiple drug chemotherapy in treatment of osteogenic sarcoma. Cancer 35:936, 1975.
100. Rosen, G., Tefft, M., Martinez, A., et al.: Combination chemotherapy and radiation therapy in the treatment of metastatic osteogenic sarcoma. Cancer 35:622, 1975.
101. Rosen, G., Wollner, N., Wu, S. J., et al.: Disease-free survival in children with Ewing's sarcoma treated with radiation therapy and adjuvant four-drug sequential chemotherapy. Cancer 33:384, 1974.
102. Rowland, S. A., Dahlin, D. C., Hayles, A. B., et al.: Diagnosis and treatment of bone tumors in children. J.A.M.A. 174:489, 1960.
103. Sagerman, R. H., Cassady, J. R., Tretter, P., et al.: Radiation induced neoplasia following external beam therapy for children with retinoblastoma. Am. J. Roentgenol. 105:529, 1969.
104. Samuels, M. L., and Howe, C. D.: Cyclophosphamide in the management of Ewing's sarcoma. Cancer 20:961, 1967.
105. Schajowicz, F.: Ewing's sarcoma and reticulum cell sarcoma of bone: with special reference to histochemical demonstration of glycogen as an aid to differential diagnosis. J. Bone Joint Surg. 41-A:349, 1959.
106. Schajowicz, F., and Bessone, J. E.: Chondrosarcoma in three brothers. A pathological and genetic study. J. Bone Joint Surg. 49-A:129, 1967.
107. Schajowicz, F., Defilippi-Novoa, C. A., and Firpo, C. A.: Thorotrast induced chondrosarcoma of the axilla. Am. J. Roentgenol. 100:931, 1967.
108. Schimlee, R. N., Lowman, J. T., and Cowan, G. A. B.: Retinoblastoma and osteogenic sarcoma in siblings. Cancer 34:2077, 1974.
109. Scranton, P. E., DeCicco, F. A., Totten, R. S., et al.: Prognostic factors in osteosarcoma. A review of 20 years' experience at the University of Pittsburgh Health Center Hospitals. Cancer 36:2179, 1975.

110. Senyszyn, J. J., Johnson, R. E., and Curran, R. E.: Treatment of metastatic Ewing's sarcoma with actinomycin D. Cancer Chemother. Rep. 54:103, 1970.
111. Shifrine, M., and Fisher, G. L.: Ceruloplasmin levels in sera from human patients with osteosarcoma. Cancer 38:244, 1976.
112. Siegal, G. P., Dahlin, D. C., and Franklin, F. H.: Osteoblastic osteogenic sarcoma in a 35-month-old girl. Report of a case. Am. J. Clin. Pathol. 63:886, 1975.
113. Sim, F. H., Cupps, R. E., Dahlin, D. C., et al.: Postradiation sarcoma of bone. J. Bone Joint Surg. 54-A:1479, 1972.
114. Southam, C. M.: Immunotherapeutic trials in sarcoma patients using autogenous tumor vaccine. Front. Radiat. Ther. Oncol. 7:199, 1972.
115. Spittle, M. F., Heal, J., Harmer, C., et al.: The association of spontaneous pneumothorax with pulmonary metastases in bone tumors of children. Clin. Radiol. 19:400, 1968.
116. Suit, H. D.: Role of therapeutic radiology in cancer of bone. Cancer 35:930, 1975.
117. Suit, H. D., Martin, R. G., and Sutow, W. W.: Primary malignant tumors of the bone. Sutow, W., Vietti, T., and Fernbach, D. (Eds.): *In* Clinical Pediatric Oncology. St. Louis, C. V. Mosby Co., 1973.
118. Sutow, W. W.: Late metastases in osteosarcoma. Lancet 1:856, 1976.
119. Sutow, W. W.: Vincristine therapy for malignant solid tumors in children (except Wilms' tumor). Cancer Chemother. Rep. 52:485, 1968.
120. Sutow, W. W., Sullivan, M. P., Fernbach, D. J., et al.: Adjuvant chemotherapy in primary treatment of osteogenic sarcoma. Cancer 36:1598, 1975.
121. Swaney, J. J.: Familial osteogenic sarcoma. Clin. Orthop. 97:64, 1973.
122. Swaney, J. J., and Cangir, A.: Spontaneous pneumothorax in metastatic osteogenic sarcoma. J. Pediatr. 82:165, 1973.
123. Sweetnam, R.: Amputation in osteosarcoma. J. Bone Joint Surg. 55-B:189, 1973.
124. Sweetnam, R. D., Knowelden, J., and Seddon, H.: Bone sarcoma—treatment by irradiation, amputation or a combination of the two. Brit. J. Med. 2:363, 1971.
125. Sweetnam, R., and Ross, K.: Surgical treatment of pulmonary metastases from primary tumours of bone. J. Bone Joint Surg. 49-B:74, 1967.
126. Tachdjian, M. O.: *In* Pediatric Orthopedics. Vol. 1. Philadelphia, W. B. Saunders Co., 1972.
127. Tjalma, R. A.: Canine bone sarcoma: estimation of relative risk as a function of body size. J. Natl. Cancer Inst. 36:1137, 1966.
128. Turner, R. C.: Unusual group of tumours among schoolgirls. Brit. J. Cancer 21:17, 1967.
129. Unni, K., Dahlin, D. C., and Beabout, J. W.: Periosteal osteogenic sarcoma. Cancer 37:2476, 1976.
130. Unni, K., Dahlin, D. C., Beabout, J. W., et al.: Adamantinomas of long bones. Cancer 34:1796, 1974.
131. Unni, K. K., Dahlin, D. C., Beabout, J. W., et al.: Parosteal osteogenic sarcoma. Cancer 37:2466, 1976.
132. Upshaw, J. E., MacDonald, J. R., and Ghormenly, R. K.: Extension of primary neoplasms of bone to bone marrow. Surg. Gynec. Obstet. 89:704, 1949.
133. Van der Heul, R. O., and von Ronnen, J. R.: Juxtacortical osteosarcoma. J. Bone Joint Surg. 49-A:415, 1967.
134. Wang, C. C.: Treatment of primary reticulum-cell sarcoma of bone by irradiation. N. Engl. J. Med. 278:1331, 1968.
135. Wang, C. C., and Schulz, M. D.: Ewing's sarcoma—a study of 50 cases treated at the Massachusetts General Hospital, 1930–1952 inclusive. N. Engl. J. Med. 248:571, 1953.
136. Wilbur, J. R., Etcubanas, E., Long, T., et al.: Four-drug therapy and irradiation in primary and metastatic osteogenic sarcoma. Proc. Amer. Assoc. Cancer Res. 15:188, 1974.
137. Williams, A. O.: Tumors of childhood in Ibadan, Nigeria. Cancer 36:370, 1975.
138. Wood, W. C., and Morton, D. L.: Host immune response to a common cell-surface antigen in human sarcomas—detection by cytotoxicity tests. N. Engl. J. Med. 284:569, 1971.
139. Yamamoto, T., and Wakabuyshi, T.: Bone tumors among atomic bomb survivors of Hiroshima and Nagasaki. Acta Pathol. Jap. 19:201, 1969.
140. Young, J. L., Jr., and Miller, R. W.: Incidence of malignant tumors in U.S. children. J. Pediatr. 86:254, 1975.

Chapter Eighteen

TUMORS OF GERM-CELL ORIGIN: EMBRYONAL CARCINOMAS, EXTRAEMBRYONAL TUMORS, AND TERATOMAS

Germ-cell tumors are thought to arise from the same cells which are destined to produce the sperm and egg cells of the male and female gonads, respectively. Not all germ cell tumors arise in the gonads, however. The reason for this appears to be a consequence of the embryologic migration of the germ cells which takes them from their origin in the yolk sac to their final destination in the definitive gonad.

Primordial germ cells in man are first definitely recognized in the 4-week embryo as large, distinctive cells embedded in a restricted area of the yolk sac wall. During the fifth week of embryogenesis, these germ cells migrate from the yolk sac to the hind gut wall and then along its mesentery to the gonadal ridge, where they reach their ultimate destination in the gonadal anlage prior to its descent into the pelvis or scrotal sac.[66] It is possible that, during their migration from the yolk sac to the definitive gonad, some germ cells may be left behind or may stray too far and come to rest at various sites along the dorsal wall of the embryo near the midline. If these cells remain viable they may give rise to tumors in these locations (e.g., sacrococcygeal region, mediastinum, pineal region, and retroperitoneum). Likewise, activation of germ cells within the gonads themselves could also lead to tumor formation.

Just as tumors of germ cells may arise at any point in their migration path, so too may tumors arise at any stage of their maturation (Fig. 18–1). Thus, *embryonal carcinoma* is considered to be composed of undifferentiated, multipotential germ cells. If maturation occurs along somatic (embryonic) pathways a *teratoma* may result, whereas development along extraembryonic pathways may produce tumors of the yolk sac epithelium (*endodermal sinus tumor*) or tropho-

```
                    Primordial Germ Cell (Totipotent)
                         /              \
                        /                \
    Multipotential Undifferentiated Germ Cell    Unipotential Primitive Germ Cell
         (EMBRYONAL CARCINOMA)                      (SEMINOMA/DYSGERMINOMA)
              /           \
             /             \
  Somatic (Embryonal) Differentiation      Extraembryonal Differentiation
       /            \                          /              \
  Mature Teratoma   Immature Teratoma     Trophoblast       Yolk Sac
  (DERMOID CYST)  (MALIGNANT TERATOMA)  (CHORIOCARCINOMA)  (ENDODERMAL
                                                            SINUS TUMOR)
```

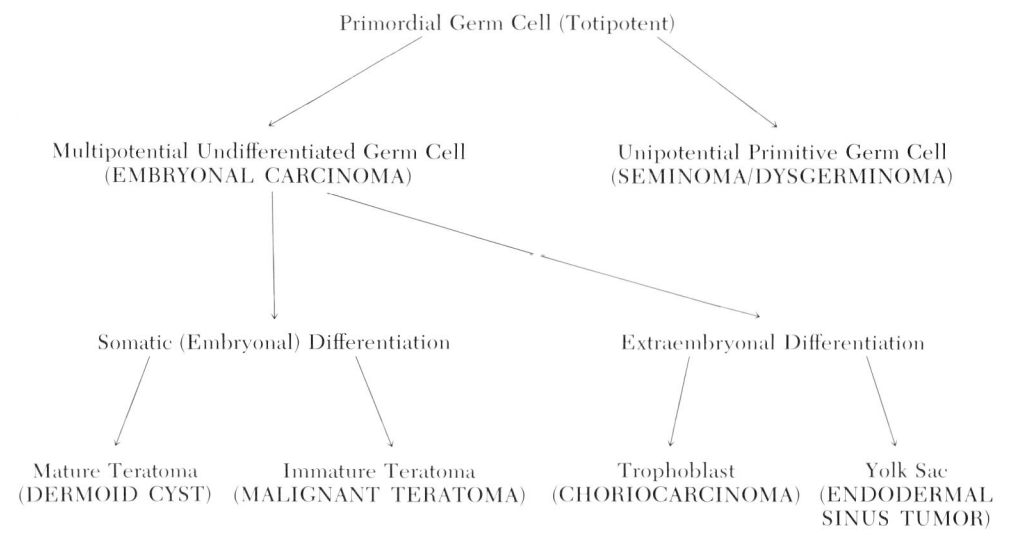

Figure 18–1 Tumors of germ cell origin.

blast (*choriocarcinoma*). Primitive germ cells may also form a distinct unicellular type tumor with very little potential for differentiation along either embryonic or extraembryonic lines; these tumors, called *seminomas* in the male and *dysgerminomas* in the female, almost always occur in the gonads and will be discussed in Chapter Nineteen.

EMBRYONAL CARCINOMA

Embryonal carcinoma is a primitive neoplasm composed of undifferentiated pluripotential germ cells (Fig. 18–2) which have the potential for differentiation along either embryonal or extraembryonal lines or even both these lines concurrently. These tumors manifest predominantly a carcinoma-

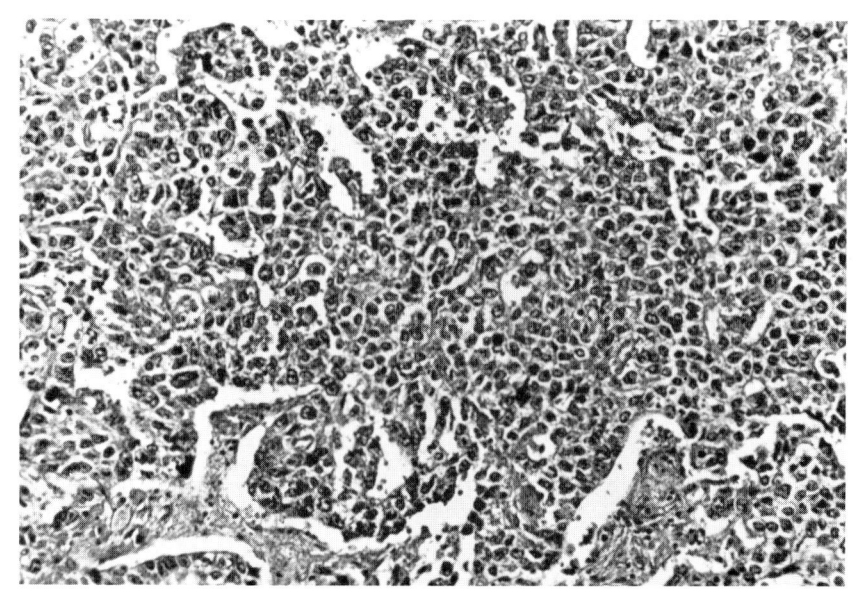

Figure 18–2 Embryonal carcinoma, showing nests of primitive undifferentiated cells. (Courtesy of Dr. Ivan Damjanov.)

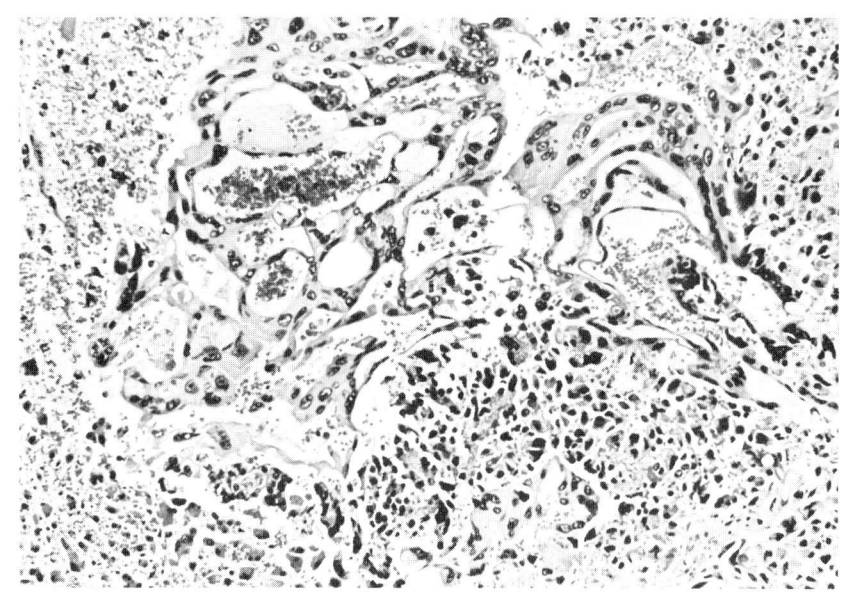

Figure 18-3 Choriocarcinoma showing syncytio- and cytotrophoblastic elements with intermingled hemorrhagic necrosis (×66). (From Johnson, D. E., et al.: Surgery 73:85, 1973.)

tous pattern with embryonal glandular, papillary, and clear cell adenocarcinomatous areas; mitotic figures are easily found.[2, 8] In some areas the cells are closely packed in solid sheets, but more characteristic is a loosely arranged reticulated network with proteinaceous fluid.[2]

EXTRAEMBRYONAL TUMORS

The extraembryonal tissues consist of the umbilical cord, the yolk sac, the amnion, the chorion (trophoblast), and the allantois. The two major malignant variants of these tissues are (1) *choriocarcinoma*, and (2) *endodermal sinus tumor (yolk sac carcinoma)*. Tumors of these extraembryonal elements may occur in pure form or may coexist with embryonal carcinoma or teratoma to form mixed germ-cell tumors. The presence of extraembryonal components in a germ-cell tumor usually significantly worsens the prognosis.[72]

Choriocarcinoma. This tumor is characterized by cellular elements resembling those of the chorion layer of the placenta (multinucleated syncytial trophoblasts and vacuolated cytotrophoblasts) (Fig. 18–3). These cellular elements are capable of producing *human chorionic gonadotropin*, and measurement of the serum or urinary concentration of this hormone provides a useful diagnostic assay as well as a means of following the patient's response to therapy.

Choriocarcinoma may arise (1) within the placenta of a pregnant female (*gestational*) or (2) within a primary germ-cell tumor in a nonpregnant individual (*nongestational*).

In the pediatric age range, choriocarcinoma usually occurs as a nongestational germ-cell tumor. In the prepubertal girl ovarian choriocarcinoma may present as precocious puberty; the opposite ovary may be enlarged due to the formation of multiple theca-lutein cysts.[37] Postpubertal girls with primary ovarian choriocarcinoma may present with the signs and symptoms of an ectopic pregnancy.[37]

Primary choriocarcinomas, as well as other tumors in which choriocarcinoma is mixed with elements such as dysgerminoma, endodermal sinus tumor, or immature teratoma, are highly malignant and have a poor prognosis. They do not respond as well to methotrexate therapy as do pure gestational choriocarcinomas of the uterus. One reason for this may be that nongestational choriocarcinoma is almost always a minor component of a mixed germ cell tumor containing other elements, such as endodermal sinus tumor or teratoma, and these may not be sensitive to methotrexate.

There are rare instances of choriocarcinoma developing in infants as a complication of maternal placental choriocarcinoma. These patients appear to present a relatively uniform and characteristic clinical picture.[71] The infant is usually 5 weeks to 7 months of age, with a history of anemia or pallor and hepatomegaly; a history of hemoptysis, hematemesis, hematuria, or melena may also be obtained. Subtle signs of gonadotropic effects (breast enlargement, pubic hair) as well as evidence of pulmonary metastases likewise may be present. When choriocarcinoma occurs in such a setting, investigation of the mother for occult choriocarcinoma should be instituted; repeat studies should be performed at frequent intervals, since occasionally the appearance of clinically overt tumor may be delayed.[71]

Endodermal Sinus Tumor. These tumors partially or completely recapitulate the structure of yolk sac;[33, 34, 35] they have a labyrinthine pattern containing tubular structures, papillary processes, and Schiller-Duval bodies supported by a loose myxoid or vascular stroma[57] (Fig. 18-4). Schiller-Duval bodies are structures consisting of a small cavity lined by a layer of endothelium-like cells containing a single papillomatous projection. When cut in cross-section, they bear a superficial resemblance to embryonal glomeruli, but actually correspond to the endodermal sinuses of the yolk sac.

Although lacking the endocrine properties of trophoblastic malignancies, yolk sac tumors are associated with elevations of serum *alpha fetoprotein* and *alpha$_1$ antitrypsin*.[48] Both of these protein markers have been demonstrated in normal human embryonic yolk sac,[26] as well as within the periodic acid–Schiff (PAS)-positive

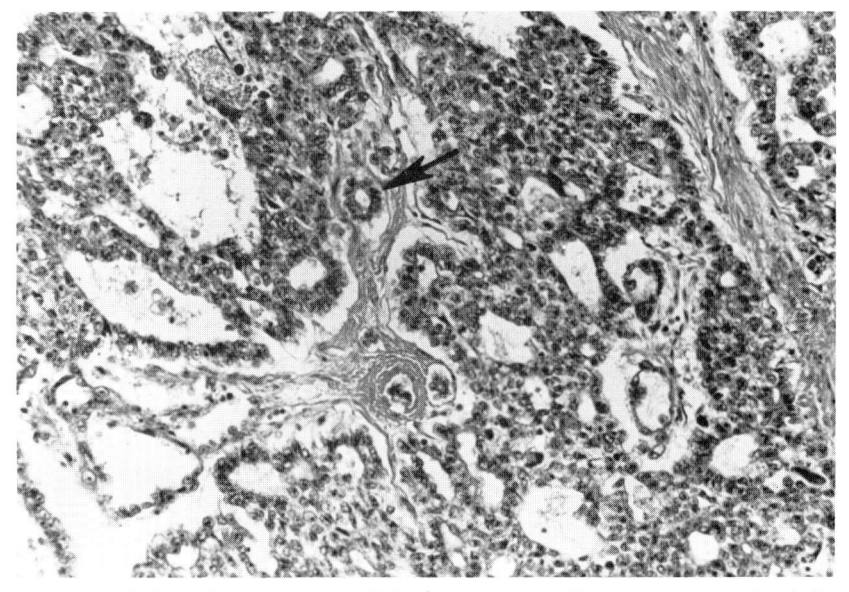

Figure 18-4 Endodermal sinus tumor with loose stroma, papillary processes, and Schiller-Duval body (arrow). (Courtesy of Dr. Ivan Damjanov.)

globules characteristic of this tumor.[48, 65] The elevated serum levels of these proteins are useful both for diagnostic purposes and for monitoring disease activity during and following therapy.[51]

Yolk sac tumors occur in both gonadal and extragonadal sites.[57] Testicular yolk sac tumors tend to occur at an early age (usually before 3 years) and the prognosis is good if orchiectomy is done prior to the age of 2 years; few patients with ovarian yolk sac tumors are under 2 years of age, and the prognosis is uniformly poor.[33] Yolk sac tumors have also been found in the sacrococcygeal region, mediastinum, and other midline areas;[34] most of these patients have unresectable tumors and a poor prognosis, but a few long-term survivors have been reported and some cases show a dramatic response to chemotherapy.[57]

TERATOMA

A teratoma is a tumor which contains multiple tissues foreign to the anatomic region in which it arises.[68] Such neoplasms contain derivatives of more than one of the three primary germ layers (ectoderm, mesoderm, endoderm) of the embryo. Ectodermal elements are represented by squamous epithelium and neuronal tissue, mesodermal elements by bone, cartilage, and muscle, and endodermal elements by gastrointestinal and respiratory tissue, as well as mucous glands. The component tissues are often arranged in a haphazard fashion and manifest asynchronous maturation; thus, cells of embryonal, fetal, or adult character may be jumbled together. Since teratomas grow and mature at a rate independent of that of the area in which they develop, they are considered to be true neoplasms. Although the biologic behavior of many teratomas is benign, one or more of the germ layer derivatives may at any time develop malignant characteristics.

THEORIES REGARDING THE ORIGIN OF TERATOMAS

Over the years many theories have been put forward to explain teratoma development. It is not likely that a single hypothesis will be adequate to explain the origin of all teratomas in view of their heterogeneous anatomic locations and biologic behavior. It is possible that some teratomas represent the frustrated development of a conjoined twin, whereas others may arise from totipotential germ cells. Teratoma formation in some areas may also represent foci of pluripotential tissue which have escaped from the influence of the "primary organizer" during fetal life.

Incomplete Twinning. Normally monozygotic twins are formed when the embryo divides completely at the blastula stage. If at this point complete separation does not occur, the twins grow instead as a fused pair of individuals (Siamese twins); in these instances, fusion usually occurs at the head, chest, abdomen, or sacrum.[7] Teratoma may represent an instance of further derangement of the twinning process whereby only a small proportion of cells separate at the blastula stage and form an incomplete embryo. This theory is attractive in that the locations of the common teratomas of early infancy—sacrococcygeal region, mediastinum, abdomen, and brain—are also sites at which Siamese twins are linked. However, it is unlikely that the teratomas of the gonads can be explained in this manner.[7]

Origin From Totipotent Germ Cells. As mentioned previously, it is possible that teratomas may arise from germ cells which have become left behind during the migration from the yolk sac to the definitive gonads, or alternatively they may arise by activation of germ cells within the gonads themselves.

There is now good evidence that benign ovarian teratomas in adults arise from parthogenetically activated oocytes following the first meiotic division. This evidence is based on homozygosity of chromosome banding and biochemical markers in the teratoma itself.[41] Testicular teratomas, on the other hand, may arise from postmeiotic fusion of two haploid germ cells, an event comparable to fertilization;[22] this concept is consistent with the observation that roughly half of testicular teratomas are sex-chromatin positive (i.e., have female nuclear sex characteristics).[22, 32]

Escape From the Influence of the "Primary Organizer." The preaxial distribution of most teratomas suggests the possibility of growth disturbances emanating from the primary axis—i.e., the notochord and contiguous structures, which are derived by invagination of tissue at Hensen's node in the early embryo.[68] Perhaps if some of these cells escape the blocking effects of primary and subsidiary organizers during early fetal life and retain totipotentiality, they would be capable of teratomatous behavior.[7, 68]

STRUCTURE AND BEHAVIOR OF TERATOMAS

Teratomas may behave as either benign or malignant lesions, and this differentiation may frequently be made on structural grounds. Benign tumors are composed wholly of mature, fully differentiated tissues, whereas malignant ones contain embryonic tissues of variable degrees of immaturity.[68] It is important to recognize that immaturity of the tissue within a teratoma per se reflects metastatic capability.[46]

Gross Appearance

Benign tumors are usually cystic, with one or more large cysts into which the solid components project; the cut surface frequently reveals fully differentiated tissues, such as skin, hair, teeth, bone, cartilage, and adipose tissue. The cysts are lined by skin, alimentary or respiratory mucosal epithelium, or central nervous tissue and contain the secretions characteristic of these tissues (sebaceous matter, mucoid secretions, or cerebrospinal fluid).

Malignant teratomas are predominantly solid, but may contain finely polycystic areas. They contain actively growing, poorly differentiated tissue mixed with some differentiated elements. Thus, spicules of bone, nodules of cartilage, and small cutaneous or mucoid cysts may be visible among the solid tissues. Areas of necrosis or hemorrhage may also be present.

Histology

Benign teratomas contain fully mature tissues which resemble the adult counterparts and are easy to recognize. Skin (including hair and sebaceous and sweat glands) is a very common component, as is nervous tissue, which usually occurs as masses of neuroglial cells (Fig. 18–5). Other mature tissues which may be seen are teeth (Fig. 18–6), thyroid, intestinal epithelium, renal tissue, cartilage, bone, and muscle. In some teratomas these tissues may form highly organized structures, such as digits, intestine, and cerebellar or cerebral cortex.

Malignant (immature) teratomas contain some fully mature tissues, as well as embryonic tissues of all degrees of immaturity; these tissues are truly embryonic in that they reproduce structures which, though neoplastic, closely correspond to all stages of embryonic and fetal development.[68] Malignant teratomas may also contain undifferentiated cells (embryonal carcinoma) and extraembryonic tissue derived from trophoblasts (choriocarcinoma) or yolk sac (endodermal sinus tumor).

Neuroectoderm is the most common form of immature tissue (Fig. 18–7); its degree of differentiation may range from primitive medullary structures, neuroblasts, and neuroblastoma-like rosettes to highly developed cerebral

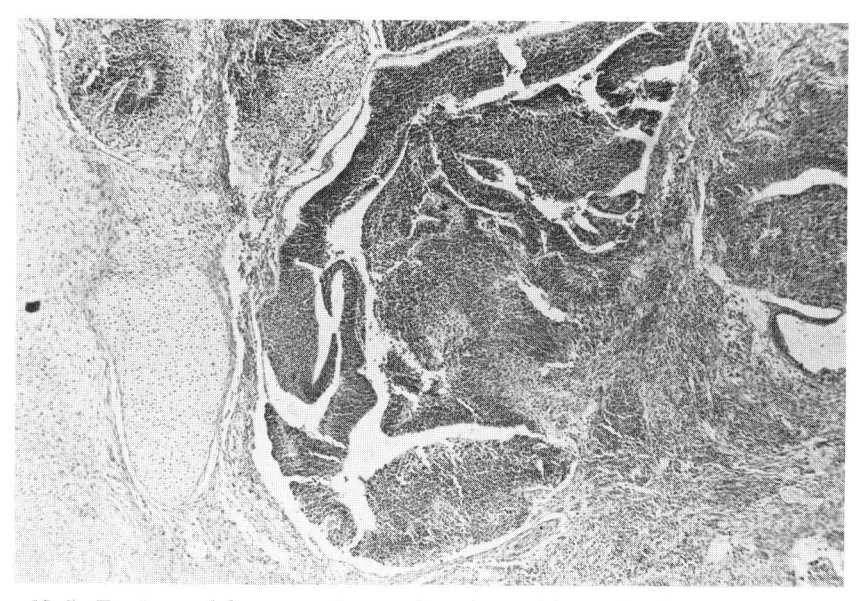

Figure 18-5 Teratoma of the ovary, showing foci of neural (center) and cartilaginous (left) tissue (×13). (Courtesy of Dr. Ronald Maenza.)

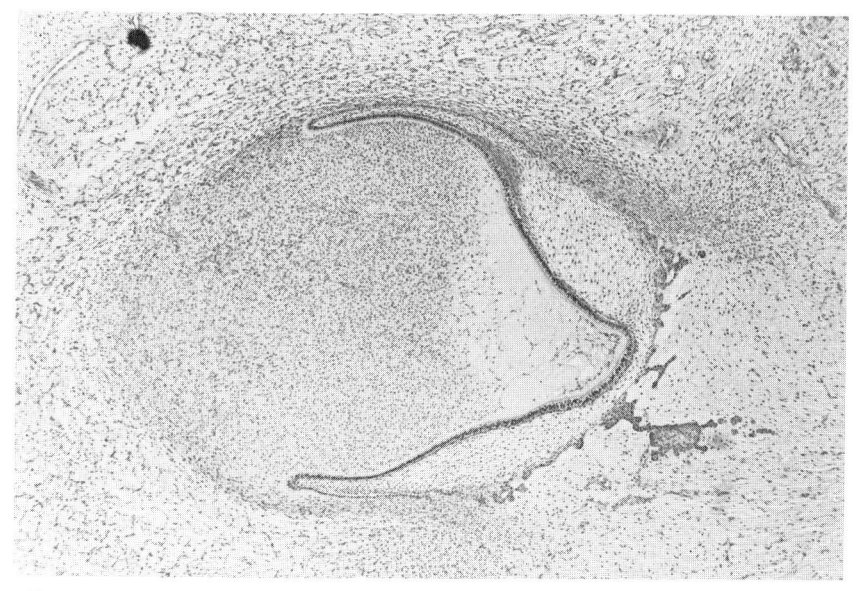

Figure 18-6 Teratoma of the ovary—tooth primordium (×13). (Courtesy of Dr. Ronald Maenza.)

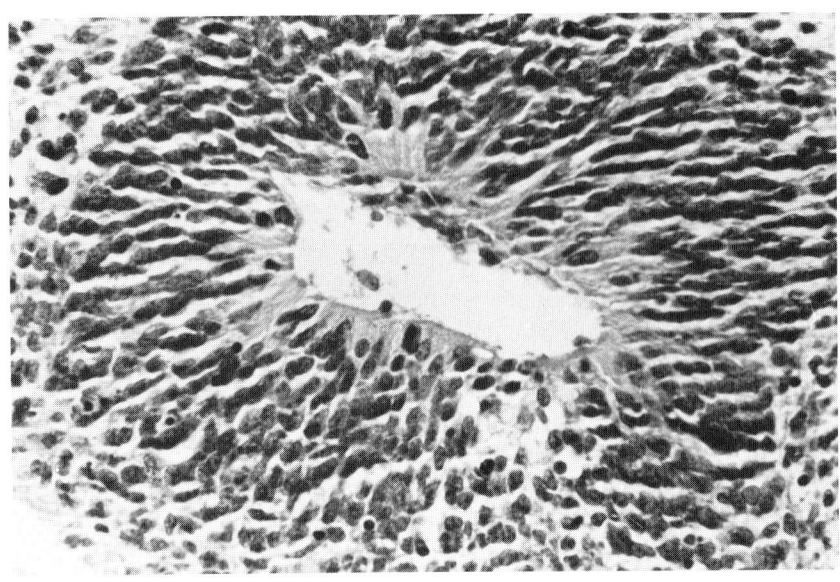

Figure 18-7 Immature teratoma of the ovary—primitive neuroectoderm (×128). (Courtesy of Dr. Ronald Maenza.)

and cerebellar tissue.[16, 72, 73] In many solid ovarian teratomas malignancy resides almost exclusively in the immature neural elements. In other tumors, the immature elements consist of epithelial formations resembling embryonic or fetal glandular structures; such tumors frequently contain extraembryonal elements (choriocarcinoma, endodermal sinus tumor) and have a poorer prognosis.[72, 73]

Robboy and Scully have graded the immature teratomas histologically according to the following criteria:[56]

Grade 0   All tissue mature; no mitotic activity
Grade 1   Minor foci of abnormally cellular or embryonal tissue mixed with mature elements; rare mitoses
Grade 2   Moderate quantities of embryonal tissue mixed with mature elements; moderate mitotic activity
Grade 3   Large quantities of embryonal tissue

CLINICAL ASPECTS OF TERATOMAS

Teratomas may arise in a wide variety of locations, but characteristically occur in close relation to the axial midline of the body. In the first year of life the sacrococcygeal region is the most common site of teratoma;[10] sacrococcygeal and other extragonadal sites (pelvis, anterior mediastinum, retroperitoneum, neck, central nervous system) predominate during childhood (Fig. 18-8). Less common extragonadal sites include kidney, liver, stomach, thyroid, and palate.[5, 10, 16] After puberty, however, teratomas occur most frequently in the gonads (particularly the ovary).

Malignant teratomas recur locally, metastasize early, and have a rapidly fatal course in most instances. In some cases, however, they may be extremely sensitive to combination chemotherapy and radiotherapy, and the early use of such adjunctive measures may be effective in prolonging and improving survival.[14, 27]

Sacrococcygeal Teratoma

Sacrococcygeal teratomas are relatively rare lesions, with an estimated incidence of 1:40,000 live births.[23] Nonetheless, they are the most common teratomas of childhood and the

TUMORS OF GERM-CELL ORIGIN

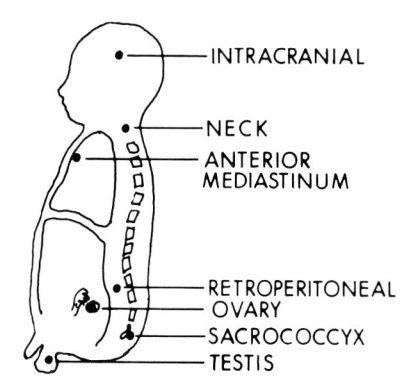

Figure 18-8 Common sites of teratoma formation during childhood.

Figure 18-9 Sacrococcygeal teratomas. Size variation of these tumors is considerable. *A*, Small (0.5 cm) benign sacrococcygeal teratoma. *B*, Large (15 × 18 × 12 cm) sacrococcygeal teratoma containing foci of malignancy. (From Lemire, R. J., Graham, C. B., and Beckwith, J. B.: Skin-covered sacrococcygeal masses in infants and children. J. Pediatr. 79:948–954, 1971.)

most common solid tumor in the newborn.[5, 29] Females are affected four times as frequently as males.[5, 55]

Most of these tumors are detected as a large swelling protruding between the coccyx and rectum (Fig. 18–9), but others may be found by rectal examination. It is important to emphasize the fact that nearly all arise at the tip or inner surface of the coccyx (an area easily palpable on rectal examination) and, consequently, could be diagnosed early in life if pediatricians would make the rectal examination a routine part of every physical evaluation.[18]

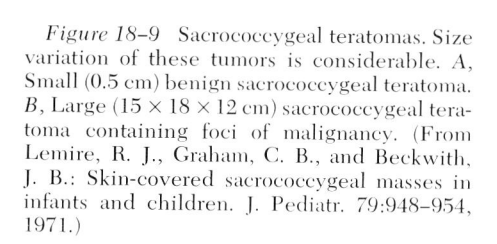

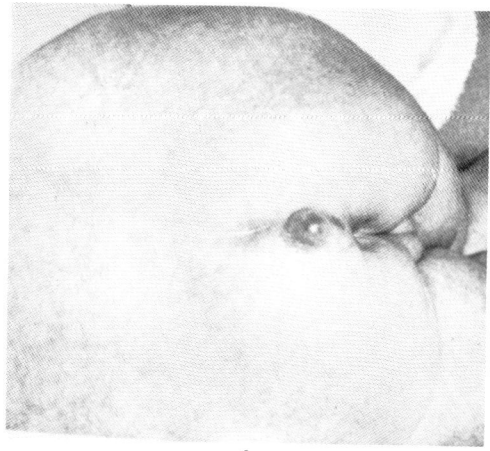

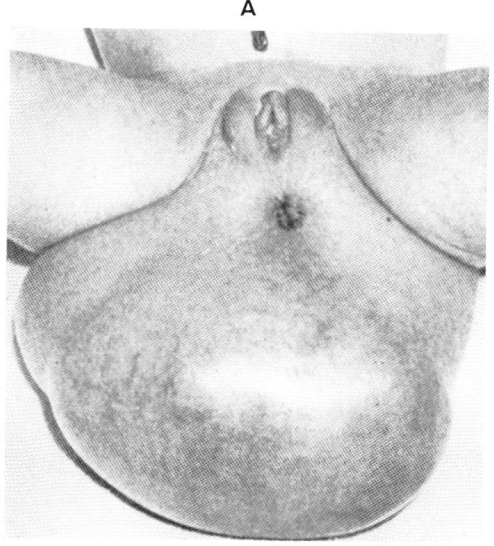

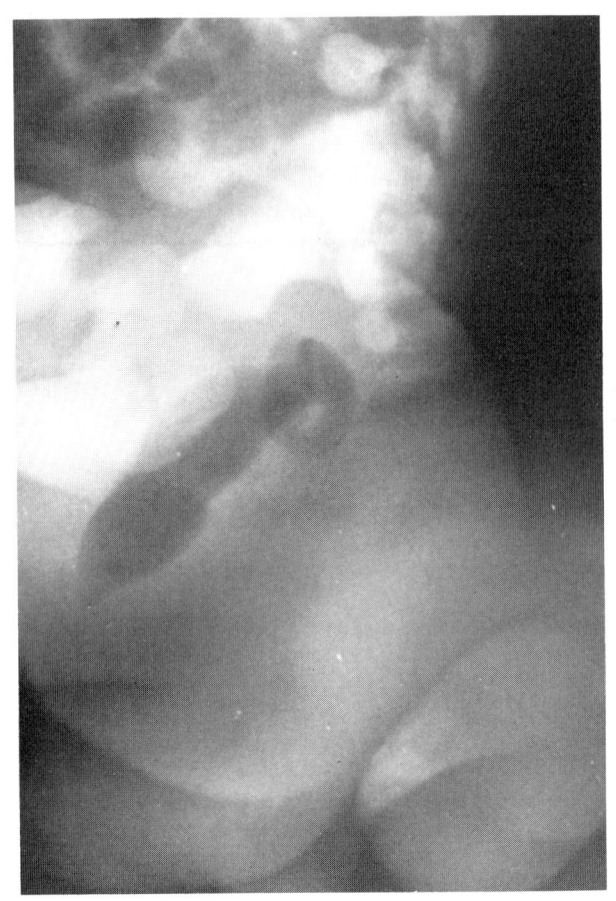

Figure 18-10 Lateral x-ray showing ventral displacement of the rectum by the presacral component of a teratoma, the only common lesion to do so. The superficial portion of the tumor is seen caudal to the sacrum. (From Lemire, R. J., Graham, C. B., and Beckwith, J. B.: Skin-covered sacrococcygeal masses in infants and children. J. Pediatr. 79:948, 1971.)

The differential diagnosis of mass lesions in the sacrococcygeal area includes: meningomyelocele, rectal abscess, neurogenic tumors of the pelvis and perineum, lymphangioma, lipoma, imperforate anus, pilonidal cyst, soft tissue sarcoma, chordoma, and giant cell tumor of the sacrum. Radiographic features of teratomas which help distinguish them from some of these lesions are: (1) anterior displacement of the gas-filled rectum; (2) calcification; and (3) presentation caudal to the sacrum on lateral radiographs[39](Fig. 18–10).

Surprisingly, the majority of benign sacrococcygeal teratomas produce no functional difficulties even when there is considerable intrapelvic extension; consequently, bowel or bladder dysfunction, pain on defecation, discomfort during standing, and vascular or lymphatic obstruction all suggest the presence of malignancy.[18]

The treatment for these tumors is primarily surgical; the techniques for removal have been discussed in detail by Gross and colleagues[28] and Donnellan and Swenson.[18] Sacrococcygeal neoplasms should be excised as soon as possible, since small, undifferentiated foci in them may proliferate and become more aggressive.[15] It is important to emphasize the attachment of sacrococcygeal teratomas to the coccyx, which *necessitates the removal of the entire coccyx as an essential part of any surgical procedure.* Failure to do so will result in a high rate of local tumor recurrence (31 to 38 per cent).[18, 28]

Prognosis. In Altman's collection

of 398 cases of sacrococcygeal teratoma, 60 per cent of patients with malignant tumors died within 10 months of operation, whereas 21 per cent were alive with residual disease, 11 per cent were alive without apparent disease, and 9 per cent were lost to follow-up.[6] By contrast, the mortality rate for patients with benign lesions was approximately 5 per cent.[6]

The incidence of malignancy for tumors diagnosed before the age of two months is approximately 10 per cent;[6, 18] however, after this age the incidence of malignancy rises to 67 per cent for males and 48 per cent for females.[6] Mortality also varies according to age:

Age	Mortality (Per Cent)
1 day	7
1 week	4.5
2–4 weeks	4
1–6 months	12
6–12 months	6
1–2 years	38
>2 years	55

Sacrococcygeal teratomas may be classified topographically, and this classification appears to be of predictive value in terms of both proclivity to metastatic behavior and potential for survival[6](Fig. 18–11). In general, internal location appears to predispose to metastatic behavior,[8] possibly because delay in diagnosis may lead to malignant transformation.

Mediastinal Teratoma

Primary intrathoracic teratomas are located in the anterior mediastinum. Most of these are benign dermoid cysts; they are usually asymptomatic and detected only as unexplained masses on chest x-ray. In general, the larger the tumor, however, the more likely it is to be malignant.[13] Other lesions of the anterior mediastinum that must be considered in the differential diagnosis include *thymoma, normal thymus, lymphoma, bronchogenic cysts,* and *intrathoracic goiter.*

The presence of calcification or anomalous bone formation helps to distinguish teratoma from these other lesions on chest x-ray.

When symptoms do occur, their onset is usually insidious; dyspnea, pleurisy, and chest pain are the most common initial complaints. Rupture of a dermoid cyst into a bronchus may result in a dramatic expectoration of hair. With malignant tumors, invasion of the lungs and mediastinal structures as well as compression and invasion of the great veins may occur. Occasionally a rapidly expanding mediastinal teratoma may be associated with respiratory distress, even in the newborn period; posterior displacement and narrowing of the trachea and the presence of calcification within such a mass will help differentiate it from the normal large benign thymus of the neonate.[61]

Surgical excision is the only effective treatment;[4, 5] postoperative irradiation may also be used for malignant teratomas.[4] However, the prognosis for malignant mediastinal teratomas in childhood is poor, as 30 to 50 per cent of these patients will develop distant metastases (bone, lung, spinal cord) and usually expire within 6 to 12 months.[4, 11, 58, 60]

Teratomas of the Head and Neck

Although teratomas are a rare cause of head and neck masses, they frequently enter into the differential diagnosis of lesions in this area because of their occurrence in a variety of sites (cranial cavity, orbit, nasopharynx, face, oral cavity, thyroid gland, soft tissues of the neck). Nearly 10 per cent of all childhood teratomas occur above the level of the clavicles,[10] and the majority of these are recognized in the newborn or very young infant. Neck teratomas may cause life-threatening airway obstruction in the neonate (Fig. 18–12); 18 to 30 per cent of these are associated with maternal hydramnios.[30, 62]

TYPE I

Predominantly external with minimal presacral component

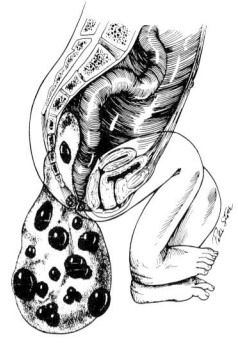

Frequency 46.6%
Metastatic rate 0%
Mortality rate 11%

TYPE II

Presenting externally, but significant intrapelvic extension

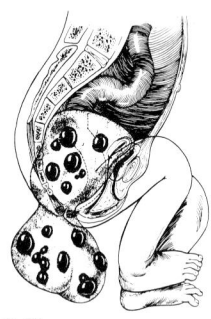

Frequency 34.6%
Metastatic rate 6%
Mortality rate 18%

TYPE III

Predominant mass pelvic with extension into abdomen

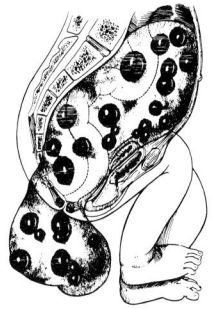

Frequency 8.8%
Metastatic rate 20%
Mortality rate 28%

TYPE IV

Entirely presacral with no external presentation

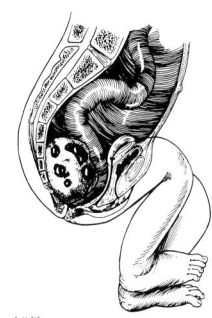

Frequency 10%
Metastatic rate 8%
Mortality rate 21%

Figure 18–11 Location of sacrococcygeal teratomas in 398 patients. (After Altman, R. P., et al.: Sacrococcygeal teratoma. J. Pediatr. Surg. 9:389–398, 1974. By permission.)

TUMORS OF GERM-CELL ORIGIN 439

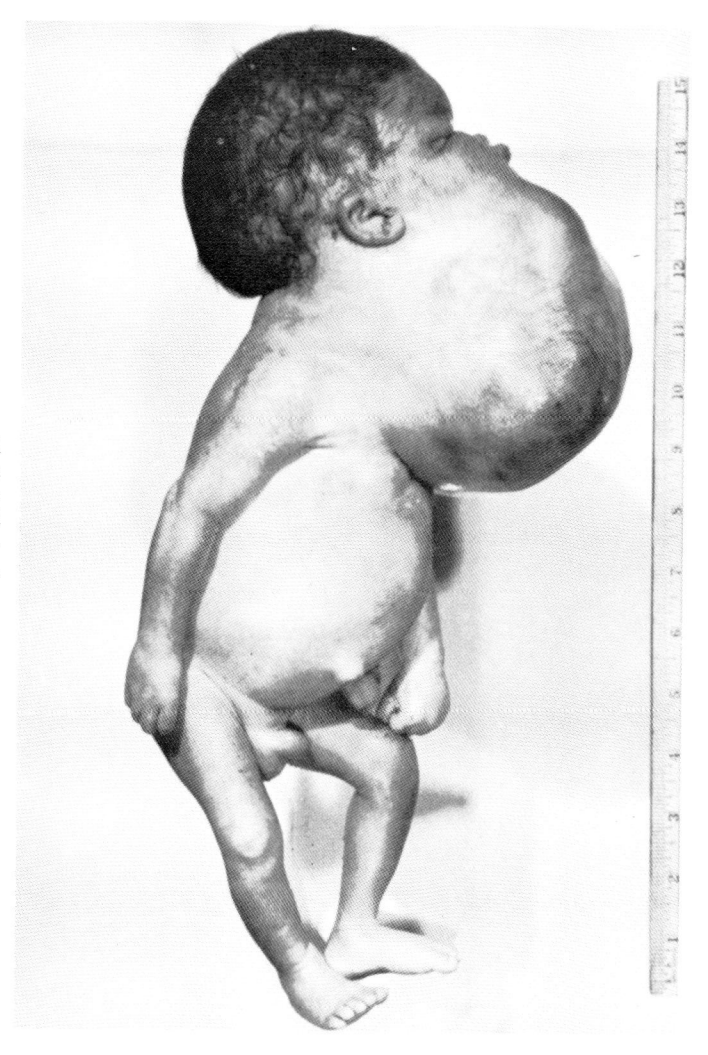

Figure 18–12 Congenital teratoma of the neck. (From Hajdu, S. I., and Hajdu, E. O.: Cytopathology of Sarcomas and Other Nonepithelial Malignant Tumors. Philadelphia, W. B. Saunders Co., 1976.)

Quick recognition of cervical teratoma is essential, since early operation can be life-saving; delay of surgery in the presence of respiratory obstruction is virtually always fatal.[30, 36, 67] In the preoperative phase, tracheal aspiration and oxygen administration are advisable; laying the infant on the side with the tumor may help to relieve the tracheal compression.[63] Surgery consists of "shelling-out" the tumor and is accompanied by a mortality rate of 17 per cent;[30] the alternative is tracheostomy, which has been found dangerous and difficult because of the large size of the tumor.[45, 62]

Intracranial teratomas behave as slow-growing mass lesions and they can cause increased intracranial pressure, Parinaud's sign, diplopia, and hearing impairment, as well as diabetes insipidus, visual field defects, hypopituitarism, and hypothalamic signs. If completely resected, they usually do not recur.

Retroperitoneal and Intraabdominal Teratomas

Unlike teratomas of the thorax, which are located arteriorly and tend to be benign cysts, abdominal teratomas are usually located posterolaterally in the retroperitoneal tissues;

about 10 per cent show malignant changes.[21, 49, 53] Although quite rare in this location, teratomas are nonetheless the third most common malignancy of the retroperitoneal space (after neuroblastoma and Wilms' tumor).[5]

Presenting symptoms are usually vague and frequently secondary to the pressure effects of the tumor on neighboring structures. Patients may thus complain of abdominal or back pain, nausea, vomiting, constipation, and urinary tract symptoms.[53]

Intraabdominal teratomas are quite unusual. Thirty two cases of gastric teratoma have been described to date; these are discussed on page 503. Teratomas of the liver and kidney have also been reported.[16]

Teratomas of the Gonads

The wide range in biologic behavior of teratomas is best exemplified by the example of ovarian and testicular tumors in pre- and postpubertal patients. In the adult, ovarian teratomas are usually benign cystic lesions filled with hair, sebum, and occasionally teeth, while testicular teratomas are usually malignant tumors composed of bizarre admixtures of various embryonal tissue elements.[22] The situation in children is exactly the reverse — ovarian teratomas in prepubertal girls are often highly malignant, whereas teratomas in prepubertal boys are uniformly benign.[22] These tumors are discussed in more detail in Chapter Nineteen.

REFERENCES

1. Abell, M. R., and Holtz, F.: Testicular neoplasms in infants and children. I. Tumors of germ cell origin. Cancer 16: 965, 1963.
2. Abell, M. R., Johnson, V. J., and Holtz, F.: Ovarian neoplasms in childhood and adolescence. I. Tumors of germ cell origin. Am. J. Obstet. Gynec. 92:1059, 1965.
3. Acosta, A. A., Kaplan, A. L., and Kaufman, R. H.: Gynecologic cancer in children. Am. J. Obstet. Gynec. 112:944, 1972.
4. Adebonojo, S. A., and Nicola, M. L.: Teratoid tumors of the mediastinum. Am. Surg. 42:361, 1976.
5. Allen, J. E.: Teratomas in infants and children. In Holland, J. F., and Frei, E., III (eds.): Cancer Medicine. Philadelphia, Lea & Febiger, 1973.
6. Altman, R. P., Randolph, J. G., and Lilly, J. R.: Sacrococcygeal teratoma: American Academy of Pediatrics Surgical Section Survey, 1973. J. Pediatr. Surg. 9:389, 1974.
7. Ashley, D. J. B.: Origin of teratomas. Cancer 32:390, 1973.
8. Bale, P. M., Painter, D. M., and Cohen, D.: Teratomas in childhood. Pathology 7:209, 1975.
9. Barnard, W. G.: Multiple teratomata of peritoneum. J. Path. Bact. 34:389, 1931.
10. Berry, C. L., Keeling, J., and Hilton, C.: Teratomata in infancy and childhood: a review of 91 cases. J. Pathol. 98:241, 1969.
11. Blades, B.: Mediastinal tumors. Ann. Surg. 123:749, 1946.
12. Bosse, M. D.: Rhabdomyosarcomatous pulmonary metastases from a teratoma testis. Am. J. Cancer 39, 343, 1940.
13. Carney, J. A., Thompson, D. P., Johnson, C. L., and Lynn, H. B.: Teratomas in children: clinical and pathologic aspects. J. Pediatr. Surg. 7:271, 1972.
14. Chretian, P. B., Mylam, J. D., Foote, F. W., et al.: Embryonal carcinomas (a type of malignant teratoma) of the sacrococcygeal region: clinical and pathological aspects in 21 cases. Cancer 26:522, 1970.
15. Conklin, J., and Abell, M. R.: Germ cell neoplasma of sacrococcygeal region. Cancer 20:2105, 1967.
16. Dehner, L. P.: Intrarenal teratoma occurring in infancy: report of a case with discussion of extragonadal germ cell tumors in infancy. J. Pediatr. Surg. 8:369, 1973.
17. Dehner, L. P.: Female reproductive system. In Kissane, J. M. (ed): Pathology of Infancy and Childhood. 2nd Ed. St. Louis, C. V. Mosby Co., 1975.
18. Donnellan, W. A., and Swenson, O.: Benign and malignant sacrococcygeal teratomas. Surgery 64:834, 1968.
19. Ein, S. H., Darte, J. M. M., and Stephens, C. A.: Cystic and solid ovarian tumors in children. A 44-year review. J. Pediatr. Surg. 5:148, 1970.
20. Emge, L. A.: Functional and growth characteristics of struma ovarii. Am. J. Obstet. Gynec. 40:738, 1940.
21. Engel, R. M., Elkins, R. C., and Fletcher, B. D.: Retroperitoneal teratoma: review of the literature and presentation of an unusual case. Cancer 22:1068, 1968.
22. Erickson, R. P., and Gondos, B.: Alternative explanations of the differing behavior of

ovarian and testicular teratomas. Lancet 1:407, 1976.
23. Gelb, A., Rosenblum, H., Jaurigue, V. G., et al.: Sacrococcygeal teratoma. Del. Med. J. 36:119, 1964.
24. Gerald, P. S.: Origin of teratomas. N. Engl. J. Med. 292:103, 1975.
25. Ghazali, S.: Presacral teratomas in children. J. Pediatr. Surg. 8:915, 1973.
26. Gitlin, D., and Perricelli, A.: Synthesis of serum albumin, prealbumin, alpha fetoprotein, alpha-antitrypsin and transferrin by the human yolk sac. Nature 228:995, 1970.
27. Grosfeld, J. L., Ballantine, T. V. N., and Baehner, R. L.: Benign and malignant teratomas in children; analysis of 85 patients. Surgery 80:297, 1976.
28. Gross, R. E., Clatworthy, H. W., Jr., and Meeker, I. A., Jr.: Sacrococcygeal teratomas in infants and children. A report of 40 cases. Surg. Gynec. Obstet. 92:341, 1951.
29. Haggard, M. E.: Miscellaneous childhood tumors. In Sutow, W. W., Vietti, T. J., and Fernbach, D. J. (eds.): Clinical Pediatric Oncology. St. Louis, C. V. Mosby Co., 1973.
30. Hajdu, S. I., Faruque, A. A., Hajdu, E. O., and Morgan, W. S.: Teratoma of the neck in infants. Am. J. Dis. Child. 111:412, 1966.
31. Houghton, J. D.: Malignant teratoma of the mediastinum. Report of a case and review of 24 cases from the literature. Am. J. Pathol. 12:349, 1936.
32. Hunter, W. F., and Lennox, B.: The sex of teratomata. Lancet 2:633, 1954.
33. Huntington, R. W., Jr., and Bullock, W. K.: Yolk sac tumors of the ovary. Cancer 25:1357, 1970.
34. Huntington, R. W., Jr., and Bullock, W. K.: Yolk sac tumors of extragonadal origin. Cancer 25:1368, 1970.
35. Huntington, R. W., Jr., and Bullock, W. K.: Endodermal sinus and other yolk sac tumors—a reappraisal. Acta Pathol. Microbiol. Scand. (Suppl. A) 233:26, 1972.
36. Hurlbut, H. J., Webb, H. W., and Moseley, T.: Cervical teratoma in infant siblings. J. Pediatr. Surg. 5:460, 1970.
37. Janovski, N. A., and Paramanandhan, T. L.: Ovarian Tumors. Philadelphia, W. B. Saunders Co., 1973.
38. Johnson, D. E., Kuhn, C. R., and Guinn, G. A.: Testicular tumors in children. J. Urol. 104:940, 1970.
38a. Krumerman, M. S., and Chung A.: Squamous carcinoma arising in benign cystic teratoma of the ovary. Cancer 39:1237, 1977.
39. Lemire, R. J., Graham, C. B., Beckwith, J. B.: Skin-covered sacrococcygeal masses in infants and children. J. Pediatr. 79:948, 1971.

40. Linder, D.: Gene loss in human teratomas. Proc. Natl. Acad. Sci. U.S.A. 63:699, 1969.
41. Linder, D., McCaw, B. K., and Hecht, F.: Parthenogenic origin of benign ovarian teratomas. N. Engl. J. Med. 292:63, 1975.
42. Luse, S. A., and Vietti, T.: Ovarian teratoma. Ultrastructure and neural component. Cancer 21:38, 1968.
43. Marcial-Rojas, R. A., Ramierez de Arellano, G. A.: Malignant melanoma arising in dermoid cyst of the ovary: Report of a case. Cancer 9:523, 1956.
44. Masson, J. C., and Ochsenhirt, N. C.: Squamous cell carcinoma arising in a dermoid cyst of the ovary. Report of three cases. Surg. Gynec. Obstet. 48:702, 1929.
45. Neustedt, J. R., and Shirkey, H. C.: Teratoma of the thyroid region: report of a case with seven-year follow-up. Am. J. Dis. Child. 107:88, 1964.
46. Norris, H. J., Zirkin, H. J., and Benson, W. L.: Immature (malignant) teratoma of the ovary. A clinical and pathologic study of 58 cases. Cancer 37:2359, 1976.
47. Oliver, H. M., and Horne, E. O.: Primary teratomatous chorionepithelioma of the ovary. N. Engl. J. Med. 239:14, 1948.
48. Palmer, P. E., Safaii, H., and Wolfe, H. J.: Alpha$_1$-antitrypsin and alpha-feto protein. Protein markers in endodermal sinus (yolk sac) tumors. Am. J. Clin. Pathol. 65:575, 1976.
49. Palumbo, L. T., Cross, S. R., Smith, A. N., and Baronas, A. A.: Primary teratomas of the lateral retroperitoneal spaces. Surgery 26:149, 1949.
50. Pantoja, E., and Rodriguez-Ibanez, I.: Sacrococcygeal dermoids and teratomas. Am. J. Surg. 132:377, 1976.
51. Perlin, E., Engeler, J. E., Jr. Edson, M., et al.: The value of serial measurement of both human chorionic gonadotropin and alpha-feto protein for monitoring germinal cell tumors. Cancer 37:215, 1976.
52. Peterson, W. F., Prevost, E. C., Edmunds, F. T., et al.: Benign cystic teratomas of the ovary: A clinico-statistical study of 1007 cases with a review of the literature. Am. J. Obstet. Gynec. 70:368, 1955.
53. Polsky, M. S., Shackelford, G. D., Weber, C. H., Jr., and Ball, T. P., Jr.: Retroperitoneal teratoma. Urology 8:618, 1976.
54. Proskauer, G. G.: Solid teratomas of the ovary with neurological metastases. Am. J. Obstet. Gynec. 52:845, 1946.
55. Ravitch, M. M., and McGoon, D. C.: Teratoid tumors and dermoid cysts. In Ariel, I. M., and Pack. G. T.: Cancer and Allied Diseases of Infancy and Childhood. Boston, Little, Brown & Co., 1960.
56. Robboy, S. J., and Scully, R. E.: Ovarian teratoma with glial implants on the peritoneum. Hum. Pathol. 1:643, 1970.
57. Roth, L. M., and Panganiban, W. G.: Gonadal

and extragonadal yolk sac carcinomas. A clinicopathologic study of 14 cases. Cancer 37:812, 1976.
58. Rusby, N. L.: Dermoid cysts and teratoma of the mediastinum. J. Thorac. Surg. 13:169, 1944.
59. Sabio, H., Burgert, E. O., Jr., Farrow, G. M., and Kelalis, P. P.: Embryonal carcinoma of the testis in childhood. Cancer 34:2118, 1974
60. Schlumberger, H. C.: Teratoma of the anterior mediastinum in group of military age: study of 16 cases and review of theories of genesis. Arch. Pathol. 41:398, 1946.
61. Seibert, J. A., Marvin, W. J., Jr., Rose, E. F., and Schieken, R. M.: Mediastinal teratoma: a rare cause of severe respiratory distress in the newborn. J. Pediatr. Surg. 11:253, 1976.
62. Silberman, R., and Mendelson, I. R.: Teratoma of the neck: report of two cases. Arch. Dis. Child. 35:159, 1960.
63. Sutton, P. W., and Gibbs, E. W.: Congenital teratoma of the thyroid: case report. Am. J. Surg. 63:405, 1944.
64. Teilum, G.: Endodermal sinus tumor of the ovary and testis. Cancer 12:1092, 1959
65. Teilum, G., Albrechtsen, R., and Norgaard-Pedersen, B.: Immunofluorescent localization of alpha-feto protein synthesis in endodermal sinus tumor (yolk sac tumor). Acta Pathol. Microbiol. Scand., Sect. A, 82:586, 1974.
66. Teilum, G.: Special Tumors of the Ovary and Testis. Comparative Pathology and Histological Identification. Philadelphia, J. B. Lippincott Co., 1976.
67. Weitzer, S.: Benign teratoma of the neck in an infant. Am. J. Dis. Child. 107:84, 1964.
68. Willis, R. A.: Teratomas in Atlas of Tumor Pathology. Section III, Fascicle 9. Washington, D.C., Armed Forces Institute of Pathology, 1951.
69. Willis, R. A.: The Borderland of Embryology. London, Butterworth, 1958.
70. Witschi, E.: Migration of the germ cells of human embryos from the yolk sac to the primitive gonadal folds. In Contributions to Embryology, Vol. 32. Washington, D.C., Carnegie Institution of Washington, 1948.
71. Witzleben, C. L., and Bruninga, G.: Infantile choriocarcinoma: a characteristic syndrome. J. Pediatr. 73:374, 1968.
72. Woodruff, J. D., Protos, P., and Peterson, W. F.: Ovarian teratomas. Relationship of histologic and ontogenic factors to prognosis. Am. J. Obstet. Gynec. 102:702, 1968.
73. Woodruff, J. D., and Jimerson, G. K.: Ovarian teratomata. Progr. Clinical Cancer 5:195, 1973.
74. Young, P. G., Mount, B. M., Foote, F. W., Jr., and Whitmore, W. F., Jr.: Embryonal adenocarcinoma in the prepubertal testis. A clinicopathologic study of 18 cases. Cancer 26:1065, 1970.

Chapter Nineteen

TUMORS OF THE SEXUAL ORGANS

Male Reproductive System

TESTICULAR TUMORS

Testicular tumors are relatively uncommon in infants and children, accounting for only 1 to 2 per cent of all pediatric solid tumors.[25, 60] Of those that do occur in the pediatric years, over half are detected before the age of 5 years. After puberty, the incidence of testicular malignancy increases significantly. In fact, testicular tumors are now the leading cause of death from solid tumors in men between the ages of 15 and 34 years.[18]

In most patients testicular tumors present as a painless scrotal swelling, and, in over half the cases, this symptom has been present at least 3 months before treatment is instituted.[8] Frequently testicular tumors are initially mistaken for testicular torsion, orchitis, epididymitis, hernia, or hydrocele; since 10 to 25 per cent of malignant testicular tumors are associated with hydrocele, successful transillumination of a scrotal mass should not be relied upon to rule out tumor.[26, 29] Rarely, a testicular tumor may be endocrinologically active and produce precocious puberty or feminizing effects. A tumor may also arise in an undescended testis and present as an abdominal mass.

Perhaps because the anatomic position of the testis affords early recognition, about 80 per cent of childhood testicular malignancies are localized at the time of diagnosis.[2, 46, 61] When metastases do occur, they appear in the retroperitoneal lymph nodes, lungs, liver, and bones.

Cancer in the Cryptorchid Testis

A cryptorchid testis is 30 to 50 times more likely to develop a malignancy than is a normal gonad;[19, 44] in fact, 10 to 20 per cent of all testicular cancers develop in the 0.23 per cent of males who are cryptorchid.[13, 15, 17] Although retroperitoneal and abdominal testes appear to be the most susceptible to malignancy (particularly of the seminoma type), 20 per cent of the tumors arising in patients with cryptorchidism actually arise in the descended testis.[15, 21] The propensity of patients with cryptorchidism to develop testicular tumors suggests that there is a basic defect in gonadogenesis that is responsible both for lack of descent and for a predilection to tumor development.

There is some question as to whether bringing an undescended testis down into the scrotal sac (orchidopexy) will reduce the subsequent risk of malignancy. Some authors feel that this procedure is useful in preventing cancer if performed prior to puberty,[21] whereas others feel that the risk of malignancy is probably not reduced.[8, 44] Most agree, however, that orchidopexy does make the testis more accessible to palpation and therefore makes possible early diagnosis of a malignant nodule; if performed prior to the age of 6 years, this procedure also permits the greatest opportunity for testicular maturation and subsequent fertility.[13] If the cryptorchidism is not detected until the age of puberty, orchiectomy should be considered in preference to orchidopexy,[28] since testicular atrophy and dysgenesis have probably rendered the gonad useless. In the situation of an intersex or phenotypically female patient with a Y chromosome and gonadal dysgenesis, both gonads should be removed prior to puberty, since the incidence of neoplasm in these gonads rises markedly at puberty.[36]

CLASSIFICATION OF TESTICULAR TUMORS

The normal testis is composed primarily of: (1) germ cells (spermatozoa), (2) supportive (Sertoli) cells, and (3) interstitial testosterone-secreting (Leydig) cells; neoplasms may arise from any of these elements (Table 19–1). In the adult, 98 per cent of testicular tumors are of germ cell origin,[7] whereas in children germ cell tumors account for approximately 60 to 80 per cent of testicular neoplasms, and nongerm cell tumors make up the other 20 to 40 per cent.

Table 19–1 A Classification of Testicular Tumors*

Tumor Type	Relative Frequency in Children (Per Cent)
I. Germ Cell	65.5
A. Seminoma	1.8
B. Embryonal carcinoma	24.6
C. Infantile adenocarcinoma (orchioblastoma)	15.8
D. Teratoma	16.0
Mature	
Immature	
E. Extraembryonal germ cell tumors	
Choriocarcinoma	
Endodermal sinus (yolk sac) tumor	
F. Mixed germ cell tumor (containing combinations of embryonal carcinoma, teratoma, and extraembryonal elements)	7.3
II. Sex Cord-Stromal	14.6
A. Leydig cell tumor	9.3
B. Sertoli cell tumor	5.3
C. Mixed Leydig and Sertoli cell tumor	
III. Gonadoblastoma	
IV. Paratesticular or Metastatic Tumors	18.4
Lymphosarcoma	7.0
Rhabdomyosarcoma and other sarcomas	11.4
V. Miscellaneous	1.5

*Based on data from 545 patients compiled by Bachmann and von Grawert.[3a]

Germ Cell Tumors

These tumors are all thought to be derived from the totipotent germ cells, which are the precursors of the spermatocytes. The histogenesis and general characteristics of tumors of this type have been discussed in Chapter Eighteen; the features specific to testicular germ cell tumors are discussed below.

Germ cell tumors can frequently be distinguished from one another at the time of surgery by their gross appearance[42] (Fig. 19–1). Seminomas are usually pale and only uncommonly contain areas of hemorrhage or necrosis. Teratomas are of varying consistency and may give a gritty sensation when cut; cystic areas may be evident. Embryonal carcinomas have irregular areas of necrosis and hemorrhage. Choriocarcinoma is characteristically associated with hemorrhage.

Local spread to the scrotal sac is unusual with these tumors because the tunicae albuginea and vaginalis act as barriers; permeation of these structures is regarded as an unfavorable prognostic sign. Metastatic spread along lymphatic or vascular routes is the usual means of dissemination. Lymphatic spread occurs via the long efferent channels, which drain into retroperitoneal lymph nodes at the level of the renal vessels; inguinal lymph node enlargement therefore is not seen with testicular tumors unless the scrotal sac has been invaded. Vascular spread most commonly produces pulmonary metastases, but the liver also may frequently be involved

Seminoma. Seminoma is considered to be derived from the germinal epithelium of the seminiferous tubules and is histologically identical to dysgerminoma of the ovary. The cells of origin may be undifferentiated germ cells, spermatogonia, or spermatocytes. These tumors rarely occur in childhood. Approximately 25 cases in males under the age of 15 years have been reported to date; ages have ranged from 2½ to 15 years.[55a]

Seminoma is a radiosensitive neoplasm. The recommended therapy is radical orchiectomy followed by radiotherapy.[9, 55a] When treated in this manner, Stage I lesions have a greater than 90 per cent 10-year survival rate. However, the prognosis is much poorer if metastases are present.

Embryonal Carcinoma. Germ cell tumors, which are composed wholly or partially of embryonal carcinomatous elements, are the most common type of testicular tumor in infancy and childhood.

Embryonal carcinoma reflects early differentiation of totipotential germ cells before definite embryonal or extraembryonal tissues are recognizable. Two major variants of this tumor are recognized: an adult form, which is highly malignant, and an infantile form, which has a relatively low degree of malignancy.

Histologically the adult form of the tumor is characterized by masses of undifferentiated cells of cuboidal, polygonal, or columnar shape arranged in large sheets or in irregular glandlike or cystic structures (Fig. 19–1D). Nests of small, closely packed hyperchromatic cells (embryonal bodies) may also be seen.

Infantile embryonal carcinoma (orchioblastoma) (infantile adenocarcinoma with clear cells) has a characteristic pattern consisting of spaces of varying size lined by flat epithelial cells alternating with more cellular areas;[37a] a glandular pattern dominates the picture and there are papillary projections and infoldings of epithelium into the lumen. This pattern is virtually identical with the endodermal sinus pattern of the extraembryonal "yolk sac" tumor of the adult testis. Orchioblastoma occurs predominantly in boys under 3 years of age, and some authors consider it to be an infantile form of embryonal carcinoma that is distinguishable by its histologic differences and by its more benign

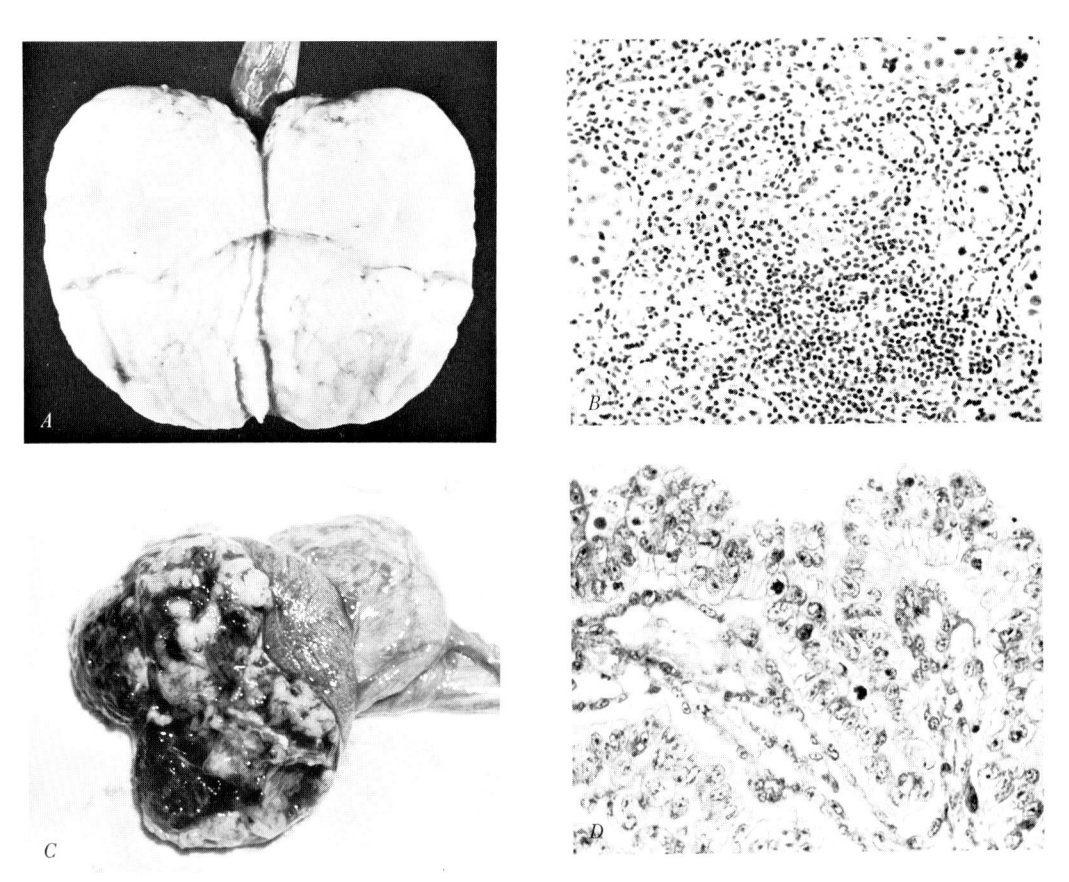

Figure 19–1 Germ cell tumors of the testis. A, Large, pale seminoma which has completely displaced the normal testis. B, Microscopic appearance of seminoma (×320). Note grouping of tumor cells with central round nuclei and clear-to-granular cytoplasm amid a fibrous stroma and a plentiful infiltrate of lymphocytes. C, Embryonal carcinoma with scattered hemorrhage and necrosis. D, Microscopic appearance of embryonal carcinoma (× 320). Note faintly papillary arrangement of undifferentiated malignant cells, with abundant mitotic activity.

TUMORS OF THE SEXUAL ORGANS 447

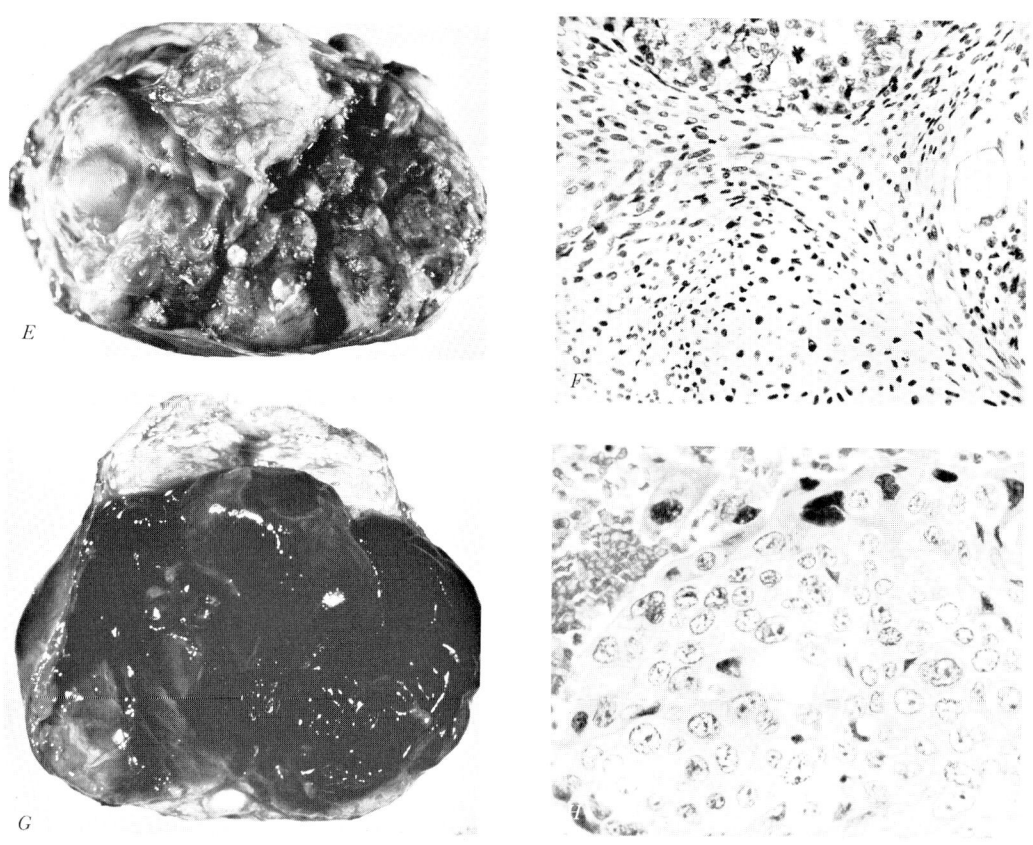

Figure 19–1 Continued E, Teratoma of testis. F, Microscopic appearance of immature testicular teratoma (× 320), showing admixture of cartilage (below) and poorly differentiated cells (above), G, Choriocarcinoma with massive hemorrhage. H, Microscopic appearance of choriocarcinoma (× 490). Note presence of syncytiotrophoblast (above) and cytotrophoblast (below). (From Prout, G. R., Jr.: Germinal tumors of the testis. *In* Holland, J. F., and Frei, E., III [eds.]: Cancer Medicine. Philadelphia, Lea & Febiger, 1973.)

course. However, the favorable prognosis of orchioblastoma may be a phenomenon of the relatively young age of the affected patients, for when patients of a similar age are considered, the prognosis is equally good for both orchioblastoma and embryonal carcinoma.[23]

TREATMENT OF EMBRYONAL CARCINOMA OF THE TESTIS IN CHILDHOOD. Ideal treatment for embryonal carcinoma of the testis in children is not yet clearly established. O3chiectomy, retroperitoneal lymphadenectomy, irradiation, and chemotherapy have all been used singly or in combination by various groups.

The initial treatment of any malignant testicular germ cell tumor, regardless of the patient's age, is radical orchiectomy with high ligation of the spermatic cord at the internal inguinal ring. Orchiectomy through the scrotum or transscrotal biopsy is contraindicated because of the danger of local tumor dissemination and subsequent scrotal or inguinal recurrence.

Complete and careful staging is then necessary to determine subsequent therapy; this would include chest x-ray, whole lung tomography, IVP (to detect deflection of the kidney or ureters by metastatic periaortic lymph nodes), liver scan, and lymphangiogram. Some groups also recommend retroperitoneal lymphadenectomy,

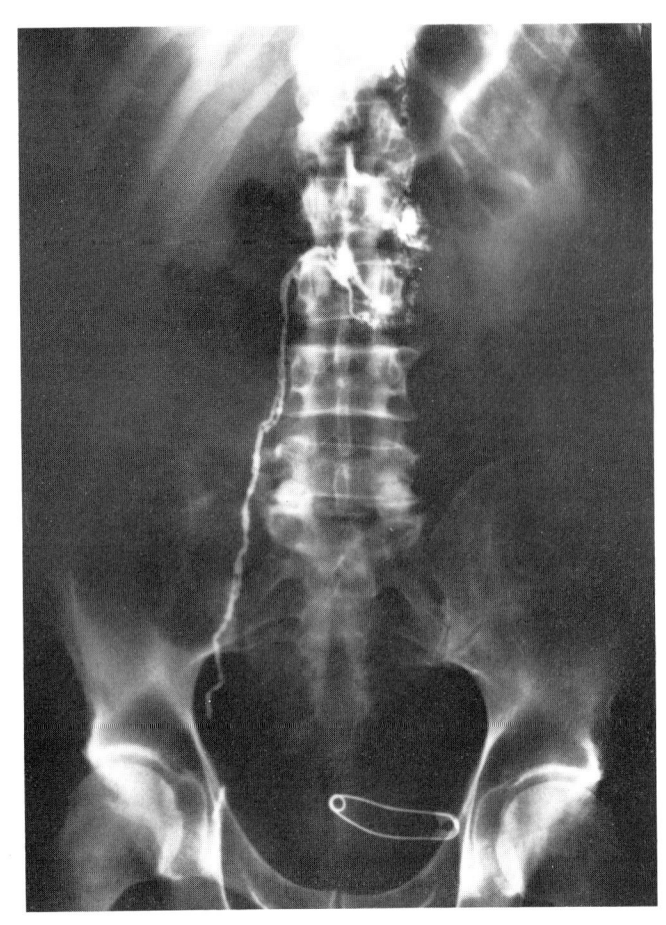

Figure 19-2 Right testicular lymphangiogram showing pathway of lymphatic drainage to periaortic lymph nodes. (From Busch, F. M., et al.: J. Urol. 93:490, 1965. © 1965 The Williams & Wilkins Co., Baltimore.)

both for staging and for therapeutic purposes. The reason for this is that, since the testes and spermatic cord are devoid of lymph nodes, their primary lymphoid drainage is through lymphatic vessels paralleling the testicular vessels up to the periaortic nodes at the level of the renal hilum (Fig. 19-2). Consequently, malignant testicular neoplasms frequently metastasize to the retroperitoneal region.

There is still disagreement as to the necessity for retroperitoneal lymphadenectomy in children, particularly since the most frequent complication of this procedure is ejaculatory impotence, which frequently results from damage to the sacral plexus, nervi erigentes, or L1 sympathetic ganglia. The failure to demonstrate metastatic disease in the removed lymph nodes in all the cases reviewed by Gangai[16] and Johnson[26] also has brought into question the routine use of this procedure in children.

In an effort to determine the effects of the various treatment modalities on the mortality rate of testicular embryonal carcinoma, Jeffs[25a] has reviewed 164 cases selected from the world literature; for the purpose of this study it was assumed that embryonal carcinoma under the age of 12 years was the same tumor as orchioblastoma.

As shown in Table 19-2, the overall survival rate was 65 per cent. However, there was great variability according to age, with the prognosis for survival decreasing as age at diagnosis increased. Prognosis was excellent for children under 12 months of age, but

Table 19-2 Prognosis of Testicular Embryonal Carcinoma in Children[25a]

AGE (MONTHS) AT DIAGNOSIS	PER CENT "ALIVE AND WELL" AFTER 12 MONTHS
0-12	85
12-24	63
24-144	41
Total	65

poor in children over 24 months of age.

When patients were evaluated according to mode of treatment (Table 19-3), it was found that retroperitoneal lymphadenectomy improved the prognosis in children over 12 months of age, but not in children younger than this. Radiotherapy to the retroperitoneal region did not appear to improve prognosis in patients 0 to 12 months and 12 to 24 months of age but may have had some value in the over-24-months group. It appears to be of particular value in patients whose tumor has spread to the retroperitoneal glands.

It is important to recognize that Jeffs' data are based on the patient being "alive and well" for a period of 12 months after operation. The justification for this is that most patients who died had evidence of metastases within this period. However, it is possible that some patients, particularly those treated less aggressively, might develop recurrent disease at a later period and eventually succumb to their tumors.

Sabio and colleagues[46] have interpreted the literature on this tumor to suggest that lymphadenectomy or radiotherapy following orchiectomy may improve the survival rate. In this study, the addition of either of these modalities to orchiectomy improved the survival rate from approximately 50 per cent to almost 85 per cent. Among a group of 10 patients treated with the combination of orchiectomy, chemotherapy, lymphadenectomy, and radiotherapy, all survived. However, the patients in the various treatment groups were not matched for age, which may be the critical factor.

A number of drugs have produced both partial and complete remissions in patients with metastatic nonseminomatous germ cell tumors; combination chemotherapy used in either a sequential or a concurrent fashion has, in general, been shown to be superior to the use of single agents.[10, 47, 59] A

Table 19-3 Analysis of Treatment of Testicular Embryonal Carcinoma in Children[25a] *

AGE (MONTHS) AT DIAGNOSIS	TREATMENT	NUMBER OF CASES	PER CENT "ALIVE AND WELL" AFTER 12 MONTHS
0-12	Orchiectomy alone	23	96
	Orchiectomy and radiation	19	79
	Orchiectomy and lymphadenectomy	10	90
12-24	Orchiectomy alone	40	60
	Orchiectomy and radiation	24	54
	Orchiectomy and lymphadenectomy	10	100
24-144	Orchiectomy alone	17	29
	Orchiectomy and radiation	8	50
	Orchiectomy and lymphadenectomy	7	71

*This analysis includes only 158 of the 164 cases collated by Jeffs; six patients treated by orchiectomy and chemotherapy are not included.

large randomized study comparing these various therapeutic approaches is still necessary before the superiority of one can be established.

Recently Einhorn and Donohue have used a three-drug regimen (cis-platinum, vinblastine, and bleomycin) to treat a group of 50 adult males suffering from disseminated germ cell tumors of the testis.[10a] They report a 74 per cent incidence of complete remission, with 64 per cent of the patients alive and disease-free at 6+ to 30+ months. These results suggest that even far-advanced testicular germ cell tumors may be treatable and perhaps even curable with an aggressive therapeutic approach.

Teratoma. When germ cell tumors differentiate along embryonal lines, the most frequently recognizable somatic tissues are neuroglia, gastrointestinal or respiratory epithelium, cartilage, bone, and smooth muscle. These tissues may be fully differentiated or may be arrested at any stage of their embryonal development; such immature elements may behave in a malignant fashion. Thus, the behavior of a teratoma is frequently determined by the most immature element present, even if this element is present in only one or two foci.

Mature teratoma of the testis is characterized by mature, well-differentiated tissue derived from all three germ layers (ectoderm, mesoderm, endoderm); this neoplasm occurs more frequently in infants and young children than in adults. Such tumors are uniformly benign and virtually never metastasize;[11, 14] even teratomas which exhibit only partial differentiation may behave in a clinically benign fashion in childhood.[16, 23, 33] This behavior is in marked contrast to testicular teratomas of adults, which must always be considered potentially malignant even when histologically "benign."[14] However, it is unjustifiable to assume that a "mature" teratoma is benign unless extensive sampling is performed to look for undifferentiated foci of embryonal carcinoma. Orchiectomy with high ligation of the spermatic cord appears to be adequate therapy for mature childhood testicular teratoma.[11, 14]

Extraembryonal Tumors. When germ cell tumors differentiate along extraembryonal lines, they may contain primitive trophoblastic tissue (choriocarcinoma) or yolk sac epithelium (endodermal sinus tumor). Tumors that contain yolk sac or trophoblastic elements have a distinctly poorer prognosis than those with "pure" embryonal carcinoma or embryonal teratoma. Such patients will frequently have elevated serum levels of *human chorionic gonadotropin* (HCG) or *alpha-fetoprotein* (AFP), particularly if the tumor is metastatic.[31, 58] Thus, these substances are extremely sensitive preoperative markers of metastatic disease. In one series, all patients who were clinically free of tumor postorchiectomy, but who had elevated serum HCG or AFP levels, were found to have retroperitoneal metastases (usually microscopic).[31] However, the greatest clinical value of these markers appears to be in monitoring the effectiveness of radiation and chemotherapy in patients with extraembryonal germ cell tumors.

Sex Cord–Stromal Tumors

The cells producing these tumors represent the hormone-producing elements of the gonads. In their primitive stage, these cells have the morphologic appearance of spindle-shaped fibroblasts; in their differentiated stage they are recognizable as Leydig and Sertoli cells in the male and as theca and granulosa cells in the female. Leydig cells are interstitial mesenchymal cells that are capable of testosterone production, while Sertoli cells are normally present in the seminiferous tubules and are capable of estrogen secretion. Most gonadal stromal tumors can be readily identified as

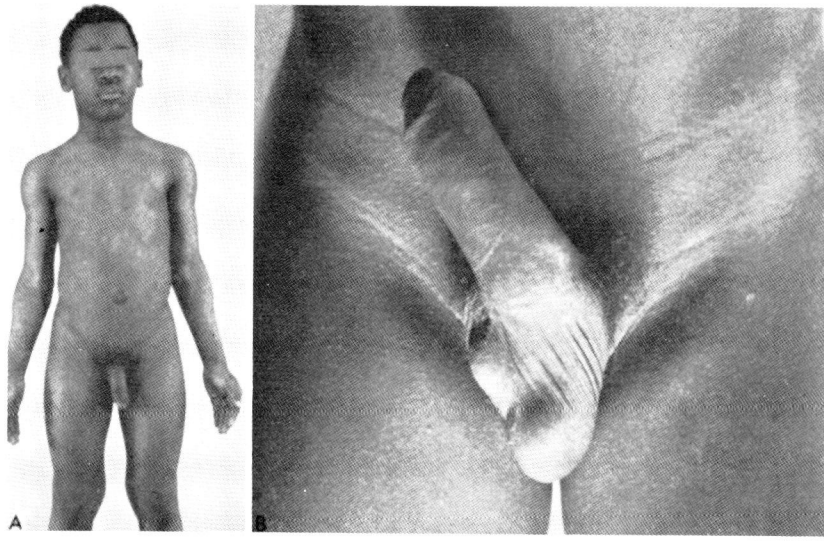

Figure 19–3 A, A 6-year-old patient with increased muscularity, pubic hair, and large penis. B, Enlarged left testis, which contained an interstitial cell tumor. (From Houser, R., et al.: Amer. J. Surg. *110*:876, 1965.)

pure Leydig cell tumors or pure Sertoli cell tumors; however, some tumors may contain mixtures of Leydig cells, Sertoli cells, and fibroblast-like cells.

Leydig Cell Tumor (Interstitial Cell Tumor). This tumor is derived from primordial mesenchyme lying within the testicular interstitial tissues. It occurs most frequently at around 4 to 5 years of age and is the most common non-germ cell tumor in both children and adults. Leydig cells are normally the source of testosterone and they are likewise capable of testosterone synthesis when they undergo neoplasia. Consequently this tumor can produce precocious puberty in the young boy (Fig. 19–3); not infrequently rapid somatic growth, enlargement of the penis, growth of pubic hair, voice change, and increase in the bone age precede the appearance of a detectable testicular mass. If treatment is delayed until adolescence, premature epiphyseal closure may occur, with resultant stunting of growth. The diagnosis in most cases may be made preoperatively by demonstration of the triad of *precocious puberty, testicular mass,* and *elevated 17-ketosteroids.* In approximately 5 per cent of cases, estrogen production with gynecomastia or feminization may occur instead of masculinization.[8]

The tumor is usually slow-growing and rarely, if ever, malignant in the prepubertal male. Consequently, simple enucleation of the tumor or orchiectomy is considered acceptable treatment.[8, 23, 41]

Sertoli Cell Tumor. Sertoli cell tumors represent 5 per cent of testicular tumors in children.[3a] Although they occur throughout childhood and after puberty, most have been discovered before the age of 2 years. The tumor may be associated with feminization or isosexual precocity, or may not produce any endocrine manifestations.

Simple high inguinal orchiectomy is usually adequate therapy, since 90 per cent are benign; however, sizable growths that have been present for long periods may warrant prophylactic retroperitoneal lymphadenectomy.

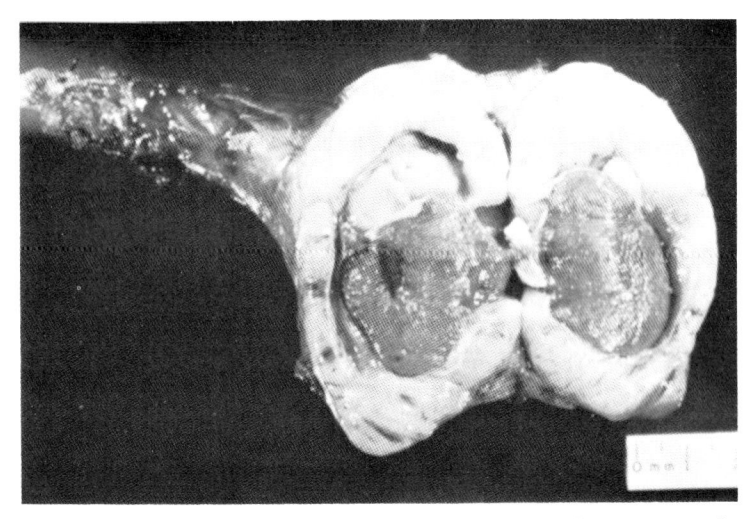

Figure 19-4 Paratesticular embryonal rhabdomyosarcoma. The pale tumor completely encircles the grayish testis. (From Hajdu, S. I., and Hajdu, E. O.: Cytopathology of Sarcomas and Other Nonepithelial Malignant Tumors. Philadelphia, W. B. Saunders Co., 1976.)

Gonadoblastoma

Gonadoblastoma is a neoplastic mixture of germinal and mesenchymal cells. It is found almost invariably in the dysplastic gonads of patients with the "testicular feminization" syndrome (phenotypic females with dysgenetic gonads, absence of sex chromatin bodies, and a 46XY or 45XO/XY karyotype);[49] 20 per cent are found in phenotypic males and 80 per cent in phenotypic females. These gonads may be situated in the inguinal canals, but more commonly one or both are in the abdomen (cryptorchid). When malignancy develops, it is due to the presence of seminomatous elements; this only occurs in gonads containing a Y chromosome.[39] Gonadoblastoma is discussed further in the section on ovarian tumors.

Paratesticular Tumors

This term refers to those intrascrotal tumors that arise from the epididymis or spermatic cord and its coverings. In childhood, these tumors are almost invariably rhabdomyosarcomas (Fig. 19-4), but lymphomas and other rare tumors, such as primary and metastatic epididymal tumors and adenocarcinoma of the appendix testis, can also occur.[8, 9, 57]

Most of these tumors occur as painless unilateral masses, arising above the testis and below the superficial inguinal ring; a hydrocele or a transilluminating mass may also be present. Benign lesions are well circumscribed and mobile, whereas sarcomas are lobulated, firm, and attached to the structure of origin.

Paratesticular rhabdomyosarcoma tends either to recur locally or to spread via the lymphatic drainage pathways to the retroperitoneal area.[3, 20, 48] Distant metastasis to bone and lung occur frequently in the late stages of the disease after local recurrence cannot be controlled or when retroperitoneal disease becomes extensive. Rhabdomyosarcoma is discussed in more detail in Chapter Sixteen.

Some authors recommend radical orchiectomy with early clamping and high ligation of the cord,[5, 9, 45] and others add retroperitoneal lymph node dissection[4, 5, 9, 56] for treatment of this lesion. Using this latter approach, Burrington achieved survival in 6 of 8 patients for periods of 1 to 20 years after definitive therapy.[5] The addition of radiation therapy and combination therapy may make possible less extensive surgical procedures as well as improve survival.[30, 43]

Female Reproductive System

Cancer of the female genital tract is relatively rare in childhood; this is fortunate because, in general, tumors in this area have a very poor prognosis. Unfortunately, the rarity of these tumors and the nonspecificity of their symptoms also frequently cause the diagnosis to be delayed past the point of potential cure. Ovarian tumors account for the majority of pediatric gynecologic malignancies; this is in marked contrast to adult gynecologic cancer, which mainly involves the vulva, vagina, cervix, and corpus uteri.

OVARIAN TUMORS

Ovarian tumors account for 1 per cent of all childhood tumors.[71] Although these neoplasms may occur at any time in the pediatric years, they tend to present most frequently at puberty (between the ages of 10 and 14 years)[68] Approximately 10 to 30 per cent of childhood ovarian tumors are malignant.[63, 68, 76, 112]

Diagnosis

Because of their anatomic position, ovarian neoplasms are less easily detected than are testicular ones. Consequently, they are usually discovered at a later age and in a more advanced state than are the corresponding testicular neoplasms.

Since the ovaries have their embryologic origin at the level of the tenth thoracic vertebra and are located within the abdomen during childhood, the most common finding with ovarian tumors is abdominal pain or mass—in about half of the patients the pain is of acute onset, is associated with nausea and vomiting, and may be related to ovarian torsion. Thus, ovarian tumor should be considered in the differential diagnosis when a girl presents with acute abdominal complaints; however, it should also be realized that in a large series of girls with abdominal complaints only 1 in 700 had an ovarian tumor, whereas 350 had acute appendicitis.[104] Gastrointestinal or urinary tract obstruction may also be presenting features of ovarian tumors. Bimanual rectal examination is thus an important part of the diagnostic approach to girls presenting with abdominal, urinary tract, or gastrointestinal complaints.

Ovarian tumors which contain stromal elements may be endocrinologically functional and may produce precocious puberty, vaginal bleeding, or masculinization. Precocious puberty due to ovarian cyst or tumor may be differentiated from that due to pituitary axis dysfunction by the fact that in the former only estrogen levels are elevated, while in the latter both pituitary hormones and estrogens are elevated.[117]

Preoperative evaluation of a girl with a suspected ovarian tumor should include a thorough physical examination with special attention paid to signs of precocious puberty or virilism. A careful search of the abdominal x-ray for calcifications or teeth within the mass should also be performed—these suggest the likelihood of a teratoma (Fig. 19–5); the presence of circumscribed, mottled, or punctate calcifications in a patient with primary amen-

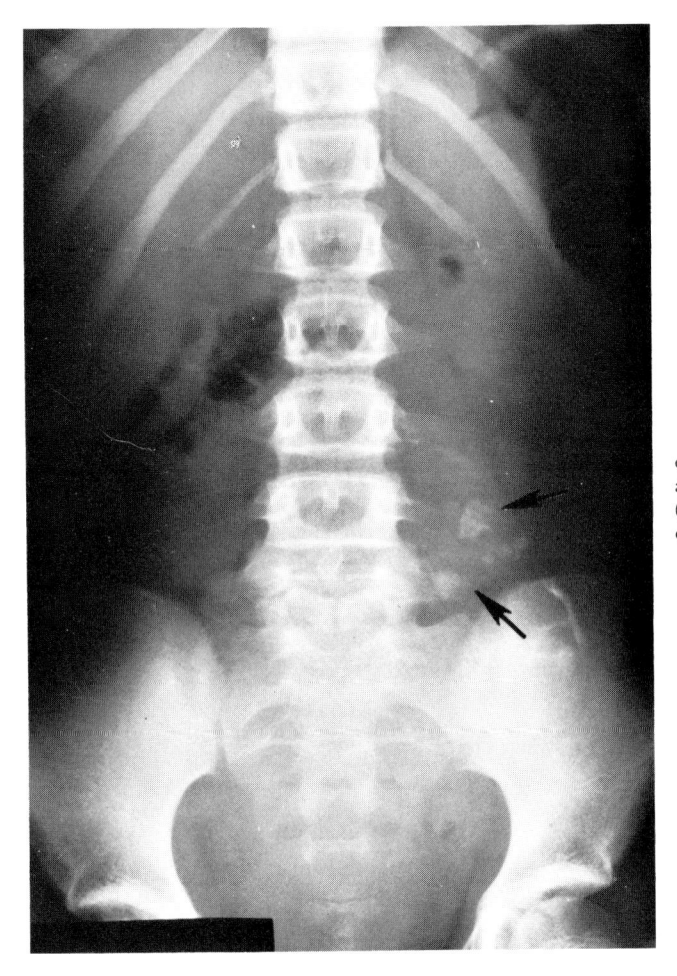

Figure 19-5 Abdominal x-ray of an ovarian immature teratoma; a mass lesion with calcifications (arrows) is evident in the left lower quadrant.

orrhea or anomalous genitalia suggests the likelihood of a gonadoblastoma.

Measurement of *alpha-fetoprotein* (AFP) and *human chorionic gonadotropin* (HCG) levels in the blood preoperatively is useful for detecting embryonal carcinoma (AFP and HCG), endodermal sinus tumor (AFP), or choriocarcinomatous (HCG) elements within the tumor. It is also useful to establish baseline values of these biochemical markers preoperatively so that they can be used to follow the patient's response to therapy and detect early recurrences.

Diagnostic ultrasound scanning may provide additional useful information, including the outline, size, location, and nature of the mass (cystic or solid), the presence of ascites, and the presence of metastatic disease within the pelvis or abdomen.

CLASSIFICATION OF OVARIAN TUMORS

Ovarian tumors arise from (1) the germ cells (oocytes), (2) the coelomic epithelium of the ovarian surface, (3) the mesenchymal ovarian stroma, (4) mesonephric rests, or (5) accessory tissues. A histogenetic classification of ovarian tumors based on their derivation from these tissues is shown in Table 19-4. In children the majority of ovarian tumors are of germ cell origin; this is in marked contrast to the situation for adult females, in whom 90 per cent of ovarian tumors are of epithelial origin.

Table 19-4 A Classification of Malignant Ovarian Tumors*

Tumor Type	Relative Frequency in Children (Per Cent)
I. Germ Cell	75.2
A. Dysgerminoma	19.2
B. Embryonal carcinoma	17.5
C. Immature teratoma	38.5
D. Extraembryonal germ cell tumor	
Choriocarcinoma	
Endodermal sinus tumor (yolk sac tumor)	
E. Mixed germ cell tumor	
F. Gonadoblastoma	
II. Stromal Mesenchyme	
A. Sex-differentiated (with potential endocrine function)	24.3
Granulosa cell tumor	11.9
Theca cell tumor	3.4
Arrhenoblastoma (Sertoli-Leydig cell tumor)	2.2
Hilus cell tumor	
Gynandroblastoma	
B. Sex-undifferentiated	6.8
Fibrosarcoma	
Neurofibrosarcoma	
Leiomyosarcoma	
Rhabdomyosarcoma	
Lymphoma	
III. Epithelial	
A. Serous cystadenocarcinoma	0.5
B. Mucinous cystadenocarcinoma	
C. Endometrioid cystadenocarcinoma	
D. Brenner tumor	

*Based on 176 malignant ovarian tumors in girls under 15 years of age compiled by Norris and Jensen[102a] and Groeber.[83]

Germ Cell Tumors

The egg cells (oocytes) of the definitive gonad are the descendants of primitive totipotential germ cells which migrate during embryonic life from the yolk sac to the urogenital ridge. Tumors derived from these cells may represent primordial germ cells (*dysgerminoma*), undifferentiated pluripotent germ cells (*embryonal carcinoma*), partially differentiated embryonal elements (*immature teratoma*) (Fig. 19-6), or partially differentiated extraembryonal elements (*endodermal sinus tumor, choriocarcinoma*). Approximately 8 per cent of malignant ovarian germ cell tumors contain combinations of one or more of these germ cell elements.[97]

While 95 per cent of all ovarian germ cell tumors are benign cystic teratomas, the younger the patient, the more likely the tumor is to be malignant. Thus, Kurman and Norris found that 84 per cent of ovarian germ cell tumors in girls under 10 years of age were malignant.[97a]

Dysgerminoma. Dysgerminoma is thought to arise from the germ cells of the sexually indifferent stage of gonadogenesis. Morphologically and histochemically, the dysgerminoma cells are identical with primordial germ cells and appear as arranged in sheets or cords separated by fibrous connective tissue stroma in which there is marked infiltration by lymphocytes. This tumor corresponds histogenetically and morphologically to seminoma of the testis. However, unlike seminoma, which occurs almost exclusively in postpubertal males, dysger-

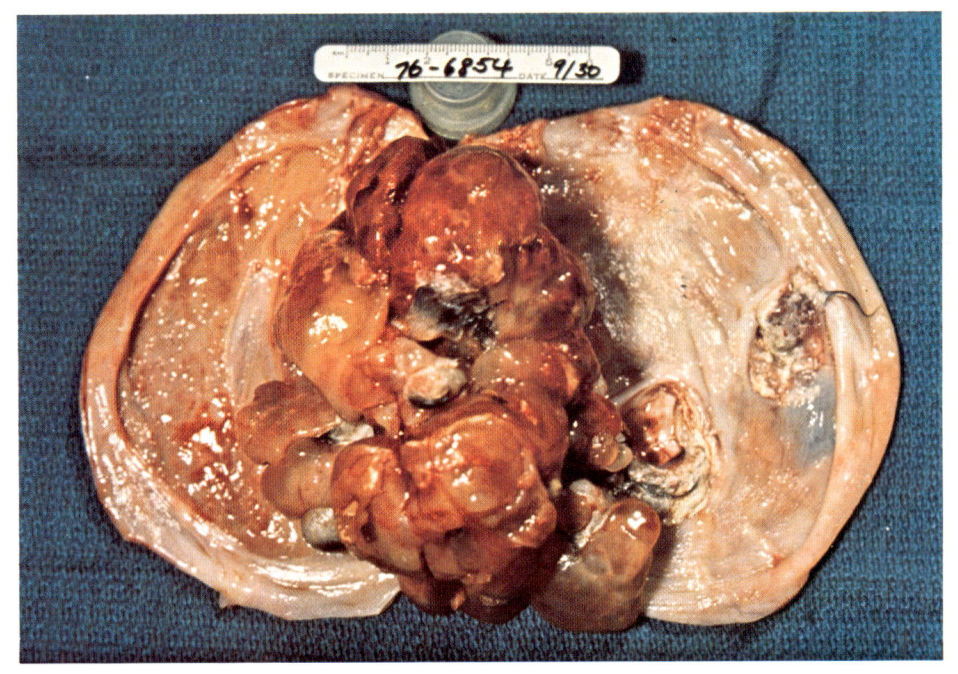

Figure 19–6 Immature teratoma of the ovary. The capsule is peeled back to show a solid, irregular mass containing hairs and immature cerebral tissue. (Courtesy of Dr. David Krugman.)

minoma not uncommonly develops prior to puberty. This may reflect the fact that meiotic events occur in the ovary during intrauterine life while meiotic events in the testis begin at puberty.[78]

Patients with unilateral tumors less than 10 cm in diameter who do not have evidence of metastases may be treated by unilateral salpingo-oophorectomy with bisection and biopsy of the opposite ovary.[68, 69, 111, 112] If the tumor is bilateral (approximately 5 to 10 per cent), larger than 10 cm, has metastasized locally or to regional nodes, or has caused bloody ascites, then total abdominal hysterectomy and bilateral salpingo-oophorectomy has been recommended.[68, 111, 112]

The tumor is very radiosensitive, and metastatic or recurrent disease will respond to radiotherapy. The role of postoperative radiotherapy is still undefined. Smith recommends treatment of the abdomen, pelvis, and para-aortic nodes with doses of 2000 to 2600 rads (3-week course), depending on the histology of the tumor and the presence and location of metastases.[111, 112]

Prognosis is excellent (over 96 per cent survival) for patients with tumor confined to the ovary.[67, 111, 112] However, extension of tumor beyond the ovary, or recurrence of the tumor during the first two years after treatment is an ominous sign; the presence of teratomatous or trophoblastic foci within a dysgerminoma likewise augurs a bad prognosis.[73]

Embryonal Carcinoma. Embryonal carcinoma of the ovary is a recently defined entity which is thought to be analogous to embryonal carcinoma of the testis in representing a primitive tumor composed of undifferentiated pluripotential germ cells.[96] These cells appear to be capable of both somatic and extraembryonic differentiation and may well be the neoplastic progenitors of embryonal and extraembryonal teratomas.

Histologically this tumor is characterized by the presence of a sheetlike proliferation of primitive cells and the absence of significant amounts of differentiated tissues; these cells are easily distinguished from the sheetlike cells of dysgerminoma by their larger size, more hyperchromatic nuclei, and tendency to form a glandular pattern.[96] Scattered among the embryonal carcinoma cells are isolated syncytiotrophoblastic giant cells (Fig. 19-7) with immunohistochemically identifiable human chorionic gonadotropin (HCG) and mononuclear embryonal cells with immunohistochemically identifiable alpha-fetoprotein (AFP).

The reported cases range in age from 4 to 28 years with a median of 14 years; nearly half were prepubertal. Two thirds of these cases presented with signs and symptoms related to hormonal stimulation (precocious puberty, amenorrhea, irregular vaginal bleeding, mild hirsutism, or a false positive pregnancy test).[96]

Teratoma. The derivation, general features, and histogenetic interrelationships of the various subtypes of teratoma have been discussed in Chapter Eighteen. Teratomas account for 40 to 50 per cent of reported ovarian masses in children.[62, 76] Of these, the majority (approximately 80 per cent) are cystic lesions (dermoid cysts) with a very low incidence of malignancy (0.8 to 3.0 per cent); however, solid teratomas, which have a much higher incidence of malignancy, are not uncommon in childhood.

IMMATURE TERATOMA. The term immature teratoma should be reserved for those germ cell tumors which are limited to somatic (embryonal) elements and do not contain dysgerminoma or extraembryonal elements (endodermal sinus tumor, choriocarcinoma). In an immature teratoma at least one of the germ cell layers lacks full differentiation; most often, the immature component is neuroepithelial, and it often forms neuroblastic rosettes.

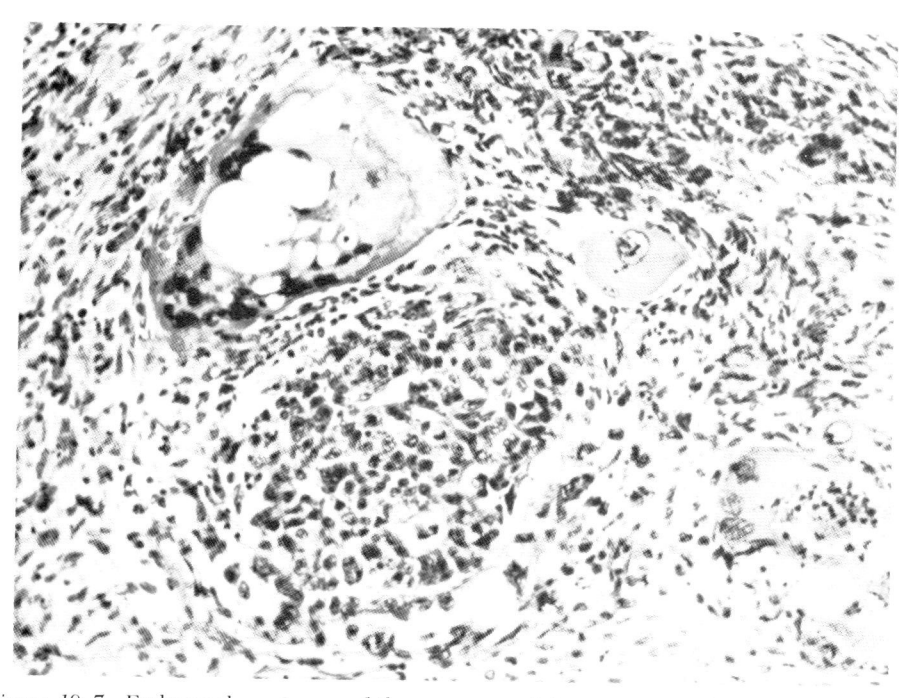

Figure 19-7 Embryonal carcinoma of the ovary containing syncytiotrophoblastic giant cells adjoining a nest of primitive undifferentiated cells. (From Kurman, R. J., and Norris, H. J.: Obstet. Gynec. 48:579, 1976. Armed Forces Institute of Pathology, Neg. No. 76-3765.)

Table 19-5 Histologic Grading of Immature Teratomas[106]

Grade 0.	All tissues mature; no mitotic activity
Grade 1.	Minor foci of abnormally cellular or embryonal tissue mixed with mature elements; rare mitoses
Grade 2.	Moderate quantities of embryonal tissue mixed with mature elements; moderate mitotic activity
Grade 3.	Large quantities of embryonal tissue present

It is important to recognize that immaturity of tissues within a teratoma reflets metastatic capability and therefore the immature elements should be considered evidence of malignancy. The grading system proposed by Robboy and Scully[106] (Table 19-5), which quantitates the degree of immaturity and the presence of neuroepithelial components, appears to correlate well with the clinical behavior of these tumors (Fig. 19-8). Thus, the histologic grade of the primary tumor appears to be one of the major determinants of the likelihood of extraovarian spread; once extraovarian spread has occurred, however, the major factor related to prognosis is the histologic grade of the metastases.[103]

Extraembryonal Germ Cell Tumors. *Endodermal sinus (yolk sac) tumor* is the most common extraembryonal germ cell tumor of the ovary. This tumor may manifest a multiplicity of histologic patterns. The Schiller-Duval body is considered to be pathognomonic for endodermal sinus tumor, but is present only in 75 per cent of cases.[95] A specific feature that may be even more useful is the presence of hyaline droplets, which represent alpha-fetoprotein synthesized by the tumor and which are present in all cases[95] (Fig. 19-9).

Clinically these tumors are characterized by rapid growth and extensive intraabdominal and intrapelvic spread with widespread involvement of peritoneal surfaces. The prognosis is generally poor even for Stage I disease, where 84 per cent of patients eventually die of metastatic disease (93 per cent of these within 2 years).[95] Survival may be improved, however, by the use of combination chemotherapy following salpingo-oophorectomy.[95]

Primary ovarian *choriocarcinoma* is a rare entity; it may be suspected in a prepubertal girl by its hormonal effects (elevated HCG level, false-positive pregnancy test, precocious puberty).

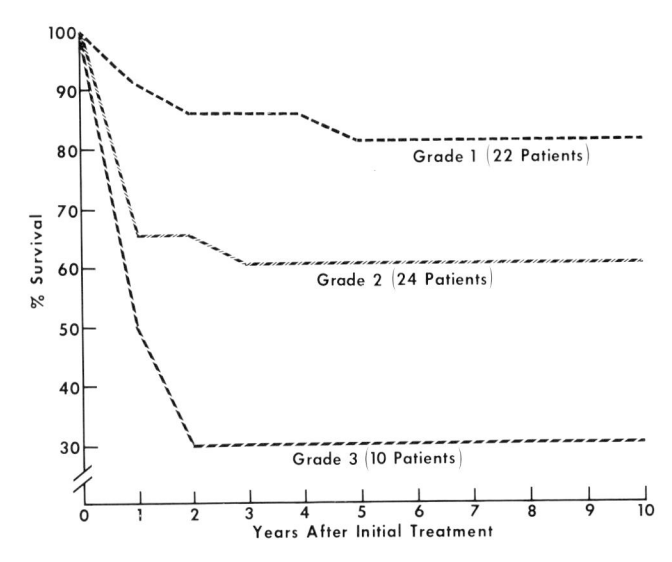

Figure 19-8 Correlation of histologic grade with actuarial survival of 56 patients with immature ovarian teratoma. (From Norris, H. J. et al.: Cancer 37:2359, 1976. Armed Forces Institute of Pathology, Neg. No. 3653.)

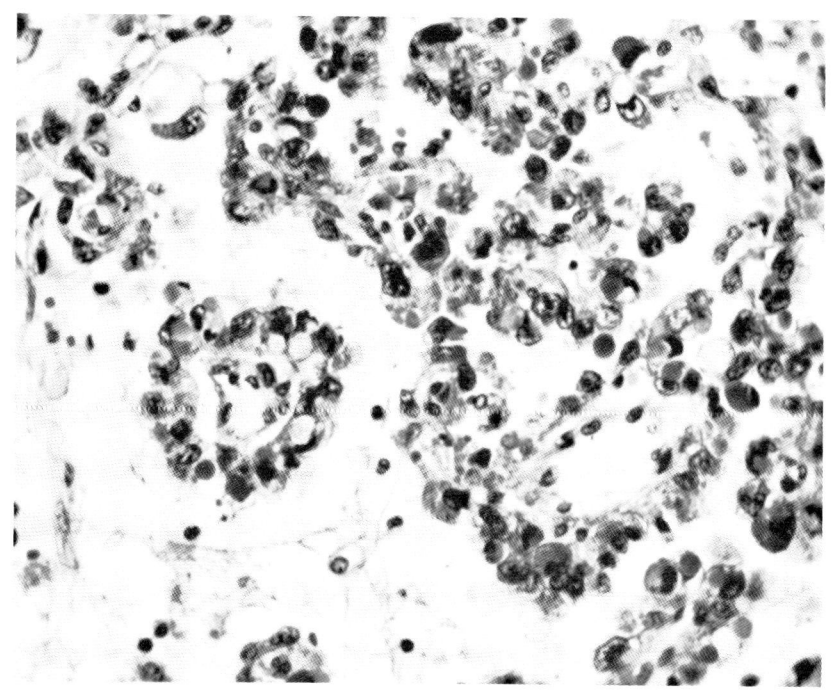

Figure 19-9 Endodermal sinus tumor of the ovary. A Schiller-Duval body associated with numerous hyaline droplets is seen to the left of center. These droplets contain alpha-fetoprotein. (From Kurman, R. J., and Norris, H. J.: Cancer 38:2404, 1976. Armed Forces Institute of Pathology, Neg. No. 74-19451.)

During the postpubertal years, an ovarian mass associated with a positive pregnancy test is more likely to be an ectopic pregnancy or a small uterine choriocarcinoma with metastasis to the ovary than primary ovarian choriocarcinoma.

METASTATIC BEHAVIOR OF OVARIAN GERM CELL TUMORS

Extraovarian spread of malignant germ cell tumors usually involves the adnexal surfaces by direct extension, the retroperitoneal lymph nodes by lymphatic spread, and the peritoneal surfaces of the abdomen and pelvis by either lymphatic or transperitoneal seeding. The peritoneal surfaces of the bladder, uterus, and sigmoid colon are probably the most frequent metastatic sites, but the peritoneal surfaces of the diaphragm, liver, and small intestine are also commonly involved. Distant sites of metastasis include lung, liver parenchyma, bone, and mediastinum.

Because of the flow pattern of ascitic fluid in the peritoneal cavity and the flow patterns of the ovarian veins, malignancies of the right ovary may spread more widely than those of the left ovary.[100] In a series of 232 patients with ovarian carcinoma (mainly adults) reported by Meleka and Rasla,[100] patients with right ovarian malignancies had extensive disease twice as frequently as those with malignancy of the left ovary. It has not been determined as yet, however, whether germ cell malignancies of the ovary in pediatric patients exhibit similar behavior.

Neoplasms that contain mixtures of different germ cell elements (dysgerminoma, embryonal carcinoma, embryonal teratoma, or extraembryonal teratoma) can metastasize as any of the malignant components; the metastases may contain complex aggregates of tissues derived from several germ layers,[74, 116] or pure carcinoma, sarcoma, or neuroepithelioma.[81, 116] Frequently only the most malignant element of the original neoplasm is evident in the metastases. When metastasis is limited to peritoneal implants composed exclusively or predominantly of mature neuroglial tissue, the implications are not nearly so grave as they are with other types of metastases, and most of such patients do well;[81, 106] the reason for this may be that these implants represent extrusion of mature glia through a defect in the primary tumor rather than true metastatic seeding.[106]

PROGNOSIS AND TREATMENT OF OVARIAN GERM CELL TUMORS

The prognosis for malignant germ cell tumors of the ovary is grave, with mortality rates ranging from 66 to 92 per cent.[75, 98, 106] Patients with endodermal sinus tumors do particularly poorly, whereas true solid embryonal teratomas may have a relatively favorable prognosis, particularly if there has not been rupture or local extension;[105, 116] in fact, some of these neoplasms may be histologically and clinically benign.[105]

Treatment of malignant ovarian germ cell tumors is still controversial and highly individualized. Some authors recommend unilateral salpingo-oophorectomy for Stage I endodermal sinus tumor (which is unilateral in 90 to 95 per cent of cases) and bilateral salpingo-oophorectomy plus hysterectomy for immature embryonal teratoma (which is frequently bilateral).[111, 112] Others feel unilateral salpingo-oophorectomy is sufficient for Stage I pure immature teratoma if a biopsy of the opposite ovary shows no involvement.[103]

These tumors will respond to chemotherapeutic combinations such as actinomycin D/5-fluorouracil/cyclophosphamide (ActFuCy) or vincristine/actinomycin D/cyclophosphamide (VAC); postoperative treatment with one of these combinations for a period of 1 to 2 years has been recommended even if the tumor appears to have been completely excised, particularly if the histologic grading shows large areas of immature tissue.[103, 111, 112, 113]

The value of radiation therapy in treatment of girls with ovarian germ cell tumors (other than dysgerminoma) is controversial. Some authors question whether radiation therapy is of any value in these patients because they consider the tumors to be radioresistant.[111, 112, 113] Other authors, on the other hand, have been successful, in a small series of cases, in preventing pelvic and abdominal recurrences by use of irradiation of the entire abdomen and pelvis; radiation therapy restricted to the pelvis appears to be inadequate treatment even for some patients with Stages I and II disease, since extension of disease within the abdominal cavity is probably as common as it is to the pelvis.[72]

An even more aggressive approach combines radical surgery (bilateral salpingo-oophorectomy, hysterectomy, retroperitoneal node dissection, and omentectomy), radiation therapy (to the entire abdomen with booster doses to para-aortic nodes and pelvis), and multiagent chemotherapy.[121] Using this approach, 6 of 10 patients with malignant teratoma, endodermal sinus tumor, or embryonal carcinoma have remained alive without evidence of recurrent disease for periods ranging from 7 to 40 months.[121] A larger series with a longer follow-up period is necessary before this approach can be fully evaluated.

Gonadoblastoma (Dysgenetic Gonadoma). Gonadoblastoma has been defined as a neoplasm containing an intimate mixture of germ cells and elements resembling immature granulosa or Sertoli cells (Fig. 19–10);

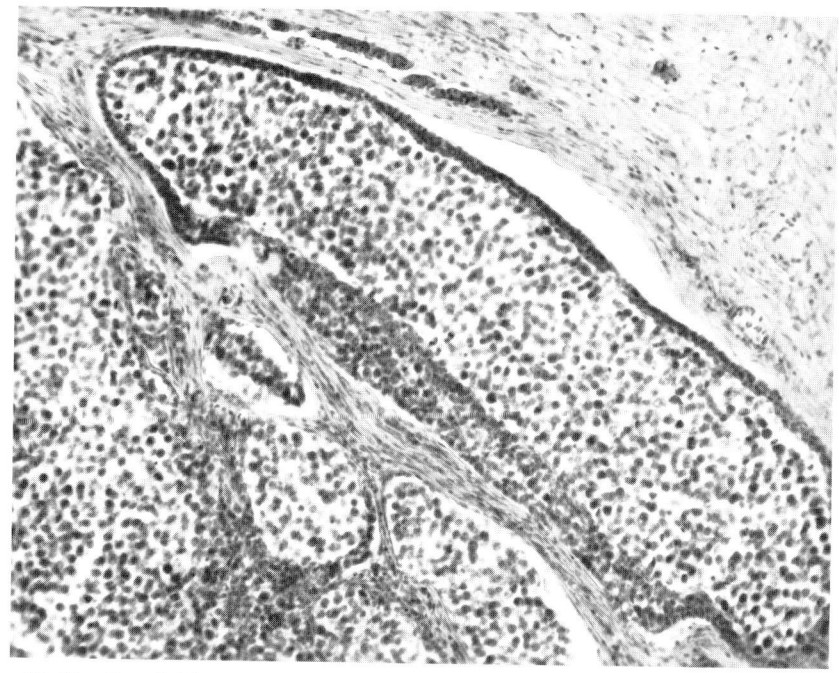

Figure 19–10 Gonadoblastoma. Sex cord–derived cells line the periphery while germ cells fill the center of an elongated nest. (From Scully, R. E.: Cancer 25:1340, 1970.)

Leydig cells or lutein-type cells may or may not be present.[108] The term gonadoblastoma was chosen for this tumor because it is felt to recapitulate gonadal development more completely than any other type of tumor.

Commonly the germ cells overgrow the other elements and the tumor resembles a dysgerminoma (seminoma) and is hormonally inert. Tumors containing granulosa cells will exert estrogenizing effects, such as precocious puberty, while Leydig cells will exert virilizing effects when they predominate.[115] The tumor may also be found fortuitously as a circumscribed mottled or punctate pelvic calcification.

This tumor develops almost exclusively in abnormal gonads. Approximately 90 per cent of the cases are sex chromatin negative, 46XY and 45XO/46XY being the most common karyotypes.[68, 69] All patients are sexually abnormal, 80 per cent appearing as phenotypic females with virilization (testicular feminization syndrome) and the remainder as phenotypic males with cryptorchidism, hypospadias, and internal female sex organs.[108] The gonad bearing the tumor is generally of indeterminate nature, but may sometimes be identified as a streak or a dysgenetic cryptorchid testis. The contralateral gonad is usually also found to be of testicular nature.

The malignant potential of the dysgenetic gonad in the intersex patient with a Y chromosome is now well documented, the commonest malignant tumor encountered in these patients being dysgerminoma (seminoma). In approximately 8 per cent of patients, more malignant germ cell tumors (endodermal sinus tumor, embryonal carcinoma, choriocarcinoma) may be present.[108]

The expectancy of tumors rises appreciably at the age of puberty in three groups of intersex patients with a Y chromosome: those with gonadal dysgenesis, asymmetric gonadal differentiation, and male hermaphroditism. It has thus been recommended that the gonads are best removed from these patients by the age of puberty.[99] In testicular feminization patients, on the other hand, delay in removing the gonads may be considered until approximately the age of 30 years, by which time the patient has spontaneously become feminized (provided that one is prepared to assume a 4 per cent risk of malignancy developing prior to age 30).[99]

Stromal Tumors

When gonadal tumors contain stromal elements they have the potential of producing hormones and exerting either feminizing or masculinizing effects. These tumors are not as common as the germ cell tumors, nor are they as malignant.

Granulosa-theca tumors are associated with feminizing effects due to the production of estrogen. These are most easily seen in the prepubertal years, when the tumor gives rise to precocious puberty with enlargement of the breasts, hemorrhagic vaginal discharge, and appearance of pubic hair; there may also be precocious body growth and osseous development.

Occasionally these tumors may be associated with ascites and hydrothorax (*Meigs' syndrome*) of a nonmalignant nature. Such manifestations should not be confused with metastases, nor should the tumor be considered inoperable.

The tumor may be bilateral in 10 per cent of cases.[91] Malignancy, which occurs in about 3 per cent of these tumors in children, is of low grade and spread is typically confined to the pelvis;[68, 69] however, recurrences beyond 5 years and as late as 15 to 20 years after resection are not uncommon. Conservative surgery (unilateral oophorectomy) is indicated when the tumor is unilateral and encapsulated;[68, 69, 117] hysterectomy and bilateral salpingo-oophorectomy with postoperative radiotherapy may be used when the tumor has spread beyond the ovary to pelvic structures.[69]

Arrhenoblastoma (Sertoli-Leydig cell tumor) may produce virilizing effects. However, many are nonfunctioning or have estrogenic effects. These tumors are rarely seen in childhood. Although this tumor bears a remarkable histologic similarity to the embryonic testis,[91] it appears to be derived directly from the ovarian stroma and to represent a mixed mesodermal tumor containing Müllerian epithelial and testicular derivatives.[90] The differential diagnosis in a female with virilization also includes adrenal hyperplasia and adrenal tumors.

Arrhenoblastomas have varying degrees of malignancy; spread is usually locally within the pelvis rather than to distant organs. Unilateral oophorectomy may be utilized if the tumor is unilateral and encapsulated.[69] However, because there is poor correlation between tumor histology and the clinical course, and because of the natural history of late recurrences, Barber has recommended total hysterectomy and bilateral salpingo-oophorectomy after the patient has completed her family.[69]

Gynandroblastoma is a gonadal stromal tumor containing a unique combination of feminizing (granulosa cells) and masculinizing (Sertoli cells, Leydig cells) elements.[66] It is thought to arise from the indifferent gonadal mesenchyme which possesses the ability to manifest bisexual potentialities. Because its constituent elements are well differentiated, its malignant potential is considered to be low; among the cases reviewed by Anderson and Reese, only one death from this tumor was found.[66]

TUMORS OF THE CERVIX, VAGINA, AND UTERUS

Rhabdomyosarcoma (sarcoma botryoides) is the only malignant tumor

TUMORS OF THE SEXUAL ORGANS

of the lower genital tract that occurs in young girls with any degree of frequency. However, all of the common types of genital tumors (and most of the unusual ones) occurring in adult women have been found in girls under 16 years of age.

Malignancy of the lower genital tract should be suspected in any child who has (1) a chronic sore, ulcer, or persistent nodule of any type on the vulva, (2) a mass protruding through the vagina, or (3) a watery, serosanguinous, purulent, or grossly bloody vaginal discharge. With the exception of a newborn baby (in whom bleeding may occur because placental hormones have been withdrawn), a neoplasm of the genitalia must be considered whenever a child less than 9 years of age has a bloody vaginal discharge or an adolescent has irregular bleeding. Other causes of vaginal discharge or bleeding in children include foreign bodies within the vagina, prolapse of the urethra, and isosexual precocity due either to constitutional factors, an intracranial lesion, or a hormone-producing ovarian tumor.

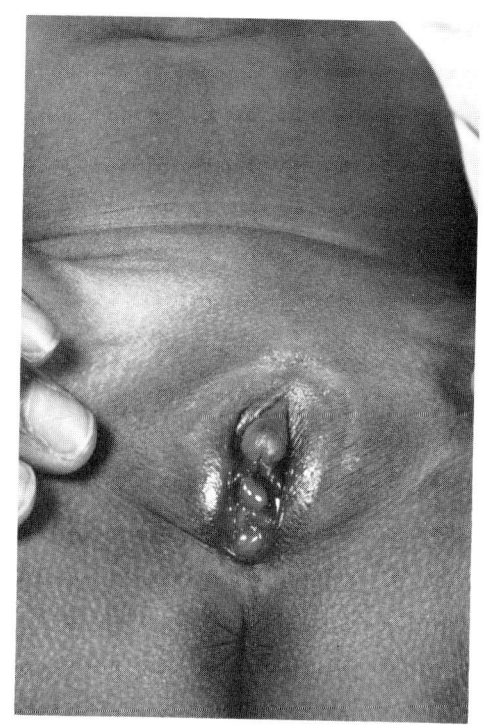

Figure 19-11 Rhabdomyosarcoma of vagina. The tumor protrudes like a "cluster of grapes" (sarcoma botryoides) through the introitus. (From Pinkel, D., and Pratt, C.: Embryonal rhabdomyosarcoma. *In* Holland, J. F., and Frei, E. III [Eds.]: Cancer Medicine. Philadelphia, Lea & Febiger, 1973.)

Rhabdomyosarcoma (Sarcoma Botryoides)

Rhabdomyosarcoma is the most common malignant tumor of the lower genital tract in children;[112] the histologic characteristics of this malignancy of striated muscle are described in Chapter Sixteen. The term sarcoma botryoides refers to the polypoid nature ("bunch of grapes") that embryonal rhabdomyosarcoma assumes when it grows within a hollow viscus.

Rhabdomyosarcoma may arise in the wall of the vagina, bladder, uterus, or cervix. Abnormal vaginal bleeding is the most common presenting complaint, although sometimes a polypoid mass lesion may actually protrude through the vaginal opening (Fig. 19-11). Spread occurs by direct infiltration of the vaginal wall and pelvic structures, by lymphatic spread to regional nodes, and by vascular routes to the lungs, bone marrow, and other distant sites.

Treatment involves a combined approach with surgery, radiation therapy, and chemotherapy (Chapter Sixteen). In the past, the surgical approach has tended to be very aggressive, entailing total pelvic exenteration, consisting of hystovaginectomy, oophorectomy, cystectomy, and occasional colon resection.[79, 112] However, the combination of high-dose irradiation and multiagent chemotherapy may permit modification of this mutilative approach and limit surgery to hystovaginectomy and oophorectomy.[94]

Carcinoma

Carcinoma has been reported, in rare instances, to involve the cervix[88, 89] and vagina[80, 85, 86, 87] in pediatric patients. When it does occur, the tumor is usually an adenocarcinoma rather than an epidermoid carcinoma. Because of its rarity in children, the diagnosis of carcinoma of the lower tract is frequently delayed for a considerable period of time after symptoms (purulent or watery vaginal discharge, genital bleeding) are noted.

Carcinoma of the cervix on gross examination appears as small growths protruding polyp-like from the cervix or as ulcerative lesions of the cervix. If the disease is far advanced, huge, fungating tumors filling the vagina and lower pelvis may be noted. This tumor usually spreads by direct extension to contiguous tissues and to nearby organs. It later spreads to the pelvic lymphatics.

Huffman,[89] after reviewing the accumulated case reports of pediatric cervical carcinoma, has suggested hysterectomy plus partial vaginectomy combined with excision of the paracervical and paravaginal connective tissues, and pelvic lymphadenectomy for early cervical carcinoma. More extensive growths require wider excision, including pelvic exenteration and total vaginectomy.

Two types of vaginal carcinoma have been described in childhood: endodermal sinus tumor and clear cell adenocarcinoma. These tumors differ in histology, age incidence, and location.

Endodermal sinus tumor of the vagina occurs mainly in infants, and few cases have been reported over the age of two years. This tumor is located in the posterior vaginal wall or the fornices. In the older literature it has been referred to as "mesonephric adenocarcinoma" or "mesonephroma"[65, 80] because of the presence of so-called "glomeruloid" structures. However, these probably are identical to the Schiller-Duval bodies seen in endodermal sinus (yolk sac) tumors of the ovary. In gross appearance some of these vaginal endodermal sinus tumors have a polypoid appearance and may simulate sarcoma botryoides. The prognosis of this tumor is poor; in the series of patients collated by Allyn and colleagues[65] and Norris and associates,[102] only 5 of 19 survived for 2 years or more.

Clear cell adenocarcinoma of the vagina occurs exclusively after the age of 2 years and is seen most frequently after menarche; its origin is thought to be from Müllerian epithelium.[86] It is most commonly located in the anterior or lateral vaginal wall. This form of adenocarcinoma appears with unusually high frequency in girls exposed prenatally before the eighteenth week of gestation to diethylstilbestrol (DES).[86, 87] DES apparently interferes with the delicately balanced interactions of Müllerian and urogenital sinus epithelium necessary for normal development of the lower female genital tract during embryogenesis.[118, 119, 120] As a result, remnants of Müllerian tissue persist beneath the squamous epithelium of the vagina and may become activated by endogenous estrogens during or after puberty; over 90 per cent of DES-associated vaginal cancers have occurred in patients 14 years of age or older.

Although it has been estimated that less than 0.1 per cent of the women at risk because of prenatal DES exposure will develop adenocarcinoma,[118] nearly all manifest some overt morphologic abnormality of the vagina or cervix. The spectrum of these abnormalities ranges from apparently inconsequential erosions about the lip of the cervix to extensive ridge- or foldlike deformities of the cervix or vagina. These lesions show the presence of nonglycogenated mucinous epithelium and benign muciparous glands instead of stratified squamous epithelium and fail to take up Schiller's iodine stain, a condition that has been called *adenosis*.

Although some patients present with abnormal vaginal bleeding or discharge, many have been asymptomatic.[86] Consequently, all females exposed to DES in utero should have screening office examinations after menarche or by the age of 14 years — this should include direct inspection of the vagina and cervix, palpation to determine the presence of submucosal lesions, cytologic sampling of the cervix and uterus, and biopsy of areas that appear red or fail to stain with Schiller's iodine solution.

Spread of disease along lymphatic pathways draining the vagina and cervix occurs early in the course; in one series, eight of 48 Stage I vaginal lesions and three of 17 Stage I cervical lesions had positive pelvic nodes.[119] Radical hysterectomy and pelvic lymphadenectomy have been recommended.[80, 110] Radiation therapy may also be useful.[111, 112, 113]

The prognosis for clear cell adenocarcinoma of the vagina is somewhat better than for endodermal sinus tumor. In Allyn and co-workers' series, eight of 17 patients were alive and without evidence of disease from 1 to 5 years after primary treatment.[65]

Breast Tumors

Breast enlargements are a common finding in infants, children, and adolescents; fortunately, however, most cases represent either normal variations in endocrine function or benign mass lesions, with malignant lesions rarely being found.[127, 137, 141, 142]

The most commonly encountered causes of breast enlargement in the infant and prepubertal female are: (1) neonatal enlargement due to transplacental hormonal stimulation, (2) premature thelarche, and (3) precocious puberty. Females with these conditions should not undergo breast biopsy, but should have careful neurologic and endocrinologic evaluation if other signs of precocious puberty are present. *Discrete mass lesions should be excised at any age, however, especially if they are hard.*[127, 144]

Discrete masses in the prepubertal or pubertal male also require excision even though malignancy is rarely found.[127] Diffuse hypertrophy of breast tissue (gynecomastia) in the prepubertal male should raise the suspicion of an underlying neurologic or endocrine problem, especially when it is bilateral. Gynecomastia in the pubertal male requires that attention be paid to evaluation of body habitus, testicular size, and buccal smear for sex chromatin examination.

DIFFUSE ENLARGEMENT OF THE BREAST

NEONATAL PERIOD

The breast of the newborn is composed of a nipple and areola overlying a bud of breast tissue containing the primary mammary ducts and a loose fibrous stroma; this bud, which is not palpable before 34 weeks, measures about 3 mm at 36 weeks and 4 to 10 mm at 40 weeks.[126] In approximately 60 per cent of normal neonates (both male and female), this bud may enlarge further to form a soft, uniform, subareolar mass (Fig. 19–12) not fixed to the chest wall, which frequently secretes a milk-like substance ("witch's milk"). Histologically, the mass consists of ductal hypertrophy and increase in vascular stroma.

Neonatal breast hypertrophy is thought to be a result of stimulation by

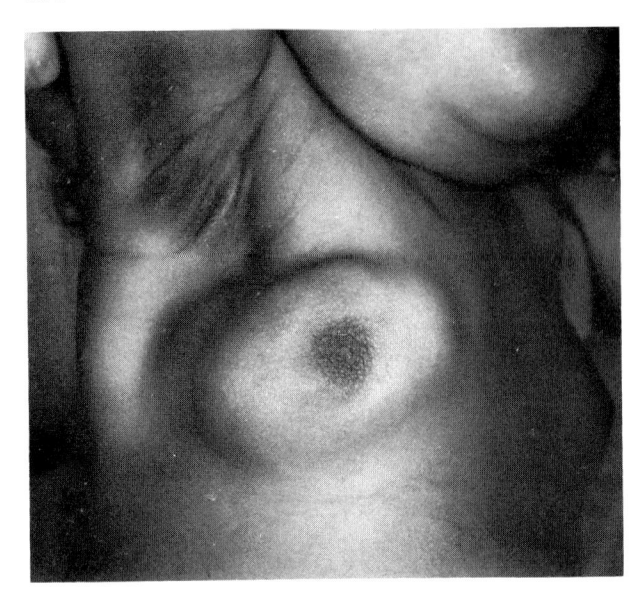

Figure 19-12 Neonate with marked hypertrophy of breast bud. (From Seashore, J. H.: Pediatr. Ann. 4:542, 1975.)

maternal hormones and, indeed, once the excessive hormonal stimulus is withdrawn, the swelling subsides (usually within a month after delivery if the infant is not breast-fed). These swellings should not be a cause for alarm, even when they are asymmetric, and no treatment other than reassurance is needed. Massage and other manipulations should be discouraged, since they may predispose to cellulitis or abscess formation.

PREPUBERTAL PERIOD

Nodular enlargement of one or both breasts may occur at any time during childhood, but is most common around the eighth year. The mass is usually subareolar, firm, and mobile, and may be slightly tender; it is composed of increased periductal fibrous tissue and slight duct hypertrophy. There are no measurable hormonal changes or clinical findings of generalized precocious sexual development.[132] Most of these lesions regress spontaneously within 6 to 12 months, but some may persist and grow slowly until puberty.[144, 149]

In some prepubertal girls, well-developed breasts may appear as early as 8 or 9 years of age; since breast development is usually asynchronous, one side may occasionally be well developed before the other has even begun to mature. This should not necessarily give rise to concern since breast development beginning after 8 years of age is considered within the normal range of puberty and, by the end of puberty, virtually all of these girls have normally developed, symmetrical breasts.[144]

Premature thelarche is defined as the growth of normal breast tissue before the age of 8 years in the absence of other signs of sexual maturation. A wrist film for bone age may be useful in distinguishing this condition from precocious puberty, where bone age advancement is present. This is a relatively common clinical problem which does not require extensive evaluation other than continued observation for other signs of precocious puberty.

Precocious puberty refers to generalized sexual development in girls under 8 years of age. Although breast growth is commonly the first manifestation, it is soon followed by pigmentation of the areola, growth and pigmentation of the labia and clitoris, appearance of pubic and axillary hair, and menstruation. In pseudoprecocious puberty (usually associated with ovarian and adrenal tumors), the gonads remain immature or develop only partially whereas true precocious puberty is associated with gonadal maturation, ovulation, and the possibility of pregnancy; this occurs most commonly on an idiopathic basis, but may also be seen in McCune-Albright's syndrome (polyostotic fibrous dysplasia of bone) and certain intracranial lesions.

Prepubertal breast enlargement is less common in males than in females, but a greater percentage of males with this abnormality will be found to have underlying endocrine, neurologic, or other abnormalities. Among the conditions which may produce this are true sexual abnormalities (hermaphroditism, Klinefelter's syndrome), adrenal, testicular, and hepatic tumors, thyroid disease, and exogenous hormones or drugs.

PUBERTY

Juvenile (Virginal) Hypertrophy

This is characterized by normal onset of breast development at puberty, followed by massive bilateral diffuse growth of the breasts over the next few years. The histology is essentially an exaggeration of the normally developing adolescent female breast and suggests a marked hypersensitivity of breast tissue to the hormonal stimuli of puberty.[129, 130, 144] Endocrine studies yield normal results. There may be some regression of the hypertrophy towards the end of adolescence.

Gynecomastia

Gynecomastia is the hypertrophy of mammary tissue in the male; it is the histologic analogue of juvenile hypertrophy in the female and is characterized by proliferation of ductal tissue and an increase in connective tissue (Fig. 19–13). It is important medically for two main reasons: (1) a mistaken diagnosis of cancer of the male breast may be made, and (2) it may be the result of some other systemic symptom complex, such as endocrine imbalance, liver disease, testicular abnormalities and tumors, or adrenal tumors.

At least 70 per cent of normal adolescent boys have palpable breast tissue; usually this is limited to 1 to 2 cm in size, appearing at about the age of 13 years, and disappearing by 18 to 21 years of age.[135, 144] Breast enlargement of a greater degree is considered gynecomastia (Fig. 19–14).

In most cases, gynecomastia occurs predominantly during puberty and ad-

Figure 19–13 Gynecomastia. Photomicrograph shows proliferation and increased branching of ducts without lobule formation, as well as marked hypertrophy of periductal fibrous tissue. (From Seashore, J. H.: Pediatr. Ann. 4:542, 1975.)

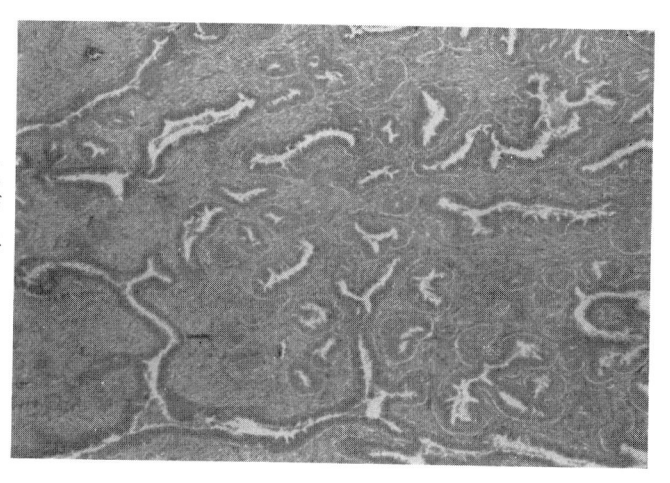

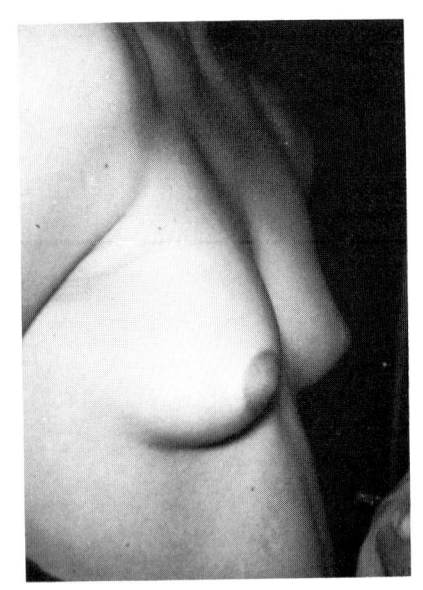

Figure 19-14 Extreme gynecomastia in a teenage boy. (From Seashore, J. H.: Pediatr. Ann. 4:542, 1975.)

olescence. When it is idiopathic and self-limited the hypertrophy is usually centrally located in the breast and predominantly unilateral. Any disease process that seriously affects the testis can lead to a hormonal imbalance sufficient to cause gynecomastia; thus, it is seen in mumps orchitis, cryptorchidism, testicular hypoplasia, and nearly every type of testicular neoplasm. Gynecomastia has also been found in association with a number of other diseases, including adrenal neoplasms, tumors of the pituitary, thyroid disease, liver disease, and endocrine imbalance.

Gynecomastia can be distinguished from cancer of the male breast by its location and other physical characteristics. In gynecomastia, the mass appears as a concentric ring of hypertrophied mammary tissue beneath or around the areola, whereas in cancer of the male breast the lesion is usually eccentric.[145] In gynecomastia the mass is rarely firm on palpation but is usually soft or moderately elastic, whereas cancer of the male breast is hard or firmly resistant to the touch. Nipple abnormalities, especially retraction and encrustation, are rare in gynecomastia and frequent in cancer. Bloody discharge from the nipple is more likely to be associated with breast cancer, since only about 1 per cent of those with gynecomastia show this finding. Thus, cancer must be ruled out whenever a patient has an eccentric, firm, localized breast lesion, a nipple discharge, or a retracted or encrusted nipple.

Antecedent or concurrent gynecomastia in males with breast cancer has been reported in from 0 to 20 per cent of cases.[138] Patients with Klinefelter's syndrome are particularly susceptible to the combination of gynecomastia and breast cancer. Patients with this syndrome are known to have altered hormonal metabolism, with decreased testosterone levels and an increased incidence of gynecomastia; they also have a 20 to 67 times greater incidence of breast cancer.

DISCRETE BREAST MASSES

NON-NEOPLASTIC

Inflammatory lesions. Cellulitis or abscess formation of the breast is usually of acute onset and accompanied by swelling, tenderness, erythema, heat, and (in the case of abscess) fluctuation. Inflammatory lesions of the breast in childhood are seen most commonly at times of unusual hormonal activity — the neonatal period and adolescence — reflecting the role of hormonal stimulation in their genesis.

Solitary cysts. These may appear at any age; they tend to be small, firm, or obviously cystic. They may be asymptomatic or tender and may exude a watery, milky, brownish, or even frankly bloody discharge.

Fibrocystic disease. Fibrocystic disease (cystic mastitis) is not as frequently seen in adolescent girls as it is in young adult women. It is never seen in males or prepubertal females. Clinically it is characterized by diffuse bilateral lumpiness, cordlike thickenings, distinct enlarged cystic areas, and pain and tenderness, which increase before each menses. Physical findings fluctuate from month to month as a result of enlargement or collapse of cysts.

NEOPLASTIC

Benign Tumors

Fibroadenoma is the most common discrete breast mass of adolescence, occurring more frequently than all other breast masses combined;[144] it has rarely been reported in girls a year or two before the onset of puberty, but is then seen with increasing frequency throughout the teenage years. The lesion is usually detected accidentally as a nontender, firm, freely mobile mass. Histologically it appears as a compact, encapsulated proliferation of periductal and perilobular fibrous tissue and of branching ducts. These tumors are benign and can be treated by simple excision;[144, 149] if lesions are bilateral, multiple, and recurrent (fibroadenomatosis), careful observation with removal of only those tumors that are growing rapidly has been recommended.[144]

Cystosarcoma Phyllodes. This tumor is similar to fibroadenoma, but has greater hypertrophy and more marked cellularity of the fibrous tissue stroma.[146] The term "sarcoma" in this regard refers to the fleshy appearance of the tumor and does not necessarily imply malignancy, although malignancy can occasionally develop in the connective tissue elements. Cystosarcoma phyllodes tends to be benign in over 80 per cent of adolescent girls;[124, 131, 134] by contrast, 23 to 27 per cent of the overall population of patients with cystosarcoma phyllodes will have histologically malignant tumors, and 6.6 to 37.5 per cent of these will develop metastases.[136]

Cystosarcoma phyllodes can grow very rapidly and should be treated by wide local excision, including a generous margin of normal breast tissue, to prevent local recurrence.[124, 144] If malignancy is present, simple mastectomy has been recommended as preferable to radical mastectomy since the malignant elements are sarcomatous and tend to metastasize mainly to the lungs and skeleton by hematogenous rather than by lymphatic dissemination.[136, 139, 144]

Other Benign Tumors. These include fibroma, lipoma, papilloma, hemangioma, lymphangioma, and intraductal papilloma. Granular cell myoblastoma is a benign tumor of neural origin which characteristically appears as a rock-hard, irregular soft-tissue mass whose unusual histologic appearance on frozen section may lead to an erroneous diagnosis of malignancy and an unnecessary mastectomy.[144, 147] The lesion should be treated by wide local excision and diagnosis should be deferred until permanent sections can be reviewed.[144]

Malignant Tumors

Malignant breast lesions occur very rarely in childhood or adolescence; they account for less than 1 per cent of cancers of childhood[148] and less than 0.1 per cent of all breast cancer cases.[137] In most cases the main finding was a painless, hard nodule almost always found near (although discrete from) the nipple.[137, 142]

Adenocarcinoma. Most of these lesions have a histologic pattern and clinical course similar to that of adult breast cancer. However, McDivitt and Stewart[137] have described a group of patients whose tumors could be discriminated morphologically from cancer of the mature breast by virtue of the presence of homogeneous eosinophilic, PAS-positive, secretory material within the cytoplasm of individual tumor cells and in rudimentary duct-like spaces formed by the tumor; these patients appear to run a relatively indolent course and have an excellent prognosis.[137, 141] In Seashore's collation of 33 cases,[144] survival also appeared to be closely related to age — 92 per cent of children under the age of 12 years survived, while only 36 per cent of teenagers lived.

Several recent reviews have recommended prompt excisional biopsy as the initial approach to a discrete mass lesion if it is hard or in the developed breast of an adolescent female.[127, 144] The diagnosis of carcinoma should be made and further therapy instituted only after examination of permanent histologic sections, preferably by several pathologists. Seashore[144] has recommended simple mastectomy as the procedure of choice for most patients, but has also suggested that no therapy other than generous excisional biopsy might be necessary for prepubertal patients and patients with the pattern of prominent eosinophilic secretory material. Radiation therapy might also be considered in older children and for those who refuse mastectomy.

Sarcoma. Primary sarcomas of the breast occur even less frequently than adenocarcinomas; fibrosarcoma and liposarcoma are the most common types. Rhabdomyosarcoma may occur as a metastatic lesion or a primary lesion.[128]

REFERENCES

Testicular Tumors

1. Abell, M. R., and Holtz, F.: Testicular neoplasms in infants and children. I. Tumors of germ cell origin. Cancer 16:965, 1963.
2. Allen, J. E.: Teratomas in infants and children. In Holland, J. F., and Frei, E., III (eds.): Cancer Medicine. Philadelphia, Lea & Febiger, 1973.
3. Arlen, M., Grabstald, H., Whitmore, W. F., Jr.: Malignant tumors of the spermatic cord. Cancer 23:525, 1969.
3a. Bachmann, K. D., and von Grawert, H.: Tumoren des hodens in Kindesalter. Monatsschr. Kinderheilk. 120:40, 1972.
4. Banowsky, L. H., and Shultz, G. N.: Sarcoma of the spermatic cord and tunics: review of the literature, case report and discussion of the role of retroperitoneal lymph node dissection. J. Urol. 103:628, 1970.
5. Burrington, J. D.: Rhabdomyosarcoma of the paratesticular tissues in children. Report of eight cases. J. Pediatr. Surg. 4:503, 1969.
6. Campbell, H. E.: The incidence of malignant growth of the undescended testicle: a reply and re-evaluation. J. Urol. 81:663, 1959.
7. Dixon, F. J., and Moore, R. A.: Tumors of the male sex organs. In Atlas of Tumor Pathology. Section VIII. Washington, D.C., Armed Forces Institute of Pathology, 1952.
8. Donaldson, M. H., Duckett, J. W., and Mulholland, S. G.: Malignant genitourinary tumors. In Sutow, W. W., Vietti, T. J., Fernbach, D. J. (eds.): Clinical Pediatric Oncology. St. Louis, C. V. Mosby Co., 1973.
9. Duckett, J. W., Jr, Cromie, W. B., and Bongiovanni, A. M.: Genitourinary tumors in children. Semin. Oncol. 1:71, 1974.
10. DuPriest, R. W., Jr., and Fletcher, W. S.: Chemotherapy of testicular germinal tumors. Oncology 28:147, 1973.
10a. Einhorn, L. H., and Donohue, J.: Cis-diaminedichloroplatinum, Vinblastine, bleomycin combination chemotherapy in disseminated testicular cancer. Ann. Intern. Med. 87:293, 1977.
11. Erickson, R. P., and Gondos, B.: Alternative explanations of the differing behavior of ovarian and testicular teratomas. Lancet 1:407, 1976.
12. Ewing, J.: Teratoma testis and its derivatives. Surg. Gynec. Obstet. 12:230, 1911.
13. Fonkalsrud, E. W.: Current concepts in the management of the undescended testis. Surg. Clin. N. Amer. 50:847, 1970.
14. Fraley, E. E., and Ketcham, A. S.: Teratoma of testis in an infant. J. Urol. 100:659, 1968.
15. Gallager, H. S.: Pathology of testicular and paratesticular neoplasms. In Johnson, D. E. (ed.): Testicular Tumors. 2nd Ed. Flushing, N.Y., Medical Examination Publishing Co., 1976.
16. Gangai, M. P.: Testicular neoplasms in an infant. Cancer 22:658, 1968.
17. Gilbert, J. B., and Hamilton, J. B.: Studies in malignant testis tumors: incidence and nature of tumors in ectopic testes. Surg. Gynec. Obstet. 71:731, 1940.
18. Grabstald, H.: Germinal tumors of the testis. CA 25:82, 1975.
19. Hausfeld, K. F., Schrandt, D.: Malignancy of the testis following atrophy. J. Urol. 94:69, 1965.

20. Hays, D. M., Mirabal, V. Q., Patel, H. R., Jr., et al.: Rhabdomyosarcoma of the spermatic cord. Surgery 65:845, 1969.
21. Hogan, J. M., and Johnson, D. E.: Etiology of testicular tumors. *In* Johnson, D. E. (ed.): Testicular Tumors. 2nd Ed. Flushing, N.Y., Medical Examination Publishing Co., 1976.
22. Holtz, F., and Abell, M. R.: Testicular neoplasms in infants and children. II. Tumors of nongerm cell origin. Cancer 16:982, 1963.
23. Houser, R., Izant, R. J., and Persky, L.: Testicular tumors in children. Amer. J. Surg. 100:876, 1965.
24. Huntington, R. W., Jr., Morgenstern, N. L., Sargent, J. A., et al.: Germinal tumors exhibiting the endodermal sinus pattern of Teilum in young children. Cancer 16:34, 1963.
25. Ise, T., Ohtsuki, H., Matsumoto, K., and Sano, R.: Management of malignant testicular tumors in children. Cancer 37:1539, 1976.
25a. Jeffs, R. D.: Management of embryonal adenocarcinoma of the testis in childhood: an analysis of 164 cases. *In* Gooden, J. A. (ed.): Cancer in Childhood. Toronto, The Ontario Cancer Treatment and Research Foundation, 1972.
26. Johnson, D. E. (ed.): Testicular Tumors. 2nd Ed. Flushing, N.Y., Medical Examination Publishing Co., 1976.
27. Johnson, D. E., Kuhn, C. R., and Guinn, G. A.: Testicular tumors in children. J. Urol. 104:940, 1970.
28. Johnson, D. E., Woodhead, D. M., Pohl, D. R., and Robison, J. R.: Cryptorchism and testicular tumorigenesis. Surgery 63:919, 1968.
29. Karamehmedovic, O., Woodtli, W., Plüss, H. J.: Testicular tumors in childhood. J. Pediatr. Surg. 10:109, 1975.
30. Kilman, J. W., Clatworthy, H. W., Jr., Newton, W. A., Jr., and Grosfeld, J. L.: Reasonable surgery for rhabdomyosarcoma. Ann. Surg. 178:346, 1973.
31. Lange, P. H., McIntire, K. R., Waldmann, T. A., et al.: Serum alpha fetoprotein and human chorionic gonadotropin in the diagnosis and management of nonseminomatous germ-cell testicular cancer. N. Engl. J. Med. 295:1237, 1976.
32. Laskowski, J.: Feminizing tumors of testis, general review with case report of granulosa cell tumor of testis. Endokrynol. Pol. 3:337, 1952.
33. Magner, D.: Pathology of tumors of the testis in children. *In* Gooden, J. A. (ed.): Cancer in Childhood. Toronto, The Ontario Cancer Treatment and Research Foundation, 1972.
34. Magner, D., Campbell, J. S., and Wiglesworth, F. W.: Testicular adenocarcinoma with clear cells occurring in infancy: a distinctive tumor. Can. Med. Assoc. J. 86:485, 1862.
35. Maier, J. G., and Van Buskirk, K.: Treatment of testicular germ cell malignancies. J.A.M.A. 213:97, 1970.
36. Manuel, M., Katayama, K. P., and Jones, H. W., Jr.: The age of occurrence of gonadal tumors in intersex patients with a Y chromosome. Am. J. Obstet. Gynec. 124:293, 1976.
37. McCullough, D. L., Carlton, C. E., and Seybold, H. M.: Testicular tumors in infants and children. Report of 5 cases and evaluation of different modes of therapy. J. Urol. 105:140, 1971.
38. Mostofi, F. K., Theiss, E. A., and Ashley, D. J. B.: Tumors of specialized gonadal stroma in human male patients; androblastoma, sertoli cell tumor, granulosatheca cell tumor of the testis, and gonadal stromal tumor. Cancer 12:944, 1966.
39. Mulvihill, J. J., Wade, W. M., and Miller, R. M.: Gonadoblastoma in dysgenetic gonads with a Y chromosome. Lancet 1:863, 1975.
40. Podis, A. D.: Malignant testis tumors of infancy. Southern Med. J. 59:1415, 1966.
41. Pomer, F. A., Stiles, R. E., and Graham, J. H.: Interstitial cell tumors of the testis in children. Report of a case and review of the literature. N. Engl. J. Med. 250:233, 1954.
42. Prout, G. R., Jr.: Germinal tumors of the testis. *In* Holland, J. F., and Frei, E., III: Cancer Medicine. Philadelphia, Lea & Febiger, 1973.
43. Rivard, G. E., Ortega, J., Hittle, R., et al.: Intensive chemotherapy as primary treatment for rhabdomyosarcoma of the pelvis. Cancer 36:1593, 1975.
44. Robson, C. J., Bruce, A. W., and Charbonneau, J.: Testicular tumors. J. Urol. 94:440, 1965.
45. Rosas-Uribe, A., Luna, M. A., and Guinn, G. A.: Paratesticular rhabdomyosarcoma: a clinicopathologic study of seven cases. Am. J. Surg. 120:787, 1970.
46. Sabio, H., Burgert, E. O., Jr., Farrow, G. M., and Kelalis, P. P.: Embryonal carcinoma of the testis in childhood. Cancer 34:2118, 1974.
47. Samuels, M. L., Lanzotti, V. J., Holoye, P. Y., et al.: Combination chemotherapy in germinal cell tumors. Cancer Treatment Rev. 3:185, 1976.
48. Satter, E. J., Heidner, F. C., II, and Wear, J. B.: Primary sarcoma of the spermatic cord and epididymis. J. Urol. 82:148, 1959.
49. Scully, R. E.: Gonadoblastoma, a review of 74 cases. Cancer 25:1340, 1970.
50. Staubitz, W. J., Magross, I. V., Grace, J. T., and Schenk, W. G., III: Surgical man-

agement of testis tumors. J. Urol. *101*: 350, 1969.
51. Sulak, M. H.: Cancer of the urogenital tract: testicular tumors. Classification of different pathologic types. *In*: Rubin, P. (ed.): Current Concepts in Cancer. Chicago, American Medical Association, 1974.
52. Tefft, M., Vawter, G. F., and Mitus, A.: Radiotherapeutic management of testicular neoplasms in children. Radiology *88*:457, 1967.
53. Teilum, G.: Classification of testicular and ovarian androblastoma and Sertoli cell tumors; survey of comparative studies with consideration of histogenesis, endocrinology and embryological theories. Cancer *11*:769, 1958.
54. Teilum, G.: Endodermal sinus tumor of the ovary and testis. Cancer *12*:1092, 1959.
55. Teoh, T. B., Steward, J. K., and Willis, R. A.: The distinctive adenocarcinoma of the infant's testis; an account of 15 cases. J. Pathol. Bacteriol. *80*:147, 1960.
55a. Viprakasit, D., Navarro, C., Guarin, U. K., and Garnes, H. A.: Seminoma in children. Urology *9*:568, 1977.
56. Weissman, M. J., Gaeta, J. F., and Albert, D. J.: Childhood urogenital sarcoma. J. Surg. Oncol. *4*:100, 1972.
57. Williams, G., and Banerjee, R.: Paratesticular tumors. Brit. J. Urol. *41*:332, 1969.
58. Wilson, J. M., and Woodhead, D. M.: Prognostic and therapeutic implications of urinary gonadotropin levels in the management of testicular neoplasia. J. Urol. *108*:754, 1972.
59. Wittes, R. E., Yagoda, A., and Silvey, O.: Chemotherapy of germ cell tumors of the testis. Induction of remissions with vinblastine, actinomycin-D, and bleomycin. Cancer *37*:637, 1976.
60. Wöckel, W., and Unger, R.: Zum Problem der bösartigen Geschwülste des Sauglings- und Kindesalters. Dtsch. Med. Wochenschr. *94*:1080, 1969.
61. Young, P. G., Mount, B. M., Foote, F. W., Jr., and Whitmore, F. W., Jr.: Embryonal adenocarcinoma in the prepubertal testis. A clinicopathologic study of 18 cases. Cancer *26*:1065, 1970.

Tumors of the Female Genital Tract

62. Abell, M. R., Johnson, V. J., and Holtz, F.: Ovarian neoplasms in childhood and adolescence. I. Tumors of germ cell origin. Am. J. Obstet. Gynec. *92*:1059, 1965.
63. Acosta, A., Kaplan, A. L., and Kaufman, R. H.: Gynecologic cancer in children. Am. J. Obstet. Gynec. *112*:944, 1972.
64. Allen, J. E.: Teratomas in infants and children. *In* Holland, J. F., and Frei, E., III (eds.): Cancer Medicine. Philadelphia, Lea & Febiger, 1973.
65. Allyn, D. L., Silverberg, S. G., and Salzberg, A. M.: Endodermal sinus tumor of the vagina. Report of a case with seven-year survival and literature review of so-called "mesonephroma." Cancer *27*:1231, 1971.
66. Anderson, M. C., and Rees, D. A.: Gynandroblastoma of the ovary. Brit. J. Obstet. Gynec. *82*:68, 1975.
67. Asadourian, L. A., and Taylor, H. B.: Dysgerminoma: an analysis of 105 cases. Obstet. Gynec. *33*:370, 1969.
68. Barber, H. R. K.: Ovarian cancer in children—guide for a difficult decision. CA *23*:334, 1975.
69. Barber, H. R. K., and Kwon, R. H.: Current status of the treatment of gynecologic cancer by site: ovary. Cancer *38*:610, 1976.
70. Bernstein, P.: Tumors of ovary: study of 1101 cases of operations for ovarian tumor. Am. J. Obstet. Gynec. *32*:1023, 1936.
71. Bronsther, B., and Abrams, M. W.: Ovarian tumors in childhood. Pediatr. Ann. *4*:565, 1975
72. Cham, W. C., Wollner, N., Exelby, P., et al.: Patterns of extension as a guide to radiation therapy in the management of ovarian neoplasms in children. Cancer *37*:1443, 1976.
73. Dehner, L. P.: Female reproductive system. *In* Kissane, J. M. (ed.): Pathology of Infancy and Childhood. 2nd Ed. St. Louis, C. V. Mosby Co., 1975.
74. Dempster, K. R., Pinninger, J. L., Rickford, R. B. K.: Malignant ovarian teratoma with complex extra-ovarian deposits. J. Obstet. Gynaec. Brit. Emp. *63*:589, 1956.
75. DiZerega, G., Acosta, A. A., Kaufman, R. H., and Kaplan, A. L.: Solid teratoma of the ovary. Gynec. Oncol. *3*:93, 1975.
76. Ein, S. H.: Malignant ovarian tumors in children. J. Pediatr. Surg. *8*:539, 1973.
77. Einsel, I. H., Bowman, R. E., and Koletsky, S.: Unusual malignant ovarian tumor in a young child. Am. J. Dis. Child. *86*:568, 1953.
78. Erickson, R. P., and Gondos, B.: Alternative explanations of the differing behavior of ovarian and testicular teratomas. Lancet *1*:407, 1976.
79. Exelby, P. R.: Management of embryonal rhabdomyosarcoma in children. Surg. Clin. North Am. *54*:849, 1974.
80. Fawcett, K. J., Dockerty, M. B., and Hunt, A. B.: Mesonephric carcinoma and adenocarcinoma of the cervix in children. J. Pediatr. *69*:104, 1966.
81. Geist, S. H.: Ovarian Tumors. New York, Paul B. Hoeber, 1942.

82. Green, G. H.: Solid malignant teratomas of the ovary. Am. J. Obstet. Gynec. 79:999, 1960.
83. Groeber, W. R.: Ovarian tumors during infancy and childhood. Am. J. Obstet. Gynec. 86:1027, 1963.
84. Helmke, K.: Gliomatose des Bauchfells bei Teratoma ovarii. Virchows. Arch. 302:509, 1938.
85. Herbst, A. L., and Scully, R. E.: Adenocarcinoma of the vagina in adolescence. Cancer 25:745, 1970.
86. Herbst, A. L., Scully, R. E., and Robboy, S. J.: Effects of maternal DES ingestion on the female genital tract. Hosp. Pract. 10:51, 1975.
87. Herbst, A. L., Ulfelder, H., and Poskanzer, D. C.. Adenocarcinoma of the vagina: Association of maternal stilbestrol therapy with tumor appearance in young women. N. Engl. J. Med. 284:878, 1971.
88. Huffman, J. W.: The Gynecology of Childhood and Adolescence. Philadelphia, W. B. Saunders Co., 1966.
89. Huffman, J. W.: Tumors of the genitalia. Clin. Obstet. Gynec. 1:663, 1974.
90. Hughesdon, P. E., and Fraser, I. T.: Arrhenoblastoma of the ovary. Acta Obstet. Gynec. Scand. 32(Suppl. 4):1, 1953.
91. Janovski, N. A., and Paramanandhan, T. L.: Ovarian Tumors. Philadelphia, W. B. Saunders Co., 1973.
92. Kelly, J. A.: Gynecologic cancer in children. J. Pediatr. 15:354, 1939.
93. Kosloske, A. M., Favura, B. E., Hays, T., et al.: Management of immature teratoma of the ovary in children by conservative resection and chemotherapy. J. Pediatr. Surg. 11:839, 1976.
94. Kumar, A. P. M., Wrenn, E. L., Jr., Fleming, I. D., et al.: Combined therapy to prevent complete pelvic exenteration for rhabdomyosarcoma of the vagina or uterus. Cancer 37:118, 1976.
95. Kurman, R. J., and Norris, H. J.: Endodermal sinus tumor of the ovary. A clinical and pathologic analysis of 71 cases. Cancer 38:2404, 1976.
96. Kurman, R. J., and Norris, H. J.: Embryonal carcinoma of the ovary. A clinicopathologic entity distinct from endodermal sinus tumor resembling embryonal carcinoma of the adult testis. Cancer 38:2420, 1976.
97. Kurman, R. J., and Norris, H. J.: Malignant mixed germ cell tumors of the ovary. A clinical and pathological analysis of 30 cases. Obstet. Gynec. 48:579, 1976.
97a. Kurman, R. J., and Norris, H. J.: Malignant germ cell tumors of the ovary. Hum. Pathol. 8:551, 1977.
98. Lisa, J. R., Hinton, J. W., Wimpfheimer, S., and Gioia, J. D.: Malignant ovarian teratomas in the first two decades of life. Am. J. Surg. 81:453, 1951.
99. Manuel, M., Katayama, K. P., and Jones, H. W., Jr.: The age of occurrence of gonadal tumors in intersex patients with a Y chromosome. Am. J. Obstet. Gynec. 124:293, 1976.
100. Meleka, F., and Rasla, S.: Variation of spread of ovarian malignancy according to site of origin. Gynec. Oncol. 3:108, 1975.
101. Nielsen, O. V.: Ovarian tumors in children. Acta Obstet. Gynec. Scand. 47:119, 1968.
102. Norris, H. J., Bagley, G. P., and Taylor, H. B.: Carcinoma of the infant vagina. A distinctive tumor. Arch. Pathol. 90:473, 1970.
102a. Norris, H. J., and Jensen, R. D.: Relative frequency of ovarian neoplasms in children and adolescents. Cancer 30:713, 1972.
103. Norris, H. J., Zirkin, H. J., and Benson, W. L.: Immature (malignant) teratoma of the ovary. A clinical and pathologic study of 58 cases. Cancer 37:2359, 1976.
104. Orr, P. S., Gibson, A., and Young, D. G.: Ovarian tumours in childhood: a 27-year review. Brit. J. Surg. 63:367, 1976.
105. Peterson, W. F.: Solid, histologically benign teratomas of the ovary. Am. J. Obstet. Gynec. 72:1094, 1956.
106. Robboy, S. J., and Scully, R. E.: Ovarian teratoma with glial implants on the peritoneum. Hum. Pathol. 1:643, 1970.
107. Scully, R. E.: Gonadoblastoma. A gonadal tumor related to dysgerminoma (seminoma) and capable of sex-hormone production. Cancer 6:455, 1953.
108. Scully, R. E.: Gonadoblastoma. Cancer 25:1340, 1970.
109. Siegel, H. A., Sagerman, R., Berdon, W. E., and Wigger, H. J.: Mesonephric adenocarcinoma of the vagina in a 7-month-old infant simulating sarcoma botryoides. Successful control with supervoltage radiotherapy. J. Pediatr. Surg. 5:468, 1970.
110. Smith, F. R.: Primary carcinoma of the vagina. Am. J. Obstet. Gynec. 69:525, 1955.
111. Smith, J. P., and Rutledge, F.: Malignant gynecologic tumors. In Sutow, W. W., Vietti, R. J., Fernbach, D. J. (eds.): Clinical Pediatric Oncology. St. Louis, C. V. Mosby Co., 1973.
112. Smith, J. P., Rutledge, F., and Sutow, W. W.: Malignant gynecologic tumors in children: current approaches to treatment. Am. J. Obstet. Gynec. 116:261, 1973.
113. Smith, J. P., and Rutledge, F.: Advances in chemotherapy for gynecologic cancer. Cancer 36:669, 1975.
113a. Sternberg, W. H., and Dhurandhar, H. N.: Functional ovarian tumors of stromal and sex cord origin. Hum. Pathol. 8:565, 1977.
114. Sulak, M. H.: Cancer of the urogenital tract:

testicular tumors. Classification of different pathologic types. *In* Rubin, P. (ed.): Current Concepts in Cancer. Chicago, American Medical Association, 1974.

115. Teter, J.: A new concept of classification of gonadal tumours arising from germ cells (gonocytoma) and their histogenesis. Gynaecologia (Basel) *150*:84, 1960.

116. Thurlbeck, W. M., and Scully, R. E.: Solid teratoma of the ovary: a clinicopathologic analysis of nine cases. Cancer *13*:804, 1960.

117. Towne, B. H., Mahour, G. H., Woolley, M. M., and Isaacs, H., Jr.: Ovarian cysts and tumors in infancy and childhood. J. Pediatr. Surg. *10*:311, 1975.

118. Ulfelder, H.: Stilbestrol, adenosis, and adenocarcinoma. Am. J. Obstet. Gynec. *117*:794, 1973.

119. Ulfelder, H.: The stilbestrol-adenosis-carcinoma syndrome. Cancer *38*:426, 1976.

120. Ulfelder, H., and Robboy, S. J.: The embryologic development of the human vagina. Am. J. Obstet. Gynec. *126*:769, 1976.

121. Wollner, N., Exelby, P. R., Woodruff, J. M., et al.: Malignant ovarian tumors in childhood. Prognosis in relation to initial therapy. Cancer *37*:1953, 1976.

122. Woodruff, D. J., and Jimerson, G. K.: Ovarian teratomata. Progr. Clin. Cancer *5*:195, 1973.

Breast Tumors

123. Altchek, A.: Premature thelarche. Pediatr. Clin. North Am. *19*:543, 1972.

124. Amerson, J. R.: Cystosarcoma phyllodes in adolescent females. Ann. Surg. *171*:849, 1970.

125. August, G. P., Chandra, R., and Hung, W.: Prepubertal male gynecomastia. J. Pediatr. *80*:259, 1972.

126. Behrman, R. E.: The fetus and the newborn infant. *In* Vaughan, V. C., III, and McKay, R. J. (eds.): Nelson's Textbook of Pediatrics. 10th Ed. Philadelphia, W. B. Saunders Company, 1975.

127. Bower, R., Bell, M. J., and Ternberg, J. L.: Management of breast lesions in children and adolescents. J. Pediatr. Surg. *11*:337, 1976.

128. Farrow, J. H., and Ashikari, H.: Breast lesions in young girls. Surg. Clin. North Am. *49*:261, 1969.

129. Fisher, W., and Smith, J.: Macromastia during puberty. Plast. Reconstr. Surg. *47*:445, 1971.

130. Geschickter, C. F.: Diseases of the Breast. Philadelphia, J. B. Lippincott Co., 1943.

131. Gibbs, B. F., Doe, R. D., and Thomas, D. F.: Malignant cystosarcoma phyllodes in a prepubertal female. Ann. Surg. *167*:229, 1968.

132. Handelman, C. C.: The breasts. Pediatr. Clin. N. Amer. *8*:337, 1961.

133. Harrington, S. W.: Results of radical mastectomy in 5026 cases of carcinoma of the breast. Pa. Med. J. *43*:413, 1939.

134. Hoover, H. C., Trestioreanu, A., and Ketcham, A. S.: Metastatic cystosarcoma phyllodes in an adolescent girl: an unusually malignant tumor. Ann. Surg. *181*:279, 1975.

135. Jung, F. T., and Shafton, A. L.: Mastitis, mazoplasia, mastalgia and gynecomastia in normal adolescent males. Ill. Med. J. *73*:113, 1938.

136. Kessinger, A., Foley, J. F., Lemon, H. M., and Miller, D. M.: Metastatic cystosarcoma phyllodes: a case report and review of the literature. J. Surg. Oncol. *4*:131, 1972.

137. McDivitt, R. W., and Stewart, F. W.: Breast carcinoma in children. J.A.M.A. *195*:388, 1966.

138. Meyskens, F. L., Jr., Tormey, D. C., and Neifeld, J. P.: Male breast cancer: a review. Cancer Treatment Rev. *3*:83, 1976.

139. Norris, H. J., and Taylor, H. B.: Relationship of histologic features to behavior of cystosarcoma phyllodes: analysis of 94 cases. Cancer *20*:2090, 1967.

140. Norris, H. J., and Taylor, H. B.: Carcinoma of the breast in women less than thirty years old. Cancer *26*:953, 1970.

141. Oberman, H. A., and Stephens, P. J.: Carcinoma of the breast in childhood. Cancer *30*:470, 1972.

142. Ramirez, G., and Ansfield, F. J.: Carcinoma of the breast in children. Arch. Surg. *96*:222, 1968.

143. Sandison, A. T., and Walker, J. C.: Diseases of the adolescent female breast. Brit. J. Surg. *55*:443, 1968.

144. Seashore, J. H.: Breast enlargements in infants and children. Pediatr. Ann. *4*:542, 1975.

145. Treves, N.: Gynecomastia. The origins of mammary swelling in the male: an analysis of 406 patients with breast hypertrophy, 525 with testicular tumors, and 13 with adrenal neoplasms. Cancer *11*:1083, 1958.

146. Treves, N., and Sunderland, D. A.: Cystosarcoma phyllodes of the breast: a malignant and benign tumor. Cancer *4*:1286, 1951.

147. Umansky, C., and Bullock, W. K.: Granular cell myoblastoma of the breast. Ann. Surg. *168*:810, 1968.

148. Williams, I. G.: Cancer in childhood. Brit. J. Radiol. *19*:182, 1946.

149. Wulsin, J. H.: Breast lesions in children. Hosp. Med. *4*:54, 1968.

Chapter Twenty

LYMPHOEPITHELIOMA, SALIVARY GLAND TUMORS, AND THYROID TUMORS

LYMPHOEPITHELIOMA

This tumor is an undifferentiated transitional epidermoid carcinoma of the nasopharynx, which generally arises in Waldeyer's ring. It differs from other types of nasopharyngeal epidermoid carcinomas by the presence of: (1) conspicuous lymphocytic infiltration and (2) syncytial strands or bands of isolated separate transitional cells (nonkeratinizing epidermoid cells)[68] (Fig. 20–1). Most pathologists consider the presence of the lymphocytes (largely T-cells) to be evidence of a cellular immune response rather than an integral part of the malignancy.[59, 63]

Nasopharyngeal carcinoma is the only tumor besides Burkitt's lymphoma to show a strong association with Epstein-Barr virus (EBV). The virus is found only in poorly differentiated or anaplastic nasopharyngeal tumors, and the EBV genome is carried by the carcinoma cells themselves rather than by the infiltrating lymphocytes; the carcinoma cells also express the EBV-determined nuclear antigen.[34a]

Unlike carcinomas at other sites, lymphoepithelioma occurs in relatively young patients. In white populations, 6 per cent of cases occur before 30 years of age, and 50 per cent before the age of 50 years;[3] patients as young as 10 months of age have been reported.[48]

Presenting symptoms include weight loss, severe trismus, throat pain, epistaxis, painful torticollis, voice change, rhinorrhea, otitis media, and tender cervical adenopathy. The most common physical sign is tender cervical adenopathy (usually unilateral); a palpable nasopharyngeal mass or depression of the soft palate may also be present.[17, 48]

Lymphoepithelioma exhibits early spread to regional structures and cervical lymph nodes (particularly in the superior posterior cervical triangle). Later distant metastases to lungs, bone, and central nervous system may appear, auguring a poor prognosis.

These tumors, despite their name,

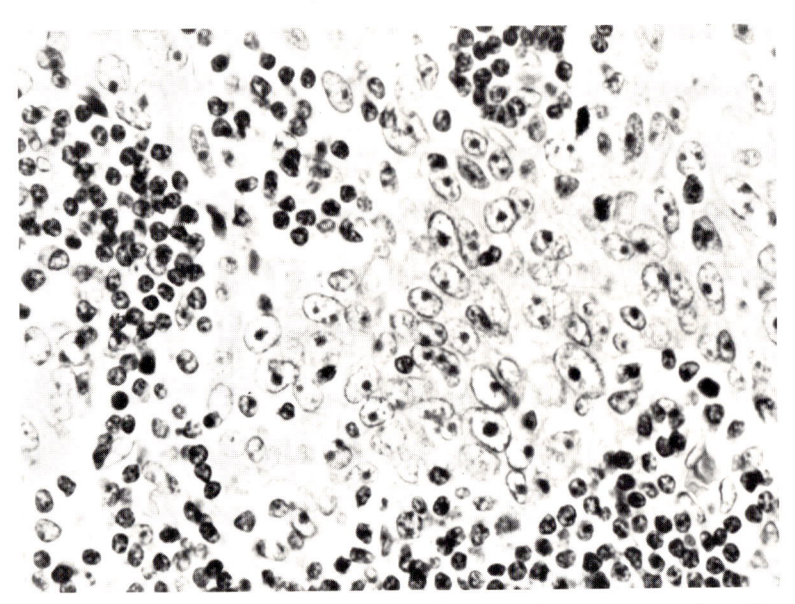

Figure 20–1 Histologic appearance of lymphoepithelioma, showing a nest of undifferentiated or transitional cells arranged in syncytial fashion without distinctive cell borders. Outside this nest are lymphoid and plasma cells (H&E, ×920). (From Pick, T., et al.: J. Pediatr. 84:96, 1974.)

should be managed as carcinomas rather than as lymphomas, and attention should be focused primarily on regional rather than systemic control. Since the primary tumor is almost always unresectable, surgery plays little, if any, role in the initial management. The primary mode of therapy is irradiation, which should be delivered to the primary tumor-bearing area of the nasopharynx and to both sides of the neck (whether there is clinically demonstrable cervical metastasis or not).[17, 44, 48, 59]

Some authors recommend eradication by radical neck dissection of any clinically palpable cervical metastases remaining after radiation therapy; this should only be attempted after there is evidence that the primary lesion has been controlled.[59] Others feel that this procedure does not play an important role in nasopharyngeal cancer since it does not attack the first line of neck node metastases in the retropharyngeal space, particularly the spinal accessory nodes and high lateral jugular nodes.[44]

In view of the fact that a significant proportion of patients (approximately 66 per cent) develop local recurrence or distant metastases, or both, within a year of diagnosis, adjuvant chemotherapy also appears warranted.[48] Cyclophosphamide, Adriamycin, and methotrexate (high-dose) have shown some effects against this malignancy.[38, 48, 59]

The overall 5-year survival rate for this tumor ranges from 35 to 62.5 per cent.[48, 59] The prognosis depends on location (posterior-superior vault lesions have a better prognosis than do lesions of the lateral wall), age (younger individuals have a higher survival rate), and extent of disease.[37, 59]

SALIVARY GLAND TUMORS

Salivary gland swellings may be caused by (1) *inflammatory lesions* (mumps, sialadenitis), (2) *congenital anomalies* (cyst or fistula of the first branchial pouch), or (3) *neoplastic processes.* Salivary gland swellings in childhood usually result from inflammations; primary tumors are rare in children.

Schneider and co-workers[56a] have found a marked increase in the occurrence of salivary tumors in patients who receive radiation to the tonsils and nasopharynx during childhood. This risk (77 cases/10^5 subjects/year) is estimated to be 13 to 40 times the risk for the unirradiated population. An especially disturbing finding in this study is the fact that the incidence of salivary gland tumors does not seem to be declining even after 35 years.

Of the major salivary glands (parotid, submandibular, and sublingual), the parotid is more commonly associated with tumor formation than are the other two combined.[64] There are also a number of smaller salivary glands (minor salivary glands) lying within the submucosa of the mouth, the interior of the lips, and the oropharynx, which may be the site of tumor formation.

It is important to realize that not all chronic salivary gland swellings are caused by neoplasms. *Chronic sialadenitis* (which is the result of repeated bouts of inflammation, congenital stenosis of the ducts, or obstruction of the duct by a stone) may produce firm, sometimes slightly tender, progressive enlargement of the salivary glands. Contrast sialography, a technique by which a radiopaque material is injected into the salivary gland duct, will produce a pathognomonic radiographic appearance in chronic sialadenitis—the acini are dilated and the contrast material collects and persists in them. Sialography can also be used to determine whether a given parotid gland swelling is benign or malignant: benign tumors produce a sharply delimited filling defect within the gland and all the ducts fill normally; malignant tumors, on the other hand, produce an irregular filling defect within the gland and the ducts are absent or distorted[55] (Fig. 20–2).

Of the salivary tumors that do occur (Table 20–1), the majority are benign and of a vascular nature—hemangioendothelioma, cystic hygroma, lymphangioma.[33, 41] Such tumors are usually recognizable by the fact that they have been present since infancy or from the first year of life, give the skin a bluish cast, and are soft, spongy, and compressible. Solid lesions may also be benign, the most common example being the mixed tumor (pleomorphic adenoma). However, carcinomas also occur and mucoepidermoid carcinoma heads the list of malignant neoplasms. Malignant lymphomas and other malignant mesenchymal tumors (rhabdomyosarcoma, fibrosarcoma) are rare, but should also be considered in the differential diagnosis of a salivary gland enlargement. A general rule of thumb for neoplasms involving the parotid area is *approximately 50 per cent are vascular and 50 per cent are solid; of those that are solid, 50 per cent are malignant.*[40, 41] Tumors that cause facial nerve paralysis are virtually always malignant.

Parotid masses must be differentiated from: (a) lymph node enlargement, (b) underlying bony tumors with erosion into the parotid area, and (c) metastases from internal sites (e.g., nasopharynx). This can be done by x-rays of the mandible and maxilla, nasopharyngeal examination, sialography, and scanning with the radionuclide ^{99m}technetium pertechnetate (*radiosialography*), which will identify a parotid tumor as a "cold" filling defect;[21] lymph node metastases, by contrast, produce external compression. Warthin's tumor gives a "hot" nodule, but this tumor does not occur in children.[30]

Recognizing the high incidence of malignancy in solid parotid gland tumors, May has recommended that any solid, nontender, firm parotid mass in a child that has been present for 3 months or longer, is increasing in size, and for which no other cause (e.g., infection) can be found, should be treated by surgical removal of the parotid gland.[41] Other authors recom-

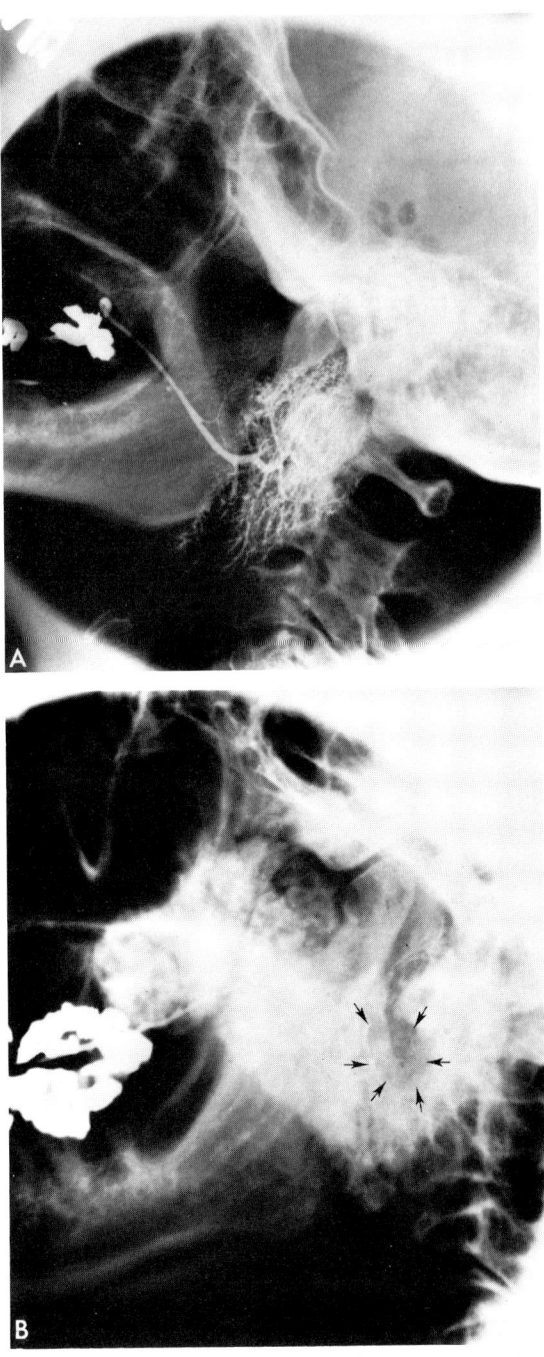

Figure 20-2 A, A normal parotid sialogram, showing the extensive, delicate arborizations of the gland (lateral view). B, An abnormal parotid sialogram. Arrows depict a mixed tumor within the gland which is displacing the opacified ducts and lobules (lateral view).

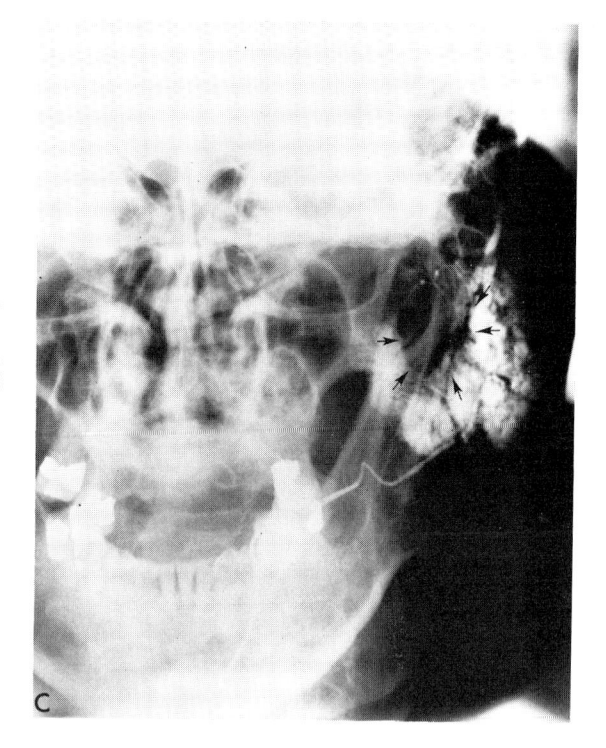

Figure 20–2 Continued. C, Anterior view of sialogram of same patient as in *B.* (From Scanlan, R. L.: *In* Steckel, R. J., and Kagan, A. R.: Diagnosis and Staging of Cancer: A Radiologic Approach. Philadelphia, W. B. Saunders Co., 1976.)

mend a complete superficial lobectomy as the minimal procedure for all parotid solid tumors; further surgery should be then performed as indicated if the frozen section shows malignancy.[40]

Table 20–1   Salivary Gland Tumors

Benign
   Hemangioma
   Benign mixed tumor
   Lymphangioma
   Hemangioendothelioma
   Papillary adenoma
Malignant
   Mucoepidermoid carcinoma
   Undifferentiated carcinoma
   Malignant mixed tumor
   Adenocarcinoma
      Adenocystic carcinoma (cylindroma)
      Acinous cell carcinoma
Metastatic
   Lymphosarcoma
   Rhabdomyosarcoma
   Fibrosarcoma

SOLID TUMORS

Mixed Tumor (Pleomorphic Adenoma)

This lesion is so named because it contains both epithelial and mesenchymal (myoepithelial) components in a variable chondromyxoid stroma.[45] It is the most common benign solid salivary gland tumor in both adults and children, but is, nonetheless, quite rare in the pediatric age range (fewer than 3 per cent of cases of mixed salivary gland tumors occur in childhood).[20] When seen in children, this tumor usually occurs in the second decade of life, and its slow asymptomatic growth frequently goes unnoticed or unheeded.

The benign histologic appearance correlates with its slow growth pattern; however, some authors recommend that it be considered malignant because of its location and capacity to infiltrate and to recur locally (local recurrence rates vary from 4 to 50 per cent).[4, 20, 36, 45] Recurrence may result in facial nerve paralysis and even death from extension into the brain.[33] Recurrences after a 10-year (or longer) quiescent period are common.[20] One reason for recurrence is inadequate initial surgery, since it may be tempting to treat an encapsulated, mobile, innocuous-appearing lesion by enucleation alone. Most authors recommend a total parotid lobectomy following identification of the facial nerve; if the tumor is broken in the process, the entire wound must be excised.[4, 20, 36, 45]

Mucoepidermoid Carcinoma

This is the most frequently encountered malignant salivary gland tumor of childhood, representing over half of the malignant salivary gland tumors in the pediatric age group.[31, 33] The parotid gland is involved 60 to 70 per cent of the time, the submaxillary gland in 10 per cent, and the minor salivary glands in 15 to 20 per cent.[19] Although it has been reported in a 1 year old patient,[31] the tumor rarely affects infants and is found more frequently later in childhood.

Mucoepidermoid carcinoma arises from salivary duct epithelium and contains both mucus-secreting and epidermoid cells, as well as intermediate types of basal or nonmucus-secreting cells (Fig. 20–3). Stewart and colleagues have divided these tumors into high- and low-grade malignancy groups on the basis of histology; epidermoid and intermediate cells predominate in the high-grade malignancies, while mucus-secreting and intermediate cells are found in low-grade tumors. There is a two thirds incidence of regional node metastases and a one third incidence of distant metastases in the high-grade group.[62] Low-grade tumors, on the other hand, follow a much more benign course. In children, however, histologic features correlate poorly with biological behavior and it seems best to regard all mucoepidermoid carcinomas as potential metastasizers.[33]

Like the mixed-cell tumor, this lesion may be deceptively well circumscribed and easy to "shell out." However, the high recurrence rate (30 to 50 per cent) makes complete removal of the affected gland (or the involved lobe if in the parotid) advisable;[4, 36] Galich recommends total parotidectomy with preservation of the facial nerve for such lesions with radical neck dissection added if the lesion is of high-grade malignancy.[20] Other authors suggest examination of regional nodes by frozen section and radical neck dissection performed if they demonstrate metastatic disease.[36] These tumors are not considered to be radiosensitive.

Undifferentiated Carcinoma

This tumor makes its appearance in infancy and early childhood and is the second most frequent salivary tumor in the pediatric group. It is by far the most malignant of the pediatric salivary gland tumors and is characterized by rapid growth, local invasion, widespread metastases, and an ominous prognosis regardless of mode of therapy.[20, 33] Management should be the same as that for an infiltrating carcinoma in any other part of the body — i.e., wide radical excision of the primary site combined with prophylactic radical neck dissection and postoperative radiotherapy.[4]

Adenocarcinoma

There are two major variants of this tumor: *adenocystic carcinoma* (cylindroma) and *acinous cell carcinoma*. Cylindroma is seen mostly in submaxillary and minor salivary glands.[19] It is distinguished by its tendency to invade perineural spaces, and the presence of facial paralysis is an ominous sign. *Cylindroma* is characterized by repeated recurrences (sometimes after

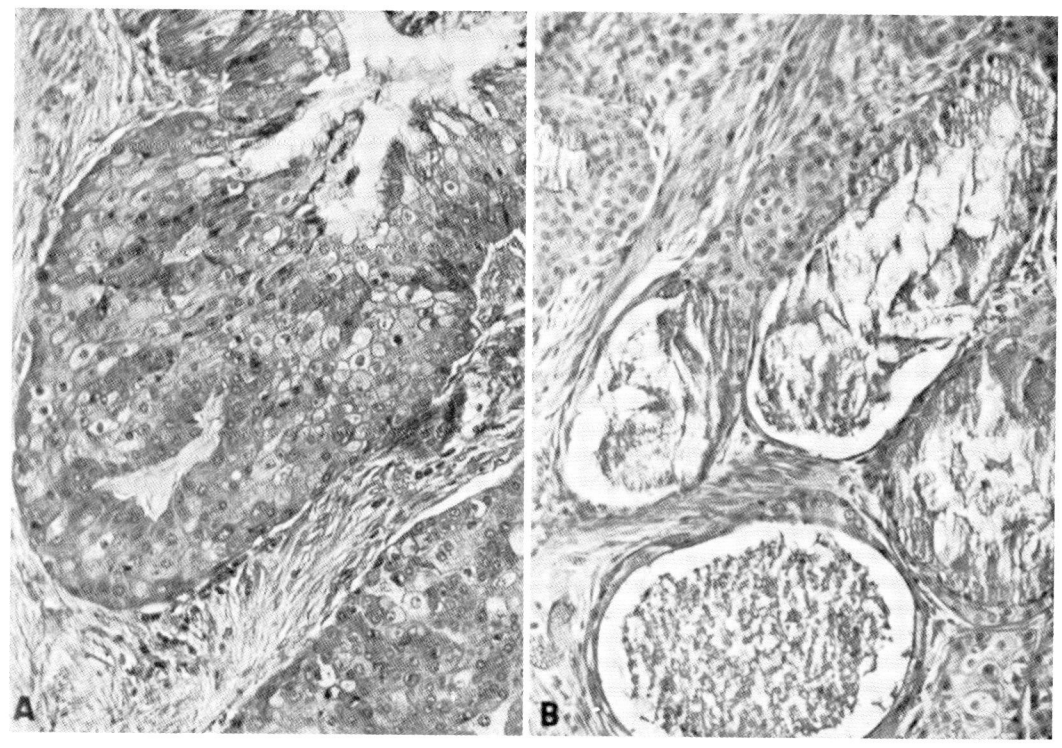

Figure 20–3 Mucoepidermoid carcinoma of the parotid gland. *A*, The bulk of the tumor consists of sheets of squamous cancer cells with occasional mucous cells lining cavities (×180). *B*, The first recurrence—there are many mucus filled cavities lined by both basal and mucous cells (× 180). (From Kauffman, S. L., and Stout, A. P.: Cancer *16*:1317, 1963.)

years of quiescence), widespread metastases, and eventually death in 75 per cent of patients. The surgical approach is essentially the same as that for mucoepidermoid carcinoma.[20, 30] Postoperative irradiation therapy may also be of value in preventing recurrence.[32]

Acinous cell carcinomas appear to be almost exclusive to the parotid. They are very uncommon in children[33] and should be treated in the same manner as other salivary gland malignancies.[36]

THYROID CARCINOMA

There is a strong correlation between radiation exposure at a young age and consequent development of thyroid carcinoma. The thyroid gland appears to be more highly susceptible to ionizing irradiation during infancy and early childhood than in adulthood;[7, 10] this may reflect the far greater rate of mitosis in the young thyroid or the small size of the gland, resulting in a greater rad exposure per gram of tissue.

At a time when radiation therapy was routinely used for treatment of benign conditions of the head and neck (cystic hygroma, hemangioma, cervical adenopathy, and tonsillar, adenoidal, or thymic enlargement), almost three fourths of young patients with thyroid carcinoma had a history of anterior neck irradiation delivered anywhere from 3.6 to 14 years prior to the development of malignancy.[67]

Favus and associates, in their study of 1056 subjects following irradiation to the tonsil-nasopharynx region, found a significant incidence of nodular thyroid disease, including benign and malignant tumors, for at least 35 years after treatment.[16] Palpable nodular thyroid disease was found in 16.5 per cent and nonpalpable lesions were detected by [99m]technetium pertechnetate thyroid imaging in an additional 10.7 per cent for a *total incidence* of 27.2 per cent. Thyroid cancer was found in 33 per cent of those with nodular disease who underwent surgery. The thyroid cancer incidence reported by Favus in tonsil-irradiated patients is identical to the 33 per cent incidence found in thymus-irradiated patients operated on for nodular thyroid disease in Hempelmann's most recent study.[25]

Although the average latent period after radiation to the discovery of thyroid carcinoma is 10 to 20 years, the period of risk may extend indefinitely; even after an average period of 25 years, there was a 7 per cent incidence of thyroid carcinoma in an unselected group of 100 adult patients with a history of such therapy.[49] Since it has been estimated that 71,000 patients in the Chicago area alone had similar neck irradiation, these individuals pose a significant public health challenge.[7] Fortunately most of the thyroid malignancies found in these patients have been well-differentiated papillary or follicular neoplasms, which grow slowly, metastasize late, and are curable if diagnosed while still localized.

There has also been a high incidence of thyroid carcinoma following the atomic bomb explosions at Hiroshima and Nagasaki[60] and in individuals exposed to radioactive iodine in fallout over the Marshall Islands in 1954.[11] On the other hand, the role of therapeutic or diagnostic doses of ^{131}I as a possible etiologic factor in pediatric thyroid carcinoma has not been established.[10] The occurrence of thyroid carcinoma after ^{131}I therapy for Graves' disease is rare and no greater than that seen following surgery or antithyroid drug therapy.[12, 54] However, the period of follow-up (12.3 years) may not be sufficiently long to detect long-term carcinogenic effects. Also, the high doses of ^{131}I used to treat Graves' disease (10 times the rad exposure to the thyroid that induced cancer in the Marshall Islanders)[11] may so severely damage the gland that all cellular proliferation is impaired.[7] Lower-dose ^{131}I regimens appear to produce thyroid nodules[12] and may possibly induce malignant transformation.[7]

Experimental studies on laboratory animals have suggested that radiation alone is incapable of inducing thyroid carcinoma; there must also be prolonged stimulation of the gland by thyrotropin (TSH).[39] Constant TSH stimulation of the thyroid gland may also be relevant to the production of thyroid carcinoma in humans with enzymatic defects in the synthesis of thyroxine.[14, 65]

CLINICAL MANIFESTATIONS

The most common presenting complaint is the presence of multiple palpable lymph nodes on the side of the neck;[15, 50] in many of these cases, careful palpation of the thyroid gland will reveal a solitary nodule. These nodules are usually firm and irregular, but may be smooth and circumscribed. Pulmonary metastases may also be present at the time of diagnosis in 12 to 30 per cent of patients.[10, 67]

The presence of a solitary nodule in the thyroid gland of a child is a matter of concern. In the past, 39 to 50 per cent of such nodules were found to be malignant;[1, 23, 35] however, this incidence has declined since the dangers of low-dose radiation have been recognized. A recent series of 36 children evaluated since 1961 for thyroid nodules showed only a 17 per cent incidence of carcinoma.[57]

The differential diagnosis of a unilateral thyroid mass in childhood includes *Hashimoto's thyroiditis, subacute nonsuppurative thyroiditis, thyroid abscess, thyroid dysgenesis, benign adenoma, thyroid cyst,* and *thyroid cancer.*

Evaluation of the patient should include the following:

History. Especially significant is information regarding familial thyroid or endocrine disease, previous radiation therapy to the cervical area, and rate of growth of the nodule.

Physical Examination. Particular attention should be paid to the cervical lymph nodes and thyroid tissue surrounding the nodule. Painful thyroid enlargement with prominent local manifestations or marked thyroid tenderness suggests acute or subacute nonsuppurative thyroiditis. Search for mucosal neuromas, Marfanoid habitus, and hypertension should also be performed.

Laboratory Examination. This should include x-rays of the chest and neck and tests of thyroid function (serum thyroxine level, serum T_3 level by radioimmunoassay, and serum TSH level). A serum calcitonin measurement should be performed to detect patients with medullary carcinoma.

Thyroid Scan. Malignant thyroid nodules usually do not concentrate the radioisotopes commonly used for thyroid scans (^{131}I, ^{123}I, [99m]technetium pertechnetate); consequently, they appear as "cold" nodules. The likelihood of malignancy in a discrete "cold" nodule in an otherwise normal thyroid gland in a child or adolescent approaches 40 per cent.[66] On the other hand, most nodules that show increased concentration of the above radioisotopes ("hot" or "functional" nodules) are not malignant. However, if such a nodule is autonomous (i.e., fails to recede after long-term therapy with supplemental thyroid hormone), then surgical excision should be considered, since carcinoma is occasionally seen in this setting.[27]

In general, carcinoma is more likely than a benign lesion if: (1) there is a history of prior irradiation, (2) the nodule is hard, (3) adjacent lymph nodes are enlarged, (4) there is evidence of tracheal invasion or vocal cord paralysis, (5) the nodule has grown rapidly, (6) the nodule is "cold" on scan, and (7) distant metastases are present.

CLASSIFICATION

Thyroid cancer may be classified into three distinct clinical and histological patterns: (1) differentiated forms (papillary and follicular carcinomas); (2) anaplastic forms, and (3) medullary carcinoma. Each of these will be discussed separately.

Differentiated Forms of Thyroid Carcinoma

These are the types most commonly seen in children; they consist of four histologic subtypes: pure papillary, pure follicular, mixed papillary-follicular, and Hürthle cell. These lesions are characterized by indolent biological behavior, with survival usually measured in decades.

Usually the most common presenting sign is a midline neck mass or palpable cervical nodes. Although malignant nodules cannot be distinguished from benign ones by physical examination, a feeling of hardness as well as the presence of ipsilateral enlarged anterior cervical node(s) suggests malignancy. Cervical metastases are more common in the papillary group than in the follicular type, while the latter has a greater tendency to pulmonary metastasis.

Surprisingly, the presence of lymph node metastases does not appear to adversely affect the prognosis for differentiated thyroid carcinoma. Indeed, there is evidence that lymph node metastases may exert a protective effect, which is directly related to the number of lymph node metastases present; of the 22 patients in one series who displayed more than 10 node metastases, not one died of the disease.[7a]

Surgery is the treatment of choice for localized disease; this has ranged from removal of the involved lobe plus the thyroid isthmus to total thyroidectomy.[10, 26] However, lack of evidence that total thyroidectomy significantly improves the cure rate for papillary and follicular carcinoma of the thyroid has led some surgeons to advise strongly against total thyroidectomy in children, especially in view of its possible serious consequences (in 5 to 10 per cent there has been inadvertent sectioning of the recurrent laryngeal nerve and 20 per cent have developed permanent hypoparathyroidism).[15, 36a] Radical neck dissection has no place in treatment of this tumor in children.[10]

Recurrent or metastatic disease is also treated surgically if possible because of the characteristically slow growth of these lesions. Disease that is not amenable to surgery may be treated with radioactive iodine, external beam radiotherapy, or Adriamycin.[22, 26] Late in the disease widespread pulmonary metastases may occur; these may regress with thyroxine therapy.

Thyroxine in doses somewhat greater than physiologic requirements should always be given after surgical or radioiodine therapy has been given because complete inhibition of TSH secretion by the pituitary may eliminate the stimulus for further growth of those cancers that are hormone dependent. The papillary type is generally the most hormone dependent and therefore the most likely to be favorably affected by this form of therapy.

Anaplastic Forms of Thyroid Carcinoma

Although seen most frequently in adults, anaplastic thyroid cancer also constitutes approximately 9 per cent of pediatric thyroid carcinomas.[61] This form of thyroid cancer is histologically undifferentiated, lacking follicles and papillary structures; microscopically it consists of a mixture of spindle and giant cells. Since such lesions may develop within a preexisting well-differentiated thyroid tumor, it is essential for the pathologist to study many sections from various portions of any large, bulky, rapidly growing tumor of the thyroid. Whenever an anaplastic component is detected, the tumor almost invariably behaves aggressively.

The highly malignant nature of this tumor requires a much more aggressive therapeutic approach than do the more differentiated forms. Tumors localized to the neck have been treated with operative removal of the tumor, radiation (6000 rads) to the neck, both supraclavicular areas, and upper mediastinum (as soon as wound healing permits), and actinomycin D.[51]

Medullary Carcinoma of the Thyroid

Medullary carcinoma of the thyroid (MCT) makes up less than 10 per cent of thyroid malignancies.[42] Unlike other tumors arising within the thyroid gland, this tumor is not derived from follicular epithelium, but originates instead from a second epithelial cell system, which migrates from the neural crest to the thyroid during embryogenesis and forms the parafollicular or C-cells of Nonides. These parafollicular cells are thought to be the source of thyrocalcitonin, a hormone which lowers blood calcium levels.

MCT is of an intermediate degree of malignancy; metastases to lymph nodes occur early and are seen in 50 per cent of patients. Wide-ranging metastases resulting in death may occur in mediastinal nodes, lung, liver, and bone.

Histologically, MCT is composed of sheets of polyhedral cells interspersed with connective tissue septa containing amyloid (it is the only thyroid tumor to contain amyloid).[24, 28] These neoplastic cells contain intracytoplasmic secretory granules and closely resemble normal thyroid parafollicular cells. This histologic resemblance is of particular relevance, since very high levels of thyrocalcitonin-like activity have been found in this tumor.[43]

MCT may occur in both sporadic (90 per cent) and familial (10 per cent) form; the latter is usually transmitted in an autosomal dominant fashion and is invariably associated with multifocal bilateral involvement of the gland.[26]

The familial (but not the sporadic) form of MCT has been associated with other tumors; the combination of MCT, pheochromocytoma (frequently bilateral), and parathyroid hyperplasia has been designated as *Sipple's syndrome or multiple endocrine neoplasia (MEN), type 2*. The parathyroid hyperplasia appears to represent not a primary neoplastic process but a compensatory response for maintaining calcium homeostasis in the face of elevated calcitonin production.

Pheochromocytoma accounts for significant mortality in the MEN type 2 syndrome; 29 to 32 per cent of patients with this condition have died of intracranial hemorrhage, hypertensive crisis, hypotensive episodes, or pulmonary metastases attributable to pheochromocytoma.[8, 9] Accordingly, primary *bilateral* total adrenalectomy has been recommended for patients with concurrent MCT and adrenal medullary disease.[9] Removal of the adrenal disease should probably precede the thyroid surgery.[26]

Another accompaniment of MCT is the *mucosal neuroma syndrome*,[18] also known as *multiple endocrine neoplasia, type 3*.[34] Patients with this syndrome have a characteristic physical appearance: they are tall, with arachnodactyly, and a Marfanoid habitus, scoliosis, pectus excavatum, pes cavus, and muscular hypotonia are also frequently present. The facies simulate acromegaly, with thickened eyelids, "bumpy" lips, and soft-tissue prognathism (Fig. 20–4A). Mucosal neuromatoma may occur on the eyelids, lips, tongue (Fig. 20–4B), buccal mucosa, and myenteric and submucosal plexus of the intestinal tract (causing both megacolon and severe diarrhea). About 30 per cent of patients with MCT have severe, unexplained diarrhea, which may precede the diagnosis; the presence of this symptom in a patient with a thyroid nodule should therefore raise

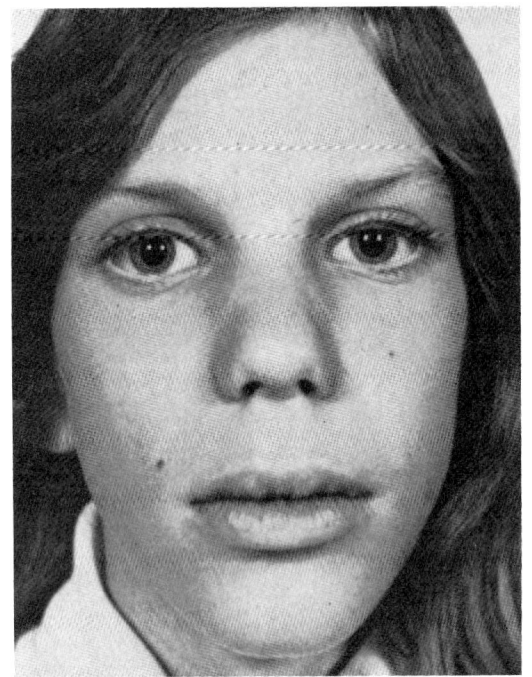

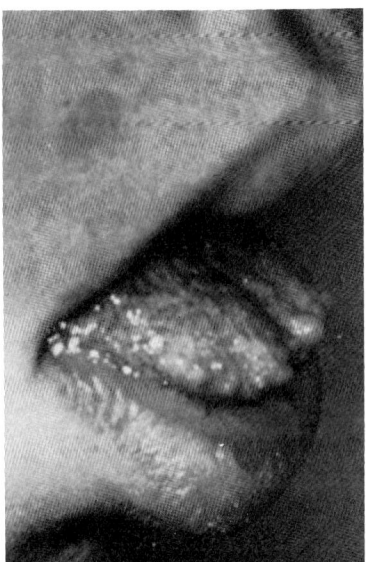

Figure 20-4 Mucosal neuroma syndrome. *A*, Characteristic facies, with thickened, "bumpy" lips and acromegalic appearance. *B*, Neuromas of the anterior third of the tongue. Similar neuromas may be seen on the gingiva, nasal mucosa, and palpebral conjunctiva. (From Brown, R. S., et al.: J. Pediatr. 86:77, 1975.)

strong suspicions that the nodule is malignant.[26] The diarrhea may be related to the secretion of calcitonin, prostaglandins, serotonin, other humoral substances, or neural abnormality.[8]

Since the neural crest is thought to be the embryonic origin for both the parafollicular cells, which give rise to MCT, and the adrenal medullary cells, which yield pheochromocytoma, these multiple endocrine neoplasia syndromes appear to represent a generalized disorder of neural crest derivatives (*"neurocristopathies"*).[6]

The familial form of MCT is multicentric in origin and the C-cells are diffusely spread throughout the thyroid gland; consequently, only total thyroidectomy will reliably remove all possible foci of tumor formation and is probably the treatment of choice for this disease.[10, 24, 36a, 42, 56] Pheochromocytoma must be ruled out before thyroid surgery is contemplated because of the risk of precipitating a hypertensive crisis under the stress of general anesthesia. Thyroidectomy is associated with significant risk to the recurrent laryngeal nerves and parathyroid glands and should be undertaken only by surgeons who are well trained in thyroid surgery. Replacement therapy with thyroid hormone is necessary after this procedure.

REFERENCES

1. Adams, H. D.: Carcinoma in nodular goiter of childhood. Postgrad Med. 43:136, 1968.
2. Arnold, J., Pinsky, S., and Ryo, U. Y.: ^{99m}Technetium pertechnetate thyroid scintigraphy in patients predisposed to thyroid neoplasms by prior radiotherapy to the head and neck. Radiology 115:653, 1975.
3. Bailar, J. C.: Nasopharyngeal cancer in white populations—a worldwide survey. *In* Muir, C. S., and Shanmigaratnam, K. (eds.): Cancer of the Nasopharynx. Flushing, N.Y., Medical Examination Publishing Co., 1967.

4. Baum, R. K., and Perzik, S. L.: Tumors of the parotid gland in children. Am. Surg. 31:719, 1965.
5. Birdsell, D. C., and Lindsay, W. K.: Malignant tumors of the head and neck in children. Plast. Reconstr. Surg. 44:255, 1969.
6. Bolande, R. P.: The neurocristopathies: a unifying concept of disease arising in neural crest maldevelopment. Hum. Pathol. 5:409, 1974.
7. Braverman, L.: Consequences of thyroid radiation in children. N. Engl. J. Med. 292:204, 1975.
7a. Cady, B., Sedgwick, C. E., Meissner, W. A., et al.: Changing clinical, pathologic, therapeutic, and survival patterns in differentiated thyroid carcinoma. Ann. Surg. 184:541, 1976.
8. Carney, J. A., Go, V.L.W., Sizemore, G. W., and Hayles, A. B.: Alimentary tract ganglioneuromatosis. A major component of the syndrome of multiple endocrine neoplasia, type 2b. N. Engl. J. Med. 295:1287, 1976.
9. Carney, J. A., Sizemore, G. W., and Sheps, S. G.: Adrenal medullary disease in multiple endocrine neoplasia, type 2. Pheochromocytoma and its precursors. Am. J. Clin. Pathol. 66:279, 1976.
10. Clayton, G. W.: Tumors of the endocrine glands. In Sutow, W. W., Vietti, T. J., and Fernbach, D. J. (eds.): Clinical Pediatric Oncology. St. Louis, C.V. Mosby Co., 1973.
11. Conrad, R. A., Dobyns, B. M., and Sutow, W. W.: Thyroid neoplasia as late effect of exposure to radioactive iodine in fallout. J.A.M.A., 214:316, 1970.
12. Dobyns, B. M., Sheline, G. E., Workman, J. B., et al.: Malignant and benign neoplasms of the thyroid in patients treated for hyperthyroidism: a report of the cooperative thyrotoxicosis therapy follow-up study. J. Clin. Endocr. Metab. 38:976, 1974.
13. Duffy, B. J., Jr., and Fitzgerald, P. J.: Cancer of the thyroid in children: a report of 28 cases. J. Clin. Endocr. Metab. 10:1296, 1950.
14. Elman, D. S.: Familial association of nerve deafness with nodular goiter and thyroid carcinoma. N. Engl. J. Med. 259:219, 1958.
15. Exelby, P. R., and Frazell, E. L.: Carcinoma of the thyroid in children. Surg. Clin. N. Amer. 49:249, 1969.
16. Favus, M. G., Schneider, A. B., Stachura, M. E., et al: Thyroid cancer occurring as a late consequence of head and neck irradiation: evaluation of 1056 patients. N. Engl. J. Med. 294:1019, 1976.
17. Fernandez, C. H., Cangir, A., Samaan, N. A., and Rivera, R: Nasopharyngeal carcinoma in children. Cancer 37:2787, 1976.
18. Forsman, P. J., and Jenkins, M. E.: Medullary carcinoma of the thyroid with Marfanlike body habitus Pediatrics 52:188, 1973.
19. Friedman, E. W., and Schwartz, A. E.: Diagnosis of salivary gland tumors. CA 24:266, 1974.
20. Galich, R.: Salivary gland neoplasms in children. Arch. Otolaryngol. 89:878, 1969.
21. Gates, O.: Radiosialographic aspects of salivary gland disorders. Laryngology 82:115, 1972.
22. Gottlieb, J. A., and Hill, C. S., Jr.: Adriamycin (NSC-123127) therapy in thyroid carcinoma. Cancer Chemother. Rep. 6:283, 1975.
23. Hayles, A. B., Johnson, M. L., Beahrs, O. H., and Woolner, L. B.: Carcinoma of the thyroid in children. Amer. J. Surg. 106:735, 1965.
24. Hazard, J. B., Hawk, W. A., and Crile, G., Jr.: Medullary (solid) carcinoma of the thyroid. A clinicopathologic entity. J. Clin. Endocr. Metab. 19:152, 1959.
25. Hempelmann, L. H., Hall, W. J., Phillips, M., et al.: Neoplasms in persons treated with x-rays in infancy: fourth survey in 20 years. J. Natl. Cancer Inst. 55:519, 1975.
26. Hill, C. S., Jr.: Thyroid cancer—iatrogenic and otherwise. CA 26:160, 1976.
27. Hopwood, N. J., Carroll, R. G., Kenny, F. M., and Foley, T. P., Jr.: Functioning thyroid masses in childhood and adolescence. J. Pediatr. 89:710, 1976.
28. Ibanez, M. L., Cole, V. W., Russell, W. O., and Clark, R. L.: Solid carcinoma of the thyroid gland: analysis of 53 cases. Cancer 20:706, 1967.
29. Jaffe, B. F.: Pediatric head and neck tumors. Laryngoscope 83:1644, 1973.
30. Jaffe, B. F., and Jaffe, N.: Head and neck tumors in children. Pediatrics 51:731, 1973.
31. Jaques, D. A., Krolls, S. O., and Chambers, R. G.: Parotid tumors in children. Am. J. Surg. 132:469, 1976.
32. Kagan, A. R., Nussbaum, H., Handler, S., et al.: Recurrences from malignant parotid salivary gland tumors. Cancer 37:2600, 1976.
33. Kauffman, S. L., and Stout, A. P.: Tumors of the major salivary glands in children. Cancer 16:1317, 1963.
34. Khairi, M. R. A., Dexter, R. N., Burzynski, N. J., and Johnston, C. C., Jr: Mucosal neuroma, pheochromocytoma, and medullary thyroid carcinoma: multiple endocrine neoplasia type 3. Medicine 54:89, 1975.
34a. Klein, G.: The Epstein-Barr virus and neoplasia. N. Engl. J. Med. 293:1353, 1975.
35. Kirkland, R. T., Kirkland, J. L., Rosenberg, H. S., et al.: Solitary thyroid nodules in 30 children and report of a child with a thyroid abscess. Pediatrics 51:85, 1973.
36. Lane, D. M., and Lonsdale, D.: Tumors of the gastrointestinal tract. In Sutow, W. W.,

Vietti, T. J., and Fernbach, D. J. (eds): Clinical Pediatric Oncology. St. Louis, C. V. Mosby Co., 1973.
36a. Leape, L. L., Miller, H. H., Graze, K., et al.: Total thyroidectomy for occult familial medullary carcinoma of the thyroid in children. J. Pediatr. Surg. 11:831, 1976.
37. Lederman, M.: Cancer of the nasopharynx — its natural history and treatment. Springfield, Ill., Charles C Thomas, 1961.
38. Leone, L. A., Albala, M. M., and Rege, V. B.: Treatment of carcinoma of the head and neck with intravenous methotrexate. Cancer 21:828, 1968.
39. Lindsay, S., Sheline, G. E., Potter, G. D., and Chaikoff, I. L.: Induction of neoplasms in the thyroid gland of the rat by x-irradiation of the gland. Cancer Res. 21:9, 1961.
40. Marlowe, J. F., and Hora, J. F.: Parotid mucoepidermoid carcinoma in children. Laryngoscope 78:68, 1968.
41. May, M.: Neck masses in children: diagnosis and treatment. Pediatr. Ann. 5:517, 1976.
42. Melvin, K. E. W., Tashjian, A. H., Jr., and Miller, H. H.: Studies in familial (medullary) thyroid carcinoma. Rec. Progr. Hormone Res. 28:399, 1972.
43. Meyer, J. S., and Abdel-Bari, W.: Granules and thyrocalcitonin-like activity in medullary carcinoma of the thyroid gland. N. Engl. J. Med. 278:523, 1968.
44. Million, R. R.: Management of neck node metastases. J.A.M.A. 220:402, 1972.
45. Naeim, F., Forsberg, M. I., Wariman, J., and Coulson, W. F.: Mixed tumors of the salivary glands. Arch. Pathol. Lab. Med. 100:271, 1976.
46. National Cancer Institute: Information for physicians on irradiation-related thyroid cancer. CA 26:150, 1976.
47. Newstedt, J. R., and Shirkey, H. C.: Teratoma of the thyroid region: report of a case with seven-year follow-up. Am. J. Dis. Child. 107:88, 1964.
48. Pick, T., Maurer, H. M., and McWilliams, N. B.: Lymphoepithelioma in childhood. J. Pediatr. 84:96, 1974.
49. Refetoff, S., Harrison, J. Karanfilski, B. T., et al.: Continuing occurrence of thyroid carcinoma after irradiation to the neck in infancy and childhood. N. Engl. J. Med. 292:171, 1975.
50. Roeher, H. D., Daum, R., Pieper, M., and Rudolph, H.: Juvenile thyroid carcinoma. J. Pediatr. Surg. 7:27, 1972.
51. Rogers, J. D., Lindberg, R. D., Hill, C. S., and Gehan, E.: Spindle and giant cell carcinoma of the thyroid: a different therapeutic approach. Cancer 34:1328, 1976.
52. Rubin, P. R.: Cancer of the head and neck. Nasopharyngeal cancer. J.A.M.A. 220:390, 1972.
53. Rush, B. F., Jr., Chambers, R. G., and Ravitch, M. M.: Cancer of the head and neck in children. Surgery 53:270, 1963.
54. Safa, A. M., Schumacher, O. P., and Antunez, A. R.: Long-term follow-up results in children and adolescents treated with radioactive iodine (^{131}I) for hyperthyroidism. N. Engl. J. Med. 292:167, 1975.
55. Scanlan, R. A.: Head and neck. In Steckel, R. J., and Kagan, A. R.: Diagnosis and Staging of Cancer: A Radiologic Approach. Philadelphia, W. B. Saunders, 1976.
56. Schimke, R. N.: Phenotype of malignancy: the mucosal neuroma syndrome. Pediatrics 52:283, 1973.
56a. Schneider, A. B., Favus, M. J., Stachura, M. E., et al.: Salivary gland neoplasms as a late consequence of head and neck irradiation. Ann. Int. Med. 87:160, 1977.
57. Scott, M. D., and Crawford, J. D.: Solitary thyroid nodules in childhood: is the incidence of thyroid carcinoma declining? Pediatrics 58:521, 1976.
58. Skolnik, E. M., Friedman, M., Becker, S., et al.: Tumors of the major salivary glands. Laryngoscope 87:843, 1977.
59. Snow, J. B., Jr.: Carcinoma of the nasopharynx. In Sutow, W. W., Vietti, T. J., and Fernbach, D. J. (eds.): Clinical Pediatric Oncology. St. Louis, C.V. Mosby Co., 1973.
60. Socolaw, E. L., Hashizume, A., Neriishi, S., and Niitani, R.: Thyroid carcinoma in man after exposure to ionizing irradiation. A summary of the findings in Hiroshima and Nagasaki. N. Engl. J. Med. 268:406, 1963.
61. Steiner, A. L., Goodman, A. D., and Powers, S. R.: Study of a kindred with pheochromocytoma, medullary thyroid carcinoma, hyperparathyroidism, and Cushing's disease: multiple endocrine neoplasia, type 2. Medicine 47:371, 1968.
62. Stewart, F. W., Foote, F. W., and Becker, W. F.: Mucoepidermoid tumors of salivary glands. Ann. Surg. 122:820, 1945.
63. Svoboda, D. J.: Cancer of the head and neck. Nasopharyngeal cancer. Pathologic classification and fine structure. J.A.M.A. 220:394, 1972.
64. Swenson, O.: Diseases of the thyroid gland. In Swenson, O. (ed.): Pediatric Surgery. New York, Appleton-Century-Crofts, 1969.
65. Thieme, E. J.: A report of the occurrence of deaf-mutism and goiter of four of six siblings of a North American family. Ann. Surg. 146:941, 1957.
66. Thomas, C. G., Jr., Buckwalter, J. A., Staab, E. V., and Kerr, C. Y.: Evaluation of dominant thyroid masses. Ann. Surg. 183:463, 1976.
67. Winship, T., and Rosvoll, R. V.: Childhood thyroid carcinoma. Cancer 14:734, 1961.
68. Yeh, S. A.: Histological classification of carcinomas of the nasopharynx with a critical review as to the existence of lymphoepitheliomas. Cancer 15:895, 1962.

Chapter Twenty-One

TUMORS OF THE LIVER

Primary tumors of the liver are uncommon in children. The majority of young patients with malignant disease of the liver have a neuroblastoma or Wilms' tumor as their primary neoplasm with the hepatic involvement due to metastases. Although the primary tumor is usually evident in the case of Wilms' tumor, the neuroblastoma often presents with a hepatic mass as the only sign of tumor, especially when diagnosed during the first few months of life. This often makes it clinically indistinguishable from a primary liver tumor.

A survey conducted by the Surgical Section of the American Academy of Pediatrics in 1974 (Table 21–1) revealed that 252 of 375 primary hepatic tumors were malignant,[22] confirming earlier reports of smaller series that malignant liver neoplasms were more common than benign ones.[11, 18] Primary malignant liver tumors occur at a rate of 1.9 per million in United States white children under 15 years of age;[87] they are found less frequently in United States black children. The great majority of primary hepatic neoplasms that occur in children are carcinomas of hepatic cell origin, the hepatomas. Of the primary malignant liver neoplasms collected in a survey by the American Academy of Pediatrics, 227 of 252 were hepatomas.[22] Primary malignant vascular tumors[12, 44] or those composed mainly of mesenchymal tissue[77] with no malignant vascular elements have been described but are very rare.

Table 21–1 Malignant Hepatic Tumors (From 1974 Survey of the Surgical Section of the American Academy of Pediatrics[22])

Hepatoblastoma	129
Hepatocellular carcinoma	98
Other:	
Mixed mesenchymal	9
Rhabdomyosarcoma	6
Angiosarcoma	4
Undifferentiated sarcoma	3
Teratocarcinoma	1
Cholangiosarcoma	1
Malignant histiocytoma	1

HEPATOMAS

Hepatomas occur more frequently in both children and adults in Asia and Africa than in the United States and Europe.[19] Carcinoma of the liver is the third most common form of abdominal cancer in Japanese children and has a much higher incidence rate in Japan than in other countries.[42] In one series from Japan, hepatomas were the most frequently observed malignant tumors in patients less than 1 year of age.[42] In Taiwan, hepatomas constitute 20 per cent of all malignant abdominal tumors in children.[50] The incidence of hepatic tumors in young Nigerian children is far less than that found in adults, but there appears to be a steep increase in the incidence of hepatocellular carcinomas in late adolescence.[86a] Fraumeni and associates[26] found the highest incidence of white children younger than 5 years of age dying from liver carcinoma in the United States to be in the north central portions of the country, whereas no significant geographic variation could be shown among affected children 5 to 14 years of age. These geographic variations in the incidence of liver cancer are believed to reflect an etiologic role of environmental conditions rather than a genetic predisposition.[74] Reports of hepatomas in siblings are extremely rare.[27] The association of exposure to vinyl chloride and later development of hepatic angiosarcomas,[49] and a relationship between aflatoxin content in food and the frequency of hepatoma in Uganda[2] indicate that, at least in some instances, exposure to hepatotoxins may result in liver cancer in adults. Since childhood hepatomas apparently originate in utero in many instances, prenatal extrinsic factors may possibly play an etiologic role. However, no definite etiologic agents have been implicated in younger children with hepatomas.

PATHOLOGY

Hepatomas, or liver-cell carcinomas, are divided into two major histologic types, hepatoblastomas and hepatocarcinomas (hepatocellular carcinomas).[39] Both types occur more frequently in males.[22, 39, 43]

Hepatoblastomas appear largely in the infant population and are seldom seen after 3 years of age. They occur in otherwise normal livers, and affected children appear to have a better prognosis following resection than do those with hepatocarcinomas. Histologically, hepatoblastomas consist of tumor cells that are smaller than normal liver cells and often contain osteoid and immature fibrous tissue. They have been further classified into two epithelial types, a fetal and embryonal form, based on the cellular pattern and degree of differentiation, and a mixed epithelial-mesenchymal type.[39] Patients with the fetal form appear to have the best prognosis;[39, 43] 6 of 23 children reported by Kasai and Watanabe having this histologic pattern survived for more than 2 years.[43]

Allison and Willis[1] have suggested that hepatoblastomas arise from a multipotential blastema derived from both endodermal and mesodermal elements, with both elements having the potential of becoming malignant. In one form, a mixed epithelial and mesenchymal hepatoblastoma results, and in the other a pure epithelial hepatoblastoma or a pure liver sarcoma (such as an embryonal rhabdomyosarcoma[32] or osteogenic sarcoma of the liver)[64] results.

Hepatocellular carcinomas are histologically identical to the hepatomas found in adults,[39, 43] and have been referred to as the "adult type" liver-cell carcinoma in children.[43] A significant number of these children have cirrhotic changes[41] in the liver, but cirrhosis is much less commonly found in association with childhood hepatocellular carcinoma than in adult liver cancer. A number of reports indicate that this tumor nearly always occurs in children over the age of 5 years.[39, 43, 45, 76] All 13 cases reported by Kasai and Watanabe[43] were in children over the age of 6 years. However, one recent large survey demonstrated two age peaks in children with hepatocellular carcinoma, one in very young patients under 4 years of age and a second in youths between 12 and 15 years of age.[22]

CLINICAL PRESENTATION AND EVALUATION

The most common complaint of the parents of a child with hepatic tumor is of an upper abdominal mass or generalized abdominal enlargement. Of 23 patients reported by Exelby and co-workers, 21 presented with these findings.[21] In addition, anorexia, weight loss, pain, and vomiting are often present.[22] On physical examination an upper abdominal mass is usually palpated. Jaundice and ascites are infrequently observed. Laboratory studies of liver function are rarely helpful in establishing a diagnosis. Bilirubin, transaminase, cholesterol, and alkaline phosphatase levels are often normal with both histologic types, but more commonly are abnormally elevated in children with hepatocellular carcinoma than in those with hepatoblastoma.[22] Anemia is a common finding. Both thrombocytopenia[22] and thrombocytosis[37] have been noted.

Biochemical Abnormalities

Alpha-fetoprotein (AFP), an alpha-1 globulin that is produced in the fetus by embryonic hepatocytes, rapidly decreases in level in the first few weeks of life and is not normally detected in the serum of children and adults. Elevated serum levels have been documented in 40 per cent of children with hepatocellular carcinoma and in two thirds of those with hepatoblastoma.[22] Although AFP levels have also been found to be elevated in some cases of malignant teratomas, nonhepatic carcinomas, and other forms of liver disease,[17] the presence of this oncogenic marker is one of the most helpful preoperative diagnostic tests in determining the presence of a primary hepatic malignancy. The serum levels have been shown to decrease after the use of effective chemotherapy.[53] Surgical tumor resection produces an immediate fall in the serum levels that parallels the catabolic decay rate for AFP;[57] recurrence of tumor in AFP-positive patients is associated with a rise in serum levels, often preceding clinical discovery of relapse.[53, 57] If there is no therapeutic intervention or response to chemotherapy, serum AFP levels usually gradually increase.[53, 57] Thus, AFP determinations appear to be useful in the diagnosis, the monitoring of therapeutic response, and the discovery of tumor recurrence.

Cystathionine, a sulfur-containing amino acid not normally found in the urine, has been reported to occur in the urine of a number of children with hepatoblastoma.[29, 31] If present, cystathioninuria may permit differentiation between hepatoblastoma and a number of benign and other malignant disorders. However, this amino acid is also found in the urine of many patients with neuroblastoma,[30] a neoplasm which commonly metastasizes to the liver in the young child and may clinically mimic a primary hepatic tumor.

Other laboratory abnormalities occasionally have been reported in adolescents and young adults with hepatocellular carcinomas, including extraordinary elevations of serum vitamin B_{12} content and binding protein,[85] and acquired dysfibrinogenemia with delayed fibrin monomer aggregation.[84] The incidence of these abnormalities in patients with hepatic malignancies is presently unknown.

Radiologic Evaluation

Roentgenographic examination of the abdomen usually reveals enlargement of the liver shadow. The right side is more commonly involved than the left. There may be displacement of the stomach or colon, and an elevation or a localized deformity of the diaphragm. Hepatic calcifications are sometimes found, but their occasional presence in metastatic neuroblastoma,[70] hepatic hemangiomas,[18, 60] hydatid cysts,[18] and malignant teratomas[10] limits the diagnostic significance of this finding. Pulmonary metastases are demonstrated on initial chest roentgenogram in about 10 per cent of cases.[10, 22]

An intravenous pyleogram, nearly always performed on the child with an abdominal mass, usually can differentiate between a hepatic and renal tumor by the normal function, shape, and position of the kidneys. Marked renal displacement, as seen with neuroblastoma, is not usually found, but compression and downward displacement of the right kidney has been noted in a significant number of patients.[10]

Radioisotopic scanning of the liver usually shows the location and size of the tumor, which appears as a "cold," space-occupying mass because of diminished uptake of the isotope. The most commonly used radionuclide is ^{99m}technetium sulfur colloid. Scanning is one of the most useful methods of demonstrating the presence of an intrahepatic tumor, although it cannot usually differentiate one type of neoplasm from another. Of 109 preoperative scans performed in one survey, 104 were positive.[22] Tonami and associates[83] reported 22 of 27 cases to have a positive scan, and, when combined with AFP radioimmunoassay, an overall diagnostic accuracy of 93 per cent for detecting the tumor was achieved. Liver scanning is also useful postoperatively to assess the rate of hepatic regeneration in patients who have had liver resections and to diagnose tumor recurrence. More recent studies using ^{67}gallium scintigraphy[15a] have shown increased uptake in the tumor rather than a cold spot (Fig. 21–1). This will differentiate a neoplasm from a cyst, which will appear as a cold spot.

Hepatic arteriography has become a procedure of major importance in both

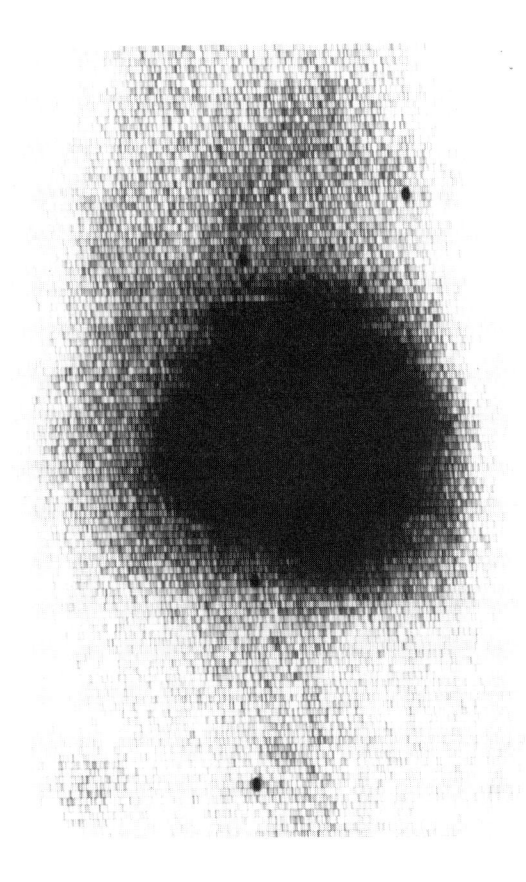

Figure 21–1 Gallium-67 citrate scan of a child with hepatoblastoma of the medial segment of the left hepatic lobe extending across the anterior surface of the right lobe. There is a markedly increased uptake of the isotope within the tumor. (Courtesy of the Nuclear Medicine Department, Johns Hopkins Hospital.)

Figure 21-2 Arteriogram of a child with a hepatoblastoma found to be confined to the medial segment of the left hepatic lobe. The child was treated by left hepatic lobectomy and has remained clinically free of disease 4 months following surgery. (Courtesy of Dr. Robert J. White, Johns Hopkins Hospital.)

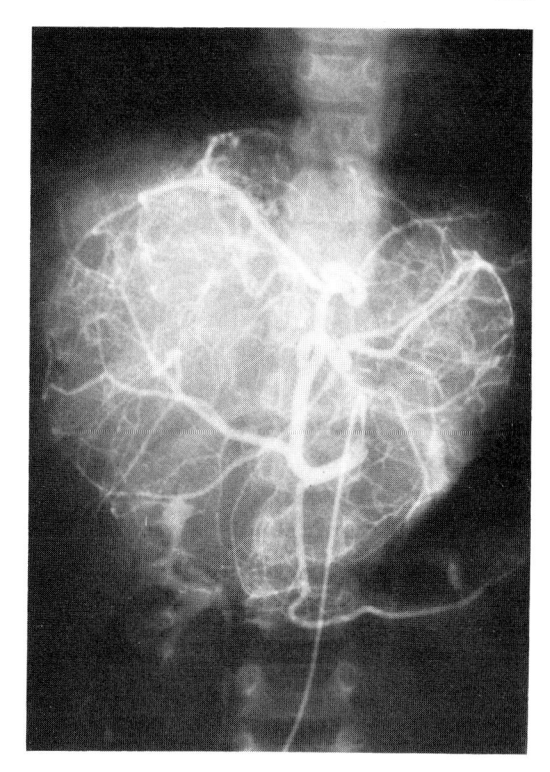

making the diagnosis and determining whether or not a tumor is surgically resectable. The typical angiographic appearance of malignant hepatic tumors in children has been described[22, 28, 56] and is similar to the findings reported in adults.[4, 88] The angiograms demonstrate abnormal neovascularity (Fig. 21-2) and a diffuse parenchymal blush, which persists late into the hepatic venous phase. Feeding arteries appear enlarged and stretched. The contrast medium is usually seen to flow preferentially into the tumor, with only a minimal amount going to the normal portion of the liver.

ASSOCIATED ABNORMALITIES

There is a striking association of cirrhosis with primary liver carcinoma in adults. In one series of 1073 patients with primary carcinomas of the liver, 658 (61.3 per cent) had cirrhosis.[34] In contrast, liver disease almost never accompanies hepatoblastoma in children. It is found in a small but significant number of children with hepatocellular carcinoma. In their study in Japan, Kasai and Watanabe[43] found four of 13 children with hepatocellular carcinoma to have cirrhosis. Among 76 children with liver cancer reported by Fraumeni and co-workers,[26] five had associated liver disease, including two with cirrhosis in early childhood who developed hepatomas at 11 and 13 years of age, one with cirrhosis accompanying the de Toni-Fanconi syndrome, one with a history of neonatal hepatitis, and one with congenital bile duct atresia and biliary cirrhosis. The association of liver cancer with giant cell hepatitis, followed by cirrhosis,[71] congenital biliary atresia,[14, 24, 62] and the de Toni-Fanconi syndrome,[79] has been noted by others.

In addition to the de Toni-Fanconi syndrome, children with other inherited metabolic disorders that result in hepatic damage may develop liver neoplasia, including patients with von Gierke's disease,[52] galactosemia,[16] and the chronic form of hereditary tyrosinemia.[86] Weinberg and colleagues[86] reported that among children with one form of hereditary tyrosinemia who survived beyond 2 years of age, hepatoma developed in 10 of 29 cases with well-documented tyrosinemia and in six of 14 whose diagnoses were presumptive. Death from these tumors occurred between 4 and 35 years of age, and all the patients had cirrhosis. The investigators who reported these findings believe that this extremely high incidence of malignant disease indicates that factors other than cirrhosis are present in the induction of tumors in patients with tyrosinemia.

It has been suggested that the marked array of liver diseases associated with hepatic neoplasms indicate that a variety of hepatic insults—hereditary, environmental, or both—may predispose an individual to develop liver cancer.[26]

Nonhepatic abnormalities have also been reported in association with primary hepatic malignancies. A number of children with hepatoblastoma have had congenital hemihypertrophy,[26, 29, 39, 51] a growth disorder also reported in association with Wilms' tumor, adrenal cortical neoplasms, and focal nodular hyperplasia of the liver.[20] A few children with hepatomas and extensive hemangiomas,[26] renal anomalies,[26] or demineralization of the bone with hypercholesterolemia[26, 35, 82] have also been described. Isosexual precocity has been reported in a number of males with hepatomas,[6, 26, 38, 39, 51] but, rather than being an associated finding, this is related directly to the production of a gonadotropin by the tumor, which stimulates testosterone production by the Leydig cells of the testes. Following tumor removal, the precocious puberty has been seen to regress and the gonadotropins have disappeared from the serum.[38]

A number of children and adults with both acquired and congenital aplastic anemia have developed hepatic carcinomas while receiving C-17 alkylated anabolic androgen therapy.[59] A causal relationship between the androgenic agents and liver cancer is still questioned,[75] because liver neoplasia has not been reported among athletes who use androgenic anabolic steroids, and hepatocellular carcinoma has been reported in at least one patient with Fanconi's anemia who received no androgens but who had severe transfusional hemosiderosis and postnecrotic cirrhosis.[8] In addition, patients with Fanconi's anemia have an increased incidence of leukemia[15] and squamous cell carcinoma,[81] suggesting that their underlying illness may be responsible for the development of the hepatic malignancy rather than the androgen therapy. However, a number of patients taking androgens for disorders other than aplastic anemia have developed hepatocellular carcinoma.[23, 89] In at least three patients the tumors have regressed after drug administration was discontinued.[40, 89] These observations and the fact that the majority of these tumors grow slowly and seldom metastasize have led to the postulation that the tumors are androgen-related but are usually clinically benign.[40, 61, 80] Similar cases have been noted following the use of oral contraceptives,[55] but the majority of tumors have been reported to be histologically benign (see below).

TREATMENT AND PROGNOSIS

The major progress in the treatment of primary hepatic tumors in children has been the result of aggressive surgery. Cure has seldom been achieved unless the tumor is localized to one lobe of the liver, is completely resected, and there is no evidence of extrahepatic spread. The size of the primary tumor does not appear to correlate with survival.[22] In one large

Table 21-2 Excision and Survival in Primary Hepatic Malignancies[22]

	LIVING	DEAD	ALIVE WITH DISEASE
Hepatoblastomas			
Complete excision	45	29	3
Not excised	0	47	2
Hepatocellular Carcinomas			
Complete excision	12	21	0
Not excised	0	61	1

survey, 45 of 77 patients with hepatoblastoma who had complete excision survived, but all 49 patients who had incomplete excision or biopsy alone died or were living but still had the disease at the time of the survey. Of those with hepatocellular carcinoma, 12 of 33 from whom the tumor was excised survived, but none of those survived in whom total removal could not be performed (although one patient was alive with disease at the time of the report) (Table 21-2).[22] The definitive surgical procedures are usually hepatic lobectomy or extended lobectomy. When the tumor is confined to one lobe, the right lobe is more commonly involved. Unfortunately, many tumors involve both lobes or are multicentric and therefore are inoperable. Surgery of the magnitude required to remove all tumor is not without risk; operative and postoperative mortality rates have been reported to range from 15 to 33 per cent.[21, 24, 25, 43] Infants and children tolerate massive liver resection well, and the liver regenerates rapidly to its original volume in a few months.[72] At the present time, liver transplantation following total hepatectomy must still be considered very experimental, and the results to date have not been promising.[78]

Although hepatomas occasionally respond to radiotherapy with a decrease in tumor size,[10] this form of therapy does not totally destroy viable tumor tissue, possibly because of the limited amount of radiation the normal liver can tolerate. Two of seven patients reported by Exelby and coworkers[21] with inoperable tumors treated with radiation therapy alone survived for 2 years, but ultimately expired. The remaining five died within 6 months of the diagnosis.

A number of chemotherapeutic agents have been used in the treatment of liver tumors, including vincristine sulfate, 5-fluorouracil, Adriamycin, methotrexate, cyclophosphamide, chlorambucil, and actinomycin D.[36, 37, 63, 66, 73, 89] There have been isolated reports of tumor regression, but chemotherapeutic cures are extremely rare. One 4 month old child with probable hepatoblastoma reported by Lascari[48] was cured following vincristine therapy. However, in most instances chemotherapy offers only brief palliation at best. In the large series collected by Exelby and associates,[22] there was no evidence that radiation therapy or chemotherapy controlled disease which could not be totally resected. However, neither is there evidence to indicate whether or not additional therapy can prevent clinical recurrence of tumor following total tumor resection by destroying undetectable residual disease. The practice of using adjunctive combination chemotherapy following total tumor resection certainly seems logical, and preliminary reports suggest that such an approach may increase survival.[37] A number of cases have been reported in which initially inoperable tumors could be removed and the patient cured by a second surgical procedure following the use of chemotherapy and radiation therapy, which resulted in a reduction in the size of the tumor.[22, 36, 67]

BENIGN TUMORS

Benign liver tumors may cause significant diagnostic and clinical problems and, not uncommonly, may result in death. It is sometimes difficult, preoperatively, to determine whether or not a liver mass is malignant or benign, and liver function studies seldom help make the distinction. Angiographic studies are usually helpful in making the diagnosis but may not always differentiate between the two.[60] Despite its limitations, angiography is often very useful in localizing the lesion for the surgeon to help determine whether the tumor can be excised. If angiography demonstrates an avascular mass, a benign cyst or hydatid disease is often found at laparotomy. Nonparasitic cysts may sometimes grow to great size before they are diagnosed. Occasionally, the diagnosis may be difficult even at the time of surgery. There have been instances reported of large benign hamartomas that grossly appear malignant,[18] focal nodular hyperplasia misdiagnosed as a hepatoma on frozen section,[18] and a well differentiated carcinoma mistakenly diagnosed as an adenoma.[11]

VASCULAR TUMORS

Hemangiomas and hemangioendotheliomas, the most common benign tumors of the liver, are neoplasms of mesodermal origin. They may be multiple, and often involve extrahepatic organs, such as skin, spleen, and bone. A clear distinction between hemangiomas and hemangioendotheliomas often is not made in the reports of these tumors found in the literature. Histologically, hemangiomas are composed of large vascular structures lined by flat epithelial cells and separated by cellular, fibrous septa. Hemangioendotheliomas have both dilated and compressed vascular spaces lined by one or more layers of thick endothelial cells which can completely fill the vascular spaces. Both histologic types may occur in the same individual or even in the same tissue specimen.[12] It has been proposed that hemangiomas may be one of the regressive pathways for infantile hemangioendotheliomas.[7] These benign neoplasms are not believed to give rise to the extremely rare malignant vascular tumors which may occur in children.

Hepatic hemangiomas in the neonate usually present as an upper abdominal mass, and occasionally may rupture, causing hemoperitoneum and shock.[46] Arteriovenous fistulae within the tumor may result in massive peripheral arteriovenous shunting, with high output congestive heart failure.[68] The classical clinical triad of hepatomegaly, heart failure, and cutaneous hemangiomas should suggest the presence of hemangiomatous involvement of the liver. Unfortunately, cutaneous lesions are not always found, making the diagnosis more difficult.[7] One of the most misleading findings is the presence of cardiac murmurs, which are usually due to excessive blood flow across cardiac valves secondary to the increased cardiac output. However, the size of the liver is often much greater than one would expect from congestive heart failure alone, the enlarged liver often feels nodular, and a bruit may sometimes be heard over the liver. Although these signs strongly suggest an extracardiac etiology as the cause of the congestive failure, the definitive diagnosis is usually made by angiographic studies.

A hemorrhagic diathesis may be associated with giant hemangiomas. This may be secondary to isolated thrombocytopenia or a more profound disturbance in the coagulation system due to intravascular coagulation, with resultant consumption of coagulation factors.[69] The exact mechanism that initiates the coagulopathy is not clearly understood.

Symptomatic hepatic hemangiomas are potentially lethal lesions. Only 10 of 31 infants reported in a review by McLean and co-workers[58] who developed cardiac failure survived. Medical therapy with digitalis and diuretics for congestive heart failure is often ineffective. A number of investigators have advocated the use of a variety of therapeutic modalities, including prednisone, which may cause involution of the hemangiomas,[68] radiation therapy,[65] ligation of the hepatic artery,[13, 54] local excision, and hepatic lobectomy.[33] In contrast to the reports of poor survival noted in many series, Braun and co-workers[7] summarized the histories of seven patients, six of whom survived. Of the four patients in their series who had congestive heart failure, three who were treated conservatively, with medical management alone, survived without the need for radiation therapy or surgery. These authors advocate surgery only if nonsurgical treatment fails and believe that the natural course of spontaneous involution will eventually occur, and the patient will experience cure without being exposed to the risks of surgery.

The problems with diagnosis and treatment of the infant with a vascular tumor of the liver are illustrated by the following case:

A 12 hour old infant was transferred to the Yale-New Haven Hospital with congestive heart failure that was diagnosed soon after birth. The child had marked tachypnea and tachycardia, and the liver edge was palpated 6 cm below the level of the umbilicus. A loud systolic murmur was heard at the base of the heart. No cutaneous hemangiomas were noted, but a vascular bruit was heard over the liver. Because a cardiac lesion was suspected, cardiac catheterization was performed. No intracardiac defect was detected, but a large vascular tumor was discovered in the liver (Fig. 21-3). Following cardiac catheterization the child began to bleed from venipuncture sites. Laboratory values revealed a markedly prolonged partial thromboplastin time and prothrombin time, a low fibrinogen level, thrombocytopenia, and elevated levels of fibrin/fibrinogen degradation products. A diagnosis of intravascular coagulation with resultant consumption of coagulation factors and platelets was made. Heparin therapy was initiated, and within 24 hours there was a marked decrease in bleeding and partial correction of the coagulation studies. Despite the use of digitalis, diuretics, prednisone, and radiation therapy to the liver the clinical condition deteriorated due to the severe congestive heart failure. Hepatic artery ligation was performed while the coagulopathy was controlled with heparin, fresh plasma, and platelets. Although bleeding from the surgical procedure was minimal, the child died within 48 hours of surgery with intractable congestive heart failure. At postmortem examination, a massive hemangioendothelioma of the liver was found. No intracardiac lesion was present.

OTHER BENIGN TUMORS

In addition to hemangiomas and hemangioendotheliomas, a variety of benign hepatic masses have been reported in children. These include hamartomas, adenomas, parasitic and nonparasitic cysts, lymphangiomas, and a number of other uncommon neoplasms (Table 21-3). These tumors seldom lead to a fatal outcome. In one series of 19 children with benign liver tumors and cysts, the only three who did not survive were in the group of eight patients with vascular tumors.[18]

Hamartomas may be fixed or pedunculated masses composed of multiple cysts up to 2 to 3 cm in diameter. They contain large amounts of connective tissue and occasionally have foci of hematopoiesis. The growth of these benign mesenchymal tumors is attributed more to the accumulation of fluid in the cysts than to proliferation of cells.

The origin of nonparasitic cysts is not known. These benign lesions may produce symptoms by pressure on adjacent structures and can be treated by resection or drainage.

Focal nodular hyperplasia grossly resembles a localized area of cirrhosis. The mass may be pedunculated or lie in the liver parenchyma. Localized focal nodular hyperplasia is not uncommon in a cirrhotic liver.

Benign hepatic adenomas are composed of uniform normal or slightly

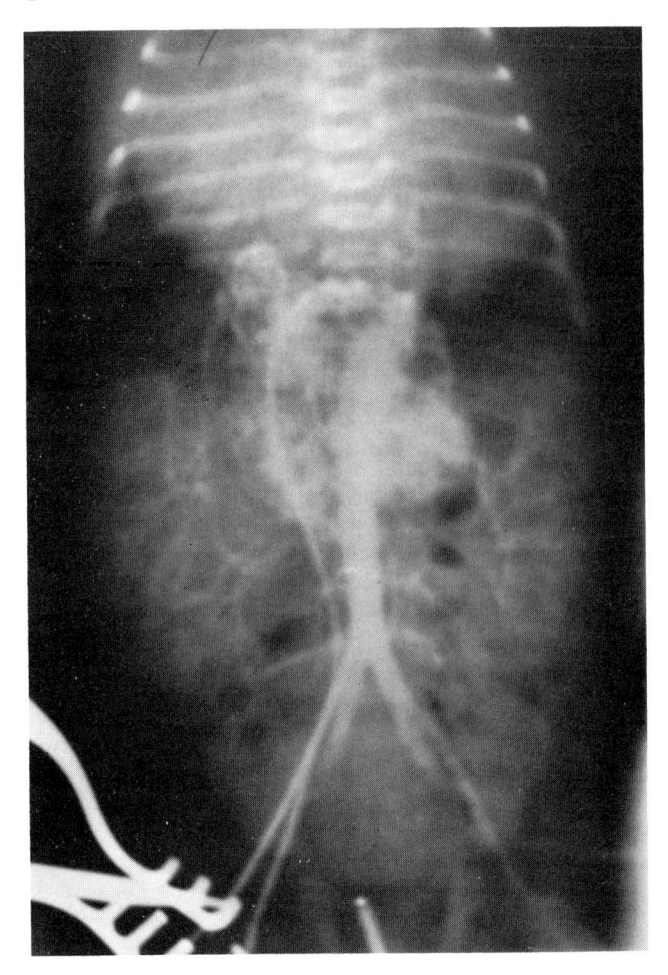

Figure 21-3 Cardiac catheterization performed in a neonate presenting with congestive heart failure. Note the massive size of the heart and evidence of a vascular tumor of the liver. (See text.)

atypical hepatic cells arranged in cords, sometimes forming pseudoacini about secreted and retained bile. There are usually no portal tracts or central veins to suggest the usual portal architecture. These tumors are rare and most of the so-called benign "hepatomas" or adenomas found in cirrhotic livers are actually areas of regenerative nodular hyperplasia.

A number of reports have suggested that the use of oral contraceptive steroids may be related to the development of benign hepatic adenomas, hamartomas, and focal nodular hyperplasia.[3, 5, 17, 55] These tumors may present as an abdominal mass noted by the patient or by the physician during a routine examination. The patient is often asymptomatic but may have upper abdominal pain or discomfort. However, a significant number are first diagnosed following sudden life-threatening intraabdominal hemor-

Table 21-3 Benign Hepatic Tumors (From 1974 Survey of the Surgical Section of the American Academy of Pediatrics[22])

Hemangioma	38
Hamartoma	37
Hemangioendothelioma	16
Adenoma	7
Focal hyperplasia	4
Cholangiohepatoma	1
Epithelial epithelioma	1
Benign cyst	10
Hydatid cyst	6
Eosinophilic granuloma	1
Lymphangioma	2

rhage, which may result in death, and rare cases of hepatocellular carcinoma have been reported following the use of oral contraceptives.[55]

REFERENCES

1. Allison, R. M., and Willis, R. A.: Ossifying embryonic mixed tumor of an infant's liver. J. Pathol. Bacteriol. 72:155, 1956.
2. Alpert, M. E., Hutt, M. S. R., Wogan, G. N., et al.: Association between aflatoxin content of food and hepatoma frequency in Uganda. Cancer 28:253, 1971.
3. Ameriks, J. A., Thompson, N. W., Frey, C. F., et al.: Hepatic cell adenomas, spontaneous liver rupture, and oral contraceptives. Arch. Surg. 110:548, 1975.
4. Bartley, O., Edlund, Y., and Helander, C. G.: Angiography in primary hepatic carcinoma. Acta Radiol. Diag. 6:81, 1967.
5. Baum, J. K., Holtz, F., Bookstein, J. J., et al.: Possible association between benign hepatomas and oral contraceptives. Lancet 2:926, 1973.
6. Behrle, F. C., Mantz, F. A., Jr., Olson, R. L., et al.: Virilization accompanying hepatoblastoma. Pediatrics 29:265, 1963.
7. Braun, P., Ducharme, J. C., Riopelle, J. L., et al.: Hemangiomatosis of the liver in infants. J. Pediatr. Surg. 10:121, 1975.
8. Cattan, D., Vesin, P., Wautier, J., et al.: Liver tumours and steroid therapy. Lancet 1:878, 1974.
9. Clatworthy, H. W., Jr., Boles, E. T., Jr., and Newton, W. A.: Primary tumors of the liver in infants and children. Arch. Dis. Child. 35:22, 1960.
10. Clatworthy, H. W., Jr., Schiller, M., and Grosfeld, J. L.: Primary liver tumors in infancy and childhood: 41 cases variously treated. Arch. Surg. 107:143, 1974.
11. Cleland, R. S.: Benign and malignant tumors of the liver. Pediatr. Clin. North Am. 6:427, 1959.
12. Dehner, L. P., and Ishak, K. G.: Vascular tumors of the liver in infants and children. A study of 30 cases and review of the literature. Arch. Pathol. 92:101, 1971.
13. deLorimier, A. A., Simpson, E. B., Baum, R. S., et al.: Hepatic artery ligation for hepatic hemangiomatosis. N. Engl. J. Med. 277:333, 1967.
14. Deoras, M. P., and Dicus, W.: Hepatocarcinoma associated with biliary cirrhosis. A case due to congenital bile duct atresia. Arch. Path. 86:338, 1968.
15. Dosik, H., Hsu, L. Y., Todaro, G. J., et al.: Leukemia in Fanconi's anemia: cytogenetic and tumor virus susceptibility studies. Blood 36:341, 1970.
15a. Edling, C. J.: Tumor imaging in children. Cancer 38:921, 1976.
16. Edmonds, A. M., Hennigar, G. R., and Crooks, R.: Galactosemia: report of case with autopsy. Pediatrics 10:40, 1952.
17. Edmondson, H. A., Henderson, B., and Benton, B.: Liver-cell adenomas associated with the use of oral contraceptives. N. Engl. J. Med. 294:470, 1976.
18. Ein, S. H., and Stephens, C. A.: Benign liver tumors and cysts in childhood. J. Pediatr. Surg. 9:847, 1974.
19. el-Domeri, A. A., Huvos, A. G., Goldsmith, H. S., et al.: Primary malignant tumors of the liver. Cancer 27:7, 1971.
20. Everson, R. B., Museles, M., Henson, D. E., et al.: Focal nodular hyperplasia of the liver in a child with hemihypertrophy. J. Pediatr. 88:985, 1976.
21. Exelby, P. R., el-Domeri, A., Huvos, A. G., et al.: Primary malignant tumors of the liver in children. J. Pediatr. Surg. 6:272, 1971.
22. Exelby, P. R., Filler, R. M., and Grosfeld, J. L.: Liver tumors in children in particular reference to hepatoblastoma and hepatocellular carcinoma: American Academy of Pediatrics Surgical Section survey. J. Pediatr. Surg. 10:329, 1975.
23. Farrell, G. G., Joshua, D. E., Uren, R. F., et al.: Androgen-induced hepatoma. Lancet 1:430, 1975.
24. Fish, J. C., and McCary, R. G.: Primary cancer of the liver in childhood. Arch. Surg. 93:355, 1966.
25. Foster, J. H.: Survival after liver resection for cancer. Cancer 26:493, 1970.
26. Fraumeni, J. F., Jr., Miller, R. W., and Hill, J. A.: Primary carcinoma of the liver in childhood: an epidemiologic study. J. Natl. Cancer Inst. 40:1087, 1968.
27. Fraumeni, J. F., Jr., Rosen, P. J., Hull, E. W., et al.: Hepatoblastoma in infant sisters. Cancer 24:1086, 1969.
28. Fredens, M.: Angiography in primary hepatic tumors in children. Acta Radiol. Diag. 8:193, 1969.
29. Geiser, C. F., Baez, A., Schindler, A. M., et al.: Epithelial hepatoblastoma associated with congenital hemihypertrophy and cystathioninuria: presentation of a case. Pediatrics 46:66, 1970.
30. Geiser, C. F., and Efron, M. L.: Cystathioninuria in patients with neuroblastoma and ganglioneuroblastoma. Cancer 22:856, 1968.
31. Gjessing, L. R., and Mauritzen, K.: Cystathioninuria in hepatoblastoma. Scand. J. Clin. Lab. Invest. 17:513, 1965.
32. Goldman, R. L., and Friedman, N. B.: Rhabdomyosarcohepatoma in an adult and embryonal hepatoma in a child. Am. J. Clin. Pathol. 51:137, 1969.

33. Graivier, L., Votteler, P., and Dorman, G. W.: Hepatic hemangiomas in newborn infants. J. Pediatr. Surg. 2:299, 1967.
34. Greene, J. M.: Primary carcinoma of the liver. A ten-year collective review. Int. Abstr. Surg. 69:231, 1939.
35. Hansen, A. E., Ziegler, M. R., and McQuarrie, I.: Disturbances of osseous and lipid metabolism in a child with primary carcinoma of the liver. J. Pediatr. 17:9, 1940.
36. Hermann, R. E., and Lonsdale, D.: Chemotherapy, radiotherapy, and hepatic lobectomy for hepatoblastoma in an infant: report of a survival. Surgery 68:383, 1970.
37. Holton, C. P., Burrington, J. D., and Hatch, E. I.: A multiple chemotherapeutic approach to the management of hepatoblastoma. A preliminary report. Cancer 35:1083, 1975.
38. Hung, W., Blizzard, R. M., Migeon, C. J., et al.: Precocious puberty in a boy with hepatoma and circulating gonadotropin. J. Pediatr. 63:895, 1963.
39. Ishak, K. G., and Glunz, P. R.: Hepatoblastoma and hepatocarcinoma in infancy and childhood: reports of 47 cases. Cancer 20:396,1967.
40. Johnson, F. L., Feagler, J. R., Lerner, K. G., et al.: Association of androgenic-anabolic steroid therapy with development of hepatocellular carcinoma. Lancet 2:1273, 1972.
41. Jones, E.: Primary carcinoma of the liver with associated cirrhosis in infants and children. Arch. Path. 70:5, 1960.
42. Kasai, M., Kimura, S., and Watanabe, I.: Primary carcinoma of the liver in infancy and childhood. Z. Kinderchirurg. 4:347, 1967.
43. Kasai, M., and Watanabe, I.: Histologic classification of liver-cell carcinoma in infancy and childhood and its clinical evaluation: a study of 70 cases collected in Japan. Cancer 25:551, 1970.
44. Kauffman, S. L., and Stout, A. P.: Malignant hemangioendothelioma in infants and children. Cancer 14:1186, 1961.
45. Keeling, J. W.: Liver tumours in infancy and childhood. J. Pathol. 103:69, 1971.
46. Kissinger, C. C., Sternfeld, E., and Zuker, S. D.: Rupture of a cavernous hemangioma of the liver as a cause of death in a newborn infant. Ohio State Med. J. 36:383, 1940.
47. Kohn, J., and Weaver, P. C.: Serum alpha$_1$-fetoprotein in hepatocellular carcinoma. Lancet 2:334, 1974.
48. Lascari, A. D.: Vincristine therapy in an infant with probable hepatoblastoma. Pediatrics 42:109, 1968.
49. Lee, F. I., and Harry, D. S.: Angiosarcoma of the liver in a vinyl-chloride worker. Lancet 1:1316, 1974.
50. Lin, T., Chen, C., and Lui, W.: Primary carcinoma of the liver in infancy and childhood: report of 21 cases with resection in 6 cases. Surgery 60:1275, 1966.
51. MacNab, G. H., Moncrieff, A. A., and Bodian, M.: Primary malignant hepatic tumours in childhood. British Empire Cancer Campaign Ann. Rep. 30:168, 1952.
52. Mason, H. H., and Anderson, D. H.: Glycogen disease of the liver (von Gierke's disease) with hepatoma: case report with metabolic studies. Pediatrics 16:785, 1955.
53. Matsumoto, Y., Suzuki, T., Ono, H., et al.: Response of alpha-fetoprotein to chemotherapy in patients with hepatomas. Cancer 34:1602, 1974.
54. Mattioli, L., Lee, K. R., and Holder, T. M.: Hepatic artery ligation for cardiac failure due to hepatic hemangioma in the newborn. J. Pediatr. Surg. 9:859, 1974.
55. Mays, E. T., Christopherson, W. M., Mahr, M. M., et al.: Hepatic changes in young women ingesting contraceptive steroids. J.A.M.A. 235:730, 1976.
56. McDonald, P.: Hepatic tumors in childhood. Clin. Radiol. 18:74, 1967.
57. McIntire, K. R., Vogel, C. L., Primack, A., et al.: Effect of surgical and chemotherapeutic treatment on alpha-fetoprotein levels in patients with hepatocellular carcinoma. Cancer 37:677, 1976.
58. McLean, R. H., Moller, J. H., Warwick, W. J., et al.: Multinodular hemangiomatosis of the liver in infancy. Pediatrics 49:563, 1972.
59. Meadows, A. T., Naimain, J. L., and Valdes-Dapéna, M.: Hepatoma associated with androgen therapy for aplastic anemia. J. Pediatr. 84:110, 1974.
60. Moss, A. A., Clark, R. E., Palubinskas, A. J., et al.: Angiographic appearance of benign and malignant hepatic tumors in infants and children. Am. J. Roentgenol. Radium Ther. Nucl. Med. 113:61, 1971.
61. Mulvihill, J. J., Ridolfi, R. L., Schultz, F. R., et al.: Hepatic adenoma in Fanconi anemia treated with oxymetholone. J. Pediatr. 87:122, 1975.
62. Okuyama, K.: Primary liver cell carcinoma associated with biliary cirrhosis due to congenital bile duct atresia. J. Pediatr. 67:89, 1965.
63. Olweny, C. L. M., Toya, T., Katongole-Mbidde, E., et al.: Treatment of hepatocellular carcinoma with Adriamycin: Preliminary communication. Cancer 36:1250, 1975.
64. Pang, L. S. C.: Bony and cartilaginous hepatoblastoma. J. Pathol. Bacteriol. 82:273, 1961.
65. Park, W. C., and Phillips, R.: The role of radiation therapy in the management of hemangiomas of the liver. J.A.M.A. 212:1496, 1970.

66. Pratt, C., Jones, D., Holton, C., et al.: Combination therapy including vincristine (MSC-67574) for malignant solid tumors in children. Cancer Chemother. Rep. 52:489, 1968.
67. Remischovsky, J., Schnaufer, L., and Gloebl, H.: Treatment of primary liver tumors. Semin. Oncol. 1:65, 1974.
68. Rocchini, A. P., Rosenthal, A., Issenberg, H. J., et al.: Hepatic hemangioendothelioma: hemodynamic observations and treatment. Pediatrics 57:131, 1976.
69. Rodriguez-Erdmann, F., Button, L., Murray, J. E., et al.: Kasabach-Merritt syndrome: coagulo-analytical observations. Am. J. Med. Sci. 261:9, 1971.
70. Ross, P.: Calcification in liver metastases from neuroblastoma. Radiology 85:1074, 1965.
71. Roth, D., and Duncan, P. A.: Primary carcinoma of the liver after giant-cell hepatitis of infancy. Cancer 8:986, 1955.
72. Samuels, L. D., and Grosfeld, J. L.: Serial scans of liver regeneration after hemihepatectomy in children. Surg. Gynec. Obstet. 131:453, 1970.
73. Selawry, O. S., Holland, J. F., and Wolman, I. J.: Effect of vincristine (NSC-67574) on malignant solid tumors in children. Cancer Chemother. Rep. 52:497, 1968.
74. Shanmugaratnam, K., and Tye, C. Y.: Liver cancer differentials in immigrant and local born Chinese in Singapore. J. Chron. Dis. 23:443, 1970.
75. Silverman, F. N., D'Angio, G. J., Ertel, I. J., et al.: Is liver cancer induced by treating aplastic anemia with androgenic agents? Pediatrics 53:764, 1974.
76. Sinniah, D., Campbell, P. E., and Colebatch, J. H.: Primary hepatic cancer in infancy and childhood: a survey of 20 cases. Progr. Pediatr. Surg. 7:141, 1974.
77. Stanley, R. J., Dehner, L. P., and Hesker, A. E.: Primary malignant mesenchymal tumors (mesenchymoma) of the liver in childhood. Cancer 32:973, 1973.
78. Starzl, T. E., Brettschneidner, L., Penn, I., et al.: Clinical liver transplantation. Transplant. Rev. 2:3, 1969.
79. Stowers, J. M., and Dent, C. E.: Studies on the mechanism of the Fanconi syndrome. Quart. J. Med. 16:275, 1947.
80. Sweeney, E. C., and Evans, D. J.: Liver lesions and androgenic steroid therapy. Lancet 2:1042, 1975.
81. Swift, M., Zimmerman, D., and McDonough, E. R.: Squamous cell carcinomas in Fanconi's anemia. J.A.M.A. 216:325, 1971.
82. Teng, C. T., Daeschner, C. W., Jr., Singleton, E. B., et al.: Liver disease and osteoporosis in children. J. Pediatr. 59:684, 1961.
83. Tonami, N., Aburano, T., and Hisada, K.: Comparison of alpha$_1$-fetoprotein radioimmunoassay method and liver scanning for detecting primary hepatic cell carcinoma. Cancer 36:466, 1975.
84. von Felten, A., Straub, P. W., and Frick, P. G.: Dysfibrinogenemia in a patient with primary hepatoma. N. Engl. J. Med. 280:405, 1969.
85. Waxman, S., and Gilbert, H. S.: A tumor-related vitamin B$_{12}$ binding protein in adolescent hepatoma. N. Engl. J. Med. 289:1053, 1973.
86. Weinberg, A. G., Mize, C. E., and Worthen, H. G.: The occurrence of hepatoma in the chronic form of hereditary tyrosinemia. J. Pediatr. 88:434, 1976.
86a. Williams, A. O.: Tumors of childhood in Ibadan, Nigeria. Cancer 36:370, 1975.
87. Young, J. L., and Miller, R. W.: Incidence of malignant tumors in U.S. children J. Pediatr. 86:254, 1975.
88. Yu, C.: Primary carcinoma of the liver (hepatoma): its diagnosis by selective celiac arteriography. Am. J. Roentgenol. Radium Ther. Nuclear Med. 99:142, 1967.
89. Ziegenfuss, J., and Carabasi, R.: Androgens and hepatocellular carcinoma. Lancet 1:

Chapter Twenty-Two

TUMORS OF THE GASTROINTESTINAL TRACT

Cancer of the gastrointestinal tract is very uncommon in children. Therefore, the diagnosis is seldom considered when early, nonspecific symptoms occur and the possibility of surgical cure exists. Although malignant gastrointestinal disease rarely develops during the first two decades of life, a number of premalignant lesions occur in children. For these reasons the pediatrician should be aware of the existence of malignant gastrointestinal tumors in children, and the more common associated lesions and predisposing factors which often present during the childhood years.

THE ESOPHAGUS

Esophageal tumors, the majority of which are benign, are extremely rare in children. Most polypoid tumors occur in the upper third of the esophagus and are usually lipomas, hamartomas, or myxofibromas.[34] One review of benign esophageal tumors and cysts revealed that the lesions in children were usually intramural cysts, while solid intramural and polypoid intraluminal tumors were seldom diagnosed during the first two decades of life.[84]

Smooth muscle tumors of the esophagus are rarely encountered in children.[98] One case of a submucosal leiomyoma involving the entire esophagus was treated by excision and later replacement with a segment of colon.[59] A review by Moore[57] described only one case of esophageal squamous cell carcinoma occurring in a child. Esophageal leukemic infiltrates, however, are not uncommon, but usually these are asymptomatic. Sometimes they have caused dysphagia and chest pain, symptoms which are usually relieved by radiation therapy.[2]

Achalasia, a motor abnormality of the esophagus characterized by failure of the lower esophageal sphincter to relax with swallowing, may be associated with an increased incidence of esophageal carcinoma later in adult life.[45] The occasional occurrence of carcinoma in achalasia has been attributed to chronic irritation resulting from stagnant food within the esophageal lumen. However, Williams found that in carcinoma of the esophagus complicating achalasia of the cardia, the tumor was found in the middle third of the esophagus in 80 per cent of cases and in the lower third in only 7.7 per cent.[94] Esophageal stricture as a result of lye burns appears to predispose to the later development of esophageal cancer in 3.5 to 5 per cent of patients.[8, 45] The usual latent period between the original stricture formation and the malignant transformation is at least 20 years. Esophageal carcinoma often occurs in patients with sideropenic dysphagia (Plummer-Vinson syndrome or Paterson-Kelly syndrome), a disorder characterized by atrophy of the mucous membranes of the mouth and pharynx, and stenoses or webs of the upper esophageal mucosa.[26, 45] This condition, usually reported in middle-aged women, is thought to be the result of severe, chronic, iron-deficiency anemia in which mucous membranes generally show degeneration and inflammatory changes. There is at present no evidence that iron deficiency during the childhood and adolescent years, even when associated with the symptoms of esophagitis, predisposes to the later development of esophageal cancer.

THE STOMACH

Although they are more frequent than neoplasms of the esophagus, tumors of the stomach in children are still uncommon and are usually the subjects of single case reports. Benign tumors include carcinoids, hemangiopericytomas, glomus tumors, lymphangiomas, lipomas, neurofibromas, eosinophilic granulomas, teratomas, inflammatory and adenomatous polyps, ectopic pancreatic tissue, and leiomyomas.[29, 48] The differential diagnosis prior to surgery should also include bezoars, gastric duplications, and foreign body granulomas.

Gastric teratomas are found mainly in infants, although rare cases have been reported in adults.[33] Of the 32 tumors reported to date, all have occurred in males.[51, 60] These large tumors in the neonate may cause the mother to have premature labor or dystocia. The usual finding is a left upper quadrant mass. Other signs and symptoms include respiratory difficulty, vomiting, or hemorrhage. Roentgenograms of the abdomen often demonstrate calcifications due to the bony structures within the tumor. The tumors are benign, and the prognosis after excision or partial gastrectomy is excellent. One case, diagnosed when the infant was 6 hours of age, involved the entire stomach; this was treated by total gastrectomy and the patient was reported to be doing well at the age of 2 years.[17]

A review of the world literature by Wurlitzer and co-workers[96] of gastric smooth muscle tumors in children and adolescents revealed only 34 cases, 14 of which were believed to be benign and 20 malignant. Roentgenographic findings were of little value in distinguishing benign from malignant tumors. The most common presentations were due to gastrointestinal bleeding, as manifested by hematemesis, melena, hematochezia, or anemia. Bleeding occurred in 88 per cent of malignant cases and 85 per cent of benign ones. The authors stressed the fact that interpretation of microscopic pathology of this group of tumors was often inaccurate in view of the subsequent clinical course. This was illustrated by one of their own cases and by a previous report of a 3½ year old girl with a tumor judged initially to be benign.[98] Over a year after the original diagnosis the latter child developed progressive jaundice and was found to have a large leiomyosarcoma diffusely infiltrating the liver.[76] Of particular interest was the fact that a review by 113 pathologists in preparation for a cancer seminar led to 52 diagnoses of leiomyoma and only 15 of the leiomyosarcoma.[76] Because of the difficulty in determining whether these tumors are benign or malignant, especially by frozen-section examination, it has been recommended that a wide resection or subtotal gastrectomy be done.[96] When a subtotal or more radical surgical procedure was employed in those with malignant disease eight of nine patients were alive at 1 year and four of five whose follow-up data were available were alive at 5 years.[96]

Carney and associates[10a] reported an association of multiple gastric leiomyosarcomas, functioning extraadrenal paragangliomas, and pulmonary chondromas in females between the ages of 12 and 24 years. Their four cases all had evidence of excessive production of pressor amines. The authors noted three previously reported cases in girls between the ages of 12 and 20 years and expressed the belief that the association of this triad of uncommon tumors constitutes a new syndrome.

Carcinoma of the stomach is an extremely rare neoplasm during the childhood years. A review of the records of the Mayo Clinic from 1935 to 1973 revealed no cases in patients under 16 years of age.[43] McNeer's review of the literature published in 1941 of 501 cases of gastric cancer in patients under the age of 30 years uncovered one case of adenocarcinoma in a child less than 5 years of age, one in the 6 to 10 year age group, and 17 cases in persons between the ages of 11 and 15 years.[53] Subsequently, a small number of well-documented cases have been reported in children, most of whom have been over 10 years of age. Few cases have been recorded during the first decade of life, the youngest patient being a 10 day old infant.[15]

There is evidence that immunologic deficiency diseases not only predispose to the development of leukemia and lymphoreticular malignancies but also sometimes may play a role in the development of gastric carcinoma. Adenocarcinoma of the stomach occurs with an increased frequency in individuals with isolated IgA deficiency and other primary immunodeficient states,[23, 24] including children with common variable immunodeficiency[78] and ataxia-telangiectasia.[37, 81]

Gastric malignancy often presents with symptoms similar to those of a benign gastric ulcer. Since gastric ulcers are also rare in this age group, it has been suggested that any child beyond the first few years of life with an apparent primary gastric ulcer have the same diagnostic evaluation that would be given an adult.[19] Treatment of adenocarcinoma of the stomach has included surgery and various chemotherapeutic regimens, but too few reports are available for children to suggest any therapeutic programs different from those now used for adults.

THE SMALL INTESTINE

The most common malignant tumors of the small intestine in childhood are the non-Hodgkin's lymphomas. These neoplasms are discussed in Chapter 10. All other malignant diseases arising in the small bowel are rare. A small number of leiomyosarcomas and angiosarcomas have been reported in children,[25, 56, 69, 91] and a number of cases of adenocarcinoma of the small intestine have occurred in adults following chronic regional enteritis, which often had its onset in childhood.[61, 88] It has been suggested that the immunosuppressive action of corticosteroid treatment for the enteritis may have played some role in the production of this neoplasm.[88] To date, no small bowel carcinoma has appeared in a patient with regional enteritis under the age of 21 years.

Carcinoid tumors, or argentaffinomas, occasionally occur in children. They arise from the chromargentaffin cells (Kultschitzky cells) which are normally present from the cardia of the stomach to the anus. These tumors usually occur within the appendix in children. They often present as an acute appendicitis and are found incidentally in the examination of the pathologic specimens. The tumor usually is found as a small nodule in the distal portion of the appendix, but it may occur proximally, occlude the lumen, and produce obstructive appendicitis.[31] The great majority of appendiceal carcinoid tumors occur in females.[30, 70] Most are small and show no recurrence following appendectomy, regardless of size, depth of invasion, or presence of perineural involvement.[70] Metastases from a carcinoid tumor of the appendix are rare.

Extra-appendiceal carcinoid tumors in children are very uncommon. They appear to occur about equally in frequency in males and females. Most occur within the ileum, but tumors have been reported to occur in the jejunum, stomach, and in a Meckel's diverticulum.[9, 30] Those which arise in the small bowel may present with intestinal obstruction or intussusception. Multiple carcinoids are sometimes observed and are believed to be multifocal primary tumors rather than the result of local metastases from a single tumor.[68] Carcinoids arising outside of the appendix, however, may metastasize to regional lymph nodes, the liver, and other distant sites. When hepatic metastases occur, the malignant carcinoid syndrome may result. Manifestations of this syndrome include a peculiar patchy cyanosis, transient vasodilatation of the skin, tachycardia, hyperperistalsis, frequent watery stools, asthma, and valvular disease of the right side of the heart.[68] The syndrome is believed to be the result of excessive tumor production of serotonin (5-hydroxytryptamine). When this occurs, elevated levels of serotonin in the blood or elevated excretion of its metabolite, 5-hydroxyindolacetic acid (5-HIAA) in the urine can be demonstrated. The carcinoid syndrome has been reported in children.[6, 9, 30]

Because of the rarity of metastasis from appendiceal carcinoid tumors in children, appendectomy and search of the bowel for other primary tumors is all that is indicated. When a tumor of the small intestine is found, more extensive excision of the small bowel has been suggested.[44] A preoperative diagnosis is rarely made in children, however, and a definite diagnosis is seldom made before there is a final pathologic report.

Carcinoid tumors grow slowly. Some patients have had a history of symptoms of carcinoid syndrome for years before the correct diagnosis was made. Even if inoperable metastases are present at surgery, the patient may live for many years.[68] Metastatic carcinoid tumors are generally resistant to radiation therapy, and there is little evidence that chemotherapy is of benefit.[12]

Benign tumors of the small intestine include adenomas, hemangiomas, lymphangiomas, and leiomyomas. More than half of all duplications of the gastrointestinal tract involve the small intestine and may present with symptoms indistinguishable from those of a neoplasm.[48] Other conditions that may simulate malignant growths include lymphoid hyperplasia of the ileum, with pseudopolyposis caused by hyperplasia of follicles in the mucosa and submucosa, regional enteritis, or a chronic inflammatory infectious process, such as tuberculosis.

THE COLON AND RECTUM

Malignant diseases of the large bowel are uncommon in children; they include malignant lymphomas (Chapter 10), leiomyosarcomas,[98] and carcinomas. Despite the fact that the incidence of large bowel malignancy in the United States is higher than that for any other site after skin cancer,[67] only 1 per cent of malignant tumors of the large intestine arise in persons under 30 years of age.[40] A number of conditions predispose to the development of colorectal carcinoma, including ulcerative colitis, regional enteritis, various inherited polyposis syndromes (discussed below), and, rarely, nodular lymphoid hyperplasia.[3] Carcinoma of the colon may sometimes aggregate in families who do not have one of the inherited syndromes associated with polyps, but the disease seldom presents during the first two decades of life.[55]

In 1971, Devroede and associates reported a marked increased risk of colorectal cancer in patients with ulcerative colitis that began in childhood.[18] Thirty-five years after the onset of symptoms, the incidence of carcinoma was 43 per cent. Those at greatest risk had colitis that began between 5 and 9 years of age and had pancolitis by the end of the second decade. In these patients there was a cancer risk of 20 per cent per decade after the first 10 years of disease and a similar increase in the mortality rate. The sexes were equally affected. Proctocolectomy appeared to protect against the high mortality rate.

Cancer seldom develops in patients who have had ulcerative colitis less than 10 years and is therefore not commonly seen during childhood. Carcinoma developed in only 3 per cent of Devroede's patients during the first 10 years of disease.[18] Thus, one of the indications for surgical intervention in patients with ulcerative colitis is 10 years of continuous symptoms or relapses, even when symptoms have not been severe. A small number of patients with ulcerative colitis, however, have developed carcinoma during the second decade of life.[93] Some have advocated earlier surgical intervention to increase survival apart from the long-term complication of malignancy.[24] Total colectomy and proctectomy with ileostomy is usually considered to be the operation of choice.[63]

There is also evidence that there is an increase in the incidence of colonic and rectal cancer in patients with Crohn's disease of the colon.[62, 90] The incidence is not as high, however, as in patients with ulcerative colitis. Weedon and co-workers have documented a 20-fold increase in colorectal cancer when the disease had its onset at 21 years of age or younger.[90]

Although colorectal cancer in young people is rare and may be a complication of inflammatory bowel disease or inherited polyposis syndromes, most cases in children still arise in individuals with no evidence of underlying disease. Probably fewer than 200 cases have been reported, with the great majority occurring in adolescents. A review of carcinoma of the colon in children up to 15 years of age by Andersson and Bergdahl revealed only 10 of 81 patients to be under 10 years of age.[4] Pickett and Briggs determined that about 5 per cent of cases occurred in children under the age of 5 years, 15 per cent occurred between 5 and 10 years of age, and the remainder occurred between 10 and 16 years of age.[63] The youngest reported patient was a 9 month old infant.[46] The disease is twice as common in males than in females, while in adults the sex distribution is equal.

The anatomic distribution of colon carcinoma in children is the same as that observed in adults.[4] Abdominal pain and vomiting are the most common presenting symptoms. When the tumor is located in the rectum, rectal bleeding is the first and most frequent symptom, and abdominal pain is the next most common complaint. Frankly obstructing lesions seldom occur, although incomplete obstruction is often found at surgery.[63] The preoperative diagnosis in many cases has been acute appendicitis,[4, 63] and occasionally in such cases the carcinoma of the colon is not detected at the initial operation.[4, 77] Rarely, carcinoma of the colon may manifest itself as intussusception.[28]

About 50 per cent of adenocarcinomas of the large bowel found in children are mucinous adenocarcinomas,[54] which are highly invasive malignancies that metastasize early.

Fewer than 5 per cent of colorectal carcinomas in adults are of this histologic type. The overall 5-year survival rate of 79 childhood cases reviewed by Andersson and Bergdahl was 2.5 per cent,[4] a figure much lower than that for adults. This poor prognosis is probably due to the fact that the majority of tumors in young patients are poorly differentiated, highly malignant, mucus-forming adenocarcinomas. In addition, the diagnosis is usually made late because of the rarity of the tumor and the nonspecific nature of the symptoms.

Radical surgical excision is indicated, but often the surgeon can only perform a palliative procedure because of extensive tumor spread. There is controversy regarding the potential usefulness of adjuvant chemotherapy in large bowel cancer in adults, but there is evidence that some patients, including children, may benefit from 5-fluorouracil.[11, 20]

GASTROINTESTINAL POLYPS

The most common tumors of the gastrointestinal tract in children are benign, juvenile polyps. Some believe these lesions to be the result of chronic inflammation, whereas others consider them to be hamartomas. They occur more commonly in males than in females and account for over 90 per cent of intestinal polyps in children. Eighty-five per cent are solitary and 90 per cent are located in the rectum or sigmoid colon.[47] There is usually no evidence of genetic transmission. The majority of patients have symptoms during the first decade of life, usually between the ages of 3 and 6 years. The most frequent presenting symptom is painless rectal bleeding, which may sometimes recur for months or even years before the diagnosis is made. Intussusception occasionally may result, and, in some, there is a history of cramping abdominal pain. Not infrequently, a polyp may prolapse and protrude through the anus.

Most polyps lying below the sigmoid flexure can be visualized and removed through the sigmoidoscope. There is some disagreement regarding indications for surgical removal of polyps beyond the reach of the sigmoidoscope. Some have recommended that they be removed once discovered to prevent future complications,[42] but others feel that these polyps need not be removed immediately because of their benign clinical course and excellent prognosis. The polyps often undergo spontaneous auto-amputation.[80] Gryboski has suggested watchful waiting for a year and elective polypectomy through a colonoscope or by surgical colostomy if the polyp remains and symptoms persist.[35]

A number of other benign tumors of the large intestine occur much less frequently than juvenile polyps. These include lipomas, lymphangiomas, hemangiomas, and leiomyomas.[48] Patients with von Recklinghausen's disease occasionally have neurofibromas or leiomyomas involving the stomach, small bowel, or colon.[41] Sarcomatous degeneration has been reported to occur in the gastrointestinal tumors of these patients.

Ulcerative colitis and Crohn's disease of the colon may sometimes manifest roentgenographically as localized tumor-like lesions of the colon.[50] Because patients with these disorders are at higher risk than the general population for developing colonic cancer, these polypoid lesions are likely to be mistaken for a malignancy and may require biopsy to avoid unnecessary extensive surgery.

The Cronkhite-Canada syndrome, a rare disorder usually described in adults, includes gastrointestinal polyposis, alopecia, nail dystrophy, cutaneous hyperpigmentation, malabsorption, and electrolyte imbalance.[14] The polyps are benign and no patients described have had affected relatives.

In addition to these disorders, a

number of familial gastrointestinal polyposis syndromes exist. Some of these disorders have a very high incidence of malignant degeneration and are discussed in detail below.

FAMILIAL POLYPOSIS COLI

Familial polyposis of the colon is transmitted as an autosomal dominant disorder and is the most common of the inherited forms of intestinal polyposis. The incidence in the general population has been estimated to be about 1 in 8300 births.[66] About 20 per cent of cases appear to be the first in their families to be affected. This may be the result of a new mutation, incomplete penetrance, in which a generation is skipped, or inadequate evaluation of seemingly unaffected persons.[27] A history of individuals who have died of what was diagnosed as tuberculous enteritis or other forms of chronic intestinal disease is frequent in affected families,[52] indicating that the diagnosis may often be missed.

The polyps are usually limited to the colon and rectum. There have been occasional reports that gastric polyps occur in this syndrome.[39, 87] The polyps are adenomas which vary from a few scattered lesions to hundreds or thousands (Fig. 22–1). Sometimes the colon is so densely covered that no normal mucosa can be seen. Polyps usually appear in the colon at an average of about 24 years, produce symptoms at about 33 years, and are diagnosed at about 36 years.[27] The lesions are clearly precancerous, and over 80 per cent of untreated patients develop adenocarcinoma of the colon. It is probable that all untreated patients eventually would develop colon carcinoma if followed for a long enough time.[27] The majority of cases develop colon cancer by the age of 40 years, and multiple primary cancers are often present. Polyps usually do not appear before the age of 10 years, but several cases have been diagnosed during the first decade of life. Polyps have developed as early as 4 months of age.[36] Abramson noted that, of 75 children with this disease who were under 14 years of age, four already had malignant changes at the time of the initial diagnosis.[1] Malignant change may occur as early as 9 years of age.[66]

Diarrhea and rectal bleeding occur in most patients, and some have a history of abdominal pain. Sometimes there may be no symptoms. Intussusception or obstruction seldom occur unless there is evidence of cancer.

Siblings and offspring of patients should be studied periodically by sigmoidoscopy and barium enema in an effort to make a diagnosis prior to malignant change. Once a diagnosis is established, some have advised total proctocolectomy and ileostomy to remove all of the area which may undergo malignant change. Total colectomy with ileorectal anastomosis now is considered by many to be the treatment of choice because the rate of cancer in the rectum has been low. If the rectal stump is retained, it should be examined periodically. There are a number of reports of spontaneous regression of residual rectal polyps after colectomy and ileorectal anastomosis.[79, 95] The Soave technique, a procedure involving dissection and excision of the rectal mucosa, leaves a muscular tunnel that can be used in conjunction with total colectomy and attachment of the terminal ileum inside the rectal musculature and the sphincters.[73]

In addition to surgical treatment, it is important that affected families receive genetic counseling, because each child of a parent with the disease has a 50 per cent chance of inheriting the disorder.

GARDNER SYNDROME[27, 92]

The Gardner syndrome is an autosomal dominant disorder consisting of soft tissue and bone abnormalities associated with multiple intestinal polyps. It occurs in 1 of every 14,025

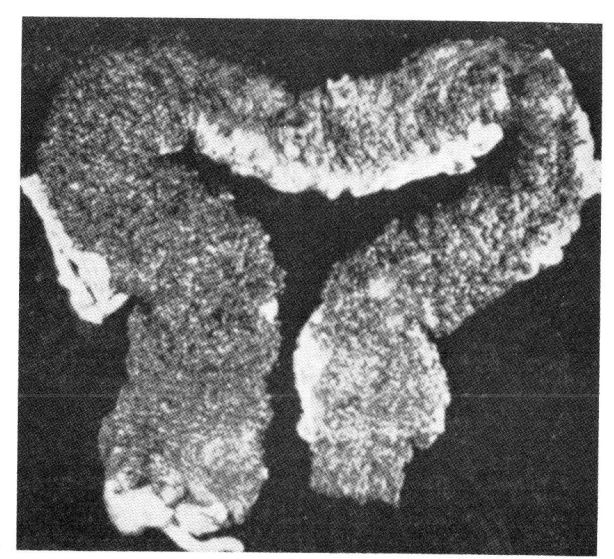

Figure 22-1 A, Multiple polyps densely covering the mucosa of the colon resected from a patient with familial polyposis coli. B, Detail of same specimen. (From McKusick, V. A.: J.A.M.A. *182*:272, 1962.)

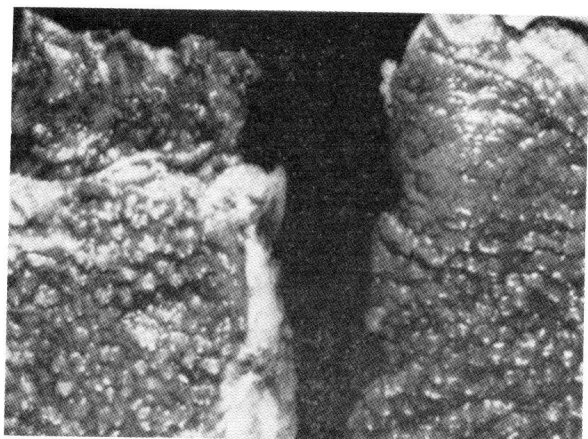

births.[64] The soft tissue abnormalities include sebaceous cysts, desmoid tumors, epidermal cysts, lipomas, and fibromatosis. The bone lesions consist of exostoses and osteomas, most often involving the mandible and resulting in dental problems (Fig. 22-2). The maxilla, orbit, calvarium, pelvis, and long bones also may be involved. Cortical thickening may occur in the long tubular bones and ribs. The intestinal polyps are adenomas which have a tendency to undergo malignant change. The number and distribution of the polyps and the mean age of both onset of symptoms and diagnosis of the intestinal tumors are similar to those described for patients with familial polyposis coli (Fig. 22-3.). The recommended surgical treatment is also the same. However, polyps that undergo malignant change may occur in areas of the gastrointestinal tract that are not usually involved in patients with familial polyposis coli. A roentgenographic examination of the upper gastrointestinal tract therefore should be obtained prior to surgery, and, if polyps are found, they should be removed. In addition, thyroid[10] and adrenal[49] carcinomas have been reported in patients with the Gardner syndrome.

Soft tissue and bone abnormalities

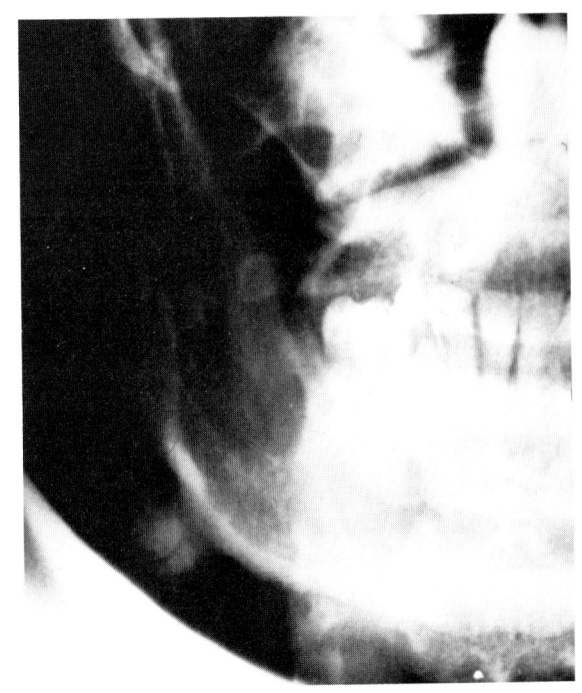

Figure 22-2 Exostosis projecting from the angle of the jaw of an adolescent patient with numerous colonic polyps who had Gardner syndrome. (Reprinted, by permission, from the New England Journal of Medicine, 295:1526, 1976.)

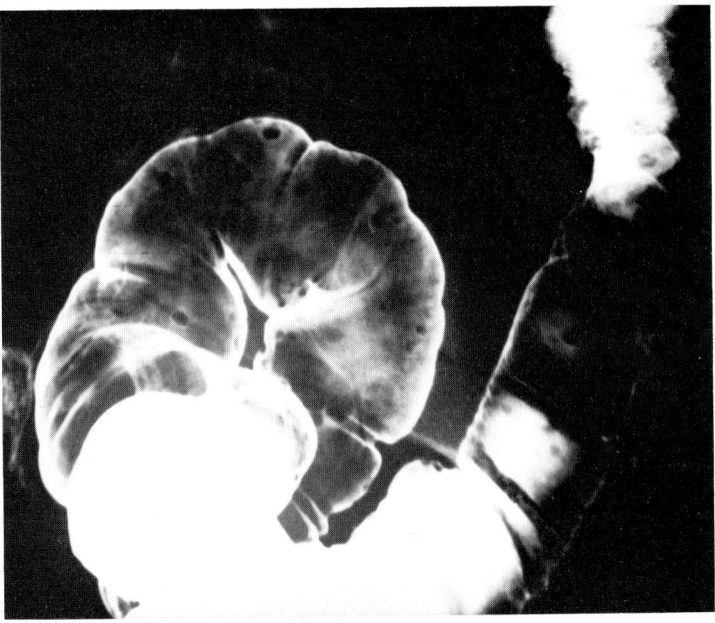

Figure 22-3 Detail view of the rectosigmoid colon from an air-contrast examination, showing numerous small polyps in a patient with Gardner syndrome. (Reprinted, by permission, from the New England Journal of Medicine, 295:1527, 1976.)

often antedate gastrointestinal symptoms.[23] Their presence in a patient should alert the physician to investigate the intestine and to examine other family members for evidence of this syndrome. Other familial disorders with only sebaceous cysts or multiple osteomas have been described and may be confused with the Gardner syndrome. Tetraploidy has been reported to be increased in skin fibroblast cultures derived from these patients and may be of value in identifying affected members in high-risk families.[16]

TURCOT SYNDROME

Familial polyposis associated with central nervous system malignant tumors was first described by Turcot and co-workers.[85] They reported a brother with a medulloblastoma and sister with a glioblastoma multiforme. Ten years later Baughman and his associates described four siblings who died with glioblastoma multiforme.[7] The three who had had autopsies or diagnostic examinations of the bowel had a small number of rectal polyps. The colon polyps were adenomas, which are considered to be precancerous lesions, and two of Baughman's patients had evidence of colon carcinoma. The syndrome is believed to be an autosomal recessive disorder because the parents in both families had no evidence of disease, and the parents in Turcot's family were third cousins.

One patient has been described with colorectal polyposis, thyroid carcinoma, and medulloblastoma,[13] and a woman has been reported with epidermal cysts, fibromas, and gastric polyps whose uncle had colonic polyps and glioblastoma multiforme.[97] In addition, a number of patients with familial polyposis coli have been reported to have primary tumors of the thyroid or brain.[82] Thus, occasionally patients or families appear to have disorders that do not clearly fit into any of the three inherited intestinal polyposis syndromes described above, and overlapping of syndromes may sometimes be seen. Smith and Kern[82] have proposed that all of the disorders of hereditary adenomatous polyposis of the intestinal tract are due to a single, autosomal dominant gene with widely variable penetrance for a number of phenotypes, and occasional gene carriers have no clinical evidence of disease. Thus, familial polyposis coli, the Gardner syndrome, and the Turcot syndrome may all be phenotypic variants of the same disease.

PEUTZ-JEGHERS SYNDROME

The Peutz-Jeghers syndrome is an autosomal dominant disorder characterized by gastrointestinal polyposis and mucocutaneous pigmentation. Well over 300 cases have been described. The polyps occur, in order of decreasing frequency, in the jejunum, ileum, colon, rectum, stomach, duodenum, and appendix.[64] The tumors are not present at birth, but develop with age. They may become very large and lead to intussusception and intestinal obstruction. Typical complaints are of brief, periodic bouts of colicky pain. Rectal bleeding may cause an iron deficiency anemia. Extrusion of a polyp is not an unusual presentation. Symptoms secondary to the polyps often develop during adolescence but have been reported to occur during the first year of life.[58]

The diagnosis is often made during childhood and adolescence before intestinal symptoms appear because of a positive family history and the presence of melanin spots on the buccal mucosa and lips. These macular lesions may also appear on the face, hands, feet, gums, palate, and intestinal mucosa (Fig. 22–4). The pigmentation is usually not present at birth, but appears during infancy and early childhood. Although the melanin deposits around the lips tend to fade during adult life, the mucosal pigmentation persists.

The typical polyp is a hamartoma

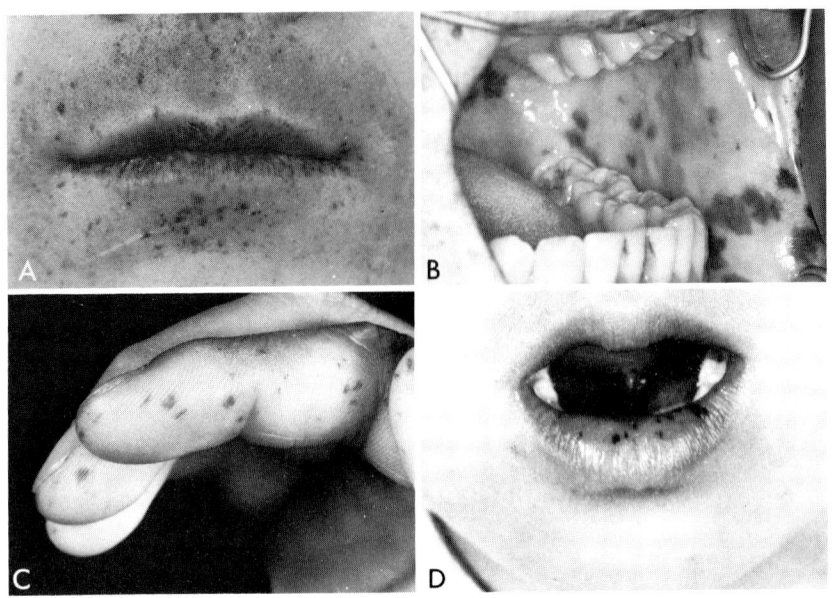

Figure 22-4 Melanin pigmentation in Peutz-Jeghers syndrome. Pigmentation of (*A*) lips and perioral region, (*B*) the buccal mucosa, and (*C*) the fingers. *D*, Pigmentation of the lower lip of the 4 year old son of the patient in *A*, *B*, and *C*. (From Utsunomiya, J., et al.: Peutz-Jeghers syndrome: Its natural course and management. Johns Hopkins Med. J., Vol. 136, No. 2, p. 79, February, 1975. © The Johns Hopkins University Press.)

which is generally believed to be without malignant potential. However, a small number of patients with frankly malignant gastrointestinal neoplasms that have resulted in metastases and death have been described.[86] Conclusive evidence of carcinoma was documented in 11 of 327 patients (3.3 per cent) reviewed by Dozois and associates.[21] The cancers seldom occur in the jejunum or ileum,[21, 86] the two areas of the intestine most commonly involved with the hamartomas. The malignant tumor may involve an area of intestine devoid of polyps, or it may appear to be anatomically unrelated to the polyps,[21] suggesting that the patient with the Peutz-Jeghers syndrome has an increased predisposition to develop gastrointestinal cancer without its being the result of malignant degeneration in a preexisting hamartoma. Adenomatous polyps have been reported to coexist with the hamartomas[21] and may be the cause of the malignancy.

Dozois and co-workers[22] found 16 of 115 women with Peutz-Jeghers syndrome to have ovarian tumors. In three the tumors were malignant. An association between ovarian tumors and Peutz-Jeghers syndrome has also been reported by Scully.[75]

Conservative management has generally been suggested unless intussusception with bowel obstruction, intractable anemia, or evidence of malignancy exists. Erbe has advocated removal of all symptomatic polyps, all gastric and duodenal polyps because of their possible tendency to develop malignancy, and all polyps greater than 2 cm in diameter.[27] Others have suggested that colonic polyps also be removed, and subtotal colectomy and cecoproctostomy be performed in the patient over 30 years of age with numerous colonic polyps because of an increased risk of developing cancer of the colon.[86]

GENERALIZED JUVENILE POLYPOSIS

This disorder consists of multiple polyps that usually involve the rectum and colon, but occasionally involve the small intestine and stomach. There usually are no extraintestinal manifestations. The genetic factors of generalized juvenile polyposis are not well understood, and the disease may represent one autosomal dominant syndrome with variable penetrance or several syndromes.[71] The disease is usually diagnosed during the first decade of life and sometimes produces symptoms or even death in infancy.[5, 72] Sachatello and Griffen believe the rare infantile form to be a clinically distinct entity with an autosomal recessive inheritance pattern, more generalized gastrointestinal involvement, and a high incidence of congenital anomalies.[71] Seven infants reported had a similar clinical course, with severe diarrhea, anemia, hypoproteinemia, and an increased susceptibility to pulmonary infections. Six of the seven died before 2 years of age.[72]

Rectal bleeding with secondary anemia, diarrhea with a mucous discharge, abdominal pain, and autoamputation of polyps or prolapse of a polyp per rectum are the usual symptoms of the disease. The polyps are hamartomas characterized by multiple cysts and large amounts of connective tissue. Although this is usually a benign condition, there appears to be an increased risk of developing carcinomas. The simultaneous occurrence of hamartomas and adenomas has been noted in some families,[83, 89] and several families have been described in which localized or generalized juvenile polyposis has been diagnosed in some members and gastrointestinal carcinoma in others.[38, 83] In the usual case, however, the management is generally conservative, with excision of polyps or local bowel resection as necessitated by the clinical course of the disease.

REFERENCES

1. Abramson, D. J.: Multiple polyposis in children: a review and a report of a case in a 6 year old child who had associated nephrosis and asthma. Surgery 61:288, 1967.
2. Al-Rashid, R. A., and Harned, R. K.: Dysphagia due to leukemic involvement of the esophagus. Am. J. Dis. Child. 121:75, 1971.
3. Ament, M. E.: Immunodeficiency syndromes and gastrointestinal disease. Pediatr. Clin. North Am. 22:807, 1975.
4. Andersson, Å., and Bergdahl, L.: Carcinoma of the colon in children: a report of six new cases and a review of the literature. J. Pediatr. Surg. 11:967, 1976.
5. Arbeter, A. M., Courtney, R. A., and Gaynor, M. F., Jr.: Diffuse gastrointestinal polyposis associated with chronic blood loss, hypoproteinemia and anasarca in an infant. J. Pediatr. 76:609, 1970.
6. Barber, D. H., and Michener, W. M.: Malignant argentaffinoma: report of a case of an eleven-year-old boy. Cleveland Clin. Quart. 32:143, 1965.
7. Baughman, F. A., Jr., List, C. F., Williams, J. R., et al.: The glioma-polyposis syndrome. N. Engl. J. Med. 281:1345, 1969.
8. Bigger, I. A., and Vinson, P. P.: Carcinoma secondary to burns of the esophagus from ingestion of lye. Surgery 28:887, 1950.
9. Biörck, G., Axén, O., and Thorson, A.: Unusual cyanosis in a boy with congenital pulmonary stenosis and tricuspid insufficiency. Fatal outcome after angiocardiography. Am. Heart J. 44:143, 1952.
10. Camiel, M. R., Mulé, J. E., Alexander L. L., et al.: Association of thyroid carcinoma with Gardner's syndrome in siblings. N. Engl. J. Med. 278:1056, 1968.
10a. Carney, J. A., Sheps, S. G., Go, V. L. W., et al.: The triad of gastric leiomyosarcoma, functioning extra-adrenal paraganglioma and pulmonary chondroma. N. Engl. J. Med. 296:1517, 1977.
11. Cline, M. J., and Haskell, C. M.: Cancer Chemotherapy. 2nd Ed. Philadelphia, W. B. Saunders Co., 1975, p. 142.
12. Cline, M. J., and Haskell, C. M.: Cancer Chemotherapy. 2nd Ed. Philadelphia, W. B. Saunders Co., 1975, p. 164.
13. Crail, H. W.: Multiple primary malignancies arising in the rectum, brain, and thyroid: report of a case. U.S. Naval Med. Bull. 49:123, 1949.
14. Cronkhite, L. W., Jr., and Canada, W. J.: Generalized gastrointestinal polyposis: an unusual syndrome of polyposis, pigmentation, alopecia, and onychotrophia. N. Engl. J. Med. 252:1011, 1955.
15. Cullingworth, C. J.: Case of cancer of the stomach in an infant five weeks old. Brit. Med. J. 2:253, 1877.
16. Danes, B. S.: The Gardner syndrome: a study in cell culture. Cancer 36:2327, 1975.
17. DeAngelis, V. R.: Gastric teratoma in a

newborn infant: total gastrectomy with survival. Surgery 66:794, 1969.
18. Devroede, G. J., Taylor, W. F., Sauer, W. G., et al.: Cancer risk and life expectancy of children with ulcerative colitis. N. Engl. J. Med. 285:17, 1971.
19. Dixon, W. L., and Fazzari, P. J.: Carcinoma of the stomach in a child. J.A.M.A. 235:2414, 1976.
20. Donaldson, M. H., Taylor, P., Rawitscher, R., et al.: Colon carcinoma in children. Pediatrics 48:307, 1971.
21. Dozois, R. R., Judd, E. S., Dahlin, D. C., et al.: The Peutz-Jeghers syndrome: is there a predisposition to the development of intestinal malignancy? Arch. Surg. 98:509, 1969.
22. Dozois, R. R., Kempers, R. D., Dahlin, D. C., et al.: Ovarian tumors associated with Peutz-Jeghers syndrome. Ann. Surg. 172:233, 1970.
23. Duncan, B. R., Dohner, V. A., and Priest, J. H.: The Gardner syndrome: need for early diagnosis. J. Pediatr. 72:497, 1968.
24. Ehrenpreiss, T., and Ericsson, N. O.: Surgical treatment of ulcerative colitis in childhood. Surg. Clin. North Am. 44:1521, 1964.
25. El Shafie, M., Spitz, L., and Ikedu, S.: Malignant tumors of the small bowel in neonates presenting with perforation. J. Pediatr. Surg. 6:62, 1971.
26. Entwhistle, C. C., and Jacobs, A.: Histological findings in the Paterson-Kelly syndrome. J. Clin. Pathol. 18:408, 1965.
27. Erbe, R. W.: Inherited gastrointestinal-polyposis syndromes. N. Engl. J. Med. 294:1101, 1976.
28. Fee, H. J., Jr., Schlater, T. L., Johnson, A. P., et al.: Adenocarcinoma of the cecum manifesting as intussusception in a 16-year-old patient: report of a case. Dis. Colon Rectum 19:680, 1976.
29. Fèvre, M., and Huguenin, R.: Malformations tumorales et tumeurs de l'enfant. Paris, Masson & Cie, 1954.
30. Field, J. L., Adamson, L. F., and Stoeckle, H. E.: Review of carcinoids in children: functioning carcinoid in a 15-year-old male. Pediatrics 29:953, 1962.
31. Foreman, R. C.: Carcinoid tumors: a report of 38 cases. Ann. Surg. 136:838, 1952.
32. Fraser, K. J., and Rankin, J. G.: Selective deficiency of IgA immunoglobulins associated with carcinoma of the stomach. Aust. Ann. Med. 19:165, 1970.
33. Gray, S. W., Johnson, H. C., Jr., and Skandalakis, J. E.: Gastric teratoma in an adult with a review of the literature. South. Med. J. 57:1346, 1964.
34. Gryboski, J.: Gastrointestinal Problems in the Infant. Philadelphia, W. B. Saunders Co., 1975, p. 97.
35. Gryboski, J.: Gastrointestinal Problems in the Infant. Philadelphia, W. B. Saunders Co., 1975, p. 708.

36. Gryboski, J.: Gastrointestinal Problems in the Infant. Philadelphia, W. B. Saunders Co., 1975, p. 712.
37. Haerer, A. F., Jackson, J. F., and Evers, C. G.: Ataxia-telangiectasia with gastric adenocarcinoma. J.A.M.A. 210:1884, 1969.
38. Haggitt, R. C., and Pitcock, J. R.: Familial juvenile polyposis of the colon. Cancer 26:1232, 1970.
39. Halsted, J. A., Harris, E. J., and Bartlett, M. K.: Involvement of the stomach in familial polyposis of the gastrointestinal tract. Gastroenterology 15:763, 1950.
40. Hardin, W. J.: Unusual manifestations of malignant disease of the large intestine. Surg. Clin. North Am. 52:287, 1972.
41. Hochberg, F. H., DaSilva, A. B., Galdabini, J., et al.: Gastrointestinal involvement in von Recklinghausen's neurofibromatosis. Neurology 24:1144, 1974.
42. Jackman, R. J., and Beahrs, O. M.: Tumors of the Large Bowel. Philadelphia, W. B. Saunders Co., 1968.
43. Johnston, D. P., Jr., van Heerden, J. A., Lynn, H. B., et al.: Carcinoma of the stomach in a 10-year-old boy. J. Pediatr. Surg. 10:151, 1975.
44. Jones, P. G., and Campbell, P. E.: Tumours of Infancy and Childhood. Oxford, Blackwell Scientific Publications, 1976.
45. Joske, R. A., and Benedict, E. B.: The role of benign esophageal obstruction in the development of carcinoma of the esophagus. Gastroenterology 36:749, 1959.
46. Kern, W. H., and White, W. C.: Adenocarcinoma of the colon in a 9-month-old infant: report of a case. Cancer 11:855, 1958.
47. Knox, W. G., Miller, R. E., Begg, C. F., et al.: Juvenile polyps of the colon: a clinicopathologic analysis of 75 polyps in 43 patients. Surgery 48:201, 1960.
48. Landing, B. H., and Martin, L. W.: Tumors of the gastrointestinal tract and pancreas. Pediatr. Clin. North Am. 6:413, 1959.
49. Marshall, W. H., Martin, F. I. R., and Mackay, I. R.: Gardner's syndrome with adrenal carcinoma. Aust. Ann. Med. 16:242, 1967.
50. Martinez, C. R., Siegelman, S. S., Saba, G. P., et al.: Localized tumor-like lesions in ulcerative colitis and Crohn's disease of the colon. Johns Hopkins Med. J. 140:249, 1977.
51. Matias, I. C., and Huang, Y. C.: Gastric teratoma in infancy: report of a case and review of world literature. Ann. Surg. 178:631, 1973.
52. McKusick, V. A.: Genetic factors in intestinal polyposis. J.A.M.A. 182:271, 1962.
53. McNeer, G.: Cancer of the stomach in the young. Am. J. Roentgenol. Radium Ther. Nucl. Med. 45:537, 1941.
54. Middelkamp, J. N., and Haffner, H.: Carcinoma of the colon in children. Pediatrics 32:558, 1963.

55. Miller, M. S., Costanza, M. E., Li, F. P., et al.: Familial colon cancer. Cancer 37:946, 1976.
56. Monheit, D. B., and Degenshein, G. A.: Leiomyosarcoma of the small bowel in a child. Ann. Internal Med. 43:903, 1955.
57. Moore, C.: Visceral squamous cancer in children. Pediatrics 21:573, 1958.
58. Morens, D. M., and Garvey, S. P.: An unusual case of Peutz-Jeghers syndrome in an infant. Am. J. Dis. Child. 129:973, 1975.
59. Nahmad, M., and Clatworthy, H. W., Jr.: Leiomyoma of the entire esophagus. J. Pediatr. Surg. 8:829, 1973.
60. Nandy, A. K., Sengupta, P., Chatterjee, S. K., et al.: Teratoma of the stomach. J. Pediatr. Surg. 9:563, 1974.
61. Nesbit, R. R., Jr., Elabadawi, N. A., Morton, J. H., et al.: Carcinoma of the small bowel: a complication of regional enteritis. Cancer 37:2948, 1976.
62. Perrett, A. D., Truelove, S. C., and Massarella, G. R.: Crohn's disease and carcinoma of the colon. Brit. Med. J. 2:466, 1968.
63. Pickett, L. K., and Briggs, H. C.: Cancer of the gastrointestinal tract in childhood. Pediatr. Clin. North Am. 14:223, 1967.
64. Pierce, E. R.: Pleiotropism and heterogeneity in hereditary intestinal polyposis. Birth Defects 8:52, 1972.
65. Pierce, E. R., Weisbord, T., and McKusick, V. A.: Gardner's syndrome: formal genetics and statistical analysis of a large Canadian kindred. Clin. Genet. 1:65, 1970.
66. Reed, T. E., and Neel, J. V.: A genetic study of multiple polyposis of the colon (with an appendix deriving a method of estimating relative fitness). Am. J. Hum. Genet. 7:236, 1955.
67. Rhoads, J. E.: The control of large bowel cancer: present status and its challenges. Cancer 36:2314, 1975.
68. Richie, A. C.: Carcinoid tumors. Am. J. Med. Sci. 232:311, 1956.
69. Roth, E., and Farinacci, C. J.: Jejunal leiomyosarcoma in a newborn. Cancer 3:1039, 1950.
70. Ryden, S. E., Drake, R. M., and Franciosi, R. A.: Carcinoid tumors of the appendix in children. Cancer 36:1538, 1975.
71. Sachatello, C. R., and Griffen, W. O., Jr.: Hereditary polypoid diseases of the gastrointestinal tract: a working classification. Am. J. Surg. 129:198, 1975.
72. Sachatello, C. R., Hahn, I. S., and Carrington, C. B.: Juvenile gastrointestinal polyposis in a female infant: report of a case and review of the literature of a recently recognized syndrome. Surgery 75:107, 1974.
73. Safaie-Shirazi, S., and Soper, R. T.: Endorectal pull-through procedure in the surgical treatment of familial polyposis coli. J. Pediatr. Surg. 8:711, 1970.
74. Schnur, P. L., David, E., Brown, P. W., Jr., et al.: Adenocarcinoma of the duodenum and the Gardner syndrome. J.A.M.A. 223:1229, 1973.
75. Scully, R. E.: Sex cord tumor with annular tubules: a distinctive ovarian tumor of the Peutz-Jeghers syndrome. Cancer 25:1107, 1970.
76. Segard, E. C.: Leiomyosarcoma (?) of the stomach. Cancer in Children. Cancer Seminar (Penrose Cancer Hospital, Colorado Springs) 2:85, 1958.
77. Sessions, R. T., Riddell, D. H., Kaplan, H. J., et al.: Carcinoma of the colon in the first two decades of life. Ann. Surg. 162:279, 1965.
78. Shackelford, G. D., and McAlister, W. H.: Primary immunodeficiency diseases and malignancy. Am. J. Roentgenol. Radium Ther. Nucl. Med. 123:144, 1975.
79. Shephard, J. A.: Familial polyposis of the colon with special reference to regression of rectal polyposis after subtotal colectomy. Brit. J. Surg. 58:85, 1971.
80. Shermeta, D. W., Morgan, W. W., Eggleston, J., et al.: Juvenile retention polyps. J. Pediatr. Surg. 4:211, 1969.
81. Siegal, S. E., Hays, D. M., Romansky, S., et al.: Carcinoma of the stomach in childhood. Cancer 38:1781, 1976.
82. Smith, W. G., and Kern, B. B.: The nature of the mutation in familial multiple polyposis: papillary carcinoma of the thyroid, brain tumor, and familial multiple polyposis. Dis. Colon Rectum 16:264, 1973.
83. Stemper, T. J., Kent, T. H., and Summers, R. W.: Juvenile polyposis and gastrointestinal carcinoma: study of a kindred. Ann. Intern. Med. 83:639, 1975.
84. Totten, R. S., Stout, A. P., Humphreys, G. H., et al.: Benign tumors and cysts of the esophagus. J. Thorac. Surg. 25:606, 1953.
85. Turcot, J., Després, J. P., and St. Pierre, F.: Malignant tumors of central nervous system associated with familial polyposis of the colon: report of two cases. Dis. Colon Rectum 2:465, 1959.
86. Utsunomiya, J., Gocho, H., Miyanaga, T., et al.: Peutz-Jeghers syndrome: its natural course and management. Johns Hopkins Med. J. 136:71, 1975.
87. Utsunomiya, J., Maki, T., Iwama, T., et al.: Gastric lesions of familial polyposis coli. Cancer 34:745, 1974.
88. Valdes-Dapéna, A., Rudolph, I., Hidayat, A., et al.: Adenocarcinoma of the small bowel in association with regional enteritis: four new cases. Cancer 37:2938, 1976.
89. Velcek, F. T., Coopersmith, I. S., Chen, C. K., et al.: Familial juvenile adenomatous polyposis. J. Pediatr. Surg. 11:781, 1976.

90. Weedon, D. D., Shorter, R. G., Ilstrup, D. M., et al.: Crohn's disease and cancer. N. Engl. J. Med. 289:1099, 1973.
91. Wells, H. G.: Occurrence and significance of congenital malignant neoplasms. Arch. Path. 30:535, 1940.
92. Wennstrom, J., Pierce, E. R., and McKusick, V. A.: Hereditary benign and malignant lesions of the large bowel. Cancer 34:850, 1974.
93. Wilcox, H. R., and Beattie, J. L.: Carcinoma complicating ulcerative colitis during childhood. Am. J. Clin. Pathol. 43:903, 1955.
94. Williams, J. L.: Carcinoma of the esophagus as a complication of achalasia of the cardia. Thorax 11:268, 1956.
95. Williams, R. D., and Fish, J. C.: Multiple polyposis, polyp regression, and carcinoma of the colon. Am. J. Surg. 112:846, 1966.
96. Wurlitzer, F. P., Mares, A. J., Isaacs, H., Jr., et al.: Smooth muscle tumors of the stomach in childhood and adolescence. J. Pediatr. Surg. 8:421, 1973.
97. Yaffee, H. S.: Gastric polyposis and soft tissue tumors: a variant of Gardner's syndrome. Arch. Dermatol. 89:806, 1964.
98. Yannopoulos, K., and Stout, A. P.: Smooth muscle tumors in children. Cancer 15:958, 1962.

INDEX

Page numbers in *italics* refer to illustrations; (t) indicates tables

Abdomen, effects of radiotherapy on, 96
Abnormalities, chromosome, tumor susceptibility and, 7, 8(t)
  congenital, tumor susceptibility and, 9, 9(t)
Abscess, brain, in cancer patients, 160
  in Hodgkin's disease, 257
Actinomycin D, 76, 76
  for Wilms' tumor, 369
Adenocarcinoma, clear cell, of vagina, 464
  of breast, 469
  of salivary gland, 480
Adenoma, pleomorphic, of salivary gland, 479
Adenosis, 465
Adrenal corticosteroids, 81
Adriamycin, 77, 77
  skin ulcers from, 77, 78
AFP. See *Alpha-fetoprotein*.
Agammaglobulinemia, infantile X-linked, 109
Age, and diagnosis of retinoblastoma, 350, 350(t)
  distribution of childhood cancer by, 1, 3
  distribution of childhood leukemia by, 169
Agents, chemotherapeutic. See *Chemotherapy, drugs for*.
Albinism, 5
Alkaloids, Vinca. See *Vinca alkaloids*.
Alkeran, 68
Alkylating agents, in cancer therapy, 64
  structural formulas of, 66
ALL. See *Leukemia(s), acute lymphoblastic*.
Alpha-fetoprotein, as marker of cancer in children, 51, 52
  in hepatoma, 491
Amethopterin, 69
AML. See *Leukemia(s), acute myeloblastic*.
AMML. See *Leukemia(s), acute myelomonocytic*.
AMoL. See *Leukemia(s), acute monocytic*.
Analgesics, in oncologic emergencies, 137
  narcotic, 137, 138(t)
Anemia, as oncologic emergency, 139
  management of, 140
  aplastic, 188
  Fanconi's, 8, 172
  hemorrhagic, 140
  in Hodgkin's disease, 244
  hypoproduction, 140

Angiography, 40, *41*
  cerebral, in brain tumors, 310
Aniridia, 9
Antibiotics, broad-spectrum, for unexplained fever, 152(t)
  in cancer therapy, 76
Antigen, carcinoembryonic, as tumor marker, 52
  in neuroblastoma, 333
  fetal, and diagnosis of cancer in children, 51
  histocompatibility, 102
  tumor, 102
Antimetabolite drugs, in cancer therapy, 68
Anus, infections of, in cancer patients, 163
Appendix, tumors of, 501
Ara-C, 72, 73
Argentaffinomas, 504
Arrhenoblastoma, 462
Aspergillus, infections from, 154(t), 157(t)
Astrocytoma, cerebellar, 313
Ataxia-telangiectasia, 8, 109
Autoimmune diseases, 112
  and thrombocytopenia, 145
5-Azacytidine, 73, 74

B-cell(s), and immune system, 106
  characteristics of, 103(t)
  humoral responses to tumors and, 106
B-cell leukemia, 179
Bacille Calmette Guérin, 113
Bacteria, infections caused by, anaerobic, 163
  in cancer patients, 150, 153(t), 154
BCG, 113
BCNU, 82, *82*
Beckwith's syndrome, 9
Bladder, effects of radiotherapy on, 98
  rhabdomyosarcoma of, 39
"Blast crisis," in leukemia, 200
Blast transformation, in chronic granulocytic leukemia, 214, 216–219
Blenoxane, 79
Bleomycin, 79
"Blocking factors," 107
Blood pressure, and coagulation, in septicemia, 145(t)
Bloom's syndrome, 7, 172, *172*

517

Bone(s), cancers of, 405–422. See also
    Sarcoma, osteogenic.
  incidence of, 405
  types of, 405. See also *Bone, tumors of.*
  Ewing's tumor of, 417. See also *Ewing's tumor.*
  fibrosarcoma of, 421
  Hodgkin's disease in, 258, 259
  leukemia in, 197, 199
  lymphoma of, malignant, 422
  tumors of, 405–422
    benign, 406(t)
    diagnosis of, 47, 48(t), 48–50, 407
    etiology of, 406
    malignant, 406(t)
Bone marrow, disease of, coagulation abnormalities and, 146(t)
  in diagnosis of leukemia, 189
  in Hodgkin's disease, 244, 245
  in neuroblastoma, 330, 331
  in rhabdomyosarcoma, 389
  suppression of, from radiotherapy, 93
  transplantation of. See *Transplantation, bone marrow.*
Bowel. See *Intestine.*
Brain. See also *Central nervous system.*
  abscess of, in cancer patients, 160
    in Hodgkin's disease, 257
  tumors of. See *Tumors, brain.*
Brain scanning, radionuclide, 309
Brain stem, gliomas of, 306(t), 314, 315
Branchial cleft cyst, 22
Breast, adenocarcinoma of, 469
  cystosarcoma phyllodes of, 469
  cysts in, 468
  diffuse enlargement of, 465
    in neonatal period, 465, 466
    in prepubertal period, 466
    in puberty, 467
  discrete masses in, 468
    neoplastic, 469
    non-neoplastic, 468
  fibroadenoma of, 469
  fibrocystic disease of, 468
  gynecomastia of, 467, 467, 468
  juvenile hypertrophy of, 467
  sarcoma of, 470
  tumors of, 465–470
Bruton's disease, 109
Burkitt's lymphoma. See *Lymphomas, Burkitt's.*
Burkitt's tumor, 279, 279. See also *Lymphomas, Burkitt's.*
Burns, x-ray, 94
Busulfan, 67

Cancer. See also *Carcinoma; Leukemia; Tumors.*
  bacterial infections in, 153(t)
  chemotherapy of, 57–84. See also *Chemotherapy.*
  diagnosis of, 17–52

Cancer (*Continued*)
  diagnosis of, methods used in, 31–52
    relationship of tumor volume and time, 17, 17, 18
  fungal infections in, 154(t), 157(t)
  immune system and, 103
    effects on, 107
  in childhood, diagnosis of, 16–52
    endocrine syndromes as presenting sign of, 50, 51(t)
    epidemiology of, 1–13
    geographic variations, 2
    high risk patients, 4, 171, 172(t)
    immunotherapy of, 112–115, 113(t). See also *Immunotherapy.*
    in immunodeficiency diseases, 108(t)
    incidence of, by age, race and sex, 1, 2, 3(t)
    irradiation as cause of, 11, 12, 12(t)
    prenatal cause of, 12
    psychological support of patient and family, 120–126
    relationship of congenital and environmental factors in, 12
    responsiveness of to chemotherapy, 58(t)
    siblings of patients and, 10
    survivors of, cancer risk in, 11
    susceptibility to, 4–10. See also *Tumors, susceptibility to.*
  in immunodeficient host, 107
  infection-related syndromes in, 151
  infectious complications in, 147
    prevention of, 148
  non-bacterial infections in, 154(t), 157(t)
  pain in, 135
  protozoal infections in, 154(t), 157(t)
  radiotherapy of, 89–100. See also *Radiotherapy.*
  unexplained fever in, 151, 151(t)
    treatment of, 152, 152(t), 153
  viral infections in, 154(t), 157(t)
Candida, endophthalmitis from, 154, 156
  infections from, 154(t), 157(t)
Candidiasis, 162. See also *Candida.*
Carcinoembryonic antigen, and diagnosis of cancer in children, 52
  in neuroblastoma, 333
Carcinogens, chemical, leukemia and, 173
Carcinoid tumors, 504
Carcinoma, 1. See also *Cancer; Leukemia; Tumors.*
  embryonal, 428, 428, 445
    of ovary, 455(t), 456, 457
    of testes, 444(t), 445, 446
      treatment of, 447, 449(t)
      prognosis of, 449(t)
  liver-cell. See *Hepatomas.*
  mucoepidermoid, of salivary gland, 480, 481
  nevoid basal cell, 5
  of cervix and vagina, 464
  of salivary gland, undifferentiated, 480
  renal cell, 374
  thyroid, 482–486. See also *Thyroid, carcinoma of.*
CAT. See *Computerized axial tomography.*

INDEX 519

Catecholamines, excretion of, in neuroblastoma, 332, 333(t)
    and survival rates, 333(t)
CCNU, 82, *82*
CEA. See *Carcinoembryonic antigen.*
Cell(s), and cell cycle, 58, *58*
  B. See *B-cells.*
  cell survival curve, radiation injury to, *91*
  growth kinetics of, Gompertzian, 59, *60*
  killer, 106
  leukemia, morphology of, *180*, 181(t)
  population dynamics, 58, *59*
  population kinetics of, 57
  radiation injury to, 89, *90*
  T. See *T-cells.*
Cellulitis, of breast, 468
Central nervous system, infections of, in cancer patients, 160
  leukemia in, 191
    prophylaxis of, 203, 205
  tumors of, 306–322. See also *Tumors, brain.*
Cerebellum, tumors of, 306(t), 316
Cerebrum, tumors of, 306(t), 316
Cervical thymus, persistent, 23
Cervix, uterine, carcinoma of, 464
  tumors of, 462
CGL. See *Leukemia, chronic granulocytic.*
Chediak-Higashi syndrome, 10
Chemotherapy, drugs for, alkylating agents, 64
    antibiotics, 76
    antimetabolites, 68
    cell-cycle nonspecific, 65(t)
    cell-cycle specific, 65(t)
    sites of action of, *64*
    Vinca alkaloids, 74
  for acute lymphocytic leukemia, 204, 204(t)
  for advanced osteogenic sarcoma, 414, *415*
  for bacterial infections in cancer, 153(t)
  for cancer, 57–84
    combination, 61
    dosage calculations and, *62*
    drug action and, 60, *64*
    drugs for, 62–84. See also *Chemotherapy, drugs for.*
    guidelines for administering, 62, 63
    interaction of with radiotherapy, 99
    pediatric malignancies, responsive to, 58(t)
  for chronic granulocytic leukemia, 218
  for histiocytosis X, response to, 301(t)
  for Hodgkin's disease, 261
    combination regimen for, 262, 262(t)
    drugs used in, 261(t)
    neurologic complications from, 257
  for non-bacterial infections, 154(t)
  for retinoblastoma, 355
  for rhabdomyosarcoma, 392
    pulse VAC, 392, 393(t)
    standard VAC, 392, 392(t)
      results of, 392(t)
  for unexplained fever, 152(t)
  for Wilms' tumor, 368
Chest, effects of radiotherapy on, 95
  x-rays of, in Hodgkin's disease, 248, *248*
Chickenpox, prophylaxis of, 150
Children, abdominal tumors in, 29, 30(t)
  brain tumors in, 305–322. See also *Tumors, brain.*
  cancer in, and cancer risk in siblings, 10
    and tumor susceptibility, 4–10
    diagnosis of, 16–52
    endocrine syndromes in, 50, 50(t)
    epidemiology of, 1–13
    high risk patients, 4
    in immunodeficiency diseases, 108(t)
    incidence of by age, race and sex, *1*, *2*, *3*, 3(t)
    relationship of congenital and environmental factors in, 12
    responsiveness of to chemotherapy, 589(t)
  gastrointestinal tract tumors in, 502–513
  head and neck tumors in, 18, 19(t), 20(t)
  hepatic tumors in, 489–499
  Hodgkin's disease in. See *Hodgkin's disease.*
  leukemia in, 169–220. See also *Leukemia(s).*
    and high risk patients, 171, 172(t)
    familial incidence of, 171
    incidence by age, sex and race, 169, 170, *170*
  neuroblastoma in, 326–389
  non-Hodgkin's lymphomas in. See *Lymphoma(s), non-Hodgkin's.*
  pelvic tumors in, 29, 31(t)
  pheochromocytoma in, 338–341
  primary bone cancers in, 405–422
  renal tumors in, 359–374
  salivary gland tumors in, 476–482
  soft tissue sarcomas in, 380–401
  teratomas in, sites of, 434, *435*
  thyroid carcinoma in, 482–486
  tumors of ear in, 21
  tumors of germ-cell origin in, 427–440, *428*
  tumors of head and neck in, 18, 19(t). 20(t)
  tumors of nasopharynx in, 21
  tumors of orbit in, 20
  tumors of oropharynx in, 21
  tumors of sexual organs in, 453–470
  Wilms' tumor in, 359(t). See also *Wilms' tumor.*
  with cancer, psychological and social support of, 121–127
    views of death of, 124
  with fibrosarcoma, prognosis for, 397
Chlorambucil, 68
Chloromas, 192
  in leukemia, 199
Chondrosarcoma, 422
Choriocarcinoma, 429, *429*
Chromosome(s), abnormalities of, and risk of leukemia, 172
  and tumor susceptibility, 7, 8(t)
  Philadelphia, in chronic granulocytic leukemia, 214, *214*, 217
Cirrhosis, hepatoma and, 493
Clonal hypothesis, of leukemia origin, 177
Coagulation, abnormalities of, in cancer patients, 146, 146(t)
  and blood pressure, in septicemia, 145(t)

Coagulation (*Continued*)
  disseminated intravascular. See *Disseminated intravascular coagulation*.
  light, in treatment of retinoblastoma, 355
Coagulation factors, abnormalities of, 146
  and blood pressure, in septicemia, 145(t)
Coagulopathy consumption. See *Disseminated intravascular coagulation*.
Colitis, Crohn's, 7, 506, 507
  ulcerative, 7
Colon, familial polyposis of, 508, 509
  tumors of, 505
Colon. See also *Gastrointestinal system*.
Compression, of spinal cord, by tumors, 131
  clinical findings in, 131
  localization of, 132(t)
  radiologic findings in, 132, 133
  treatment of, 132
Computerized axial tomography, for brain tumors, 309, 310
  in diagnosis of cancer in children, 46, 47
Congenital mesoblastic nephroma, 373, 373
Consumption coagulopathy. See *Disseminated intravascular coagulation*.
Cordotomy, 139
Corticosteroids, adrenal, in cancer therapy, 81
Corynebacterium parvum, 114
Cosmegen, 76, 76
CRAB, 57. See also *Chemotherapy*.
Craniopharyngiomas, 317, 318
Crohn's disease, 7, 506, 507
Cronkhite-Canada syndrome, 507
Cryotherapy, for retinoblastoma, 355
Cryptococcus neoformans, infections from, 160
  negative staining of, 161
Cryptorchidism, 9
  cancer and, 443
Cyclophosphamide, 67
Cylindroma, 480
Cyst, branchial cleft, 22
  of breast, 468
  thyroglossal duct, 22
Cystathionine, excretion of, in neuroblastoma, 333
Cystosarcoma phyllodes, 469
Cytomegalovirus, infections from, 157(t), 159
  treatment of, 154(t)
Cytosar, 72, 73
Cytosine arabinoside, 72, 73
Cytoxan, 67

Dacarbazine, 83
Dactinomycin, 76, 76
Daunomycin, 77, 77
Daunorubicin, 77, 77
DDP, 84, 84
Death, of child patient, psychological support of family and, 125
Deoxyuridylate, transformation of to deoxythymidylate, 68, 69
Dermatofibrosarcoma protuberans, 392, 396
Desmoids, 396. See also *Fibromatosis*.
de Toni-Fanconi syndrome, hepatoma and, 403
Diagnosis, of cancer in childhood, 16–52. See also *Cancer, diagnosis of*.

Diaminodichloroplatinum, 84, 84
Diarrhea, as complication of Wilms' tumor therapy, 372
DiGeorge syndrome, 109
DiGuglielmo's syndrome, 180, 183
Dimethyltriazeno imidazolecarboxamide, 83, 84
Disseminated intravascular coagulation, 144
  coagulation abnormalities and, 146(t)
Dosages, for drugs, calculations for, 62
Double syringe technique, for administering chemotherapeutic agents, 63
Down's syndrome, leukemia and, 172
  neonatal, 186
Doxorubicin, 77, 77
Drugs, action of, kinetics of, 60
  for cancer therapy. See *Chemotherapy*.
  mechanism of action, 61
DTIC, 83
dUMP. See *Deoxyuridylate*.
Dysgerminoma, 455
Dyskeratosis congenita, 5

Ear, tumors of, in children, 21
Ecthyma gangrenosum, 154, 155
Edema, from radiotherapy, 135
Electroencephalogram, and tumors, 308
Embryonal carcinoma. See *Carcinoma, embryonal*.
Emergencies, oncologic, 128–163. See also *Oncologic emergencies*.
Emotions, of cancer patient and family, 121
Encephalitis, 160
Enchondromatosis, 9
Endocrine syndromes, as presenting feature of cancer in children, 50, 51(t)
Endophthalmitis, *Candida*, 154, 156
Endoxan, 67
Enteritis, radiation, 97
Environment, and heredity, relationship of in cancer etiology, 12
Eosinophilic granuloma. See *Granuloma, eosinophilic; Hand-Schüller-Christian disease*.
Ependymomas, infratentorial, 315
  supratentorial, 317
Epidermoplasia verruciformis, 5
Epithelioma, cystic, multiple benign, 5
Erythroleukemia, 180, 183
Esophagitis, 162, 162
Esophagus, lesions of, in cancer patients, 162
  tumors of, 502
Ewing's tumor, 417
  clinical course of, 419
  clinical features of, 417
  diagnosis of, 47, 49, 418
  of lung, 24
  treatment for, 420
  x-rays in, 418, 418, 419
Extremities, effects of radiotherapy on, 98
  tumors of, 47, 48(t)
Eye, effects of radiotherapy on, 94
  neoplasms of, 346–357. See also *Orbit, tumors of; Retinoblastoma*.

INDEX 521

Factor, transfer, 115
Factors, blocking, 107
  coagulation, abnormalities of, 146, 146(t)
  and blood pressure, in septicemia, 145(t)
Familial polyposis coli, 508, 509
Family, leukemia incidence and, 171
  of cancer patient, psychological support of,
    120–126. See also *Psychological support of
    patient and family.*
Fanconi's anemia, 8, 172
FEL. See *Lymphohistiocytosis, familial
  erythrophagocytic.*
Female reproductive system, 453–465. See also
  Breast; Ovary.
Fever, in Hodgkin's disease, 243
  Pel-Ebstein, 244
  unexplained, 151
    broad-spectrum antibiotic regimen for,
      152(t)
    evaluation of, 151(t)
    treatment of, 152, 152(t), 153
Fibroadenoma, of breast, 469
Fibrocystic disease, of breast, 468
Fibromatosis, 392, 393, 394
  adult type, 393, 395(t)
  juvenile type, 395, 395(t)
  treatment of, 395
Fibromatosis colli, 395
Fibrosarcoma, 392, 396, 421
  in children, prognosis of, 397
  retroperitoneal, 35
  treatment of, 396
Folate antagonists, 69
Folic acid, structural formula of, 69
5-Fluorouracil, 74
5-FU, 74
Fungi, infections caused by, in cancer patients, 154(t), 157(t)
FUO. See *Fever, unexplained.*

Ganglioneuroma, mediastinal tumor in, 28
Gardner's syndrome, 6, 508, 510
Gastrointestinal system, disorders of, tumor
  susceptibility and, 6, 6(t)
  leukemia in, 197
  non-Hodgkin's lymphoma of, 278
  polyps of, 501
  tumors of, 502–513
Genitourinary system, effects of radiotherapy
  on, 98
Germ cell tumors, 427–440
  of ovary, 455, 455(t)
  of testes, 444(t), 445, 446
Glands, salivary. See *Salivary gland(s).*
Gliomas, brain stem, 314, 315
  optic nerve, 318
Gompertzian kinetics, of cell populations, 59,
  60
Gonadoblastoma, 452
  ovarian, 460, 461
Gonadoma, dysgenetic, 460
Graft rejection, in marrow transplantation, 212
Graft versus host disease, 212

Granule, Langerhans, in histiocytosis X
  cells, 293, 293
Granuloma, eosinophilic, 298, 300
  multifocal, 295
Granulosa-theca tumors, 462
Growth, kinetics of, Gompertzian, 59, 60
  of tumors, on arithmetic scale, 17, 17
    on semilogarithmic scale, 17, 18
Growth rates, fetal and childhood, versus
  leukemic cell growth, 60
Guilt, in family of cancer patient, 121
Gynandroblastoma, 462
Gynecomastia, 467, 468

Hamartomas, 5
Hand-Schüller-Christian disease, 295
Head, effects of radiotherapy on, 94
  teratoma of, 437
  tumors of, in children, 18, 19(t), 20(t)
Heart, effects of radiotherapy on, 96
Hemangioendotheliomas, 496
Hemangiomas, of liver, 496, 498
Hemorrhage, as oncologic emergency, 142
  and platelet abnormalities, 142
  and thrombocytopenia, 142
Hepatitis, radiation, 97
Hepatoma(s), 489
  abnormalities associated with, 493
  biochemical abnormalities in, 491
  calcification of, 35
  clinical presentation of, 491
  de Toni-Fanconi syndrome and, 493
  evaluation of, 491
  liver scanning for, 492, 492
  pathology of, 490
  prognosis after surgery, 494, 495(t)
  radiologic examination for, 491
  treatment for, 494
Heredity, and environment relationship of to
  cancer etiology, 12
Herpes simplex, 157(t), 162
  treatment of, 154(t)
Herpes zoster, in Hodgkin's disease, 256, 257
Histiocytes, in histiocytic medullary reticulosis,
  291
  maturation of, cell series, 290
Histiocytosis(es), 289–302. See also
  Histiocytosis X.
  classification of, 290(t)
  malignant, 289, 291
  sinus, with massive lymphadenopathy, 281
Histiocytosis X, 292–302
  "benign" vs. "malignant," 292
  cellular ultrastructure of, 293, 293, 296, 298,
    299
  Hand-Schüller-Christian disease and, 295
  immunologic function in, 299
  Letterer-Siwe disease and, 294
  prognosis of, 300
    factors associated with, 301(t)
  skeletal lesions in, 295, 297, 298, 299, 300
  skin lesions in, 294, 294, 295, 296
  survival from, and complications, 301

Histiocytosis X (*Continued*)
  teeth in, 297
  therapy of, 301
    response to, 301(t)
Histocompatibility, in bone marrow transplantation, 210
Histocompatibility antigens, 102
Histoplasma, infections from, 154(t), 157(t)
Histoplasmosis, disseminated, 37
HLA antigens, 102
Hodgkin's cells, 238, *238*
  lineage of, 238
Hodgkin's disease, 234–266
  age at diagnosis of, 235
  and incidence of second cancers, 265
  bone marrow involvement in, 244, *245*
  cell types in, 237, 238, *238*
  chemotherapy for, 261
    combination regimens for, 262, 262(t)
    drugs used in, 261(t)
  chemotherapy plus radiotherapy for, 262
  chest x-rays in, 248, *248*
  clinical presentation of, 243
  epidemiology of, 234, 235
  etiology of, 236
  exploratory laparotomy in, 251
  follow-up examination for, 264
  hematologic findings in, 244
  herpes zoster in, 256, 257
  histopathology of, 237
  Hodgkin's cells in, 238
  immunodeficiency in, 247
  immunologic testing in, 247, 247(t)
  incidence of, by stage, 253(t)
  infections in, 256
  inferior venacavography in, 249
  inflammatory cells in, 237
  intravenous pyelography in, 249
  jaundice in, 259
  laboratory features of, 244
  lacunar cells in, 240, *241*
  lymph node involvement in, 239
  lymphangiography in, 249, *250*
  lymphocyte depletion type, 242
  lymphocyte predominant type, 239(t), 240, *240*, 241(t)
  malignant cells in, 238, *238*
  mediastinal involvement in, 254
  mixed cellularity type, 242, *242*
  natural history of, 253
  neurologic complications in, 255
  nodular sclerosis type, 239(t), 240, *241*
  of bone, 258, *259*
  of liver, 258
  organ involvement in, 254
  pathogenesis of, 236
  Pel-Ebstein fever in, 244
  prognosis of, 263
  pulmonary involvement in, 254
  radiologic features of, 248
  radiotherapy of, 260
    dosage for, 260
    radiation fields for, 260, *261*
    reactive cells in, 237
  Reed-Sternberg cells in, 238, *238*
  relapses of, 265, *265*

Hodgkin's disease (*Continued*)
  serologic findings in, 246
  staging system for, 252, 253(t)
    procedure for, 249, 249(t)
  stromal cells in, 237
  subtypes of, 239, 239(t), 240(t)
    evolution of, 243
  survival rate after therapy, 262, *263*
  therapy of, 260
Homovanillic acid, excretion of, and survival in neuroblastoma, 333, 333(t)
HVA. See *Homovanillic acid*.
Hydrea, 83
Hydroxyurea, 83
Hypercalcemia, 130
  in leukemia, 190
Hypergammaglobulinemia, in sex-linked reticulohistiocytosis, 292
Hyperkalemia, in leukemia, 190
Hypernatremia, in leukemia, 190
Hyperplasia, lymphoid, and intestinal disorders, 281
Hypersplenism, 145
Hyperuricemia, 128
  in leukemia, 190
  treatment of, 129, 129(t)
Hypocalcemia, 131
  in leukemia, 190
Hypoglycemia, in leukemia, 191
Hypokalemia, 190
Hyponatremia, in leukemia, 190
Hypothalamus, tumors of, 320

IGA deficiency, selective, 110
Ileocecal syndrome, 197
Immune response, to tumors, cell-mediated, 105. See also *Immunity*.
  humoral, 106
Immune RNA, 115
Immune system, and cancer, 103
  B-cells and, 106
  deficiency in, 106. See also *Immunodeficiency*.
  effects of cancer on, 106
  T-cells and, 104
Immunity, alterations of in transplant recipients, 110
  cell-mediated, 105
    infectious complications and, 147
  humoral, 106
    infectious complications and, 147
  immunologic surveillance hypothesis and, 107
  in tumors, 102–112
  tumor-specific, suppression of, 107
Immunocompetence, suppression of, 107
Immunodeficiency, 106
  common variable, 109
  diseases of, forms of cancer associated with, 180(t)
  severe combined, 108
  in histiocytosis X, 299
  in Hodgkin's disease, 247
  infectious complications and, 147

INDEX 523

Immunodeficiency (*Continued*)
  primary diseases of, 108
  syndromes of, and tumor susceptibility, 8, 8(t)
Immunoglobulin A, deficiency of, selective, 110
Immunologic surveillance hypothesis, 107
Immunosuppression, 107
  in patients receiving therapy, 110
  in patients with malignant disease, 111
  in patients with nonmalignant disease, 111
  tumor-associated, 107(t)
Immunotherapy, adoptive, 114
  for acute leukemia, 209
  for tumors, 112–115
  of cancer, 112–115
    active, 113
    drugs for, 113
    types of, 113, 113(t)
  passive, 114
Infantile X-linked agammaglobulinemia, 109
Infants, tumors in, 30
Infections, after bone marrow transplantation, 212
  anorectal, 163
  central nervous system, in cancer patients, 160
  from anaerobic bacteria, 163
  in cancer, 147
    bacterial, 153(t)
    fever and, 151, 151(t)
    fungal, 154(t), 157(t)
    nonbacterial, 154(t)
    prevention of, 148
      patient isolation units and, 149, *149*
    protozoal, 154(t), 157(t)
    viral, 154(t), 157(t)
  in Hodgkin's disease, 256
  mechanical barriers to, 147
  pulmonary, in cancer patients, 155
  related syndromes of, in cancer patients, 151
Inferior venacavography, 39, *40*
Infratentorial, tumors. See *Tumors, brain, infratentorial.*
Intestine(s), effects of radiotherapy on, 97
  inflammatory disease of, 7. See also *Colitis.*
  leukemia in, 197, *198*
  lymphoid hyperplasia of, 281
  non-Hodgkin's lymphoma of, 278
  small tumors of, 504
Irradiation. See *Radiation; X-rays.*
  ionizing, leukemia and, 173
ITP. See *Purpura, idiopathic thrombocytopenic.*

Jaundice, in Hodgkin's disease, 259
Joints, leukemia in, 197

K-cells, 106
Kidney(s), congenital mesoblastic nephroma of, 373
  effects of radiotherapy on, 97

Kidney(s) (*Continued*)
  leukemia in, 196
  renal cell carcinoma of, 374
  tumors of, 359–374
  Wilms' tumor of, 359–373. See also *Wilms' tumor.*
Killer cells, 106
Klinefelter's syndrome, 7

Laminar air flow room, 149, *149*
Langerhans' cells, and histiocytosis X cells, 293
Langerhans' granule, in histiocytosis X cells, 293, *293*
Laparotomy, exploratory, in Hodgkin's disease, 251
L-Asparaginase, 81
Leiomyosarcoma, 400
Leptomeninges, anatomy of, *192*
Lesions, oropharyngeal and esophageal, in cancer patients, 162
Letterer-Siwe disease, 294, *294*
  Langerhans' granule in, 293, *293*
Leukemia(s), 169–220. See also *Cancer; Tumors.*
  accumulative nature of, 177
  acute, 176–213
    and clonal hypothesis, 177
    classification of, 178, 179(t)
    clinical features of, 184
    cytogenetics of, 177
    diagnosis of in childhood, 186
    differential diagnosis of, 185, 187
    "epidemics" of, 170
    immunotherapy for, 209
    in children, management of, 200
    pathogenesis of, 176
  acute lymphoblastic, 179, 179(t), *180*
    cytologic features of, *181*, 181(t)
    functional classification of, 182(t)
    immunologic classification of, 179
  acute lymphocytic, and bone marrow relapse, 206
    CNS prophylaxis in, 205
    maintenance therapy for, 205
    management of, 204
    remission induction in, 204, 204(t)
    survival rates after therapy, 207
  acute monocytic, *180*, 181
    management of, 209
  acute myeloblastic, 179, 179(t), *180*
  acute myelogenous, management of, 208
    remission induction in, 208
    survival rates after therapy, 208
  acute myelomonocytic, *180*, 181
  acute promyelocytic, management of, 209
  acute undifferentiated, 178, *180*
  basophilic, 184
  B-cell, 179, 182(t)
  "blast crisis" in, 200
  blood values in, 188
  bone marrow findings in, 189
  bone marrow transplantation in, 210, *211*. See also *Transplantation, bone marrow.*

Leukemia(s) (*Continued*)
  cell types of, *180*
  central nervous system, 191
    prophylaxis of, 203, 205
  chemical carcinogens and, 173
  chloromas in, 199
  chronic, 213–220
  chronic granulocytic, 213
    adult type, 213
      characteristics of, 220(t)
    blast cell transformation in, 217
    chemotherapy for, 218
    clinical features of, 216
    juvenile type, 219
      differentiation from adult type, 220(t)
    management of, 218
    pathogenesis of, 215
    Philadelphia chromosome in, 214, *214*
  congenital, 184, *185*
  diagnosis of, blood chemistries and, 190
  eosinophilic, 183
    management of, 209
  epidemiology of, 169
  erythroid, 180, *183*
  etiology of, 173
  extramedullary, 191
  in bones and joints, 197, *199*
  in childhood, epidemiology of, 169
    familial incidence of, 171
    incidence by age, race and sex, 169, 170, *170*
    high risk patients and, 171, 172(t)
  in children with congenital chromosomal abnormalities, 172
  in gastrointestinal tract, 197
  in identical twins, 171
  in kidneys, 196
  ionizing radiation and, 173
  life-threatening complications of, at initial diagnosis, 200
  lymphoblastic, mediastinal tumor in, 27
  neonatal, with Down's syndrome, 186
  null cell, 179, 182(t)
  ovarian, 195
  persistence of after remission, 202, *202*
  remission of, and maintenance therapy, 203
    and persistence of leukemic cells, 202, *202*
    induction of, 201
  T-cell, 179, *182*, 182(t)
  testicular, 195, *196*
  viruses and, 173, *175*
Leukemia cutis, 185
Leukemoid reaction, 188
Leukeran, 68
Leukoencephalopathy, progressive multifocal, 160
Leukoerythroblastosis, 188
Leukokoria, 350
Leydig cell tumor, 451, *451*
Lhermitte's sign, 96, 258
Life Island, 149
Light coagulation, in treatment of retinoblastoma, 355
Liposarcoma, 399, *399*
  pathology of, 400
  therapy for, 400

Listeria monocytogenes, infections from, 160
Liver, carcinoma of, intravenous pyelography of, 36
  damage to, as complication of Wilms' tumor therapy, 372
  disease of, coagulation abnormalities in, 146, 146(t)
  effects of radiotherapy on, 97
  hemangioendotheliomas of, 496
  Hodgkin's disease in, 258
  neuroblastoma involving, 330, *330*
  tumors of, 489–499. See also *Hepatoma.*
    benign, 495, 498(t)
    incidence of, 489, 489(t)
    vascular, 496, *498*
Lumbar puncture, for brain tumors, 310
Lungs, effects of radiotherapy on, 95
  in Hodgkin's disease, 254
  infections of, in cancer patients, 155
  neoplasms of, in children, 23, 24(t), *24*, *25*
  Wilms' tumor in, 366, *367*
Lymph node(s), in Hodgkin's disease, 239, 239(t), 240(t). See also *Hodgkin's disease; Lymphoma(s).*
  mucocutaneous lymph node syndrome and, 280
  rhabdomyosarcoma of, 387, *388*
Lymph vessels, swellings of, 23
Lymphadenitis, cervical, in children, 280
Lymphadenopathy, drug-induced, 280
  in non-Hodgkin's lymphoma, 277, *277*
  with sinus histiocytosis, 281
Lymphangiography, in Hodgkin's disease, 249, *250*
Lymphocytes, B, 103, 106. See also *B-cells.*
  differentiation of, pathways for, 103, *104*
  T, 103, *104*. See also *T-cells.*
Lymphocytosis, infectious, 187
Lymphoepithelioma, 475, 476
Lymphoma(s), Burkitt's, 273, *274*
  Hodgkin's. See *Hodgkin's disease.*
  malignant, of bone, 422
  non-Hodgkin's, 272–285
    clinical presentations of, 277
    differential diagnosis of, 279
    distribution of, 276(t)
    etiology of, 272
    evaluation of, 281, 283(t)
    histologic classification of, 274, 275(t)
    lymphadenopathy and, 277, *277*
    mediastinal, 277, *278*
    pathology of, 274
    primary gastrointestinal, 278
    prognosis of, 283
    therapy for, 283

Macrophages. See *Histiocytes; Histiocytoses.*
Maffucci's syndrome, 9
Male reproductive system, tumors of, 443–453
Malformation, congenital, tumor susceptibility and, 9, 9(t)
Mass(es). See *Tumors.*
Matulane, 83, *83*
MCT. See *Thyroid, carcinoma of, medullary.*

Index

Mechlorethamine hydrochloride, 65
Medulloblastoma, 306(t), 312, 313(t)
  survival rates for, 313(t)
Meigs' syndrome, 462
Melanin, deposition of, in Peutz-Jeghers syndrome, 511, 512
Melphalan, 68
Meningitis, in Hodgkin's disease, 257
  leukemic, 193, *193*, *194*
6-Mercaptopurine, 72, *72*
Mesenchyme, primitive, tumors of, 397
Mesenchymoma, 397
Methotrexate, 69
  "high dose," 71
  intrathecal, 71
    toxicity from, symptoms of, 71(t)
  structural formula of, *69*
  toxicity from, 70
Methyl-CCNU, 82, *82*
Mitosis, 58
Mithracin, 80, *80*
Mithramycin, 80, *80*
Monilia, infections with, 154(t), 157(t)
Mononucleosis, infectious, 187
MOPP regimen, for Hodgkin's disease, 262, 262(t)
Mouth, lesions of, in cancer patients, 162
  tumors of, in children, 22
6-MP, 72, *72*
Mucocutaneous lymph node syndrome, 280
Mucoepidermoid carcinoma, of salivary gland, 480, *481*
Mucosal neuroma syndrome, 485, *486*
Mucous membranes, effects of radiotherapy on, 93
Multiple endocrine neoplasia, 485
Muramidase, in leukemia, 191
Mustard, nitrogen, 65
  phenylalanine, 68
Mustargen, 65
Myerlan, 67
Myxoma, 397

Narcotics, in oncologic emergencies, 137
Nasopharynx, carcinoma of, 475
  tumors of, in children, 21
Natulan, 83, *83*
Neck, embryonic remnants in, 22
  swellings of, in children, diagnosis of, 22
  teratoma of, 437, *439*
  tumors of, in children, 18, 19(t), 20(t)
Neoplasia, multiple endocrine, 10
Neoplasms. See *Cancer; Carcinoma; Leukemia(s); Sarcoma; Tumors.*
Nephritis, radiation, 97
Nephroblastoma, congenital, 359. See also *Wilms' tumor.*
Nephroma, congenital mesoblastic, 373, *373*
Nephrotomography, in diagnosis of renal disease, 39
Nervous system, central, tumors of, 305–322. See also *Tumors, brain.*
  involvement of, in Hodgkin's disease, 255

Nervous system (*Continued*)
  peripheral, tumors of, 305–322. See also *Central nervous system.*
  sympathetic, tumors of, 326–341, *328*, *329*
Neuroblastoma, 188, 326–338
  biochemical features of, 332
  bone marrow in, 330, *331*
  carcinoembryonic antigen, levels in, 333
  catecholamine levels in, 332
  clinical manifestations of, 327, *328*, *329*
  cystathionine levels in, 333
  differentiation of from Wilms' tumor, 32, *32*
  etiology of, 326
  liver involvement by, *330*
  of adrenal, intravenous pyelography of, 38
  of lungs, 25
  pathology of, 334
  periorbital metastases from, 330, *331*
  prognosis of, 334, 335(t)
  staging system for, 334
  survival in, and secretion of VMA and HVA, 333, 333(t)
  survival rates, 335, 335(t)
  treatment for, 336
Neurocutaneous syndromes, tumor susceptibility and, 5, 6(t)
Neuroectoderm, in teratoma, 432, *433*
Neurofibromas, 321
Neurofibromatosis, 5
Neuroma, mucosal syndrome of, 485, *486*
  of tongue, 485, *486*
Neutropenia, 141
  and risk of infection, 141, *142*
  management of, 142
Nevoid basal cell carcinoma, 5
Nitrogen mustard, 65
Nitrosoureas, 82, *82*
Non-Hodgkin's lymphomas, 272–285. See also *Lymphomas, non-Hodgkin's.*
Null cell leukemia, 179

Oligodendroglioma, calcifications in, 308, *309*
Ollier's syndrome, 9
"Oncogene" hypothesis, of viral causation of leukemia, 174
Oncologic emergencies, 128–163
  anemia, 139
  hemorrhage, 142
  hypercalcemia, 130
  hyperuricemia, 128
  hypocalcemia, 131
  infections, 147
  metabolic, 128
  neutropenia, 141
  pain, 135
  spinal cord compression, 131
  superior vena cava syndrome, 134
Oncovin, 75
Opacification, total body, in diagnosis, 39
Optic nerve glioma, 318
Orbit, ecchymosis from neuroblastoma, 330, *331*

Orbit (*Continued*)
  effects of radiotherapy on, 95
  tumors of, in children, 19(t), 20
Oropharynx, tumors of, in children, 21
Osteogenic sarcoma, 408. See also *Sarcoma, osteogenic*.
Osteoporosis, in leukemia, 199
Osteosarcoma, 408. See also *Sarcoma, osteogenic*.
Ovary, arrhenoblastoma of, 462
  embryonal carcinoma of, 455(t), 456, *457*
  endodermal sinus tumor of, 458, *459*
  gonadoblastoma of, 460, *461*
  leukemia in, 196
  stromal tumors of, 462
  teratoma of, *433*, *454*, *456*, *457*
    immature, *456*, *457*, 458, *458*, 458(t)
    survival of, 458
  tumors of, 453
    classification of, 454, 455(t)
    diagnosis of, 453
    dysgerminoma, 455
    extraembryonal, 459
    germ cell, 455, 455(t)
      metastatic behavior of, 459
      prognosis of, 460
      treatment for, 460

Pain, in cancer, 135
  surgery for, 138
  treatment of, 137
PAM, 68
Parosteal osteogenic sarcoma, 415, *416*
Patient, psychological support of, 120–126. See also *Psychological support of patient and family*.
Pel-Ebstein fever, 244
Pelvis, effects of radiotherapy on, 98
Pericarditis, radiation-induced, 96
Peripheral nerve block, 138
Pertussis, 187
Peutz-Jeghers syndrome, 7, 511, *512*
Phakomatoses, tumor susceptibility and, 5, 6(t)
Phenylalanine mustard, 68
Pheochromocytoma, 338, 339(t), *340*
Philadelphia chromosome, in chronic granulocytic leukemia, 214, *214*, 217
Phycomycosis, infections from, 157(t)
Physical examination, in diagnosis of cancer in children, 31
Pigmentation, in Peutz-Jeghers syndrome, 511, *512*
Pineal, tumors of, 319
Platelets, thrombocytopenia and, 142. See also *Thrombocytopenia*.
Platinum compounds, 84
Pneumocystis carinii, infections from, 157(t), 159, *159*
  treatment of, 154(t), 160
  interstitial pneumonia from, 159, *159*
Pneumoencephalography, for brain tumors, 310, *311*, *315*
Pneumonia, *Pseudomonas*, 158, *158*
  in cancer patients, 155

Pneumonia (*Continued*)
  interstitial, from *Pneumocystis carinii*, 157(t), 159, *159*
    from Wilms' tumor therapy, 372
  radiation, 95
Pneumonitis. See *Pneumonia*.
Polydysplastic epidermolysis bullosa, 5
Polyps, gastrointestinal, 507, *509*, *510*
Polyposis, generalized juvenile, 512
Polyposis coli, 6
  familial, 508, *509*
Pregnancy, exposure to radiation in, and cancer risk, 12, 12(t)
Pressure, blood. See *Blood pressure*.
Procarbazine, 83, *83*
Progeria, adult, 5
Protozoa, infections caused by, in cancer patients, 154(t), 157(t)
Psychological support of patient and family, 120–126
  after child has died, 123
  after initial diagnosis, 120
  and dying child, 123
  and recurrence of disease, 123
  and remission of disease, 122
Puberty, precocious, 466
Pulmonary infections, in cancer patients, 155. See also *Lungs*.
Purine analogues, in chemotherapy, 72
Purinethol, 72
Purpura, idiopathic thrombocytopenic, 187
Pyelogram, intravenous, in diagnosis of cancer, 33, *36*, *37*, *38*
  in Hodgkin's disease, 249
Pyrimidine analogues, in chemotherapy, 72

Race, cancer incidence and, 2, *2*, 3(t)
  leukemia incidence and, 170
Radiation. See also *Radiotherapy; Roentgenography; X-rays*.
  absorbed doses of, in roentgenography versus scanning, 41(t)
  and risk of cancer development, 11
  as cancer therapy, in retinoblastoma, 354
    and development of osteogenic sarcoma, 356, *356*
  diagnostic, in pregnancy, cancer risk and, 12, 12(t)
  ionizing, cellular effects of, 89, *90*, *91*
Radiation edema, 135
Radiation enteritis, 97
Radiation hepatitis, 97
Radiation necrosis, of spinal cord, 258
Radiation nephritis, 97
  from Wilms' tumor therapy, 372
Radiation pneumonitis, 95
Radiation sickness, 93
Radiology. See *Roentgenography; X-rays*.
Radionuclide scanning. See *Scanning, radionuclide*.
Radionuclides, used in scanning, 41(t)
Radiotherapy. See also *Radiation; X-rays*.
  and bone marrow suppression, 93
  and radiation sickness, 93

INDEX 527

Radiotherapy (*Continued*)
  edema from, 135
  effects of, on abdomen, 96
    on extremities, 98
    on genitourinary system, 98
    on head, 94
    on orbit, 95
    on pelvis, 98
  enteritis from, 97
  for cancer, 89–100
    and damage to normal tissue, 92
    and interaction with cancer chemotherapy, 99
    fractionation of dose in, 92
    late effects of, 99
    local effects of, 94
    normal tissue tolerance of, 92
    relationship of dose and volume in, 91
    systemic effects of, 93
    time-dose relationship in, 92
  for Hodgkin's disease, 260
    neurologic complications from, 258
    radiation dosage for, 260
    radiation fields for, 260, *261*
  for rhabdomyosarcoma, 391
  for Wilms' tumor, 368
    dosages for, 368, 368(t)
  hepatitis from, 97
  nephritis from, 97
  pneumonitis from, 95
  skin and mucous membrane reactions to, 93
Rectum, infections of, in cancer patients, 163
  tumors of, 505
Reed-Sternberg cells, 238, *238*
Remission, of acute lymphocytic leukemia, 204
  of cancer, psychological support of patient and family in, 122
  of leukemia, induction of, 201
    maintenance therapy in, 203
Renal cell carcinoma, 374
Reticuloendothelioses, 289–302. See also *Histiocytoses*.
Reticulohistiocytosis, sex-linked, with hypergammaglobulinemia, 292
Reticulosis, hemophagocytic, familial, 291
  histiocytic medullary, 289, *291*
Reticulum cell sarcoma, of bone, 422
Retinoblastoma, 346–357, *348*
  abnormalities associated with, 347
  age distribution of, 350, 350(t)
  chemotherapy for, 355
  cryotherapy for, 355
  differential diagnosis of, 351
  funduscopic appearance of eye in, 350, *351*
  histology of, *349*
  incidence of, 346
  inheritance of, 346
  leukokoria in, 350
  light coagulation for, 355
  pathology of, 348
  radiation therapy for, 354
    and development of osteogenic sarcoma, 356, *356*
  retinal detachment in, *349*
  rosette formation in, 349, *349*
  signs and symptoms of, 350, 351(t)

Retinoblastoma (*Continued*)
  staging system for, 352, 352(t)
  surgery for, 354
  therapy of, 353
    results of, 355, 356(t)
Rhabdomyoblasts, 382, *383*, *384*, *389*
Rhabdomyosarcoma, 381
  alveolar, 385, *386*
  bone marrow in, *389*
  chemotherapy for, 392
    pulse VAC, 392, 393(t)
    standard VAC, 392, 392(t)
      results of treatment with, 392(t)
  clinical manifestations of, 386
  course of, 387
  embryonal, *383*, 385
  histology of, 382, *383*, *384*
  lymph node in, *388*
  mixed, 386
  of bladder, 39
  of female genital tract, 463, *463*
  paratesticular, *452*
  pathology of, 382, *383*
  pelvic, ultrasonography of, *46*
  pleomorphic, 386
  primary sites of, 387(t)
    prognosis and, 387
  prognostic factors in, 387
  radiotherapy for, 391
  rhabdomyoblasts in, 382, *383*, *384*, *389*
  staging system of, 390
  surgery for, 391
  treatment of, 390
  variants of, 385
Rheumatic diseases, 188
Rhizotomy, 138
RNA, immune, 115
RNA tumor virus, leukemia and, 174, *175*
Roentgenography, for salivary gland tumors, 477, *479*
  in diagnosis of cancer in children, 33, *35–41*
  in hepatoma, *491*, *493*
  in Hodgkin's disease, 248, *248*, *250*
  in teratoma, 436, *436*
  of bone tumors, 408
  of brain tumors, 308, *308*, *309*
  of Ewing's tumor, 418, *418*, *419*
  of osteogenic sarcoma, *411*, *412*
    parosteal, *416*
  of Wilms' tumor, 365, *366*, *367*
  radiation doses absorbed in, 43(t)
Rosettes, formation of by T-cells, 104, *105*
Rubidomycin, 77, *77*

Sacrococcygeal teratoma, 434, *435*, *438*
Saline injection, subarachnoid, 139
Salivary glands, adenocarcinoma of, 480
  pleomorphic adenoma of, *479*
  tumors of, 476–482, *479*, 479(t)
    solid, *479*
  undifferentiated carcinoma of, 480
Sarcoma(s), 1. See also *Cancer; Leukemia(s); Tumors.*
  Ewing's. See *Ewing's tumor.*

Sarcoma(s) (Continued)
  of breast, 470
  osteogenic, 408
    advanced, survival rates, 415
    clinical presentation of, 408
    clinical course of, 412
    diagnostic studies of, 409
    from radiation therapy for retinoblastoma, 356, 356
    incidence of by location and age, 410
    of distal femur, 411
    parosteal, 415, 416
    prognosis of, 412
    pulmonary, 412
    rehabilitation for, 422
    treatment for, 412
    x-rays of, 48
  reticulum cell, of bone, 422
  soft tissue, 380–401. See also specific types, such as Rhabdomyosarcoma.
    characteristics of, 380
    classification of, 381, 382
    diagnosis of, 47, 48(t)
    etiology of, 381
    incidence of, 382(t)
  synovial, 398
    pathology of, 398
    therapy for, 399
Sarcoma botryoides, 385, 385
  of bladder, 39
  of vagina, 463, 463
Scanning, brain, for tumors, 309
  radionuclide, agents used in, 41(t)
    bone, 50, 50
    for thyroid carcinoma, 483
    in diagnosis of cancer, 41, 44
    in hepatoma, 492, 492
    liver-spleen, 43, 44
    radiation doses absorbed in, 43(t)
Schiller-Duval body, 458, 459
Schwannomas, 321
SCID. See Immunodeficiency, diseases of, severe combined.
Sclerosis, tuberous, 6
Seminoma, 444(t), 445, 446
Septicemia, as oncologic emergency, 145
  blood pressure versus coagulation in, 145(t)
  in bacterial infections in cancer patients, 154, 154
Sequestration, splenic, 145
Sertoli cell tumor, 451
Sex, cancer incidence and, 2
  leukemia incidence and, 170, 170
Sex cord–stromal tumors, 444(t), 450
Sexual organs, tumors of, 443–470. See also Ovary; Testis(es).
Shingles. See Herpes zoster.
Sialadenitis, 477
Sialography, for salivary gland tumors, 477, 479
Siblings, of cancer patients, cancer risk in, 10
Sinus(es), paranasal, tumors of, in children, 21
Sinus histiocytosis, with lymphadenopathy, 281
Sipple's syndrome, 10, 485
Skeletal lesions, in eosinophilic granuloma, 298, 300

Skeletal lesions (Continued)
  in Hand-Schüller-Christian disease, 295, 297, 298, 299
  in Wilms' tumor, as result of therapy, 373
Skin, effects of radiotherapy on, 93
  lesions of, from Adriamycin, 77, 78
Skin syndromes, in Letterer-Siwe disease, 294, 294, 295, 296
  tumor susceptibility and, 4, 4(t)
Skull, x-rays of, in brain tumors, 308, 308, 309
Small intestine. See Intestine, small.
Soft tissue sarcomas. See Sarcomas, soft tissue, and specific types, such as Rhabdomyosarcoma.
Spinal cord, compression of, by tumors. See Compression, of spinal cord.
  radiation necrosis of, in Hodgkin's disease, 258
  tumors of, 320
Spleen, role in combatting infections, 148
  sequestration by, 145
Staff, medical, emotional reactions to dying child, 126
Sternomastoid tumor, 23
Steroid hormones, in cancer therapy, 81
Stilbestrol, prenatal exposure to, and cancer risk, 12
Stomach, tumors of, 503. See also Gastrointestinal system.
Subarachnoid saline injection, 139
Superior vena cava syndrome, 134, 136
  treatment of, 135
Supratentorial tumors. See Tumors, brain, supratentorial.
Surgery, for hepatoma, 494
  survival and, 495(t)
  for retinoblastoma, 354
  for rhabdomyosarcoma, 391
  for Wilms' tumor, 366
SVC. See Superior vena cava syndrome.
Sympathetic nervous system. See Nervous system, sympathetic.
Synovial sarcoma, 398
  pathology of, 398
  therapy for, 399

T-cells, 103, 104
  characteristics of, 103(t)
T-cell leukemia, 179
Teeth, in Hand-Schüller-Christian disease, 297
Telangiectasia, and ataxia. See Ataxia-telangiectasia.
Teratoma(s), 430
  clinical aspects of, 434
  cystic, benign, 26
  histology of, 432, 433, 434
  intraabdominal, 439
  malignant, 437
  mediastinal, 437
  of gonads, 440
  of head and neck, 437
  ovarian, 433, 454, 456, 457
    grading of, 458, 458(t)

INDEX 529

Teratoma(s) (Continued)
  ovarian, immature, 456, 457, 458, 458(t)
    survival of, 458
  retroperitoneal, 439
  sacrococcygeal, 434, 435, 438
  staging system for, 434
  structure of, 432, 433
  testicular, 447, 450
  theories of origin of, 431
Testis(es), cryptorchid, cancer in, 443
  embryonal carcinoma of. See Carcinoma, embryonal.
  leukemia in, 195, 196
  seminoma of, 445, 446
  teratoma of, 446, 450
  tumors of, 443
    classification of, 444, 444(t)
    extraembryonal, 444(t), 450
    germ cells, 444(t), 445. See also Carcinoma, embryonal.
    granuloblastoma, 453
    interstitial cell, 451, 451
    Leydig cell, 451, 451
    Sertoli cell, 451
    sex cord-stromal, 444(t), 450
6-TG, 72, 72
Thelarche, premature, 466
6-Thioguanine, 72, 72
13q-syndrome; 7
Thorax, tumors of, in children, 23, 24(t)
Thrombocytopenia, 142
  autoimmune, 145
  due to accelerated platelet destruction, 144
  due to platelet hypoproduction, 143
  management of, 143, 143(t)
  mechanisms of, 142, 142(t)
Thymosin, 115
Thymus, persistent cervical, 23
Thyroglossal duct cyst, 22
Thyroid, carcinoma of, 482–486
  anaplastic forms of, 484
  and multiple endocrine neoplasia, 485, 486
  classification of, 484
  clinical manifestations of, 483
  differentiated forms of, 484
  medullary, 485
  thyroid scan for, 483
  ectopic, 22
Tomography, computerized axial, 309, 310
Total body opacification, 39
Toxicity, Adriamycin, skin ulcers and, 77, 78
  methotrexate, 70
  symptoms of, 71(t)
Toxoplasma, infections from, 154(t), 157(t)
Transfer factor, 115
Transplantation, bone marrow, complications of, 212
  histocompatibility and, 210
  in leukemia, 210
  results of, 212
  technique of, 211
  organ, immunosuppression in, cancer in recipients of, 110
Trichoepithelioma, familial, 5

Tuberculosis, in cancer patients, 158
  prophylaxis of, 150
Tumor(s). See also Cancer; Leukemia.
  abdominal, calcification in, 33(t)
    in children, 29, 30(t)
  antigens of, 102
  brain, 305–322
    computerized axial tomography for, 309, 310
    electroencephalography for, 308
    infratentorial, 306(t), 311
    pathogenesis of, 305
    supratentorial, 306(t), 316
  Burkitt's, 279, 279
  carcinoid, 504
  cell-mediated response to, 105
  central nervous system, incidence of, 306, 306(t), 307(t)
  cerebellar, 306(t), 311
  embryonal, 427
  emergencies associated with. See Oncologic emergencies.
  endodermal sinus, 430
    of ovary, 458, 459
    of vagina, 464
  Ewing's, 417. See also Ewing's tumor.
  extraembryonal, 429, 429
    choriocarcinoma, 429, 429
    endodermal sinus, 429, 430
  fibrous tissue, 392, 394
  germ-cell, 444(t), 445, 446. See also Carcinoma, embryonal.
  granulosa-theca, 462
  growth curves of, logarithmic, 17, 17, 18
  humoral response to, 106
  hypothalamic, 320
  immunology of, 102–112
  immunosuppression in, 107(t)
  immunotherapy for, 112–115
  in children, diagnosis of, 16–52
  in neonates, 30
  interstitial cell, 451, 451
  intracranial. See Tumors, brain.
  intraspinal, 320
  kidney, 359–374. See also Wilms' tumor.
  Leydig cell, 451, 451
  life-threatening complications of, 128–163
  mediastinal, in children, 26, 27, 27, 28
  of bone, 405–422. See also Bone(s), tumors of.
  of breast, 465–470. See also Breast.
    benign, 469
    malignant, 469
  of central nervous system, 305–322. See also Tumors, brain.
    clinical symptoms of, 307
    diagnostic studies in, 308
    histologic types of, 306, 307(t)
  of colon, 505
  of ear, in children, 21
  of esophagus, 502
  of eye. See Retinoblastoma.
  of gastrointestinal tract, 502–513
  of germ-cell origin, 427–440, 428
  of head and neck, in children, 18, 19(t)
    incidence of, 20(t)

Tumor(s) (Continued)
  of liver, 489–499. See also Hepatoma.
    benign, 495, 498(t)
    incidence of, 489, 489(t)
    vascular, 496
  of lungs, in children, 23, 24(t), 24, 25
  of nasopharynx, in children, 21
  of orbit, in children, 20(t)
  of oropharynx, in children, 21
  of ovary, 453. See also Ovary, tumors of.
    stromal, 462
  of peripheral nervous system, 321
  of primitive mesenchyme, 397
  of rectum, 505
  of salivary glands, 476–482, 479, 479(t)
    solid, 479
  of the sexual organs, 443–470. See also Ovary; Testis(es).
  of small intestine, 504
  of stomach, 503
  of sympathetic nervous system, 326–341
  of uterine cervix, 462
  of uterus, 462
  of vagina, 463
  paratesticular, 452, 452
  pelvic, in children, 29, 31(t)
  pineal, 319
  radiosensitivity of, 91
  relationship of volume and time of diagnosis, 17, 17, 18
  renal, 359–374
  Sertoli cell, 451
  sex cord–stromal, 444(t), 450
  soft tissue, 380–401. See also Sarcomas, soft tissue.
  spinal cord, 320
  sternomastoid, 23
  supratentorial, 316
  susceptibility to, 4–10
    chromosome syndromes and, 7, 8(t)
    congenital malformations and, 9, 9(t)
    gastrointestinal syndromes and, 6, 6(t)
    immunodeficiency syndromes and, 8, 8(t)
    irradiation and, 11
    neurocutaneous syndromes and, 5, 6(t)
    of siblings of cancer patients, 10
    skin syndromes associated with, 4, 4(t)
  teratomas and, 431. See also Teratomas.
  testicular. See Testis(es), tumors of.
  Wilms', 359. See also Wilms' tumor.
  yolk sac, 429, 430, 430, 458
Turcot's syndrome, 7, 510, 511
Twins, identical, leukemia in, 171
Tylosis, 5
Typhlitis, 197, 198
Tyrosinemia, 10

Ultrasonography, in diagnosis of cancer in children, 45, 45, 46
Uterus, carcinoma of, 464
  cervical tumors of, 462
  tumors of, 462

VAC. See Chemotherapy, of rhabdomyosarcoma.
Vagina, carcinoma of, 464
  rhabdomyosarcoma of, 463, 463
  tumors of, 462
Vanillylmandelic acid, excretion of, and survival in neuroblastoma, 333, 333(t)
Varicella, prophylaxis of, 150
Varicella-zoster virus, infections from, 157(t)
  treatment of, 154(t)
Velban, 75
Venacavography, inferior, 39, 40
  in Hodgkin's disease, 249
Vinblastine, 75
Vinca alkaloids in chemotherapy, 74
  structural formulas of, 74
Vincristine, 75
Vincristine sulfate, for Wilms' tumor, 369
Virus(es), infections caused by, in cancer patients, 154(t), 157(t)
  leukemia and, 173, 175
  prenatal exposure to, and cancer risk, 12
  RNA, leukemia and, 174, 175
Vitamin K, deficiency of, coagulation abnormalities and, 146, 146(t)
VMA. See Vanillylmandelic acid.
Vomiting, as complication of Wilms' tumor therapy, 371
von Hippel-Lindau disease, 6
von Recklinghausen's disease, 5

Werner's syndrome, 5
Wilms' tumor, 359
  and age at diagnosis, 359
  and complications of therapy, 371
  associated congenital anomalies of, 360, 361(t)
  bilateral, 370, 371
  chemotherapy for, 368
  clinical manifestations of, 360
  computerized axial tomography of, 47
  differentiation of from neuroblastoma, 32, 32
  evaluation of, 365
  genetics of, 362
  hemihypertrophy and, 361, 362
  incidence of, 359
  inferior venacavography of, 40
  intravenous pyelogram of, 37
  liver scan of, 44
  metastatic recurrence of, 369, 370
  pathology of, 363
  prognosis of, after therapy, 370
  radiotherapy for, 368
    dosages for, 368, 368(t)
  staging system for, 365, 365(t)
  surgery for, 366
  survival rates, and epithelial involvement, 364, 364(t)
    and extent of disease, 365, 365(t)
    and number of tubules, 364, 364(t)
  treatment of, 366
    complications of, 371

INDEX

Wilms' tumor (*Continued*)
  ultrasonography of, 45
Wiskott-Aldrich syndrome, 110

Xeroderma pigmentosum, 5
X-rays. See also *Radiation; Radiotherapy; Roentgenography.*

X-rays (*Continued*)
  burns from, 94
  chest, in Ewing's tumor, 418, *418*
    in Hodgkin's disease, 248, *248*
    in Wilms' tumor, 366, *367*
  in bone cancers, 408
  in teratoma, *436*
  prenatal, cancer risk and, 12, 12(t)
  skull, brain tumors and, 308, *308*, *309*

NOMOGRAM

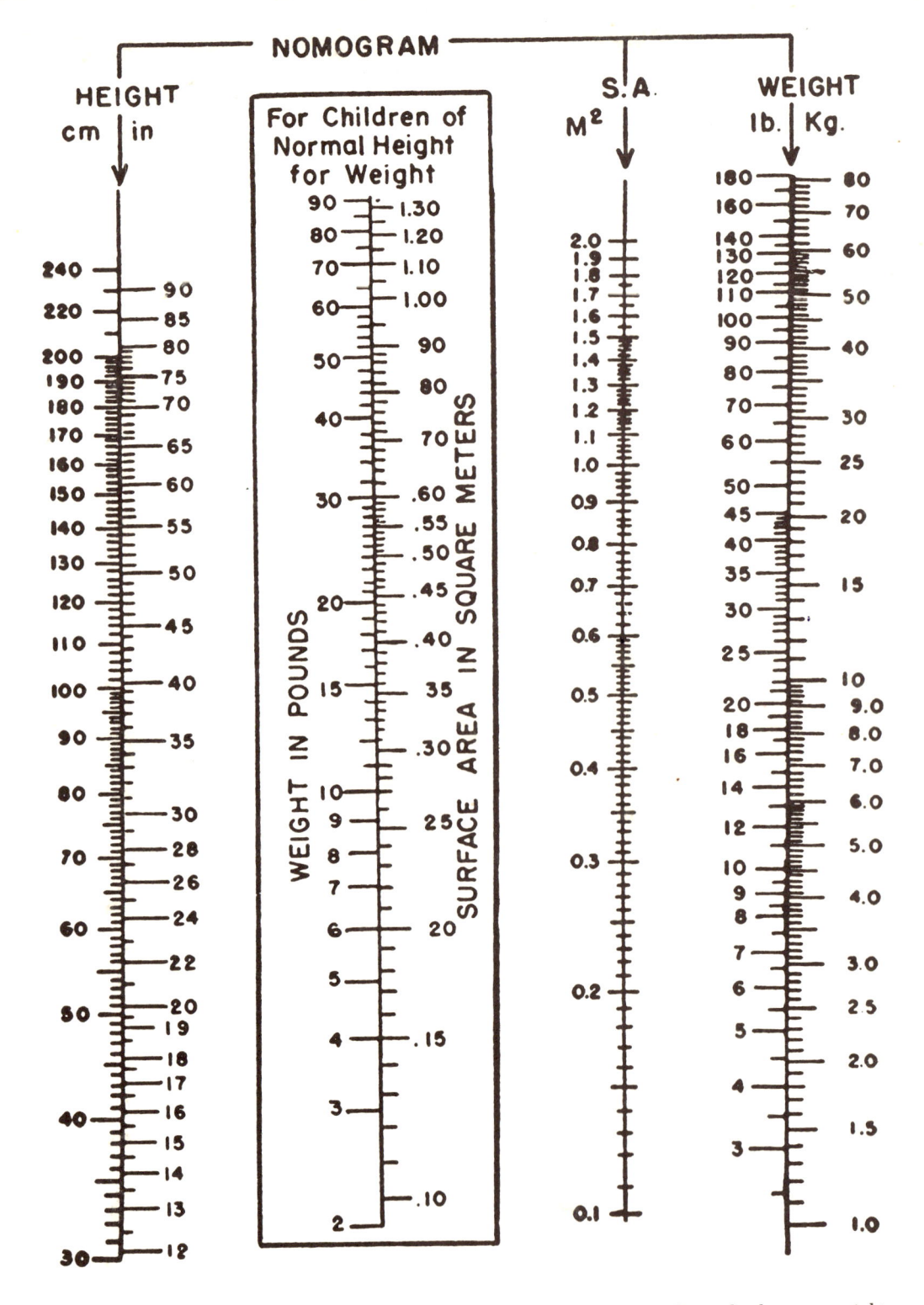

Nomogram for estimation of surface area. The surface area is indicated where a straight line which connects the height and weight levels intersects the surface area column; or the patient is roughly of average size, from the weight alone (enclosed area). (Nomogram modified from data of E. Boyd by C. D. West.)